PEDIATRIC ORTHOPAEDIC SECRETS

PEDIATRIC ORTHOPAEDIC SECRETS

LYNN T. STAHELI, MD
Professor Emeritus
Department of Orthopaedics
University of Washington
School of Medicine
Pediatric Orthopaedic Consultant
Children's Hospital & Medical Center
Seattle, Washington

HANLEY & BELFUS, INC./ Philadelphia

Publisher: HANLEY & BELFUS, INC.
                    Medical Publishers
                    210 South 13th Street
                    Philadelphia, PA 19107
                    (215) 546-7293; 800-962-1892
                    FAX (215) 790-9330

United States sales and distribution:

                    Mosby
                    11830 Westline Industrial Drive
                    St. Louis, MO 63146

Note to the reader: Although the information in this book has been carefully reviewed for correctness of dosage and indications, neither the authors nor the editors nor the publisher can accept any legal responsibility for any errors or omissions that may be made. Neither the publisher nor the editors make any warranty, expressed or implied, with respect to the material contained herein. Experimental compounds and off-label uses of approved products are discussed. Before prescribing any drug, the reader must review the manufacturer's current product information (package inserts) for accepted indications, absolute dosage recommendations, and other information pertinent to the safe and effective use of the product described.

Library of Congress Cataloging-in-Publication Data

Pediatric orthopedic secrets / edited by Lynn T. Staheli.
        p.   cm. — (The Secrets series)
     Includes bibliographical references and index.
     ISBN 1-56053-207-6 (alk. paper)
     1. Pediatric orthopedics—Examinations, questions, etc.   2. Pediatric orthopedics—Miscellanea. I. Staheli, Lynn T.   II. Series.
     [DNLM: 1. Orthopedics—in infancy & childhood—examination questions. 2. Orthopedics—in adolescence—examination questions.
WS 18.2 P3701 1997]
RD732.3.C48P43 1997
618.92'7'0076—dc21
DNLM/DLC
for Library of Congress   97-25774
                                                           CIP

PEDIATRIC ORTHOPAEDIC SECRETS   ISBN 1-56053-207-6

Last digit is the print number   9   8   7   6   5   4   3   2   1

CONTENTS

ACUTE PROBLEMS

Trauma

Sports

REGIONAL PROBLEMS

Lower Limb

Foot and Ankle

Knee and Tibia

Hip

Infections

Neuromuscular Disorders

Limb Deficiency

Miscellaneous Disorders

CONTRIBUTORS

Jon M. Aase, M.D.
Clinical Professor, Department of Pediatrics, University of New Mexico School of Medicine; University of New Mexico Hospital; Presbyterian Medical Center; St. Joseph Hospital, Albuquerque, New Mexico

Peter F. Armstrong, M.D., FRCSC, FACS, FAAP
Professor of Orthopaedic Surgery, Adjunct Professor of Pediatrics, Department of Orthopaedic Surgery, University of Utah; Active Staff, Shriners Hospitals for Children, Salt Lake City, Utah

James Aronson, M.D.
Chief of Pediatric Orthopaedics; Professor, Department of Orthopaedics, University of Arkansas for Medical Sciences, Little Rock, Arkansas

David D. Aronsson, M.D.
Associate Professor, Department of Orthopaedics and Rehabilitation, University of Vermont College of Medicine; Fletcher Allen Health Care, Burlington, Vermont

James H. Beaty, M.D.
Professor of Orthopaedics, University of Tennessee College of Medicine; Director of Orthopaedic Residency, Campbell Clinic; LeBonheur Children's Medical Center, Memphis, Tennessee

Robert M. Bernstein, M.D.
Assistant Clinical Professor of Orthopaedic Surgery, University of California, Los Angeles, UCLA School of Medicine; Pediatric Orthopaedic Surgeon, Shriner's Hospital for Children, Los Angeles, California

John G. Birch, M.D., FRCS
Associate Professor, Department of Orthopaedics, University of Texas Southwestern Medical Center; Texas Scottish Rite Hospital for Children, Dallas, Texas

Eugene E. Bleck, M.D.
Professor Emeritus, Department of Orthopaedic Surgery, Stanford University School of Medicine; Stanford University Hospital; Lucile Salter Packard Children's Hospital at Stanford, Stanford, California

J. Richard Bowen, M.D.
Professor of Orthopaedics, Department of Orthopaedics, duPont Children's Hospital of the Alfred I. duPont Institute, Wilmington, Delaware; Professor of Orthopaedics, Jefferson Medical College, Philadelphia, Pennsylvania; Professor of Orthopaedics, Georgetown University School of Medicine, Washington, D.C.

James D. Bruckner, M.D.
Assistant Professor, Department of Orthopaedics, University of Washington School of Medicine; University of Washington Medical Center; Seattle Children's Hospital; Harborview Medical Center; Veterans Affairs Medical Center, Seattle, Washington

Wilton H. Bunch, M.D., Ph.D.
Church Divinity School of the Pacific, Berkeley, California

Michael T. Busch, M.D.
Director of Sports Medicine, Department of Orthopaedic Surgery, Scottish Rite Children's Medical Center, Atlanta, Georgia

S. Terry Canale, M.D.
Professor, Department of Orthopaedic Surgery, University of Tennessee, Memphis, College of Medicine; Chief-of-Staff, Campbell Clinic; Chief of Orthopaedics, LeBonheur Children's Medical Center, Memphis, Tennessee

Norris C. Carroll, B.Sc., M.D., FRCSC
Professor of Orthopaedic Surgery, Northwestern University Medical School; Children's Memorial Hospital, Chicago, Illinois

Henry Chambers, M.D.
Assistant Professor of Orthopaedic Surgery, Department of Orthopaedic Surgery, University of California, San Diego, School of Medicine; San Diego Children's Hospital and Health Center, San Diego, California

Jack C. Y. Cheng, MBBS, FRCS Ed (Orth), FACS, FHKAM (Orth)
Professor, Department of Orthopaedics and Traumatology, Chinese University of Hong Kong; Prince of Wales Hospital, Shatin, N.T., Hong Kong

Mary Williams Clark, M.D.
Professor of Orthopaedic Surgery, Department of Orthopaedic Surgery, Medical College of Ohio; Medical College Hospital, Toledo, Ohio

N. M. P. Clarke, Ch.M., FRCS
Consultant Orthopaedic Surgeon, Southampton General Hospital, Southampton, England

Ernest U. Conrad III, M.D.
Private practice, Seattle, Washington

Kathryn E. Cramer, M.D.
Staff Physician, Department of Orthopaedics, Henry Ford Hospital, Detroit, Michigan

Alvin H. Crawford, M.D., FACS
Professor of Orthopaedics and Pediatrics, Department of Pediatric Orthopaedic Surgery, Children's Hospital Medical Center, Cincinnati, Ohio

R. Jay Cummings, M.D.
Assistant Professor and Chair, Department of Orthopaedics, Mayo School of Medicine; Nemours Children's Clinic, Jacksonville, Florida

Jon R. Davids, M.D.
Director, Motion Analysis Laboratory, Shriner's Hospital, Greenville, South Carolina

Darin Davidson
Research Associate, Division of Pediatric Orthopaedics, University of Ottawa; Children's Hospital of Eastern Ontario, Ottawa, Ontario, Canada

Jose Fernando De la Garza, M.D.
Titular Professor and Divisional Chief, Department of Pediatric Orthopaedics and Trauma Service, Universidad Autónoma de Nuevo León, Monterrey, Nuevo León

Sharon Kay DeMuth, D.P.T.
Clinical Faculty, Department of Biokinesiology and Physical Therapy, University of Southern California, Los Angeles; Physical Therapist, Children's Hospital of Los Angeles, Los Angeles, California

Mohammad Diab, M.D.
Department of Orthopaedics, University of Washington School of Medicine, Seattle, Washington

James C. Drennan, M.D.
Professor of Orthopaedics and Pediatrics, University of New Mexico Health Sciences Center; Medical Director and CEO, Carrie Tingley Hospital, Albuquerque, New Mexico

Denis S. Drummond, M.D.
Department of Orthopaedic Surgery, Children's Hospital of Philadelphia, Philadelphia, Pennsylvania

Victoria M. Dvonch, M.D.
Associate Professor, Department of Human Restoration, Stanford University, Palo Alto, California

Robert E. Eilert, M.D.
Professor of Orthopaedic Surgery, University of Colorado School of Medicine; Chair, Department of Orthopaedics, Children's Hospital, Denver, Colorado

Mark A. Erickson, M.D.
Assistant Professor of Orthopaedics, University of Colorado School of Medicine; Attending Physician, The Children's Hospital, Denver, Colorado

Marybeth Ezaki, M.D.
Assistant Professor of Orthopaedic Surgery, University of Texas Southwestern Medical School; Director, Hand Services, Texas Scottish Rite Hospital for Children, Dallas, Texas

Edilson Forlin, M.D., M.Sc.
Instructor, Orthopaedic Section, Universidade Federal do Paraná; Pediatric Orthopaedic Surgeon, Hospital Infantil Pequeno Principe, Curitiba Parana, Brazil

James R. Gage, M.D.
Professor of Orthopaedics, University of Minnesota Medical School, Minneapolis, Minnesota; Medical Director, Gillette Children's Specialty Healthcare, St. Paul, Minnesota

James Gibson Gamble, M.D., Ph.D.
Professor of Orthopaedic Surgery, Stanford University School of Medicine; Packard Children's Hospital at Stanford; Stanford University Hospital; Palo Alto, California

Mark C. Gebhardt, M.D.
Associate Professor of Orthopaedic Surgery, Harvard Medical School; Massachusetts General Hospital; Children's Hospital, Boston, Massachusetts

Robert Gillespie, M.B., Ch.B., FRCS (C), FRCS (Ed)
Professor and Chairman, Department of Orthopaedic Surgery, State University of New York at Buffalo School of Medicine and Biomedical Sciences; Head, Department of Orthopaedics, The Children's Hospital of Buffalo, Buffalo, New York

Michael J. Goldberg, M.D.
Professor and Chairman, Department of Orthopaedics, Tufts University School of Medicine; New England Medical Center, Boston, Massachusetts

Alfred D. Grant, M.D.
Clinical Professor of Orthopaedic Surgery, New York University; Hospital for Joint Diseases Orthopaedic Institute, New York, New York

Neil E. Green, M.D.
Professor, Department of Orthopaedic Surgery, Vanderbilt University Medical Center; Vanderbilt Hospital, Nashville, Tennessee

Walter Blair Greene, M.D.
James B. Luck Distinguished Professor and Chairman, Department of Orthopaedic Surgery, University of Missouri–Columbia School of Medicine, Columbia, Missouri

Richard H. Gross, M.D.
Professor, Departments of Orthopaedic Surgery and Pediatrics, Medical University of South Carolina, Charleston, South Carolina

Martin J. Herman, M.D.
Instructor, Orthopaedic Center for Children, Allegheny University of the Health Sciences MCP–Hahnemann School of Medicine; St. Christopher's Hospital for Children, Philadelphia, Pennsylvania

John Anthony Herring, M.D.
Professor of Orthopaedic Surgery, University of Texas Southwestern Medical School; Chief of Staff, Texas Scottish Rite Hospital for Children, Dallas, Texas

M. Mark Hoffer, M.D.
Lowman Professor of Children's Orthopaedics, Orthopaedic Hospital of Los Angeles, Los Angeles, California

Larry H. Hollier, M.D.
Fellow, Department of Plastic Surgery, New York University Medical Center, New York, New York

Walter W. Huurman, M.D.
Professor of Orthopaedic Surgery, University of Nebraska Medical Center; Department of Orthopaedic Surgery, Children's Memorial Hospital, Omaha, Nebraska

John Charles Hyndman, M.D., FRCS(C)
Professor of Surgery, Dalhousie University Faculty of Medicine; Head, Department of Orthopaedics, IWK Grace Health Centre, Halifax, Nova Scotia, Canada

Marci D. Jones, M.D.
Department of Orthopaedics and Rehabilitation, University of Vermont College of Medicine; Fletcher Allen Health Care, Burlington, Vermont

David Keret, M.D.
Senior Orthopaedic Surgeon, Department of Pediatric Orthopaedics, Sackler School of Medicine, Tel-Aviv University; Dana Children's Hospital; Tel-Aviv Medical Center, Tel-Aviv, Israel

Christopher K. Kim, M.D.
Department of Pediatric Orthopaedics, Children's Hospital, San Diego, California

Richard Murray Kirby, M.D.
Clinical Associate Professor, Department of Orthopaedics, University of Washington School of Medicine, Seattle, Washington

Thomas F. Kling, Jr., M.D.
Chief of Pediatrics and Professor of Orthopaedic Surgery, Indiana University Medical Center; Chief of Pediatric Orthopaedics, Riley Children's Hospital, Indianapolis, Indiana

Ken N. Kuo, M.D.
Professor and Associate Chairman of Education, Department of Orthopaedic Surgery, Rush Medical College of Rush University; Senior orthopaedic surgical attending staff, Rush-Presbyterian-St. Luke's Medical Center, Chicago, Illinois

Merv Letts, M.D., FRCSC
Professor of Surgery, Division of Pediatric Orthopaedics, University of Ottawa; Children's Hospital of Eastern Ontario, Ottawa, Ontario, Canada

Richard E. Lindseth, M.D.
Professor and Chairman, Department of Orthopaedic Surgery, Indiana University School of Medicine; Indiana University Medical Center, Indianapolis, Indiana

Randall T. Loder, M.D.
Associate Professor, Section of Orthopaedic Surgery, University of Michigan Medical School, Ann Arbor, Michigan

Scott John Luhmann, M.D.
Associate Medical Staff, Department of Orthopaedic Surgery, St. Louis Shriner's Hospital for Children, St. Louis, Missouri

G. Dean MacEwen, M.D.
Professor of Orthopaedic Surgery, Orthopaedic Center for Children, Allegheny University of the Health Sciences MCP-Hahnemann School of Medicine; St. Christopher's Hospital for Children, Philadelphia, Pennsylvania

Richard E. McCarthy, M.D.
Clinical Associate Professor of Orthopaedics, University of Arkansas for Medical Sciences; Arkansas Children's Hospital, Little Rock, Arkansas

Peter L. Meehan, M.D.
Assistant Clinical Professor, Department of Orthopaedic Surgery, Emory University School of Medicine; Egleston Children's Hospital, Atlanta, Georgia

Vincent S. Mosca, M.D.
Associate Professor of Orthopaedics and Chief of Pediatric Orthopaedics, University of Washington School of Medicine; Director, Department of Orthopaedics, Children's Hospital and Medical Center, Seattle, Washington

Colin F. Moseley, M.D.
Clinical Professor of Orthopaedic Surgery, University of California, Los Angeles, UCLA School of Medicine; Chief Surgeon, Shriner's Hospital for Children, Los Angeles, California

Jeroen G. V. Neyt, M.D.
Visiting Assistant Professor, Department of Orthopaedic Surgery, University of Iowa; University of Iowa Hospitals and Clinics, Iowa City, Iowa

Tom F. Novacheck, M.D.
Director, Motion Analysis Laboratory; Assistant Professor, Department of Orthopaedics, University of Minnesota Medical School, Minneapolis, Minnesota; Gillette Children's Specialty Healthcare, St. Paul, Minnesota

John A. Ogden, M.D.
Clinical Professor of Orthopaedics, Emory University School of Medicine; Director of Orthopaedics, Georgia Baptist Medical Center, Atlanta, Georgia

William L. Oppenheim, M.D.
Professor and Head, Division of Pediatric Orthopaedics, University of California, Los Angeles, UCLA School of Medicine; UCLA Medical Center, Los Angeles, California

Klaus Parsch, Dr. med.
Professor of Orthopaedics, Heidelberg Medical School, Olgahospital, Stuttgart, Germany

Hamlet A. Peterson, M.D., M.S.
Professor of Orthopaedic Surgery, Mayo Medical School; Chair, Division of Pediatric Orthopaedics, Department of Orthopaedic Surgery, Mayo Clinic; St. Mary's Hospital; Methodist Hospital, Rochester, Minnesota

Peter D. Pizzutillo, M.D.
Professor of Orthopaedic Surgery; Professor of Pediatrics, Allegheny University of the Health Sciences MCP-Hahnemann School of Medicine; Chief of Pediatric Orthopaedics, St. Christopher's Hospital for Children, Philadelphia, Pennsylvania

Daniel D. Ramsey, M.A., C.P.O.
Director of Prosthetics and Orthotics, Department of Prosthetics and Orthotics, Shriner's Hospital for Children, Salt Lake City, Utah

Kent Reinker, M.D.
Clinical Professor of Surgery, John A. Burns School of Medicine, University of Hawaii; Chief of Staff, Shriner's Hospital for Children, Honolulu, Hawaii

Thomas S. Renshaw, M.D.
Professor and Chairman, Department of Orthopaedic Surgery, University of South Carolina School of Medicine; Richland Memorial Hospital, Columbia, South Carolina

B. Stephens Richards, M.D.
Associate Professor, Department of Orthopaedic Surgery, University of Texas Southwestern Medical Center at Dallas; Assistant Chief-of-Staff, Texas Scottish Rite Hospital for Children, Dallas, Texas

Fay Z. Safavi, MBBS, FFARCS
Assistant Professor, Department of Anesthesiology, University of Texas Southwestern Medical Center at Dallas; Director of Anesthesiology, Texas Scottish Rite Hospital for Children, Dallas, Texas

Perry Lee Schoenecker, M.D.
Professor, Department of Orthopaedic Surgery, Washington University School of Medicine; Chief of Staff, Shriner's Hospital for Children, St. Louis, Missouri

David D. Sherry, M.D.
Associate Professor, Department of Pediatrics, University of Washington School of Medicine; Director, Pediatric Rheumatology, Children's Hospital and Medical Center, Seattle, Washington

Kit M. Song, M.D.
Assistant Professor of Orthopaedics, University of Washington School of Medicine; Assistant Director, Department of Orthopaedics, Children's Hospital and Medical Center, Seattle, Washington

Paul D. Sponseller, M.D.
Associate Professor, Department of Orthopaedic Surgery, Johns Hopkins University School of Medicine; Chief, Pediatric Orthopaedics, Johns Hopkins Hospital, Baltimore, Maryland

Lynn T. Staheli, M.D.
Professor Emeritus, Department of Orthopaedics, University of Washington School of Medicine, Seattle, Washington

Carl L. Stanitski, M.D.
Professor, Department of Orthopaedic Surgery, Wayne State University School of Medicine; Chief, Department of Orthopaedic Surgery, Children's Hospital of Michigan, Detroit, Michigan

Deborah F. Stanitski, M.D.
Associate Professor, Department of Orthopaedic Surgery, Wayne State University School of Medicine; Associate Chief, Department of Orthopaedic Surgery, Children's Hospital of Michigan, Detroit, Michigan

Peter M. Stevens, M.D.
Professor, Department of Orthopaedics, University of Utah School of Medicine, Salt Lake City, Utah

J. Andrew Sullivan, M.D.
Professor and Chair, Department of Orthopaedic Surgery and Rehabilitation, University of Oklahoma College of Medicine; Children's Hospital of Oklahoma, Oklahoma City, Oklahoma

Michael D. Sussman, M.D.
Professor, Department of Orthopaedic Surgery, Oregon Health Sciences University School of Medicine; Chief of Staff, Shriner's Hospital for Children, Portland, Oregon

Marc F. Swiontkowski, M.D.
Professor of Orthopaedic Surgery, University of Washington School of Medicine; Chief of Orthopaedics, Harborview Medical Center; Staff Physician, Children's Hospital and Medical Center, Seattle, Washington

George H. Thompson, M.D.
Professor of Orthopaedic Surgery and Pediatrics, Case Western Reserve University School of Medicine; Director of Pediatric Orthopaedics, Rainbow Babies and Children's Hospital, Cleveland, Ohio

Stephen John Tredwell, M.D., FRCS(C)
Associate Professor, Department of Orthopaedic Surgery, University of British Columbia; Head, Division of Pediatric Orthopaedic Surgery, British Columbia's Children's Hospital, Vancouver, British Columbia, Canada

Elizabeth A. Tursky, R.N.P., B.S.N.
Orthopaedic Specialty Nurse and Registered Nurse Practitioner, Department of Pediatric Orthopaedics, Arkansas Children's Hospital, Little Rock, Arkansas

Charles Douglas Wallace, M.D.
Assistant Clinical Professor, Department of Orthopaedic Surgery, University of California, San Diego, School of Medicine, San Diego, California

Peter M. Waters, M.D.
Assistant Professor, Department of Orthopaedic Surgery, Harvard Medical School; Director, Hand and Upper Extremity Clinic, Children's Hospital, Boston, Massachusetts

Hugh Godfrey Watts, M.D.
Clinical Professor of Orthopaedics, Department of Orthopaedic Surgery, University of California, Los Angeles, UCLA School of Medicine; Shriner's Hospital for Children, Los Angeles, California

Stuart L. Weinstein, M.D.
Ponseti Professor of Orthopaedic Surgery, University of Iowa College of Medicine, University of Iowa Hospitals and Clinics, Iowa City, Iowa

Dennis R. Wenger, M.D.
Clinical Professor of Orthopaedic Surgery, University of California, San Diego, School of Medicine; Director, Pediatric Orthopaedics, Children's Hospital and Health Center, San Diego, California

Shlomo Wientroub, M.D.
Professor and Head, Department of Pediatric Orthopaedics, Sackler School of Medicine, Tel-Aviv University; Dana Children's Hospital, Tel-Aviv Medical Center, Tel-Aviv, Israel

Kaye E. Wilkins, D.V.M., M.D.
Clinical Professor, Department of Orthopaedics and Pediatrics, University of Texas Health Science Center at San Antonio; Santa Rosa Children's Hospital, San Antonio, Texas

PREFACE

This volume follows the proven format of The Secrets Series®. The Socratic question-and-answer style is intuitive and a natural way of both teaching and learning.

Pediatric Orthopaedics is an important subspecialty as it deals with children and with disorders which are common in practice. Often, training in this subspecialty is limited and only when the physician encounters the child with an orthopaedic problem in their practice is this deficiency appreciated.

We hope that *Pediatric Orthopaedic Secrets* helps resolve this problem. It was designed to be authoritative, reasonably comprehensive, and useful. Recruiting outstanding authors was surprisingly easy as a need for such a book is widely recognized. The authors were selected based on their interest, experience, and reputation. The authors come from many centers and provide an approach which is scientific, child oriented, and practical.

Lynn T. Staheli, M.D.

ACKNOWLEDGMENT

I would like to express my appreciation to Charlene Butler, Ed.D., for her excellent work as Project Coordinator during the preparation of this book.

1. GROWTH AND DEVELOPMENT

John A. Ogden, M.D.

1. Name the four developmental regions of a bone.
Diaphysis—the main shaft of the bone.
Metaphysis—the flared ends adjacent to the diaphysis.
Physis—the zone of growth cartilage.
Epiphysis—the initially cartilaginous end of the bone.

2. Name the basic types of bone development.
Membranous—the direct transformation of a mesenchymal precursor into bone. This is present particularly in the skull and facial bones.
Endochondral—ossification of the mesenchymal precursor. This pattern is typical of the long bones.

3. What is an ossification center?
This is the expanding bone that replaces precursor mesenchymal or cartilaginous tissue. A primary center forms in the midportion of the bone anlage, expanding to become the initial diaphyseal and metaphyseal bone. A secondary center forms within the epiphyseal cartilage.

4. When do secondary ossification centers form?
The distal femoral epiphyseal ossification center is usually present by 40 weeks of development. It is considered indicative of a full-term pregnancy. All other epiphyseal ossification centers form postnatally.

5. What is unusual about the proximal clavicular ossification center?
It is generally the last epiphysis to ossify, around 16–18 years. It is also the last to fuse to the metaphysis, which may not occur until 25–26 years of age.

6. How many secondary ossification centers are present in the distal humerus?
Four: capitellar (appears at 7–12 months), medial epicondylar (5–7 years), trochlear (7–10 years), and lateral epicondylar (12–14 years).

7. What is unusual about trochlear ossification?
In contrast to most areas (which consist of a single focus that gradually enlarges), the trochlea forms multiple small ossification centers that eventually coalesce.

8. Name the two kinds of growth plates.
Physis—a growth plate primarily responsive to compression loading forces.
Apophysis—a growth plate primarily responsive to traction (tensile) loading forces.

9. What is unique about an apophysis?
The normal physeal cell columns of hypertrophic cartilage are replaced by fibrocartilage with the typical tensile stress patterns.

10. Where does a growth plate (physis) fail when it is fractured?
Through the hypertrophic zone, leaving the germinal and dividing zones intact and attached to their blood supply.

11. What is the filum terminale?
This is the attachment of the lower end of the spinal cord to the lumbosacral junction region. Different rates of cord and spine growth occur in the last trimester and postnatally. The filum normally separates to allow asymptomatic separate growth rates. Failure to separate leads to the tethered cord syndrome.

12. What is spinal dysraphism?
Failure of the two posterior spinal elements anlagen to fuse in the midline. This may be evident as a small radiolucent defect (spina bifida occulta), which is usually an asymptomatic radiologic observation, or as a wide defect that may be associated with spinal cord and meningeal abnormalities (myelomeningocoele) and various neurologic deficits.

13. What is the significance of the notochord?
It acts as the linear template for the elaboration of the spinal segment anlagen. It usually disappears (cellular aptosis) before birth. Remnants may become "reactivated" to form chordomas, however, usually in the sacral or basioccipital regions.

14. How does the spine form?
It forms from three anlagen for each vertebra: an anterior one known as the centrium, which forms most of the final vertebral body, and two posterior anlagen that unite to form the pedicles, facets, laminae, and spinous processes.

15. What is a neurosynchondrosis?
This is the cartilaginous tissue between each osseous posterior element and the osseous anterior centrium. It is a growth plate that allows widening of the neural canal.

16. What happens if the neurosynchondrosis fuses prematurely?
The spinal canal does not form properly, leading to spinal stenosis. A similar mechanism of retarded growth occurs in spinal dysplasias, leading to early claudication symptoms, as in achondroplasia.

17. What is epiphyseodesis?
This is the closure of a growth plate (physis) by the formation of bone bridges that connect the metaphyseal bone and the epiphyseal ossification center. It occurs normally during adolescence (physiologic epiphyseodesis). It may occur prematurely after injury or infection (pathologic epiphyseodesis) and may lead to bone shortening or angular deformity.

18. What is a ring apophysis?
This is the thin rim of marginal bone equivalent to a secondary (epiphyseal) ossification center that forms at the superior and inferior borders of the vertebral body during adolescence.

19. What is a Risser sign?
This is the gradual secondary ossification of the epiphysis along the iliac crest. It is used to stage maturation in the treatment of scoliosis.

20. What is the zone of Ranvier?
This is the peripheral margin of each growth plate. It allows circumferential expansion of the physis in conjunction with progressive elongation.

21. What are the two basic types of bone growth?
   Longitudinal—the elongation of a bone through cell proliferation, progressive hypertrophy of the new cells, and their replacement by bone at the metaphyseal interface.
   Latitudinal—the widening of the bone (more properly, circumferential enlargement)

through several mechanisms, including the periosteum (enlargement of the diaphysis and metaphysis), the zone of Ranvier (enlargement of the physis), and the perichondrium (enlargement of the epiphysis).

22. What is an osteon?
This is a longitudinally oriented tunnel surrounded by osteocytes within the diaphyseal bone. Primary osteons are present prenatally in a few bones but principally form postnatally. Biologic stresses cause remodeling and replacement of primary osteons by secondary and tertiary osteons to strengthen the diaphyseal bone.

23. How does the metaphyseal cortex differ from the diaphyseal cortex in a child?
The metaphyseal cortex lacks osteons. The surface is relatively porous (microfenestrate) compared with the solid surface of the diaphysis.

24. How does the bone of the metaphysis fail (fracture)?
The bone formed by rapid longitudinal growth is not biomechanically responsive and allows compression failure. This typically forms a buckling of the bone, referred to as a torus fracture.

25. What is the effect of minimal transition of primary osteon bone to remodeled secondary osteon bone?
The resilient bone, which has much less stiffness, may plastically deform (causing bowing rather than obvious fracturing) or may form an incomplete (greenstick) fracture.

26. How does narrowing of the foramen magnum occur in disorders such as achondroplasia?
The basiocciput forms from occipital somites, which give rise to endochondral ossification at the skull base. This forms synchondroses that allow expansion of the foramen magnum. Cartilage growth is impaired, causing less than normal expansion.

27. How does a joint form?
Cell death (aptosis) leads to initial formation of a cavity between adjacent epiphyseal anlagen. Early embryonic and subsequent fetal motion then progressively elaborates the joint. Failure to cavitate may lead to a synchondrosis and subsequent synostosis of a joint (e.g., congenital proximal radioulnar fusion in fetal alcohol syndrome or a tarsal coalition).

28. How does congenital scoliosis occur?
The mesenchymal anlagen of the somites condense irregularly to form abnormal somites, leading to the formation of abnormally suspended vertebrae (e.g., a hemivertebra).

29. When are the skeletal precursors formed?
The mesenchymal and endochondral anlagen form all the discrete skeletal elements by the end of the gestational period (approximately 8 weeks of development).

30. What is skeletal embryopathy?
The failure to form a skeletal element properly. An example is proximal femoral focal deficiency, which occurs in the gestational period.

31. What is fetopathy?
This is the progressive plastic deformation of an initially normally formed skeletal element in the fetal period. Examples are developmental hip dysplasia or clubfoot.

32. What is Klippel-Feil syndrome?
This is the failure of normal segmentation of the mesenchymal anlagen of the cervical spine. It leads to abnormal vertebral formation and fusions, often presenting as torticollis.

33. What is syringomyelias?

This is the failure of the neural canal to obliterate. Fluid accumulates and expands the canal, pushing portions of the spinal canal against unyielding osseous portions and causing variable neurologic deficits.

BIBLIOGRAPHY

1. Guidera KJ, Ganey TM, Keneally CR, Ogden JA: The embryology of lower-extremity torsion. Clin Orthop 302:17–21, 1994.
2. Guidera KJ, Grogan DP, Carey TC, Ogden JA: Biology of skeletal development and maturation. In Menelaus MB (ed): The Management of Limb Inequality. London, Churchill-Livingstone, 1991.
3. Lord MJ, Ganey TM, Ogden JA: Postnatal development of the thoracic spine. Spine 20:1692–1698, 1995.
4. Ogden JA: Development and maturation of the neuromusculoskeletal system. In Morrissy RT (ed): Lovell & Winter's Pediatric Orthopaedics, 3rd ed. Philadelphia, J.B. Lippincott, 1990, pp 1–33.
5. Ogden JA: Development of the lower limb. In Kalamchi A (ed): Congenital Lower Limb Deficiency. New York, Springer-Verlag, 1989, pp 1–45.
6. Ogden JA, Ganey TM, Ogden DA: The biologic aspects of children's fractures. In Fractures in Children, vol 3. In Rockwood CA, Wilkins KE, Beaty JW (eds). Philadelphia, Lippincott-Raven, 1996.
7. Ogden JA, Ganey TM, Sasse J, Neame PJ, Hilbelink DR: Development and maturation of the axial skeleton. In Weinstein S (ed): The Pediatric Spine: Principles and Practice. New York, Raven Press, 1994, pp 3–69.
8. Ogden JA, Neame PJ, Sasse JK, Ganey TM: Skeletal growth and development. In Chapman MW (ed): Operative Orthopaedics, vol. 4, 2nd ed. Philadelphia, J.B. Lippincott, 1993, pp 3005–3029.
9. Ogden JA: Skeletal growth and development. In Putman CE, Ravin CE (eds): Textbook of Diagnostic Imaging, 2nd ed. Philadelphia, W.B. Saunders, 1994.

2. ETIOLOGY OF ORTHOPAEDIC DISORDERS

James G. Gamble, M.D., Ph.D.

1. What does *etiology* mean?

Etiology is derived from the Greek *attia,* meaning cause. We use the term to indicate the classification and theory of the causes of disease.

2. What are the etiological categories of most pediatric orthopaedic disorders?

Congenital, developmental, genetic, traumatic, infectious-inflammatory, metabolic, and neoplastic.

3. What is the difference between a congenital and a developmental disorder?

A congenital disorder is present before or at the time of birth. A developmental disorder is a condition that appears later in the child's life.

4. What is a birth defect?

"Birth defect" is an imprecise term for a congenital disorder. It is preferrable to use the term "congenital disorder" or "congenital abnormality" when referring to a structural abnormality that is present at birth.

5. Roughly, what is the frequency of children born with some type of a structural abnormality?

One in 33 babies is born with some type of structural abnormality, ranging in severity from mild to catastrophic.

6. What is the difference between a congenital and a genetic disorder?

A genetic condition is a disorder that results from an abnormality of the genome. The genetic disorder may be present at birth, in which case it can be classified as a congenital condition, or it may appear later in life.

7. Are all congenital disorders genetic?
No. To be a congenital disorder, the condition must be present at the time of birth. Only some congenital disorders are genetic. Other congenital disorders have no genetic basis.

8. What is the genome?
The genome is the complete set of nucleic acid instructions for making a human. It is the DNA blueprint for all cellular structures and biochemical reactions. There are approximately 100,000 genes in a typical human cell, but only a small proportion of those genes is expressed in any one cell type. The expressed genes vary from one cell type to another.

9. What is a gene?
A gene is the DNA nucleotide sequence from which messenger RNA is transcribed and used to direct the synthesis of a specific protein.

10. What genes are responsible for basic body design?
Homeotic genes are responsible for basic body design. They are involved in establishing the molecular coordinate system throughout the embryo that defines the basic body plan.

11. What is the embryonic period, and why is it so important?
The embryonic period is the first 8 weeks of gestation and includes five stages: fertilization, cleavage, gastrulation, neurulation, and organogenesis. By the end of the embryonic period, all the major body systems have been established, and the basic body plan is complete. Any extrinsic perturbation during this period can result in severe structural disorders.

12. What is organogenesis?
Organogenesis is the differentiation of the three primary cell types—the ectoderm, the mesoderm, and the endoderm—to generate the early organ systems during the end of the embryonic period of gestation.

13. What is meant by the terms "growth" and "development"?
Growth is an increase in physical size of an organ or a system. Development is a change in complexity that includes both growth and differentiation. It is recognized as the sequential physical changes that occur with aging of an infant.

14. What are four major errors of normal growth and development?
Malformations, disruptions, deformations, and dysplasias.

15. What are malformations?
Malformations are structural disorders that result from an interruption of normal organogenesis during the second month of gestation. Examples include myelomeningocele, syndactyly, and preaxial polydactyly.

16. What are disruptions?
Disruptions are structural disorders that result from an extrinsic interference with normal growth and development. Examples include congenital constriction bands.

17. What are deformations?
Deformations are structural disorders caused by mechanical pressure. Examples are supple metatarsus adductus and physiologic bowing of the tibias.

18. What are dysplasias?
Dysplasias are structural disorders caused by abnormal tissue differentiation. Examples include osteogenesis imperfecta, achondroplasia, and spondyloepiphyseal dysplasia.

19. Why is it important to differentiate malformations from deformations?
Deformations can often be treated relatively easily by removing the deforming force or by providing a satisfactory counterforce, such as corrective casting or bracing.

20. What is a metameric shift?
Metameres are segmental collections of sclerotome cells, separated into cranial and caudal portions in the vertebral anlagen. In a metameric shift, the cranial portion of the inferior sclerotome recombines with the caudal portion of the directly superior sclerotome.

21. Why are renal anomalies commonly associated with congenital scoliosis and with other spinal anomalies such as Klippel-Feil syndrome?
The close temporal and spatial relationship of vertebral body formation and nephrogenesis means that an insult can affect both systems, explaining the clinical association of congenital vertebral anomalies with renal anomalies. While the spinal precursors are undergoing metameric shift to form the vertebral bodies, the renal precursors, the heart, the trachea, and the esophagus are differentiating, so a noxious influence present during this time can damage all systems.

22. Why does the cervical spine have eight nerves but only seven vertebrae?
As a result of resegmentation of the sclerotomes, the cranial portion of the first cervical sclerotome combines with the fourth occipital sclerotome to form the base of the skull. The caudal portion of C1 combines with the cranial portion of the C2 sclerotome to form the atlas. This resegmentation continues all the way down the spinal precursors.

23. What are the two major types of malformations that involve vertebral bodies?
Defects of *formation* cause wedged vertebra, hemivertebra, and butterfly vertebra. Defects of *segmentation* result in unsegmented bars, laminar synostosis, and block vertebra.

24. Why do rib anomalies commonly accompany vertebral anomalies?
Because the cells of the sclerotome become the vertebrae and the ribs, a disturbance can affect the final morphology of both ribs and vertebrae at the same level.

25. What is apoptosis, and what does it have to do with syndactyly or the presence of a medial plica in the knee?
Apoptosis is a process of programmed cell death in which a gene called REAPER produces a small peptide that causes the release of lyosomal enzymes into the cell, resulting in a form of cellular suicide. Failure of apoptosis in the human foot or hand plate causes syndactyly. Incomplete cavitation due to failure of apoptosis results in the presence of residual synovial folds, which we recognize clinically as suprapatellar, infrapatellar, and mediopatellar plicae.

26. What are the two mechanisms of normal bone formation, and how do they differ?
The skeleton is formed by two mechanisms, intramembranous and endochondral. Intramembranous bone formation, usually taking place at periosteal surfaces, results from the direct differentiation of mesenchymal cells into osteoblasts. Endochondral bone formation, occurring at the growth plate, results from the replacement of a cartilaginous precursor matrix with a mineralized matrix, which is subsequently remodeled.

27. What is the growth plate?
The growth plate, also called the physis, is the histologic site of longitudinal growth of bones. It consists of the reserve zone, the proliferative zone, the hypertrophic zone, and the metaphyseal zone.

28. How does the growth plate produce longitudinal growth of bones?
Bone length is gained by the processes of chondrocyte proliferation, maturation, and hypertrophy. Matrix production, mineralization, and subsequent ossification maintain the increased length achieved by chondrocyte hyperplasia and hypertrophy.

29. What is the Hueter-Volkmann law, and what does it have to do with progressive adolescent genu varum?

This law states that compressive forces inhibit growth and tensile forces stimulate growth. Although the factors controlling growth are much more complex than this, a varus knee results in increased compressive forces in the medial part of the physis, presumably contributing to the progressive valgus.

BIBLIOGRAPHY

1. Dunne KB, Clarren SK: The origin of prenatal and postnatal deformities. Pediatr Clin North Am 33:1277–1286, 1986.
2. Gamble JG: Development and Maturation of the Neuromusculoskeletal System. In Morrissy RT, Weinstein SL (eds): Pediatric Orthopaedics, 4th ed. Philadelphia, Lippincott-Raven, 1996, pp 1–24.
3. Gilbert SF: Developmental Biology, 4th ed. Sunderland MA, Sinauer Associates, 1994.
4. Moore KL: The Developing Human, Clinically Oriented Embryology, 4th ed. Philadelphia, W.B. Saunders Co., 1988.
5. Simon SR: Orthopaedic Basic Science, Chaps. 4 and 5. Rosemont, IL, American Academy of Orthopaedic Surgeons, 1994, pp 127–219.

3. SCREENING

John G. Birch, M.D.

1. What are the components of an ideal screening?
- A disorder that untreated or detected late results in significant morbidity or mortality. In orthopaedics, examples include undetected developmental dysplasia of the hip, which results in limp and early degenerative arthritis, and scoliosis, which can produce severe cosmetic deformity and potential pulmonary compromise.
- A cost-effective, reliable, and specific tool for identifying the disorder in question. The forward-bending test to screen for scoliosis is reliable but is in a way too sensitive, since many false-positives are detected by this method. Radiographs of the spine are highly specific for the identification of scoliosis but are not a cost-effective manner to screen the entire at-risk population.
- A cost-effective treatment that significantly alters the natural history of the disorder in question. Early detection of neonatal hip instability can result in a cure of the disorder by the use of the Pavlik harness and can prevent the need for much more costly treatment in the older child. School screening examinations for scoliosis are more controversial because well-documented evidence of the effectiveness of treatment (brace or surgery) in altering the natural history of scoliosis is lacking.

2. What conditions should be screened for as part of a musculoskeletal examination?

In the neonate, common orthopaedic conditions to look for are developmental dysplasia of the hip, evidence of spinal deformity or malformation, digital anomalies, long-bone deformity, and foot deformities. Developmental dysplasia of the hip should be screened for until after a child has developed a mature normal gait. All children should have an assessment of lower extremity alignment and general neurologic gross motor development. Children and adolescents should be screened for evidence of scoliosis, kyphosis, or limb-length inequality.

3. What measurements should be taken?

Height, weight, and head circumference should be measured and charted.

4. When should I worry about these measurements?
Further evaluation is needed if:
- Weight or height is excessively high or low (> 95th percentile or < 5th percentile)
- Weight or height is disproportionate
- Head circumference is disproportionate for height/weight
- The weight, height, or head circumference deviates from the percentile line it has been keeping

5. What should you ask to assess for delayed neuromuscular development in the infant?
Were there any problems with the pregnancy or delivery?
How much did the child weigh?
Was the child premature?
Did the child present in a vertex or breech position?
When did the child begin to: roll over? sit? crawl? pull to stand? walk independently?

6. When should a child start to do these things?
Most infants will begin to roll over at 4–6 months, sit at 6–7 months, crawl at 7–9 months, pull up to stand at 9–12 months, and walk at 12–16 months.

7. What common foot deformities are seen in infants?
The most common is the typical marked inturning of the feet resulting from the combination of internal tibial torsion and metatarsus adductus due to fetal position in the uterus. Others include rigid metatarsus adductus, clubfoot deformity (talipes equinovarus), calcaneovalgus foot, and digital anomalies (such as syndactyly or absence).

8. How do you tell the deformities apart?
Metatarsus adductus is characterized by an outward curvature of the lateral border of the foot, with the apex of this curvature usually at the base of the fifth metatarsal bone. In mild deformities, the foot can easily be held manually in a straight position, whereas in more severe cases, the foot can be held straight only with firm pressure or not at all.

Clubfoot (talipes equinovarus) superficially resembles the typical markedly inwardly rotated newborn foot. The foot resists even firm efforts at correction, however.

Calcaneovalgus feet rest in a marked dorsiflexed position and on examination have limited plantar flexion (usually they can be pulled down into a neutral plantigrade position).

The most common digital anomalies are simple syndactyly (webbing) between two toes. Occasionally, more severe webbing with toe deformity or absence occurs.

9. What is developmental dysplasia of the hip?
Developmental dysplasia of the hip (DDH) is maldevelopment of the hip joint characterized by a misshapen femoral head and acetabulum as well as hip joint ligamentous laxity, resulting in a variable degree of displacement of the femoral head out of the acetabulum. The severity of the condition varies from partial dislocation (subluxation) when the examiner attempts to dislocate the femoral head to complete irreducible dislocation of the femoral head from the acetabulum.

10. Which children should be checked for DDH?
All children are at risk. Furthermore, no symptoms occur in newborns or infants. Therefore, ALL newborn children and ALL infants should be screened by physical examination regularly until they have developed a mature, normal walking pattern. Approximately one neonate in a hundred has evidence of hip instability. Many of these will improve spontaneously, so that the incidence of DDH in infants and children is closer to 1 per 1000.

Children who are first-born females who presented in a breech position (irrespective of the method of delivery) or in whom there is a family history of DDH are at increased risk for having this condition and must be particularly carefully screened.

11. What happens if DDH goes undetected?

If the hip remains dislocated at walking age, the mechanics of the hip will be severely altered, resulting in limp and shortening of the leg. Ultimately, the hip may become painful because of excessive forces on the abnormal cartilage surfaces of the joint. If both hips are dislocated, there may be no shortening of the leg, but the child will have a waddling gait and increased lordosis of the lumbar spine.

12. How do you detect DDH?

First, is the hip dislocatable, i.e., does the femoral hip lie in the acetabulum but can be pushed out on examination? Check for this by pushing gently outwardly and posteriorly on the relaxed baby's hip with the leg flexed 90° and in neutral abduction (see Figure). If instability exists, you will feel the femoral head dislocate from the acetabulum (and then spontaneously reduce when you relax the pressure on the leg) with a distinct "clunk." No other physical findings may be apparent.

Second, is the femoral head dislocated? In this more severe situation, physical findings include limited abduction (usually the infant's hips will abduct nearly 90°), asymmetric thigh folds (extra on the affected side), and shortening of the leg compared with the normal side. In the neonate, the femoral head may still be temporarily reducible by gently abducting the hip and lifting the upper leg forward; a distinct "clunk" will be felt as the femoral head reduces. As you release the pressure, the femoral head will pop out of place again.

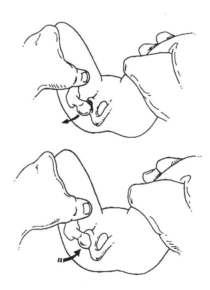

13. What should you do if the examination findings are equivocal?

The best thing to do is to reexamine the infant later, particularly if the child was crying or otherwise resisting examination. If still unsure, or particularly if the infant has any of the aforementioned risk factors, hip ultrasonography is a good imaging investigation. Radiographs of the hip should be taken only in children older than 3–4 months in whom there are physical findings or risk factors.

14. Why is it important to detect DDH early?

Children in whom the disorder is detected early will be treated with a Pavlik harness, with a high likelihood of successful outcome. After 6 months of age, and especially after walking age, surgical reduction and body casting will be required, with a less certain favorable result.

15. What problems can occur in the spine of newborns?
Torticollis, scoliosis, and spinal dysraphism.

16. How do you screen for problems in the spine?
Gently check the range of motion of the neck. With congenital muscular torticollis, the head will be held tilted to one side with the chin rotated away from the side to which the head tilts. Resistance will be felt when you try to tilt and rotate the head in the opposite direction. Examine the back by running your fingers along the spine. Look for discoloration of the skin over the middle of the spine, and palpate for stiff curvature or defects in the spinous processes.

17. How do you investigate spinal abnormality in the infant?
The next appropriate investigation is a radiograph of the spine. Any infant in whom you have identified a spinal abnormality should be evaluated by an orthopaedist, however. Patients with congenital scoliosis will require radiographs of the spine, renal ultrasonography, and careful neurologic examination and may require MRI of the spinal cord.

18. What is the best way to check for leg-length discrepancy?
The child who is not yet walking is best assessed by looking at the knee and foot levels with the child supine. Be sure that the hips are in neutral abduction and equal extension. Asymmetric positioning of the joints will make a leg look falsely longer or shorter. In the ambulatory child, look at the level of the iliac crest or the dimples over the posterior superior iliac spine. Be sure the child is standing evenly with the knees extended.

19. Can bowlegs or knock-knees be normal?
Yes. Typically at birth, the legs are slightly bowed. Normally, the legs will straighten by age 18–24 months, only to become knock-kneed. Knock-knee can be normal in a healthy child, usually between the ages of 2 and 6–7 years, by which time the legs usually look straight.

20. What should cause concern when you see a child with bowlegs or knock-knees?
    A history of injury or infection in the legs
    Inappropriate age group (> 24 months for bowlegs, < 18 months or > 7 years for knock-
        knees)
    Asymmetry in the severity of the deformity
    Extreme deformity
    Child not developing normally, appearing disproportionate, small, or unwell

21. Can flatfeet be normal?
Yes. Many newborn feet look chubby and flat. As long as the feet are flexible and the child otherwise appears normal, there is no cause for alarm or need for further investigation. Young children often will have flat-appearing feet as well. This most commonly occurs during the time period when the child is knock-kneed (18 months–7 years, usually maximum at 3–4 years).

22. How do you make sure flatfeet are not serious?
    The foot should be painless, functional, and flexible on examination. This deformity is usually most apparent in children who are in the "knock-knee" stage of lower extremity angular development, since at this stage, the feet are lateral to the weight-bearing axis of the limb and tend to roll into the flatfoot appearance with weight-bearing.
    Check to be sure the foot is flexible. There should be no tight heelcord. Both the hindfoot and the midfoot should be freely and painlessly mobile under your hands with passive movement.
    Ask the child to walk on his or her toes. With flexible flatfoot deformity, the longitudinal arch will be obvious in this position.

23. How do you check for scoliosis?
    The forward-bending test. Have the patient stand with his or her back to you. Be sure that the patient stands evenly on both legs and that the knees are straight. Ask the child to bend forward

at the waist as if touching the toes. Look at the back for elevation of one hemithorax or flank compared with the other due to the rotational deformity of scoliosis.

This is a good time to check flexibility by seeing if the child can touch the toes. Look at the spine from the side to rule out excessive thoracic kyphosis.

24. When is the best time to check for scoliosis?
Scoliosis may show up at any age and in either sex and is usually painless, so all children should be examined with the bending test. Girls, particularly in early adolescence, are at greatest risk for the development of progressive scoliosis, and should be the most carefully assessed group.

25. What problems might arise in screening for scoliosis?
Most commonly the patient is not positioned accurately, so that he or she is not standing evenly on both feet with the knees straight or bends, leaning to one side.

A true limb-length inequality will appear positive for scoliosis on screening examination, since the higher pelvis (on the longer side) will result in the entire side of the body seeming to be elevated compared with the shorter side. Look at the level of the iliac crests, or better, the dimples over the posterior superior iliac spine. If you suspect limb-length inequality, put an appropriately sized block under the shorter leg and have the patient lean forward again. Now you should see that the pelvis is level and the spine straight.

26. How can you assess a child's gross motor function?
Ask the child to heel walk, toe walk, and hop on either foot. This will allow you to assess gross strength and balance in the legs. It is also a good idea to watch the child walk briskly or run. Normal fluid movement and balance will be easily recognizable; many neuromusculoskeletal abnormalities will prevent this normal motion and function.

BIBLIOGRAPHY

1. Bunnell WP: Outcome of spinal screening. Spine 18:1572–1580, 1993.
2. Heath CH, Staheli LT: Normal limits of knee angle in white children. Genu varum and genu valgum. J Pediatr Orthop 13:259–262, 1993.
3. Mazur JM, Shurtleff D, Menelaus M, et al.: Orthopaedic management of high-level spina bifida: early walking compared with early use of a wheelchair. J Bone Joint Surg 71A:56–61, 1989.
4. Ponseti IV: Treatment of congenital clubfoot. J Bone Joint Surg 74A:448–454, 1992.
5. Salenius P, Vankka E: The development of the tibiofemoral angle in children. J Bone Joint Surg [Am] 57:260, 1975.
6. US Preventive Services Task Force: Review article: screening for adolescent idiopathic scoliosis. JAMA 269:2667–2672, 1993.

4. PHYSICAL EXAMINATION

Richard Gross, M.D.

1. What techniques are useful for gathering a history from the family of a child with a pediatric orthopaedic problem?
A printed form that can be completed by the parent is very helpful in documenting the reason for the physician visit, birth and developmental history, allergies, previous treatment, other treating physicians, referring physicians, and family physician. This is supplemented by the actual interview with the patient and family. Open-ended questions are more informative than factual inquiries. For example, "When did you feel something was wrong?" is preferable to "How long has your child had this problem?"

2. What techniques are useful for the pediatric orthopaedic examination?

The examination is performed in a manner dictated by the age of the patient and the presenting problem. A great deal of information can be gleaned by observation of the child while interviewing the parents, noting spontaneous movement, use of the limbs in undressing or moving about the room, guarding, gait, and playing with toys. A systematic examination in a child is not always possible. When observing gait, concentrate initially on the degree of toeing in. On the second pass, note the position of the patella to determine if toeing in originates above the knee or below (or both). Younger children are usually more comfortable if the examination is performed on the mother's lap, and the prone torsional profile can easily be evaluated in this position. If pain in a certain location is suspected, perform the examination of the normal limb first; once a painful site has been detected, the examination is over.

3. What is the difference between malformation, deformation, and dysplasia?

Malformations result from an interruption of normal organogenesis in fetal life and are not reversible. Deformations are abnormalities in form, shape, or position of normally formed body parts caused by mechanical molding. The effect of deforming forces is proportional to the rate of growth, so the fetus and infant are most susceptible. Dysplasias result from abnormal organization of cells into tissues.

4. Describe the normal development of the newborn.

The newborn is largely reflexive, with a predominant flexor tone that is responsible for the lack of complete hip and knee flexion. By 3 months of age, the head can be held above the plane of the body and should not lag when the baby is pulled from a supine to a sitting position. At 6 months, the baby should be able to grasp objects and sit with minimal external support. Walking is achieved at about 12 months, with wide variation.

5. At what age do some useful developmental milestones become apparent that help to determine normal or delayed development?

Development proceeds in a cephalocaudal direction; head and hand control precede the ability to control the lower limbs. Thus, at 3 months of age, the infant should be able to hold the head above the plane of the body when supported in a prone position, and by 4 months, the head should not lag when the baby is pulled from a supine to a sitting position. By 6 months, the baby should be able to grasp objects such as a bottle and sit with minimal support. At about 9 months, the lower limbs are developing, and the child can pull up to a standing position by holding on to furniture by 10 months. At 12 months, ambulation occurs, although this milestone can have a wide temporal variation. The 12-month-old can throw objects on the floor and speak a couple of words. Handedness is not evident until about 18 months. Earlier evidence of handedness should direct attention to the status of the hand and arm not being used.

6. How does one examine for leg length discrepancy?

Complaints of leg length discrepancy are fairly common. The discrepancy can be apparent, such as with lumbar scoliosis or contracture of the hips and pelvis, or real, with a true difference in leg lengths. Therefore, the child is best examined initially in the standing position, with weight evenly borne on both legs, if possible. With the examiner seated on a stool behind the patient, the iliac crests can be palpated with the extended index finger, and a visual estimate of the finger position should be noted. The ability to detect discrepancy in this manner is surprisingly acute. If a difference is noted, blocks are placed under the short leg, and the height necessary to level the pelvis is noted. In the same position, a search is conducted for lumbar scoliosis, including forward bending to test for trunk rotation. The position of the pelvis in the coronal plane is also noted. Posterior displacement of either hemipelvis resulting from infra- or suprapelvic contracture is noted. Observation of gait may reveal the presence of a trunk shift secondary to muscle weakness, which may give the impression of a leg length discrepancy.

With the patient in the supine position, the iliac crests are palpated, and the leg lengths may be measured with a tape measure. A careful assessment of joint motion is performed, since flexion contractures of hip or knee will produce apparent shortening. While hip motion can be assessed in flexion or extension, it is mandatory that this examination be performed in the extended position because the functional effects of leg length discrepancy are seen with the hip in this position. Finally, if scanograms are ordered in the presence of flexion contractures of hip or knee, the femora and tibiae must be scanned separately. The bone being measured must be flat against the cassette to eliminate apparent shortening secondary to contracture.

7. Describe the examination of the spine for deformity.
The spine is ideally examined with the patient clad only in underwear or a bathing suit. The spine is first examined in the standing position in the coronal and sagittal planes, evaluating symmetry and compensation. Decompensation is present if the occiput is not directly over the gluteal cleft, which denotes the sacral midline. This is best evaluated with the aid of a plumb hanging from the occiput, but a pencil on a string can be a quick substitute. Decompensation is recorded in centimeters. Shoulder height and scapular prominence are compared for symmetry. The position of the pelvis is noted, and a check for leg length discrepancy is quickly done at this time. In the sagittal plane, the head should be directly over the first sacral body, without excessive lordosis or kyphosis. In the presence of a right thoracic curve, the posteriorly rotated rib cage may obscure thoracic lordosis, so a visual assessment from both sides can be helpful. The patient is then asked to bend forward, with the arms hanging free. The spine is visually examined from the caudal and cephalad perspectives to note rotation, which, if present, is measured with a scoliometer. The spine is then observed from the side with the patient still bending over. A sharp "V" shape anywhere in the thoracolumbar spine signals the presence of structural kyphosis. Lumbar kyphosis in the sitting position with the legs extended is a result of tight hamstrings.

8. Are there any special techniques for evaluating forearm rotation?
Careful attention to maintaining the humerus flat against the chest wall is useful to avoid misinterpreting the trick movement of humeral adduction and abduction to augment pronation and supination.

9. How does one examine for developmental dysplasia of the hip?
The examination is performed in the supine position. The normal newborn has a hip flexion contracture of about 30°. Dislocation of the hip eliminates this flexion contracture. The goal of the examination is to detect excessive mobility of the femoral head in relation to the acetabulum. Both hips may be examined simultaneously, but examining each hip separately allows easier detection of movement. The examiner's hand grasps the thigh on the side being evaluated, with the knee flexed. The web space is over the proximal tibia, the thumb sits on the region of the lesser trochanter, and the long finger rests on the greater trochanter. The other hand stabilizes the pelvis, with the thumb on the symphysis pubis and the fingers under the sacrum. The web space exerts posterior pressure on the knee, much like the mechanism of injury in traumatic dislocation of the hip, where the knee strikes the dashboard. With a rotatory movement, the thumb exerts lateral pressure on the lesser trochanter at the same time, attempting to lever the femoral head over the posterior acetabulum. This is known as *Barlow's maneuver*. The hip is then abducted, pressure on the web space is relieved, and upward pressure is exerted with the long finger on the greater trochanter. This is known as *Ortolani's maneuver* and will reduce a displaced hip. Findings are best described as normal, subluxatable (a feeling of excess mobility is suspected, but the femoral head does not exit the acetabulum), dislocatable, or dislocated. A truly dislocated hip is very rare unless the dislocation is teratologic. The infant with a dislocatable hip has no restriction of abduction, since secondary contracture has not yet developed.

By 6 weeks to 3 months of age, if the hip is still displaced, secondary contracture will become evident. The findings related to instability will now be absent. Instead, there will be variable amounts of restriction of abduction, tested with the baby supine and the hips flexed. Attention is necessary to be sure the pelvis does not rock to one side, which may factitiously affect the measured value. With the hips still flexed but in neutral abduction-adduction and the pelvis flat on the table, shortening of the thigh segment signals posterior displacement of the hip (or a congenital short femur). Careful inspection in the supine position with the hip extended may reveal the laterally displaced location of the femoral shaft. These findings are present until walking age, at which time a waddling gait (secondary to excessive trunk shift over the dysplastic hip) makes recognition, especially by the parents, much easier.

10. How does one detect contracture of the hip?

If the patient can stand, excessive lumbar lordosis should direct special attention to the possibility of hip flexion contracture. There are two examination methods for detection of hip flexion contracture. The *Thomas test* requires both hips to be initially flexed to flatten the lumbar spine, which serves as a reference point. The hip being examined is then extended while the contralateral hip remains flexed. At the point where further extension is blocked, the angle between the thigh and the table is the degree of contracture. A hand of a coexaminer, which can be the parent, under the lumbar spine will help to denote accurately the degree of contracture because the lumbar spine will extend to compensate for restricted hip extension.

Staheli has described an alternate method. The patient is in the prone position with the legs over the end of the examination table. The flexed hip is extended with one hand while the other hand is placed on the lumbar spine, noting the angle at which the spine begins to extend.

A frequently omitted maneuver is examination for abduction contracture. Although this can be performed in the supine position, the prone position seems to render the findings more easily seen. The hip is abducted with one hand on the leg. With the other hand on the pelvis, the leg is adducted until pelvic motion is detected.

Hip rotation may be measured with the hips flexed or extended. The iliopsoas and anterior capsule are more relaxed in flexion, and the measurements may differ. Inasmuch as rotational deviations have more effect in extension (walking), the findings in this position are probably more meaningful. The method described as part of Staheli's torsional profile lends itself most readily to accurate documentation. The patient is prone, the hips are extended, and the knees flexed to 90°. The tibiae serve as markers as the hips are internally and externally rotated, which facilitates measurement. A hand on the pelvis is helpful to ascertain that the rotation noted is entirely femoral. In the presence of hip flexion contracture, examination in the prone position may not be possible. The knees may be flexed over the end of the examination table with the hips in maximum extension so that the tibiae may again serve as markets. The chart should document whether the rotational assessment was performed with the hips flexed or extended. Similarly, abduction can be performed in flexion or extension, again with greater rotation generally noted in flexion. A hand on the pelvis will more accurately determine the end point. In the presence of medial hamstring contracture, abduction is reduced when the knee is extended.

The *Ober test* for iliotibial band contracture is often useful when examining for lateral knee pain or a snapping iliotibial band on the greater trochanter. The patient is placed in a side-lying position. The hip not being examined (closest to the table) is flexed to stabilize the pelvis. The hip on the side being examined is held in a slightly flexed position, with the knee flexed 90°. The hip is then abducted and completely extended. In the presence of iliotibial band contracture, the hip cannot be adducted to neutral position. A supple iliotibial band contracture should allow about 20° of adduction.

The *Ely test* results are positive in the presence of quadriceps spasticity. The patient is prone with the hips and knees extended. The leg being examined is flexed at the knee. If hip flexion accompanies knee flexion, quadriceps spasticity is present.

11. What is the Wilson test?

The Wilson test is designed to detect osteochondral defects in their most common location, on the lateral aspect of the medial femoral condyle. The knee is flexed 90°. The tibia is internally rotated and slowly extended while internal rotation is maintained. In the presence of an osteochondral defect, pain may be detected at about 30° of flexion. If the pain is relieved by laterally rotating the tibia, an osteochondral defect is likely.

12. What are some methods to evaluate the extensor mechanism in the presence of patellofemoral pain?

The "Q" angle is formed by two lines: (1) a line from the anterior superior spine to the center of the patella and (2) a line from the center of the patella to the center of the tibial tubercle. The larger the angle, the greater the tendency for lateral displacement of the patella with quadriceps contraction. Patellar mobility is tested in the supine position, in both full extension and 30° of flexion. In extension, the patella can be displaced laterally up to half its width, but in 30° of flexion, it should be contained by the femoral condyles. If pain is felt with lateral pressure, this is known as a *positive apprehension test*. Tenderness lateral to the patella may accompany iliotibial band contracture.

The modified *Helfet test* detects dysfunction of patellofemoral mechanics. Ordinarily, as the flexed knee is extended, the femur rotates on the tibia near complete extension, the so-called "screw home" mechanism. If the flexed knee is hanging over the edge of the examination table and visualized from above, the tibial tubercle is aligned with the midpatella. As the knee completely extends, the femur and patella internally rotate, and the tibial tubercle is aligned with the lateral patella. If the tibial tubercle remains aligned with the midpatella, the mechanics are pathologically altered, generally from lateral retinacular contracture. In addition to measuring thigh circumference for quadriceps atrophy, quadriceps weakness can be assessed by placing the patient in the supine position with the contralateral hip and knee flexed. The extended knee on the side being examined is lifted to a point approximately 10 cm above the table and held for a count of three. Patients with quadriceps weakness have difficulty repeating this 10 times.

13. Describe some useful maneuvers for examination of the child's foot.

Difficulties with terminology continue to confound the description of the foot examination. Briefly, inversion and eversion describe movement of the subtalar joint. Valgus and varus are often substituted for inversion and eversion, although the movements are more multiplanar than simple valgus and varus. Pronation and supination are more complex, with supination including inversion and midfoot adduction and equinus. Pronation includes eversion with midfoot abduction and dorsiflexion. These motions are best noted with the patient in the prone position, with the knees flexed. With the knees flexed 135°, the plane of motion of the subtalar joint is parallel with the table top. The position of the subtalar joint affects midfoot mobility; pronation allows more motion of the calcaneocuboid and talonavicular joints. Many foot deformities are characterized by alterations in the position of the forefoot as compared with the hindfoot. The forefoot may be in equinus (pes cavus), supination (clubfoot), pronation (pes cavus), or abduction (congenital vertical talus). The *block test* is designed to test for forefoot pronation (plantar flexion of the first metatarsal). In the presence of a plantar-flexed first metatarsal, the first metatarsal head strikes the floor firmly and in effect tilts the hindfoot into inversion. A block placed under the lateral foot gives the first metatarsal more room to accommodate the plantar-flexed position, and the tilting effect is eliminated. Thus, the hindfoot inversion is eliminated with a block under the lateral foot, and the test is positive.

Pes planovalgus is common and is generally a normal variant. A heelcord contracture can disrupt normal subtalar mechanics, however, and this combination is more likely to be painful. To test the effect of heelcord contracture on foot posture, the patient is supine with the knee extended, and the plantar-flexed foot is supinated. This eliminates midfoot motion and maintains the calcaneus in a neutral position. A heelcord contracture will prevent dorsiflexion of a foot held in this supinated position. The lateral border of the foot must be observed to measure the degree of contracture.

BIBLIOGRAPHY

1. Baird HW, Gordon EC: Neurological evaluation of infants and children. Clin Dev Med. 84:85, 1983.
2. Bartlett MD, Wolf LS, Shurtleff DB, et al. Hip flexion contractures: a comparison of measurement methods. Arch Phys Med Rehabil 66:620–625, 1985.
3. Bleck EE: Orthopaedic Management in Cerebral Palsy. Philadelphia, J.B. Lippincott Co., 1987.
4. Bunnell WP: An objective criterion for scoliosis screening. J Bone Joint Surg [Am] 66:1381–1387, 1984.

5. Coleman SS: Complex foot deformities in children. Philadelphia, Lea & Febiger, 1983.
6. Forero N, Okamura LA, Larson MA: Normal ranges of hip motion in neonates. J Pediatr Orthop 9:391–395, 1989.
7. Greene WB, Heckman JD: The clinical measurement of joint motion. Rosemont IL, American Academy of Orrthopaedic Surgeons, 1994.
8. Hughston JC, Walsh WM, Puddu G: Patellar Subluxation and Dislocation. Philadelphia, W.B. Saunders Co., 1984.
9. Illingworth RS: The Development of The Infant and Young Child: Normal and Abnormal, 3rd ed. Edinburgh, E & S Livingstone, 1966.
10. Ober FR: The role of the iliotibial band and fascia: A factor in the causation of low back disorders and sciatica. J Bone Joint Surg 18:185, 1936.
11. Staheli LT: The prone hip extension test. Clin Orthop Rel Res 123:12–15, 1977.
12. Staheli LT, Corbett M, Wyss C, et al.: Lower-extremity rotational problems in children. Normal values to guide management. J Bone Joint Surg [Am] 67:39–47, 1985.

5. THE SICK CHILD

Thomas Kling, M.D.

1. List the common conditions that present with musculoskeletal symptoms in a sick child.

Septic arthritis (see chapter 83)   Ewing's sarcoma
Acute hematogenous osteomyelitis   Child abuse
Systemic juvenile rheumatoid arthritis   Sickle cell crisis
leukemia

2. Describe the clinical presentation of acute hematogenous osteomyelitis in a young child.

Acute osteomyelitis is characterized by fever and pain that is progressive in severity. Two thirds of young children are sick; in the remaining one third of cases, the child does not present an ill patient. The initial complaint is either a painful limp or refusal to walk when the lower extremity is involved. It is common in an infant for the pain to cause pseudoparalysis, with the patient refusing to move the extremity.

3. What are the local physical findings in an ill child with acute hematogenous osteomyelitis?

Local findings include pain, swelling, and local warmth over the affected bone. Often, there is some limitation of motion of the adjacent joint. The pain is usually severe. The swelling may involve the soft tissues over the length of the bone, and there may be an effusion of the adjacent joint. Early in the disease process, the tenderness is localized to the metaphysis of the affected bone. The most frequent site of infection is the metaphysis of long bones, although osteomyelitis can occur in any bone. Two thirds of infections occur in the lower extremity, with the femur and tibia most commonly affected.

4. What diagnostic tests are useful in acute osteomyelitis?

The white blood cell count and sedimentation rate results are elevated. An x-ray of the painful bone will reveal soft tissue swelling that obliterates the muscle planes. (It is helpful to have a comparison radiograph of the opposite extremity.) Elevated periosteum and bone changes are not seen on x-ray study for at least 10 days after the onset of symptoms. Large-bore needle aspiration of the subperiosteal space and metaphyseal bone within a centimeter of the physis performed under general anesthesia will often yield pus, which confirms the diagnosis. The pus and any other fluid should be sent immediately to the laboratory for Gram's staining and culturing. Blood cultures will yield an organism in 50% of cases.

5. Describe the presenting symptoms of an ill child with systemic-onset juvenile rheumatoid arthritis.

Fever, malaise, and joint pain suggest the diagnosis of systemic JRA. Typically, systemic-onset JRA begins between the ages of 5 and 10 years, but it can occur at any time from infancy to adulthood. Fever is the key finding, which by definition must exceed 39.3°C (103°F). Initially, the fever may be erratic, but usually there is a daily for twice-daily pattern. The peak fever is usually in the evening; by morning, the child feels better and has a normal temperature. These high fevers can be associated with intense arthralgias and myalgias, which can inhibit the child's movements. Cervical spine stiffness is common. The characteristic rash of systemic JRA is non-pruritic, pink to salmon-colored, macular or maculopapular, and evanescent. It is seen most frequently on the trunk and in the axillae when the child is febrile. The joint pain in JRA typically improves with use of the affected joint. Morning stiffness is commonly reported and improves as the day progresses. By definition, the diagnosis of JRA requires the presence of arthritis for a minimum of 6 weeks.

6. Describe the joint findings in systemic-onset JRA.

Any number of joints may be involved in systemic-onset JRA. The arthritic joints can often look worse than they feel. The only finding may be swelling, although most involved joints have some combination of heat, pain, and tenderness. As a rule, children walk on these joints despite the presence of fusiform swelling, warmth, discomfort, and limitation of motion. There is generally greater active and passive motion and less pain than is found in joint swelling caused by infection or trauma. Tenderness is diffuse and nonfocal. Atrophy and weakness of the adjacent muscles (suggesting chronicity) are often already present at the time of diagnosis.

7. What laboratory tests should be ordered in systemic-onset JRA?

Unfortunately, there is no single laboratory test that can be used to make a definitive diagnosis of JRA. The initial laboratory evaluation should include analysis of erythrocyte sedimentation rate (ESR), complete blood count (CBC), antinuclear antibody (ANA), rheumatoid factor (RF), and urine. The ESR is usually elevated. The CBC is important in screening for neoplasia. The white blood cell (WBC) count should be normal or elevated. (It can be very high in systemic onset-JRA—40,000 WBC/mm³ or greater). Low platelet count or WBC count may indicate leukemia or systemic lupus erythematosus. The hematocrit is usually normal or slightly low in chronic arthritis. The ANA and RF are only rarely positive in JRA but when positive are suggestive of the disease. A low ANA (less then 1:320) is highly suggestive of JRA and is a marker for those children at high risk for developing asymptomatic iritis.

8. Describe the radiographic findings of joints with JRA.

Early radiographs in JRA are not diagnostic. They usually show only soft tissue swelling, effusion, and osteopenia of the adjacent bone. They are, however, very helpful in ruling out other diagnoses (trauma, neoplasia, and osteomyelitis).

9. Name several other diseases that may present with features similar to systemic-onset JRA in an ill child.

Septic arthritis	Acute rheumatic fever
Osteomyelitis	Sickle cell disease
Leukemia	Systemic lupus erythematosus

10. Describe the musculoskeletal presentation of leukemia in an ill child.

Leukemia is the most common cancer of childhood and usually affects young children. Most children appear systemically ill at presentation. All organ systems are eventually involved, although the initial symptoms of leukemia often involve only the musculoskeletal system. Twenty to thirty percent of children with acute leukemia present with bone pain. The bone pain is diffuse and nonspecific and may extend to adjacent joints. It usually results from distention of the medullary cavities due to the rapid proliferation of hematopoietic tissue. Frequent sites of pain are the long bones and the spine. The pain maybe periarticular and may be associated with joint effusion, fever, and elevated leukocyte count and sedimentation rate, which mimics the diagnosis of septic arthritis or osteomyelitis.

Initially, it is difficult to make the diagnosis because symptoms are diffuse and the physical exam is nonspecific. When a child presents with obscure bone or joint pain, one should be highly suspicious of leukemia.

11. Describe the radiographic findings in a child with leukemia.

Radiographic changes may or may not be seen, depending on the duration of the disease. When radiographs are abnormal, osteopenia is seen most typically. In actively growing bones (usually the distal end of the femur and the proximal end of the tibia), metaphyseal bands (leukemic lines) appear as radiolucent transverse bands next to the growth plate. These radiolucent bands are due not to the infiltration of leukemia cells but rather a disturbance in formation of bone in the growth plate. Osteopenia is generalized, and there may be cortical thinning. With progression of the disease, lytic areas develop, which may be demarcated or moth-eaten in appearance. The lytic lesion may involve the metaphysis of long bones, the skull, the pelvis, and the tubular bones of the hands and feet. There may be associated subperiosteal new bone formation, suggesting acute osteomyelitis.

12. Describe the laboratory findings in a child with acute leukemia.

The white blood cell count may be elevated, depressed, or, in some instances, normal. Severe anemia is common. When the hemoglobin is 9 g/100 ml or less, leukemia should be ruled out. Blast forms are often seen in the peripheral blood smear, but their absence does not exclude leukemia. The erythrocyte sedimentation rate is often elevated.

13. Describe the presenting features of acute rheumatic fever.

Acute rheumatic fever (ARF) is an autoimmune reaction that occurs 2–4 weeks after a streptococcal infection in children 5–15 years of age. The joints in ARF are exquisitely tender, red, and hot, and the arthritis typically migrates from joint to joint over a period of hours. The rapid decrease in joint symptoms with aspirin therapy is almost diagnostic.

The arthritis may be associated with carditis, chorea, erythema marginatum, subcutaneous nodules, and fever. These associated features and a history of previous streptococcal infection are used to make the diagnosis.

14. Describe the clinical presentation and characteristics of Ewing's sarcoma.

Ewing's sarcoma occurs between the ages of 5 and 25 years and is usually located in the diaphysis or midshaft of a long bone. Severe pain and swelling are usually present at the site of the tumor. The presentation may mimic that of an infection, with slight to moderate fever, elevated erthrocyte sedimentation rate and white cell count, and a mottled appearance of the involved bone on x-rays. The femur is most commonly involved, followed by the tibia, the fibula, and the humerus. The flat bones of the pelvis are involved in approximately 20% of patients.

15. What is the plain radiographic appearance of Ewing's sarcoma?

Diffuse permeative or moth-eaten destruction of the diaphyseal bone, extension of the tumor through the cortex into the surrounding soft tissue, and periosteal reaction. The cortex may appear to be destroyed. The periosteal reaction typically causes an onionskin appearance but may also cause a Codman's triangle or a sunburst appearance. All these findings suggest an aggressive bone tumor that has rapidly penetrated the cortex and elevated the periosteum, but they are not pathognomonic for Ewing's sarcoma.

BIBLIOGRAPHY

1. Fink CW, Nelson JD: Septic arthritis and osteomyelitis in children. Clin Rheum Dis 12:423, 1986.
2. Green NE, Edwards K: Bone and joint infections in children. Orthop Clin North Am 18:555, 1987.

3. Hugos HG: Bone Tumors: Diagnosis, Treatment, and Prognosis, 2nd ed. Philadelphia, W.B. Saunders Co., 1991.
4. Rogalsky RJ, Black GB, and Reed MH: Orthopaedic manifestations of leukemia in children. J Bone Joint Surg 68A:494, 1986.
5. Schaller JG: Chronic arthritis in childhood. Juvenile rheumatoid arthritis. Clin Orthop 182:79, 1984.
6. Stollerman GH: Rheumatic Fever and Streptococcal Infection. New York, Grune & Stratton, 1975.

6. DISPROPORTIONAL MUSCULOSKELETAL PAIN

David D. Sherry, M.D.

1. What is disproportional musculoskeletal pain?
Every child suffers musculoskeletal pain from time to time. A child with disproportional musculoskeletal pain has an amplified pain response so that the pain he or she experiences is much greater than one would expect. Additionally, most of these children have disproportional dysfunction. A child with knee pain will not bend the knee, will be completely non-weightbearing, and will not even tolerate bedcovers touching the knee. Because of the pain, the child will miss school for weeks at a time and will even need help dressing.

2. Who gets disproportional musculoskeletal pain?
Most (80%) are females between 9 and 18 years old, with the average being 12 years old. It is rare before the age of 6 years.

3. What causes disproportional pain?
These pains can be initiated by trauma or inflammation, such as tendinitis or arthritis; however, they seem to be related to psychologic factors in the majority of children.

4. If it is due to psychologic factors, is the pain "just in the child's head"?
No. Pain is a personal experience, and these children suffer tremendously. Each person's psychologic makeup influences the way in which he experiences and copes with pain.

5. Are there different kinds of disproportional musculoskeletal pain?
There are several patterns of disproportional musculoskeletal pain, depending on the location of the pain, associated symptoms, and physical findings. The names used to describe the clinical variations are legion, and all are somewhat unsatisfactory. It may not be useful to label each variation, but when confronted with a child in pain, delineating the pattern in your own mind may help you make the diagnosis. The most common patterns are:
- **Psychogenic or idiopathic musculoskeletal pain.** This is the most common form. It may be constant or intermittent, may be well localized or diffuse, and may involve multiple sites. The pain is disproportionate and is characterized by hyperesthesia, marked dysfunction, an incongruent affect, and an absence of signs of overt autonomic dysfunction.
- **Reflex neurovascular dystrophy, reflex sympathetic dystrophy, or complex regional pain syndrome, type 1.** It usually involves a single site. Lower extremities are more com-com-monly involved than upper extremities, and the pain is usually constant. The characteristics of the pain are identical to those of psychogenic musculoskeletal pain, but there are signs of overt autonomic dysfunction. The limb is cold and cyanotic and can be edematous.

Less common signs are perspiration changes or dystrophic skin changes (thickened, waxy, hairy skin).

- **Fibromyalgia.** This is characterized by widespread pain (involving more than half the body) that lasts more than 6 months. On examination, 11 of 18 possible trigger points are reported to be painful to digital palpation. These children report more feelings of depression, have unrestful sleep, and have other associated pain symptoms such as headaches, chest pains, and abdominal pains.
- **Hypervigilance.** This is relatively uncommon. These children seem to pay too much attention to normal body sensations and interpret these sensations as painful. These pains are usually short lived and do not significantly interfere with function but cause the child great anxiety.

6. What are some clues in the history of disproportional musculoskeletal pain?

Frequently, the patient has a minor injury that subsequently becomes increasingly painful. Commonly, the child presents in an emergency room days after the injury because the parents suspect a fracture. The pain is either minimally responsive or not responsive to conservative management with pain or anti-inflammatory medications. Immobilization frequently makes it worse. There may be a history of color changes (purple) and temperature changes (cold). The pain may be so intense that clothing or bedcovers are intolerable. The pain prohibits activities of daily living such as attending school, interferes with mental concentration, and is reported to be much more severe than the pain experienced by children with organic disorders such as arthritis.

On a 10-point scale, most patients will report their pain to be near 10 or even higher. There is an absence of symptoms that would suggest infection. Interestingly, those with lower extremity pain frequently crawl around their homes rather than walk; this is exceedingly rare, if not completely absent, in children with arthritis.

7. Is there anything to be learned from the past history?

These children are described as slow healers (possibly taking 6 months or more to recover from an uncomplicated fracture) or have had similar prolonged painful experiences in the past. An occasional child will report hundreds of musculoskeletal injuries, such as spraining his or her ankle every week or even every day.

8. What should one inquire about in the family history?

Similar pain or chronic pain in family members or even friends.

9. Is there anything to be learned from the social history?

Most of these children are in the midst of multiple traumatic life events, such as parental divorce, a change in schools, a change in family membership, and loss of significant people in their lives. Physical and sexual abuse needs to be discussed in the appropriate setting.

10. What physical examination findings should one seek?

Important things to look for include inappropriate child/parent (usually the mother) interactions, incongruent affect, belle indifférence, hyperesthesia, signs of autonomic dysfunction, compliance, and fibromyalgia tender points. Rule out inflammation, infection, or neurologic dysfunction.

11. What do you mean by mother/daughter interaction?

Most of the mothers and daughters are inappropriately close and overinvolved in the emotional life of the other.

12. What do you mean by incongruent affect?

Most, but not all, of these children report that the pain rates a 10 on a scale of 1–10 (or even a 20) yet will be smiling and manifest no pain behaviors.

13. What do you mean by belle indifférence?

The child has the appearance of being unconcerned about the amount of pain and dysfunction she has.

14. What do you mean by hyperesthesia?

Severe pain in response to a stimulus that normally is not interpreted as being noxious. Test for this by either lightly touching the skin or gently pinching the skin between your thumb and forefinger. During either maneuver, the child will report severe pain, with or without pain behaviors such as wincing. Repeatedly check the location of the border of the area of skin that is hyperesthetic. Commonly, the border will vary by as much as 6–8 cm.

15. What are the signs of autonomic dysfunction?

- Cyanosis
- Coolness
- Edema
- Increased perspiration
- Dystrophic skin

Autonomic signs need to be checked both before and after exercising the limb, since they may become manifest after use. The limb will be cool and cyanotic, purple, or ruddy in color and can be quite mottled. Sometimes the pulse is decreased. Occasionally, the limb will be diffusely edematous; the joints are not swollen. Rarely is it clammy or are there dystrophic skin changes (waxy, hairy, thick skin).

16. What are the fibromyalgia tender points?

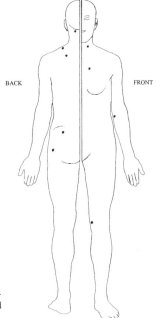

The insertion of the suboccipital muscle at the base of the occiput

The lateral transverse cervical processes of C6 or C7

The mid-upper border of the trapezius

Above the medial border of the scapula spine

The second costochondral junction

2 cm distal to the lateral epicondyle

The gluteal muscle fold

1 cm posterior to the greater trochanter

1 cm proximal to the medial knee joint mortise

In addition to the trigger points, you should check control points such as the center of the forehead, the muscles of the midforearm, the left thumbnail, and the midshin.

Tender points in children with the fibromyalgia variant of disproportional musculoskeletal pain. Tenderness in 11 of 18 points is required for diagnosis.

17. How does one know if a trigger point is truly tender?

One applies 4 kg of pressure with the flat surface of the thumb, held perpendicular to the body. The patient may or may not wince but needs to indicate verbally that the pressure caused definite pain, not just discomfort.

18. What are other signs of fibromyalgia?

Fibromyalgia is widespread body pain for longer than 6 months involving more than half the body in which 11 of 18 trigger points are painful to digital palpation. Children with fibromyalgia also frequently report feeling depressed and unrested in the morning, even if they sleep late.

19. What components of the neurologic examination are recommended?

Motor function is hard to assess accurately because strength, muscle bulk, and tone may be diminished owing to the pain and disability. Some children will voluntarily give way when tested.

Deep tendon reflexes are normal. Focus on findings of sensory testing using sharp-dull, two-point discrimination, proprioception, and light touch tests. Rarely, Fabry's disease can mimic disproportional pain.

20. What tests are indicated?

If you are sure of the diagnosis, no tests are indicated. If you are unsure, make certain that acute-phase reactant levels are not elevated (erythrocyte sedimentation rate or C-reactive protein) and that the CBC and radiographs are normal. If still unsure, obtain a three-phase bone scan. This can confirm the diagnosis by showing decreased blood flow to the involved limb and decreased uptake in the delayed images. The bone scan can be normal, in which case it is reassuring that one is not missing a small, hidden osteoid osteoma or an occult fracture. Rarely, the bone scan will show increased spotty uptake, which is characteristic of reflex neurovascular dystrophy in adults.

21. What is the treatment for disproportional musculoskeletal pain?

The treatment is intense exercise therapy that is focused on function and desensitizing hyperesthetic skin. We administer 5–6 hours of aerobic therapy (1:1 physical therapy and occupational therapy plus pool therapy) daily. Exercises focus on the disability. Stairs, jumping activities, biking, and walking are used for those with leg involvement; wall washing, writing, typing, throwing, and gripping are used for those with upper extremity involvement. What hurts the most is what we emphasize. We acknowledge the pain but encourage the child to complete the exercises in much the same way a coach motivates a player. Changing the activity frequently helps keep the child interested, along with having specific goals of performance (beating her last time or number of repetitions). We reinforce the idea that the pain does not indicate tissue damage but is an abnormal amplified response and needs to be worked through.

22. What about other modalities, medications, and surgery?

We do not recommend any modalities such as transcutaneous nerve stimulation, ultrasound, nerve blocks, sympathectomies, or medications. We have found that if the child is dependent on us to fix the pain, the recurrence rate is much higher.

23. How does one desensitize hyperesthetic skin?

Rub it with a towel or lotion, possibly with cornmeal added, for 2 minutes at a time. Repeat this 2 or 3 times during the day. Care needs to be taken to assure that there is no skin breakdown.

24. How long does it take for improvement to be seen?

Within a few days, most children will have a significant increase in function, although the pain may increase. It will gradually decrease over time. The intense exercise program is usually followed daily for the first week and, in most, can be decreased to 2–3 days a week the following week. Thereafter the child graduates to a daily home program that takes about 40 minutes to complete. Some require 2 full weeks of daily therapy, and the rare child requires more than a month. For most, the daily home program can be stopped after a month, after which the child is encouraged to participate in normal activities such as sports, dance, and physical education class. This helps decrease the emphasis on illness and promotes the idea that he or she is healthy.

25. What about the psychologic aspects?

Stresses may be caused by family, school, or friends. Marital discord may be covert, so the parents may not report strife.

School can be another source of stress, since most of these children work hard to be excellent students and relate to others competently. They may be overachievers. Many have an average IQ but are in gifted and accelerated courses. As the work becomes more difficult, they find it very stressful to keep up with truly gifted students.

26. Are these children depressed?
Few of these children are clinically depressed. About half of children with the fibromyalgia variant are depressed, however, which is one of the distinguishing features of that condition.

27. What is the outcome?
The vast majority (80%) are completely without symptoms within a month or two. Another 15% have only mild or intermittent pain and are fully active. About 5% continue to have disabling pain and require psychotherapy before they can become better. About half of such children, in our experience, do seek appropriate psychologic care and eventually are free of pain.

28. How can they prevent a recurrence?
It is most important to recognize that a recurrence is happening. The pain may or may not feel like the first episode and may be at a different site. Clues are hyperesthesia, marked dysfunction, and increasing pain over time. The second episode may not necessarily have the same manifestations as the first episode. It is imperative to exercise the limb as soon as a recurrence is thought to be starting, even if it was initiated by injury. Desensitization early on is helpful for those with hyperesthesia. Most children will not want to repeat an intense exercise program and will work hard on their home program to avoid a full recurrence.

29. Can disproportional musculoskeletal pain involve the back or jaw?
Yes. It is harder to diagnose, but the basic principles are the same.

30. What signs does one find in those with disproportional musculoskeletal pain of the back?
- Distracted straight-leg-raising (back pain when hip is flexed to 90° with knee extended when supine but not when seated; rarely positive in children)
- Axial loading (with patient standing, pressure on the head causes back pain)
- Passive rotation (back pain is reported while twisting the patient at the ankles and knees while keeping the back in one plane, causing no real back rotation)
- Nonanatomic tenderness or regional pain (half the back)
- Nonanatomic hyperesthesia (common in children)
- Overreaction (exaggerated wincing, loud ouches, or collapsing)

31. How do those with intermittent disproportional musculoskeletal pain present, and how does one treat it?
They look entirely well and are without pain or dysfunction. The history reveals that after activity, there is such pain that the child cannot function for hours to days. Often, there is a history of hyperesthesia while the pain lasts, and rarely there is a history consistent with overt autonomic dysfunction.

The treatment is the same, that is, intense exercise daily. Most do very well after exercising daily for a week and suffer no further episodes of postactivity disproportional musculoskeletal pain.

32. How does one treat children with hypervigilance?
Recognizing the diagnosis, avoiding any further testing, and offering reassurance are all that are needed in most cases. Occasionally, a home exercise program is prescribed, which is to be carried out when the child is feeling the pain. It is important to evaluate these children a few months later to reaffirm the diagnosis.

33. What if the child has an underlying illness or injury?
A child with an underlying condition needs that condition addressed while the exercise program is started. If the underlying condition is active, such as arthritis, it should be aggressively treated. If it is inactive without organic sequelae, such as reactive arthritis, it should be ignored.

If it is associated with musculoskeletal sequelae, such as cerebral palsy or destructive arthritis, the exercise program will have to be modified but should still focus on regaining baseline function and desensitization. Pool therapy is quite helpful for children who are normally nonambulatory.

34. How do I explain disproportional musculoskeletal pain to the child and parents?
The child should be told that the nerves going to the blood vessels are working too much, and that is causing the amplification of the pain. The exercise therapy retrains these nerves so that blood flow is restored. Function comes back first, then the pain subsides. Occasionally, the pain will stop instantaneously.

BIBLIOGRAPHY

1. Malleson PN, al-Matar M, Petty RE: Idiopathic musculoskeletal pain syndromes in children. J Rheumatol 19:1786–1789, 1992.
2. Sherry DD, Weisman R: Psychological aspects of children reflex neurovascular dystrophy. Pediatrics 81:572–578, 1988.
3. Sherry DD, McGuire T, Mellins E, Salmonson K, Wallace CA, Nepom B: Psychosomatic musculoskeletal pain in childhood: clinical and psychological analyses of 100 children. Pediatrics 88:1093–1099, 1991.
4. Waddell G, McCulloch JA, Kummel E, Venner RM: 1979 Volvo award in clinical science. Nonorganic physical signs in low-back pain. Spine 5:117–125, 1980.
5. Wolfe F, Smythe HA, Yunus MB, et al: The American College of Rheumatology 1990 criteria for the classification of fibromyalgia. Report of the multicenter criteria committee. Arthritis Rheum 36:160–172, 1990.

7. DIAGNOSTIC RADIOLOGY

Dennis R. Wenger, M.D., and Christopher Kim, M.D.

1. Are x-rays generally necessary for diagnosis? What should the physician say when parents express concern about the risk of x-rays?
The need for a radiograph depends on the clinical circumstances and findings and also on the degree of certainty with which you want to clarify a diagnosis. For a minor limb injury, particularly on the first encounter with a primary care physician, a clinical exam alone may suffice. If the child is seeing an orthopaedic specialist, a radiograph is more often required. The parents should be told that modern x-ray methods use low-dose radiation. The ordering physician should be certain to use a facility that uses low-dose techniques. Parents should be told that there is a risk-benefit ratio for all diagnostic studies and that in the physician's opinion, the benefit to the child outweighs the risk.

2. Should x-rays be ordered for all musculoskeletal complaints?
No. If a child has mild musculoskeletal complaints, an x-ray is not required. If there is acute trauma or swelling, fever, or prolonged symptoms, an x-ray is usually required. The experience of the examining physician determines whether an x-ray is ordered. Often, the less experienced physician should order an x-ray to help in clarifying the diagnosis.

3. Are AP and lateral views required to assess potential bone injury?
Yes. To study a bone carefully, two views taken at right angles to each other are required. This is particularly important when assessing for a possible fracture. Many oblique fracture lines are missed if one performs only an AP view.

4. Will x-rays demonstrate early osteomyelitis?

No. Osteomyelitis begins as a small nidus of infection within the metaphysis of the bone. It takes some time (often 7–10 days) for a lytic area to be radiographically apparent.

5. Will x-rays help in determining if a child has joint sepsis?

Possibly. Joint sepsis does not show true radiographic changes in its early stages. Eventually, the infection will produce swelling within the joint, and soft tissue shadows can be analyzed, particularly about the hip (capsular swelling), knee, and elbow. Aspiration of the joint is the definitive study to clarify diagnosis.

6. Should all children who have failed a scoliosis screening examination in school have spine x-rays?

No. School screening is usually performed by a nurse, and sometimes overly sensitive methods are used. The so-called angle of trunk rotation, as measured with a scoliometer, is defined as being abnormal with an angle as small as 5°. To minimize radiation exposure, a child who has failed the school screening examination should first have an examination by an orthopaedic surgeon. If it is determined that the angle of trunk rotation is 7° and the child has clinical deformity, a standing spine x-ray should be performed. The first film needs only to be a PA radiograph of the spine; lateral views and bending views are not required.

7. Should all infants with suspected hip dysplasia (or hip clicks that might be caused by developmental dysplasia of the hip) have hip radiographs?

No. Hip radiographs are difficult to interpret in early infancy because the ossific nucleus does not usually appear until the age of 4–8 months. The cartilaginous femoral head and its relationship to the acetabulum are much better assessed with an ultrasound examination up to the age of 3 months.

8. Do children with a complaint of thigh and knee pain always require knee x-rays?

No. A careful physical exam is required to clarify a history of thigh and knee pain. In many cases, these symptoms are due to an occult hip disorder, such as Legg-Calvé-Perthes disease or slipped capital femoral epiphysis. Many times only knee films are taken when the patient in fact has hip disease.

9. Is an AP view of the pelvis adequate to assess complaints of hip pain or thigh pain in an adolescent?

Both an AP and a frog-leg view of the pelvis is required, particularly in slipped capital femoral epiphysis, in which movement of the femoral epiphysis posteriorly on the femoral neck is apparent only on the frog-leg lateral view in the early stages. Similarly, a frog-leg lateral view can help clarify the diagnosis of Perthes' disease.

10. If a child has hip pain, should one order only AP and lateral views of the affected hip?

No. Hip disorders are difficult to clarify in children. One should always perform an AP view of the pelvis, which allows comparison of both the symptomatic hip and the normal hip. Similarly, if a lateral view is needed, a frog-leg view of the pelvis is ordered, which allows comparison of the normal with the symptomatic hip.

11. Do children with hip pain require only films of the hip?

No. Surprisingly, spinal conditions such as spondylolysis can cause radiating pain to the greater trochanter and can present as hip pain. If hip films are normal in a child with puzzling hip pain, one should consider performing a lateral view of the lumbosacral spine to assess for possible spondylolysis or spondylolisthesis.

12. Are x-rays always needed to assess bowleg and knock-knee in young children?

No. An experienced orthopaedist will simply observe a bowleg deformity so long as it is not asymmetric or severe. Generally, bowlegs with a clinical tibiofemoral angle of less than 20° in children younger than age 2 can be observed without radiographs being performed. As the child gets older, the lower limb evolves toward a natural genu valgum. Thus, radiographs are usually not performed unless the valgus is greater than 20° in children aged 3–8.

13. Will standing x-rays of both legs always allow one to measure and quantitate accurately the degree of knock-knee (genu valgum)?
No. Commonly, knee valgus is underestimated by radiographs because the child stands with the knees together and tends to prop one knee against the other. For accurate x-ray documentation of the severity of genu valgum, the child must stand for the radiograph with a space of a few centimeters between the knees.

14. How does one read an x-ray to rule out metabolic bone disease?
The classic finding is thickening, widening, and irregularity of the physis (growth plate).

15. In a child with a suspected knee problem (once hip disease has been ruled out), what x-rays should be ordered?
Initially, one should order only AP and lateral views of the knee. If the history is more complex and the findings puzzling, one should consider the tunnel or notch view, which allows one to assess more clearly the posterior portion of the condyle, where osteochondritis dissecans is likely to occur. If patellar instability is suspected, bilateral Merchant (sunrise) views are performed to assess patellofemoral alignment. (Both knees are studied to allow comparison.)

16. What is the differential diagnosis in a child with hip x-ray findings that suggest avascular necrosis (increased density or collapse of femoral head)?

Legg-Calvé-Perthes disease
   (idiopathic avascular necrosis)
Steroid medication
Prior treatment of hip dysplasia
Sickle cell disease

Leukemia
Prior hip sepsis
Prior treatment of slipped capital femoral
   epiphysis
Gaucher's disease

BIBLIOGRAPHY

1. Morrisy RT, Weinstein SL (eds): Lovell and Winter's Pediatric Orthopaedics, Vol. I. Philadelphia, Lippincott-Raven, 1996.
2. Orthopaedic Knowledge Update 5. Rosemont, IL, American Academy of Orthopaedic Surgeons, 1966.
3. Resnick D: Bone and Joint Imaging. Philadelphia, W.B. Saunders Co., 1989.
4. Rockwood CA Jr, Wilkins KE, Beatty JH (eds): Fractures in Children, Vol. 3. Philadelphia, J.B. Lippincott Co., 1996.

8. SPECIAL IMAGING

Christopher K. Kim, M.D., and Dennis R. Wenger, M.D.

1. Are tomograms an important part of the work-up of a musculoskeletal problem in children's orthopaedics?
Although conventional tomography can be useful for assessing certain spine conditions, osteoid osteoma, or delayed union, many hospitals no longer keep tomography equipment in repair and available because CT (computer tomography) scans have for the most part replaced conventional tomography.

2. When is fluoroscopy useful?

The most common uses are intraoperative for performance of an arthrogram, assessment of joint motion, reduction of fractures, assessment of hip and other complex osteotomies, monitoring internal fixation, and removal of foreign bodies.

New, small, portable low-radiation units are used in clinics and emergency departments to reduce fractures.

3. What are some common uses of an arthrogram?

The most common use is documentation of the adequacy of arthrocentesis for joint sepsis. (Radiopaque dye is injected to confirm that the joint has been entered.) Another common use is the study of closed reduction of developmental dysplasia of hip (DDH). Other uses include documenting the nature of intra-articular fractures and the adequacy of reductions (especially for fractures of the lateral condyle of the elbow). An arthrogram can also be used to study the joint congruency and coverage in Legg-Calvé-Perthes disease. Although not strictly an arthrogram, the injection of dye into a simple bone cyst to document its extent (prior to steroid injection as treatment) is common.

4. What is the imaging method of choice for assessing potential DDH in an infant younger than the age of 3 months?

Hip ultrasonography is gaining wide acceptance as the method of choice for imaging the infant hip. The use of hip sonography to diagnose hip dysplasia in infancy was developed by Dr. Graf. His method emphasized angular measurement of acetabular landmarks in addition to assessment of hip position. Dr. Harcke developed a dynamic approach that assesses the hip in several positions.

5. What are the most common uses of diagnostic ultrasound in children's orthopaedics?

Ultrasonography is the method of choice in detecting early DDH before ossification of the femoral head. It is also a valuable study for evaluation of a possible imbedded foreign body, detection of joint effusion (especially the hip joint), and evaluation of soft tissue masses. Ultrasonography can also be used to evaluate physeal fractures in young children.

6. When is a bone scan ordered?

In osteomyelitis, the plain films may be negative until 7–10 days after the onset of symptoms. Early diagnosis is greatly aided by use of a 3-phase bone scan. The study is also a good screening tool for the child with occult back or limb complaints.

7. How can osteomyelitis be differentiated from cellulitis with a bone scan?

On the 3-phase bone scan, cellulitis demonstrates increased uptake in the immediate phase (perfusion images) and the blood pool images. Normal activity is demonstrated on delayed images. Osteomyelitis often has abnormal activity in all three phases but is most specifically positive on the delayed image.

8. Are bone scans useful in the diagnosis of spondylolysis?

A bone scan has been shown to be an effective method for identifying acute spondylolysis. AP, lateral, and oblique views of the lumbosacral spine should be obtained first. In many cases, even the oblique views are not clear, and then the bone scan is needed.

9. When is SPECT used?

A single-photon emission computed tomography (SPECT) scan can be used in conjunction with a bone scan. With this technique, sectional images of the body can be obtained in the sagittal, coronal, and axial planes. The SPECT scan is used effectively to detect spondylolysis and to search for small lesions such as osteoid osteoma.

10. Should bone scans be routinely ordered for Legg-Calvé-Perthes disease?

No. In most cases, the decisions required for treating this disease can be made by careful study of plain films. A bone scan rarely changes one's treatment plan.

11. What are some of the most common uses of CT scans in children's orthopaedics?
The most common use is to determine torsional alignment of the lower limbs. To assess accurately femoral anteversion and tibial torsion, the hip, knee, and ankle must be measured in the transverse plane. Also, exact limb-length measurement and assessment of benign and malignant bone lesions can be done.

The CT scan is also used document physeal injury with closure and bar formation. In complex pelvic and acetabular fractures, CT scanning helps to document the exact nature of the injury and also helps in treatment planning. In patients with foot pain with inconclusive plain films, the CT scan can help identify a tarsal coalition.

12. When is three-dimensional CT useful?
The addition of orthogonal planar sections and 3-D reconstruction to routine axial CT imaging enhances the imaging of complex structures. The edit function allows removal of any structure in the image for direct visualization of a single part (e.g., removing the hip so that the acetabulum can be seen directly). These capabilities aid in the evaluation of hip dysplasia in children (especially those older than the age of 4 years). Three-dimensional CT scans are also helpful for assessment of femoral head deformity in avascular necrosis and for the evaluation of complex congenital spine deformities.

13. What children's orthopaedic conditions are best studied by MRI?
Spine: Hydromyelia (syringomyelia), Chiari malformation, tethered cord, bifid spine conditions (diastematomyelia), intraspinal neoplasm, herniated disk and diskitis (infectious spondylitis). If a child with scoliosis has an unusual curve pattern (especially a left-sided thoracic curve), one should consider further evaluation with an MRI. Children who have unexplainable unilateral deformity of an upper or lower extremity (shoulder weakness, unilateral cavus deformity of the foot) should have a screening spinal MRI to rule out intraspinal disease.

Marrow system: Avascular necrosis of the femoral head, assessment of the presence and extent of osteomyelitis and soft tissue abscesses, detection of nondisplaced femoral neck fractures, and early diagnosis of bone marrow tumors.

Knee: Meniscal tears, cruciate ligament injuries, and other soft tissue lesions can be diagnosed with an accuracy close to 95%. More important, occult bone lesions and osteochondral injuries, which are not detectable radiographically, can be diagnosed. In young children, MRI allows diagnosis of a discoid meniscus.

Ankle: Osteochondral lesions, tendon tears, and ligament injuries. MRI can also be used to detect tarsal coalition; however, a CT scan is the preferred method.

BIBLIOGRAPHY

1. Morrisy RT, Weinstein SL (eds): Lovell and Winter's Pediatric Orthopaedics, Vol. I. Philadelphia, Lippincott-Raven, 1996.
2. Orthopaedic Knowledge Update 5. Rosemont, IL, American Academy of Orthopaedic Surgeons, 1996.
3. Resnick D: Bone and Joint Imaging. Philadelphia, W.B. Saunders Co., 1989.
4. Rockwood CA Jr, Wilkins KE, Beatty JE (eds): Fractures in Children, Vol. 3. Philadelphia, J.B. Lippincott Co., 1996.

9. GAIT LABORATORY

Tom F. Novacheck, M.D., and James R. Gage, M.D.

1. What is a gait laboratory, who works there, and what type of information can be obtained from it?

A gait lab is an area where an individual's gait can be assessed. In its simplest sense, gait analysis may consist of study of a videotape of an individual walking, perhaps reviewed in slow motion. When this information is coupled with the physical exam, the practitioner begins to have some understanding of the individual's gait.

A modern-day gait lab generally includes some type of marker set and camera system that can be used to evaluate three-dimensional joint movement. The study of joint movement is called kinematics. If this information is combined with force-plate data, joint moments and powers can be studied. This is called *kinetics*. It provides insight into the "how" and "why" of the movement we observe. Dynamic EMG provides the timing of muscle activation. EMG data can be gathered for some muscle groups by use of surface electrodes applied to the skin. For others, fine wire needle electrodes may be needed. Some gait labs use the pedobarograph to measure plantar pressure distribution in the foot. Gait efficiency can be measured with an oximeter. A computer system allows collection, storage, manipulation, and evaluation of the data.

The space and computer equipment would be useless without the trained technical and professional staff who know how to use it. At bare minimum, this includes a physical therapist or kinesiologist and a computer technician. Most gait labs also employ an engineer (or computer system administrator) and clerical support. A physician trained in this area of expertise completes the team.

2. Describe the normal walking gait cycle.

A complete gait cycle or stride can be considered the basic unit of measurement of gait (see Figure). It begins when one foot strikes the ground and ends when the same foot strikes the ground again. The gait cycle is divided into two major phases, stance and swing. Stance phase begins with "initial contact," which in normal gait is with the heel, and ends at "toe off," when swing phase begins. Toe off typically occurs at about 60% of the gait cycle in normal walking. Swing phase is the period of time from "toe off" until the foot hits the ground again.

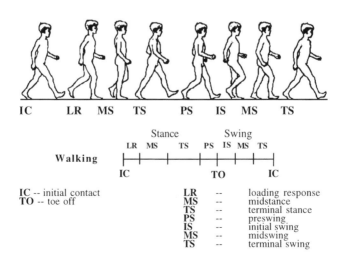

The Normal Walking Gait Cycle

29

3. Describe the normal running gait cycle.

In running, toe off occurs before 50% of the gait cycle. Stance and swing phases are subdivided into two periods, absorption and generation. In stance phase, the shock of contact with the ground is initially absorbed by the stance phase limb while body weight is being accepted. Stance phase reversal (StR) marks the end of the absorption period, when the muscles begin to generate power and the joints extend. The muscles continue to generate power into swing phase as the leg is propelled forward. As in stance, there is a reversal point, swing phase reversal (SwR), after which the joints extend. The purpose of the absorption period in swing phase is to decelerate the leg in preparation for contact with the ground.

The Running Gait Cycle

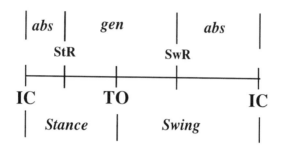

| absorption | -- | from SwR through IC to StR |
| propulsion | -- | from StR through TO to SwR |

The Running Gait Cycle

4. How do walking and running differ?

Walking and running differ in several ways.

1. Although they share the same basic principle of maintaining energy efficiency, they differ in the speed of locomotion.

2. By the most basic definition, greater than 50% of the gait cycle is spent in stance during walking. Therefore, there are two periods of double support during each gait cycle. Because toe off occurs before the midpoint of the gait cycle in running, the two periods of double support seen in walking give way to two periods of double float in running, during which neither foot is in contact with the ground (see Figure).

3. The third basic difference is in the way that potential and kinetic energy are related. During walking, potential and kinetic energy are out of phase; i.e., when potential energy is high, kinetic energy is low, and vice versa. During running gait, potential and kinetic energy are in phase. They are both low during the midportion of stance, and both are highest during double float. En-

Double Support(DS)/Double Float(DF)

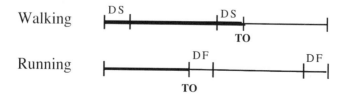

Double Support(DS)/Double Float(DF)

ergy efficiency during walking can be effectively maintained by the interchange between kinetic and potential energy. This cannot occur during running. Instead, potential energy is stored as elastic potential energy in the tendons, and the two joint muscles act as energy straps transferring energy between body segments.

5. What is kinematics?

Kinematics is a description of movement, including joint angles, displacement, velocities, and accelerations, without consideration of the forces responsible for creating those movements. The results are plotted on a graph as a function of time.

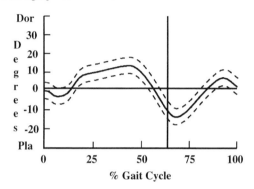

Ankle Motion (sagittal plane). This graph of the ankle shows one complete walking cycle plotted along the X axis, or abscissa, as a percentage of the gait cycle. The graph begins and ends at initial contact with the vertical line (at about 60%), representing toe off. The degree of motion of the joint is plotted along the Y axis, or ordinate. At initial contact, the ankle is at a 90° angle (neutral position). As the foot moves to being flat on the floor, the ankle plantar flexes (below the zero line). During the period of increasing dorsiflexion, the tibia advances over the stationary foot. A maximum of 12° of dorsiflexion is reached. A period of plantar flexion follows as the heel rises from the floor at the time of push-off. During swing phase, the ankle dorsiflexes to avoid dragging the toe and to prepare for the next heel strike.

6. What is kinetics?

Kinetics studies the cause of movement. The parameters include ground reaction and inertial forces, muscle and ligament forces, joint moments, and joint powers. By combining joint motion

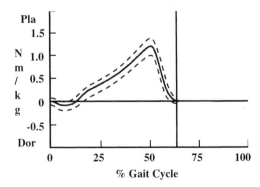

Ankle Moment (sagittal plane). As in the kinematic graph, the X axis depicts the percentage of the gait cycle, beginning at initial contact. The vertical line represents toe off. The ordinate or Y axis is the joint moment standardized for body weight. Below the zero line is a net dorsiflexor moment (the forefoot is being lowered to the ground under the control of the dorsiflexors). Above is a net plantar flexor moment (the plantar flexors dominate for the remainder of the stance phase).

and force-plate information, moments and powers can be calculated using a process called *inverse dynamics*. A moment of force (see Figure) is a force acting at a distance from the axis of rotation, causing the body to rotate. It is expressed as M = F × d and is expressed in newton-meters (Nm). The joint power (see Figure) is the product of the joint's net moment times the joint's velocity of movement (P = F × d × angular velocity).

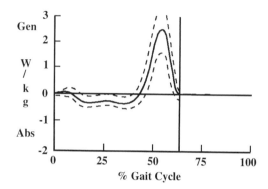

% Gait Cycle

Ankle Joint Power (sagittal plane). Power output is displayed on the Y axis of the power graph. It is also standardized for body weight and is expressed in watts/kg. Power generation is positive, above the zero line, and represents a concentric muscle contraction. Power absorption is negative, representing an eccentric or lengthening contraction. During midstance, the position of the tibia is controlled by the eccentric contraction of the plantar flexors. During preswing (just prior to toe off), the plantar flexors contract concentrically to gen-erate power, driving the heel off the floor and propelling the leg into swing phase.

7. What are the five prerequisites of normal gait?
1. Stability in stance
2. Clearance in swing
3. Adequate step length
4. Appropriate prepositioning for initial contact
5. Energy conservation

8. What are the main sources of power in normal walking?
The center of mass rises to its zenith twice during each gait cycle, in midstance and again in midswing. As the body's center of mass falls, *potential energy is converted to kinetic energy* to provide the momentum necessary for forward movement. The lowest point of the center of mass occurs during the two periods of double support, loading response and preswing. It is from these two lowest points that energy from muscle contraction must be input into the system. A pulling of the body by the *hip extensors* (gluteus maximus and hamstrings) of the forward limb occurs at the beginning of stance during loading response. During preswing, the *gastrocsoleus* and the *il-iopsoas* contract to propel the trailing limb into swing.

9. In which situations might a patient be appropriately referred to a gait lab?
Abnormal gait is a frequent presenting complaint. The astute clinician can frequently deter-mine the cause by evaluating the history, physical exam and x-rays. Occasionally, the cause or nature of the abnormality remains elusive. In this situation, the gait laboratory, can be thought of as a dynamic assessment tool. A better understanding of the consequences of a deformity such as leg length discrepancy can also be assessed.

The most frequent use of the gait lab is to aid in decision-making in the management of neu-romuscular conditions. The effects of arthrodesis, lower extremity deformity, orthotics, or pros-thetics can also be assessed.

10. Wouldn't the clinical examination of such individuals in conjunction with appropriate roentgenograms and videotaping of gait be sufficient to treat the majority of patients with neuromuscular problems? Why is gait analysis necessary?
During the clinical examination, the person being examined is usually either sitting or lying down. Muscle tone in cerebral palsy varies a great deal with position and activity. During walking, a trained observer can see many gait disorders, but he or she will miss many more, since the human eye frames at only 16 hertz (sees 16 separate events per second). Videotaping a patient is better since it can be viewed repetitively and in slow motion, but the motions of the hip and ankle are difficult to observe. Even if one could accurately assess the motion of each of the lower extremity joints during gait, one would still know nothing about the forces that drive that motion. Gait analysis examines the patient dynamically during the act of walking and accurately measures the three-dimensional motions at each of the major lower extremity joints. In addition, gait analysis can estimate the moments that are being produced around the hip, knee, and ankle joints during gait and can also estimate the net muscle moments that must be produced to resist those moments. Since the masses of the various segments can be calculated and the distances between the points of application of the muscle forces and the joint centers are known, the net muscle forces can be calculated through a process known as *inverse dynamics*.

11. Why is posttreatment gait analysis obtained? What specific information does it provide?
Posttreatment gait analysis provides a great deal of information. For example, oxygen cost (mlO_2/kg/m) provides us with information about the efficiency of gait. If this is compared with the presurgical oxygen cost, we can assess the benefits of the patient's surgery in terms of energy consumption. Kinematic and kinetic parameters can also be assessed and compared with both normal values and the patient's preoperative state. This allows us to critique surgery accurately, which is extremely useful, particularly if multiple procedures are done during a single operative session. Postoperative gait analysis will also frequently demonstrate persistent abnormalities of gait that can be corrected but that were not appreciated at the time of the original analysis because they were masked by other problems.

12. If gait analysis is so useful, why isn't it accepted more widely?
Gait analysis is not as "user friendly" as some of the other new technologies, like MRI or CT. For example, most physicians can employ their knowledge of anatomy when they look at CT or MRI images and so can immediately see the disorder that is present. Gait analysis is more like electrocardiography. The graphs and charts that are generated do not mean anything to the observer unless he or she has been trained to interpret them. In addition, gait analysis requires a lot of background information, such as an understanding of the principles of normal and pathologic gait. Unfortunately, this type of training is not included in most orthopaedic residency programs.

13. Can you demonstrate the usefulness of clinical gait analysis with a specific clinical example?
Yes. A.B. is a patient who had a cerebrovascular accident at the age of 2, which left him with a right spastic hemiplegia. Although on clinical examination and observation of gait, he appeared to have involvement of both lower extremities, gait analysis (which included dynamic EMG, kinematics, and kinetics) demonstrated that all his fixed deformities were on the right side and that the abnormalities on the left were dynamic in nature. That is, they were adaptive or "coping" responses to the right-sided deformities. On the right, he had contractures of the psoas, medial hamstrings, rectus femoris, and gastrocnemius (but not the soleus). He also had excessive femoral anteversion on the right. He compensated for this by retracting the right side of his pelvis during walking. This gait adaptation made the rotation of the right lower extremity appear normal to observational gait analysis but produced an apparent internal rotation deformity of the left lower extremity. Once all the structural abnormalities of gait had been identified with certainty, we could correct them surgically. Consequently, the patient underwent the following procedures on the right side: intertrochanteric derotational femoral osteotomy, intramuscular psoas tenotomy, me-

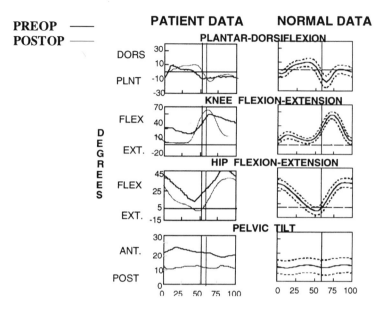

Kinematics—sagittal plane

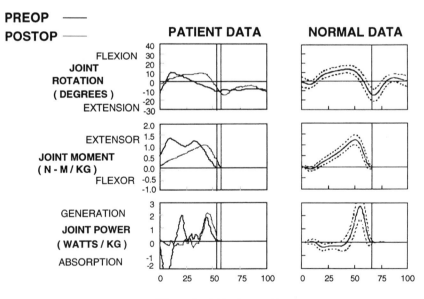

Kinematics & kinetics—ankle

dial hamstring lengthening, transfer of the distal end of the rectus femoris to the intramuscular tendon of the gracilis, and recession of the gastrocnemius on the soleus (Strayer procedure). The pre- and postoperative sagittal plane kinematics (see Figure) are shown here along with the pre- and postoperative ankle kinetics (see Figure). Normal values are included on the graphs so that the reader can see the changes that occurred as a result of the surgery and can compare the pre- and postoperative values with the normal curves.

14. Should insurance be expected to pay for this type of complex, expensive testing?

Most major insurance carriers state that they are interested in quality (optimal outcomes) and cost. Gait analysis allows accurate assessment of the patient's preoperative status as well as the outcome of the intervention. The former allows optimal correction of the gait abnormalities, and the latter allows an accurate critique of the outcome. Over the long term, gait analysis will allow us to identify treatments that are ineffective or harmful. This should have the effect of improving outcomes and reducing the long-term cost of care. Since gait analysis is a general term that can cover a multitude of assessments, however, it is reasonable for insurance companies to ask that national standards be set up and monitored so that treatment centers that are using gait analysis assessments appropriately can be reimbursed and frivolous or unnecessary tests can be avoided.

15. Computerized gait analysis has been available at some centers for more than a decade. Can you point to specific clinically useful information that has come about through the use of gait analysis?

The treatment of cerebral palsy has changed dramatically as a result of knowledge gleaned from pre- and postoperative gait analysis. For example, psoas tenotomy or recession of the psoas tendon to the hip capsule has been replaced by intramuscular psoas tenotomy because the former procedures excessively weaken hip flexion. We have learned that the hip adductors perform an extremely important function during walking and that excessive adductor weakening must be avoided. Consequently, in an ambulator, we rarely do more than release the adductor longus from its pelvic origin in conjunction with an intramuscular gracilis tenotomy, and we *never* perform an obturator neurectomy. The rationale for transfer of the distal end of the rectus femoris to the sartorius or gracilis came about as a result of information gained from gait analysis, and this procedure has proved to be very useful in restoring knee motion during the swing phase of gait. Gait analysis has demonstrated that the soleus is almost never contracted in spastic diplegia, and as such tendoachilles lengthening is rarely indicated, since it lengthens both the gastrocnemius and the soleus. As a result, at our center, this procedure has largely been replaced by gastrocnemius recession (Strayer procedure).

Finally, we now have a much better understanding of pathologic gait and the interactions between muscle, ground reaction, and inertial forces. All these forces act on skeletal levers to produce moments on the joints of the lower extremities. We now know that these skeletal levers are often deformed by the abnormal growth forces induced by the patient's neuromuscular condition. Hip subluxation, torsional deformities of the femur or tibia, or pes varus or valgus are all examples of this. Consequently, we have coined the term "lever-arm dysfunction" to describe the skeletal malformations that produce gait abnormalities. It is worth noting that once identified, most of these abnormalities can be corrected with appropriate orthopaedic procedures.

16. Is it necessary to utilize gait analysis routinely in the treatment of all or most individuals with neuromuscular impairment of locomotion, or would it be better to utilize it in certain centers as a research tool?

We feel that to obtain and measure optimal patient outcomes, some form of gait analysis will be necessary at all centers that treat cerebral palsy. Clinical centers probably will not require measurement tools as extensively as those centers that are involved in research, however. For example, specific treatment protocols for each of four distinct subtypes of hemiplegia in cerebral palsy could not have been developed without the use of comprehensive gait analysis, including kinetics (moments and powers). Now that the patterns have been described and their characteristics are known, however, a clinical center could easily identify the patterns and could apply the treatment protocols with the aid of a laboratory that only generated kinematic information.

17. What happens if gait analysis is not employed routinely in neuromuscular conditions such as cerebral palsy?

There are three major problems that occur when gait analysis is not routinely employed.

1. In general, physicians who do not make use of gait analysis usually have not studied ambulation and so have little or no knowledge of the principles of normal and pathologic gait. As such, their treatment decisions are almost always empiric and based on inadequate knowledge. Consequently, the results of their treatment are usually inadequate.

2. Even if the physician were to understand fully the principles of normal and pathologic gait, he or she would probably not be able to obtain an optimal treatment result without gait analysis because the subtleties of the gait disorder could not be determined.

3. Without gait analysis, there is no way to assess accurately the results of treatment.

18. Is there any objective evidence of improved outcomes with the use of gait analysis? If not, how can this be obtained?

Gait laboratory outcome studies are starting to appear. Many of these are critiques of individual procedures such as selective dorsal rhizotomy, tendoachilles lengthening or rectus femoris transfer.

The problem is that the question that needs to be answered definitively is, "What is the outcome of treatment of patients with gait analysis compared with treatment of patients without it?" Consequently, what is really needed is a study in which two groups of patients have gait analysis pre- and postoperatively. In the first group, gait analysis would be used to document the initial and final states only, and no preoperative gait information would be provided to the treating physician. In the second group, gait analysis would be fully employed in the decision-making process. The dilemma at present is that centers that utilize gait analysis are unwilling to subject patients to treatment without it, and those that do not use motion analysis will not send their patients to a gait analysis center for pre-and posttreatment assessment.

19. How can one insure that children who require gait analysis have access to it?

This is probably the most difficult question to answer. I think that this can only be accomplished when physicians, consumers, and payers are aware of the benefits of gait analysis and of the harm that can occur when the tool is not used.

20. What is the future of gait analysis?

The technology of gait analysis is improving rapidly. Currently, software is being rewritten to make the output of the analysis much more "user friendly." Within the next few years, motion analysis reports will probably be delivered in a CD-ROM format, which will include the actual video of the patient, the roentgenograms, and results of the static examination plus the entire gait analysis presented in an easily understood style. For example, to view the kinetics about the knee, the user might just double click with the mouse on the knee joint of the patient and then would be presented with the data for that joint in a variety of user-friendly formats. New technology will allow better modeling of the foot and other parts of the anatomy with multiple articulations in close proximity that are now difficult to assess. Gait analysis will therefore come into routine use in the design and evaluation of prosthetics, orthotics, and running shoes. Faster cameras and more portable equipment will bring gait analysis out onto the sports field, where it will find great use in the evaluation of elite performance. Best of all, we can expect that with improvements in technology, the cost of the equipment will continue to fall, which should bring gait analysis into much wider use.

BIBLIOGRAPHY

1. Boscarino LF, Ounpuu S, Davis RB, et al.: Effects of selective dorsal rhizotomy on gait in children with cerebral palsy. J Pediatr Orthop 13:174–179, 1993.
2. Gage JR, Perry J, Hicks RR, et al.: Rectus femoris transfer to improve knee function of children with cerebral palsy. Dev Med Child Neurol 29:159–166, 1987.
3. Gage JR: Gait Analysis in Cerebral Palsy. New York, MacKeith Press, 1991.
4. Gage JR: Gait analysis: An essential tool in the treatment of cerebral palsy. Clin Orthop 288:126–134, March 1993.
5. Gage JR: The clinical use of kinetics for evaluation of pathological gait in cerebral palsy. J Bone Joint Surg 26A(4):622–631, 1994.
6. Gage JR, DeLuca PA, Renshaw TS: Gait analysis: principles and applications. J Bone Joint Surg 77A:1607–1623, 1995.
7. Novacheck TF: "Running and Sprinting: A Dynamic Analysis" (video). St. Paul, MN, Motion Analysis Lab, Gillette Children's Hospital, 1996.
8. Novacheck TF: Walking, running, and sprinting: A three-dimensional analysis of kinematics and kinetics. Instructional Course Lecture. Am Acad Orthop Surg 44:497–506, 1995.
9. Winters TF, Hicks R, Gage JR: Gait patterns in spastic hemiplegia in children and young adults. J Bone Joint Surg 69A:437–441, 1987.

10. PHILOSOPHY OF CARE

Klaus Parsch, Dr. med.

1. What factors go into a treatment decision?
- The treatment must be necessary. The condition being treated must have a potential to produce disability.
- Treatment should be effective in altering the course of the disease.
- The benefits of the treatment should not exceed the risks and negative psychologic effects.

2. What are the major responsibilities of the physician?
- Establish a correct diagnosis by an exact examination of the problem area and a general musculoskeletal screening examination.
- Discover conditions that are treatable and have the potential to cause disability.
- Explain your findings in understandable words to the parents and, if the child is old enough, to the patient as well.

3. What are some of the pediatric orthopaedic red flags?
- A neonate with a painful paralyzed-looking arm or leg. You must rule out septic arthritis and neonatal osteomyelitis of the shoulder or the hip in this infant.
- Asymmetry of the spine, the neck, or the legs or a foot deformity of small infant. You must rule out developmental dysplasia by doing an ultrasound examination of the hips.
- A kindergarten or school-aged child with minor discrete limb complaints on physical activity. An exact clinical examination of knees and hips must be performed. An effusion of the hip or Legg-Calvé-Perthes disease may be present.
- Knee pain, especially in the adolescent. Always examine the knees and the hips to discover clinically a possible slip of the capital femoral epiphysis.
- Knee pain at rest or at night in children and adolescents. Take an x-ray to look for osteosarcoma of the distal femur.
- A child refusing to walk and play, complaining about the back, and showing signs of obstipation. Clinical, laboratory, and possibly MRI examinations must be done to rule out spondylodiskitis.

4. What must you know about the natural history?
Do not suggest active treatment if the natural history will allow spontaneous resolution.

5. What do you do if spontaneous correction cannot be expected?
You *may* discuss active treatment if spontaneous resolution is improbable. If the only effective treatment would be surgical correction, the potential for disability must be weighed against the risks of correction.

You *must* suggest active surgical or other treatment if the spontaneous evolution of this condition has proven disadvantages for the child.

6. What should you do if the primary care doctor or your orthopaedic colleague has overlooked an important diagnosis?
Try to find out all the background information before expressing a negative opinion. Talk to the involved colleague. Such sensitive matters should be handled with great care.

7. What are the main reasons that parents choose *not* to change doctors?
- **Good human relations**. The doctor has explained enough. The patient and the family have felt themselves to be the center of interest.
- **Competence, good service.**

8. Is there a risk of overtreatment?

With an oversupply of doctors, the risk of overdiagnosis and overtreatment is growing. Instead of an exact clinical examination being performed, more expensive tests such as radiography and MRIs are ordered and billed.

9. How do I avoid just "doing something"?

Relatives and friends can cause a parent to wonder whether a condition is normal or not and whether this needs treatment. It may be helpful to have photos of similar cases demonstrating that many conditions do well without "doing something."

10. Did I follow the right timing for treatment?

Knock-knees or bow knees is a good example of the effectiveness of good timing. A mild knock-knee in a 3-year-old child needs simple observation. The same deformity in a 10-year-old girl might require medial epiphyseodesis to straighten out the legs during residual growth.

If fixation of a unilateral slipped capital femoral epiphysis is done in a boy aged 10 years, something will need to be planned on the contralateral side, because the risk is about 50% that slipping of that side will develop as well.

11. What are some examples of the risk-benefit ratio?

Radiographs taken of mobile flatfeet or asymptomatic spines that are clinically straight are a waste of money and bear the risk of radiation exposure.

Clinical, ultrasound, or radiographic screening programs for hip dysplasia can have a positive risk-benefit ratio. If such programs are run by a constantly changing team with little experience, the risk-benefit ratio may become negative, however, because too many normal hips may be rated as dysplastic and treated by harness or splinting which carries the risk of avascular necrosis.

12. What must the parents be told about certain fractures?

Proximal tibial metaphyseal fractures have the potential risk of resulting in genu valgum if certain precautions are not taken. Even if valgus can be prevented, there will be overgrowth.

Distal tibial metaphyseal fractures need a cast in equinus position to prevent crus recurvatum. The parents and the child will accept better the uncomfortable application if they have received instruction before application of the cast.

Proximal humeral fractures do not need anatomic reduction, heal quickly, and remodel even after major malunion. If this is explained to the parents, they will not demand anatomic reduction under general anesthesia.

Displaced midshaft fractures of the forearm are difficult to reduce and even more difficult to retain in satisfactory position. Repeated manipulations under anesthesia might follow the initial reduction. Provision of simple but complete information to the parents will make it easier for them to accept surgical treatment, such as insertion of intramedullary wires.

All *Salter-Harris grade 4 fractures* and some *grade 2 and 3 fractures* bear the risk of late epiphyseal disturbance, even if they are reduced anatomically. Regular follow-ups are essential to discover such problems. The family must know about the risk right from the start. They must know about the potential complications if they miss a follow-up appointment.

13. How do I instill confidence in the child's family?

Accept the child as a partner. If the child is very unhappy in consultation, try to find a diversion before concentrating on your examination. A chat about a doll or a football team can break the ice.

If you have pictures of similar cases ready, this is helpful for the parents (for example, a lengthening procedure with an Ilizarov apparatus). If you know families who have gone through the same procedure, you might ask them to contact each other. Parent associations are the most important factor in establishing confidence in your medical and surgical abilities.

BIBLIOGRAPHY

1. Rang M: Children's Fractures. Philadelphia, J.B. Lippincott Co., 1974.
2. Staheli LT: Philosophy of Care. Pediatr Clin North Am 33:1269, 1986.

11. PHYSICIAN-PARENT RELATIONSHIP

G. Dean MacEwen, M.D.

1. When should you see parents again after an initial serious discussion?
Arrangements should be made to have a follow-up discussion, preferably face-to-face, within 1–2 weeks of the initial evaluation for a serious problem. A telephone conversation should be used only when a direct discussion is not possible.

2. When should you make specific recommendations for surgery?
It is usually best to have the family and the patient return for a second visit so that questions can be answered before surgery is scheduled. Often, the families feel rushed and believe that they have inadequate information to make a final decision after only one visit with the doctor.

3. When should this follow-up visit be?
An ideal time, in my experience, is 1–3 weeks after the first appointment. I often ask the parents to return with their questions in written form. In this way, they will be more likely to have all their concerns and questions answered.

4. How do you handle parents and patients that live a long distance away when a significant treatment program is necessary?
Although it is ideal to see the patient and the parents back within 1–3 weeks, this may not be practical. Speaking on the telephone with both parents on extensions or using a speaker phone is a possibility. Again, I think this is usually preferable to setting up the surgery date at the first visit.

5. How do you speak to families with a language barrier?
The ideal situation is to find someone who has a medical background to translate. Sometimes people can read English better than they can understand the spoken word. Therefore, some written material or drawings can be very helpful.

6. How much should you tell parents?
Parents need a good deal of information; however, I think it is most important to end consultations with a positive attitude and with some optimism.

7. How do I deliver bad news?
If at all possible, bad news should be delivered at a person-to-person level. Even though you may not feel comfortable delivering bad news face-to-face, it is the best way to do it. Telephone conversations can be perceived as impersonal and unsatisfying.

8. How do you talk with a grandparent who bring the child alone?
This can be a potentially hazardous situation. This is an excellent time to do a little extra listening and a little less talking, so as not to interfere with the relationship you have with the parents.

9. How do you talk to a mother who arrives with the grandmother?
Speak to the mother as much as possible, even if the grandmother dominates the conversation.

10. What is the significance of both the mother and the father showing up?
It is important to direct some of your questions to each parent rather than only to the parent that dominates the conversation. In many cases, both parents attending the conference suggests that the family has a greater than usual concern for a problem that may seem of relatively little consequence to you. In other words, it may take a longer-than-usual interview to determine why both parents are there in come cases. Hear out both parents.

11. What situations can arise with a single parent?
Sometimes one parent thinks that the other parent is not taking good care of the child or has not received good medical advice. You need to get more than the usual amount of history in this situation. If possible, try to hear the other side by involving the other parent. The information in this situation may be very biased. Listen a great deal and be careful about specific recommendations. Try not to take sides or make judgments, at least until you hear from both sides.

12. How do you handle a parent who is hypercritical of treatment by other physicians?
This is the time to slow the consultation down, get the history and the exact names of the physicians who have treated the child, and offer to evaluate the records from the other physician or, better yet, call the other physician directly to see what treatment has been done or offered. It may be flattering to think that the family wants to see *you,* but you can very easily be added to the list of physicians who have displeased the parents. Therefore, finding out the details is most important.

13. What words and sentences should be avoided?
"This problem always corrects with time." I think one should say that the problem *usually* corrects itself but that there are some exceptions; if the exceptions exist, the family and patient may need to return.

Avoid the word "fix." To an orthopaedic surgeon, this often means to stabilize or to improve the immediate problem. To the family, however, this often means that the underlying problem is corrected permanently.

The other word to avoid is "suffered." Rather than writing, "He/she suffered a fracture," the more objective statement would be, "He/she sustained a fracture" or "Fracture is seen on x-ray."

14. What about x-rays?
In almost all instances, the x-rays should be shown to the family and explained. X-rays can easily be obtained for review by others, so it is better for you to explain the details that the family needs to see and understand. If you do not show them the x-rays, they are sometimes concerned that there is a major problem that you do not want them to see. Also, comparison with x-rays that were previously taken can help demonstrate the healing process of a fracture, any change in alignment of a bone after a fracture, and so forth.

15. Should you encourage parents to read about their child's problem?
I think that they should be encouraged to read, but you should encourage them to return with the information they have obtained so that you may help them to interpret it. This avoids confusion, especially when the new information may cause skepticism of your treatment program.

16. Should you try to settle problems on the telephone?
A problem that is a real concern to a family should probably be dealt with face-to-face. Minor problems can be settled on the telephone, but many times a few minutes of direct observation are necessary to show the degree of seriousness of the problem.

17. Should you keep records of telephone calls?
All telephone calls concerning follow-up of a patient, especially postoperative calls or those after application of a stabilizing cast, should be recorded, with a copy placed in the patient's chart. This prevents forgetting or misinterpreting what has been said.

18. How can you tell if the parents want another opinion?
Offering parents an opportunity to come back and discuss the case before surgery many times will reduce the concern that the family has and will reduce the need for a second opinion. If you have a hint that the family would like a second opinion, discuss it openly with them and offer to make your notes and x-rays available. If this is not discussed and the second opinion is different from yours, the family will be reluctant to come back and discuss the situation with you. If you have already brought up the subject, they will feel more comfortable returning to you.

19. What should you do if parents leave in a very obviously agitated condition?
Call them that evening or no later than the next morning to see what the problem is. Showing your concern and interest is probably the best thing that you can offer them at such a time. It is most undesirable to have parents leave very upset, because the unhappiness may lead to a very poor plan for their child's care.

12. ETHICS

Wilton H. Bunch, M.D., Ph.D., and Victoria M. Dvonch, M.D.

1. What is ethics?
Ethics is the system of problem solving that has the goal of answering the question, "What would the good person do in this situation?" It is concerned with the questions of what is the good and how is the good achieved. Ethics is a philosophic system, not a religious one.

2. Why isn't there one ethical answer?
Different people make different assumptions about the reality of the situation, and there are different ethical systems with which to solve the problem.

3 How many ethical systems exist?
There are at least a half-dozen ethical systems, and because some people tend to be "splitters," we could probably double this number. We will consider only three, which are the most commonly used: rule- or duty-based ethics, consequential- or utilitarian-based ethics, and principle-based ethics.

4. What is rule- or duty-based ethics?
This system of ethics looks for rules that we have a duty to follow. The rules and laws of society provide us with the basis for deciding what is good. These may change quite dramatically over time. In the early 1970s, society considered it acceptable for high-level myelomeningocele babies to receive comfort care only; however, in the later years of that decade, the rules changed dramatically and society determined that there was a duty to treat. The physician who did not change with society was at personal and professional risk.

Implicit in rule-based ethics is the notion that what is legal is what is moral and that the will of the majority (legislators) creates morality and defines ethical behavior. Certainly, there was a great change in the percentage of people who approved of abortion after the Supreme Court ruled that it was legal. This is thought to be at least in part due to the fact that abortion was legal, therefore, in many minds, moral.

The concept of duty to a law is entirely independent of who is the lawgiver. People who believe in God may feel an obligation to obey what they perceive to be the rules and laws of God. This is the ethical system of many, whether or not they recognize it as ethics.

5. What is consequentialist- or utilitarian-based ethics?
This system of ethics focuses on the results of actions (consequences) rather than the actions themselves. In thinking this way, one must consider the value that is placed on achieving a certain outcome and the likelihood of achieving such a result. The ethical person will take those actions that result in providing the maximum amount of "goodness" to the most people.

Consider a child with a somewhat short femur for whom the choices are lengthening it or arresting the epiphyses on the opposite side. The value of achieving normal length is very high, but in this particular child, the probability is low of arriving there without major complications and an extended period of treatment. This is compared with the lower desirability of short but equal femurs obtained with little likelihood of complications and a short treatment course. Consequentialist thinking would lead to a comparison of these outcomes (and others) and would choose the one that offered the best (greatest good) expected outcome. This illustration shows that consequentialist thinking is identical, in many cases, with medical decision-making.

The emphasis on the consequences of actions rather than the actions themselves can lead to serious arguments. For example, an infant has multiple congenital anomalies that are not consistent with life. Is allowing this child to die the same as assisting in the death of such an infant? After all, the end (consequence) is the same, death.

6. What is principle-based ethics (bioethics)?

Principle-based ethicists argue that you will never get people to agree on rules or the values of outcomes, so we should try to agree on some basic ideas that everyone can support. This system of ethics has become the dominant system in medicine since the late 1960s. In this system, there are four principles that should govern moral actions.

- **Autonomy.** Autonomy is the right of the individual to exercise the capacity of rational choice. It is the personal rule of self, free from control by others and free from external or internal constraints. In theory, this requires the cognitive capacity to collect and process information in order to arrive at a decision for personal choice. In pediatric practice, the autonomy is exercised on behalf of the child by the parent.

An occasional physician demonstrates confusion with regard to this ethical principle. It is concerned with the autonomy of the patient and family, not the autonomy of the physician.

- **Beneficence.** A physician, nurse, or other health care professional should always try to prevent evil, remove evil when present, and promote good. There is nothing in principle-based ethics that defines what is evil and good, however. It is usually necessary to use another system to reach the decision about the good.
- **Nonmaleficence.** One ought never to inflict evil or harm on any person. This principle specifies an omission of actions that would result in harm. Clearly, it is the other side of the coin from beneficence.
- **Justice.** The principle of justice requires that equals be treated equally. Thus, two children with identical diseases should, in justice, receive treatment that anticipates the identical result. This principle demands that technically complex procedures should be done by the most experienced surgeon regardless of the source of the payment.

Justice is also concerned with the distribution of essential services to members of a community. Pediatric orthopaedists have long worried about performing expensive surgery on a severely retarded child that would be paid for by the state when the same money could provide immunizations or dental care for thousands of children. In general, even after worrying, the surgery was performed because the surgeon knew that not doing the surgery would not insure the alternative benefits. If there is any silver lining to the cloud of capitated care, it is that a large, comprehensive pediatric group can now make such ethical choices and determine that the preventative care would be given to the many.

7. Is one system better than another?

No. "Different strokes for different folks" contains a great deal of truth. The personality type who chooses an ethical system based on law is very different from one who thinks consequentially. In many cases, the final conclusion will be the same, even if the process starts from a different point. The major reason for recognizing the different systems is that the physician must be sensitive to the ethical system of the patient's family and work within this scheme.

8. Can I switch from system to system as the occasion changes?

Yes, so long as you know what you are doing. For example, physicians are usually quite comfortable working out of a consequentialist system, and the authors find that this is frequently useful in identifying what is the good. A weakness of this system, however, is that it does not separate letting die from assisting in dying (euthanasia), since the end result is the same.

9. If justice is "treating equals equally," does this mean that all patients must have identical treatment plans?

No!! All patients must receive a treatment plan that anticipates the same functional result, but there may be many ways to achieve this. Consider a 14-year-old girl with 60° right thoracic scoliosis, moderate hypokyphosis, and a 30° flexible left lumbar curve. The correction obtained with a Harrington-Drummond construct, with a Cotrel-Dubousset device, or with an Isola device is slightly greater with increasing implant complexity, but it has never been shown that there is a functional difference. The possible cosmetic differences are still being argued, so it can be assumed that this difference is not great either. Justice requires that the patient be treated with the maximum skill of the surgeon but not necessarily with the same implant.

The hospital deserves justice also. Assume that the surgery is funded by some type of fixed-fee contract. The cost to the hospital of the Harrington-Drummond construct is approximately $750, the Cotrel-Dubousset instrumentation for the same curve would cost about $3500, and the Isola system would cost approximately $5500. It is more than likely that the hospital cannot afford to have the surgeon use the more expensive devices except in unusual cases where the degree of correction is so different that the results are not equal. "Treating equals equally" is not an excuse for rigidly using the most expensive implant system in all cases. On the other hand, it also means that one should not use an inexpensive option that has never been shown to produce comparable results.

10. Will all physicians who use the same ethical system come to the same conclusions?

Frequently not. There are a number of assumptions made by the physician that are as important as the ethical system he or she finds most natural. This is where religion intersects with ethics. Religious beliefs create assumptions about what it means to be a person and the nature of good and evil. Philosophic systems, such as feminism or environmentalism, and the spectrum of political thought also provide assumptions that may enter into ethical thinking.

Other assumptions that physicians make concern natural history of the disease, costs, and the risks of intervention. They also include quality-of-life issues, the support for the family during the treatment plan, the support by the family for this intervention, and the physician's previous experience with similar problems. No doubt other unrecognized personal factors also strongly influence the final ethical decision.

Imagine the problem of a severely retarded 10-year-old child with a 50° scoliosis. One physician may assume that curve progression is not a priority when everything else concerning this person's life is considered. Another physician may assume that increasing curvature will cause care problems that have an impact on quality of life and therefore must be prevented. Yet another physician will assume that all progressive spinal curves must be fused and that the other disabilities of the child are irrelevant. These different assumptions lead to different conclusions about what is good for this child.

In this case, all the physicians may think in terms of an ethical system of duty and obligation. Two feel an obligation to intervene in the natural history, and the other recognizes an obligation not to intervene but to let nature take its course, even if the patient were to die earlier owing to respiratory complications. The difference is not ethics, but assumptions.

These three physicians may be thinking in terms of a consequentialist ethical system. Two place a high negative value on the consequence of curve progression, while the other may place little value on a curve increase owing to other factors, such as the physician's assessment of the patient's quality of life, which are deemed more important.

11. Is ethics more than just personal opinion?

Yes, much more. Some people try to equate ethics with emotions and feelings, but this approach contains no objective consideration of good or evil and no systematic appreciation of the consequences of action. This view is summarized, "If it feels good, do it."

Some attempt to equate ethics with preferences or choices, but this establishes values that are arbitrary. This is summarized by the statement of a famous film producer, "The heart wants what the heart wants."

Some try to equate ethics with intuition. For these, the knowledge of good and evil is essentially mysterious, and their deeds are based on isolated acts of insight. There is no continuity or ability to communicate these insights. This view is expressed as, "Trust me, I know that we should do this."

13. INTEGRATING THE CHILD WITH A DISABILITY INTO SOCIETY

Mary Williams Clark, M.D.

1. Why is this chapter necessary?
Without some help from medical professionals, many children with disabilities will not achieve their maximum potential for participation in society.

2. What are the everyday issues facing the young person with a significant physical difference?
Communication, mobility, independence in self-care (ADL's, or activities of daily living: getting in and out of bed, dressing, hygiene, eating, etc.), and *access* to buildings, to public and private transportation, to educational and vocational opportunities, and recreation. It is important to ask patients and their families about the above practical concerns, and to note any problems.

3. Who can help with communication?
Evaluation and recommendation of appropriate devices is usually arranged through speech and language specialists, with the help of rehabilitation engineers and sometimes occupational therapists (usually part of the team in rehabilitation programs in medical or rehabilitation centers; most of these centers have outpatient programs to which you can refer.) If your patients are having problems getting help, start with the closest department of speech pathology.

4. Who can help with mobility aids?
Crutches and walkers are most easily obtained from physical therapists, orthotists, or DME (durable medical equipment) vendors. Therapists can fit and train in use of the equipment.

Braces (orthoses) are necessary for many young people with disabilities. They almost always need to be custom-made and rechecked for fit and any skin reactions. Therapists should teach function with the braces, including using steps and ramps and getting up and down from chairs and the floor.

Wheelchairs and cushions need to be ordered with the particular patient's size, ability to push, necessary height, etc., in mind. Therapists and DME vendors can help you and the patient select appropriate options.

For special needs, adaptive seating specialists are available, usually at medical or rehabilitation centers. These specialists offer evaluation for power chairs and scooters and custom supportive seating. Power chairs are now lighter, quieter, and easier to maneuver than before, and the controls are programmable.

5. Who can help with ADL's?
Occupational therapists and rehabilitation nurses. Children need "tune-ups" as they reach different ages and stages. Some children with significant disabilities will need on-going therapy for ADL function and mobility as outpatients; this therapy is usually available in the community. Therapists are also available through school systems for monitoring education-related functions

(mobility, communication, bathroom use, etc.), but it is difficult to accomplish actual training in the school setting, as most school districts have a limited number of therapists.

6. Who can help with education?
Special education teachers and psychologists can evaluate children with appropriately-mod-ified-if-necessary IQ testing for learning disabilities, and to determine other aspects of appropriate school placement. Early intervention units and developmental clinics can be found through pediatricians. Physical accessibility is mandated for all publicly funded schools. Parents have the right to be present and have input into Individual Education Plans (IEP's) if their child is eligible for special education.

Public Law 94-142 was enacted in 1975 and became effective in late 1977. It was the first U.S. federal law to mandate appropriate education in "the least restrictive environment" for all children with disabilities. In 1986, P.L.99-457 mandated Early Intervention services for infants and children under three years. P.L.101-476 further updated and specified the provisions of 94-142, and is titled Individuals with Disabilities Education Act (IDEA).

These laws are still necessary and important: many obstacles exist, and openness to students with differences varies among school districts, often relating directly to the principal's attitude.

7. Are there any specific school-related problems?
Inappropriate placement: a child in a setting that is too restrictive for his/her intellectual or physical capabilities; children mainstreamed into a situation beyond their capabilities.

Inappropriate "solutions": e.g., football players carrying a student up and down the stairs, instead of an elevator or reorganization of room and floor class assignments.

Inappropriate fears: children not allowed to go out for recess with their classmates, forbidden from climbing gyms or swings, not allowed to try out for a sport, etc.

Inappropriate rewards: A's "because she works so hard," or "it's hard for him," don't help prepare them for the real world.

8. Who can help with vocational rehabilitation?
All states have an Office or Division of Vocational Rehabilitation (OVR). Counselors are available to evaluate and help patients 16 and older. There are many Independent Living units and organizations, and they may have more help available than some OVR's, which may be overworked and understaffed.

9. Who can help with social and recreational opportunities?
Therapeutic recreation specialists, or "recreation therapists," and adapted physical educators. Community recreational activities ranging from camping to wheelchair basketball to adaptive skiing are also available. The appendix contains a list of national organizations; information is also becoming available through the Internet.

10. What is the Americans with Disabilities Act (ADA)?
The ADA is a complex law that was enacted in 1990. It has five "titles" or sections, as follows: *Title I* covers *employment*, prohibiting discrimination in terms or conditions of employment for qualified disabled individuals; *Title II* covers *public service* and requires that services offered by public entities (including public transportation) be available and accessible to everyone; *Title III* covers *public accomodation*—"goods, services, privileges, benefits and accomodations offered to the general public." Any new construction open to the public occupied after January 26, 1993 must be accessible. *Titles IV* and *V* address *telecommunication* and *miscellaneous* provisions respectively.

Quote the ADA to individual business owners, local government officials, school boards, etc. Advocate for and with those who need better access wherever you see a need.

11. Define *impairment, disability,* and *handicapped.*
In 1980, the World Health Organization published the International Classification of Impairments, Disabilities, and Handicaps, in which they defined the following terms. *Impairment* as "any

loss or abnormality of psychological, physiologic, or anatomic structure or function"; *Disability* as any restriction or lack of ability [resulting from an impairment] to perform an activity in the manner or within the range considered normal for a human being"; under federal law in the U.S., an individual is *Handicapped* if he or she "has an impairment that substantially limits one or more of life's activities . . . ", and the 1993 AMA Guide to the Evaluation of Permanent Impairment states that "an impaired individual who is able to accomplish a specific task with or without accomodation is *neither* handicapped nor disabled with regard to that task." [emphasis author's]

12. How can I avoid saying things that will offend people who have differences?
People who have physical differences vary in opinion about the use of the words "handicapped," "disabled," and "impaired." Some of them think that some or even all of these words are insulting or demeaning, and would prefer more neutral terms such as "a difference." The WHO and AMA guidelines are very useful for written communication, but they are not much help for spoken language.

The first rule is to think of and mention the person as a person first, and then, if necessary and relevant, his/her condition: they are people who happen to have a certain condition—a young woman with cerebral palsy or a young man who uses a wheelchair (Never say "wheelchair-bound." In reality, people who use wheelchairs move in and out of them; they use them like using a car.) Do not define people by their impairment.

The United Cerebral Palsy Association points out that "People with cerebral palsy and other disabilities have the same rights as everyone else in this world—the right to fall in love, to marry, to hold down a competitive job, to acquire an adequate and appropriate education. Above all, they have a right to self-esteem. Please insure these rights by referring to people with disabilities in terms that acknowledge ability, merit, dignity."

PERIODICALS/NEWSLETTERS

Avenues (arthrogryposis)
P.O. Box 5192
Sonora, CA 95370
avenues@sonnet.com

Exceptional Parent
P.O. Box 3000, Dept EP
Denville, NJ 07834-9919

In Motion
Amputee Coalition of America
P.O. Box 2528
Knoxville, TN 37901-2528

Insights
Spina Bifida Assoc. of America
4590 MacArthur Blvd NW, Suite 250
Washington, DC 20007-4226
spinabifda@aol.com

Mainstream
P.O. Box 370598
San Diego, CA 92137-0598
publisher@mainstream-mag.com
http://www.mainstream-mag.com

New Mobility
P.O. Box 15518
North Hollywood, CA 91615-9773
sam@miramar.com
http://www.newmobility.com

Sports 'n Spokes (sports, wheelchair users)
2111 Highland Ave, Suite 180
Phoenix, AZ 85016-4702

SuperKids (limb differences)
60 Clyde St
Newton, MA 02160

ORGANIZATIONS

Association of Disabled American Golfers
7700 E. Arapahoe Rd, Suite 350
Englewood, CO 80112
303-220-0921

Disabled Sports USA
451 Hungerford Dr, Suite 100
Rockville, MD 20850
301-217-0960

National Foundation for Wheelchair Tennis
940 Calle Amanecer, Suite B
San Clemente, CA 92673
714-361-3663
nfwt@aol.com
www.nfwt.org

National Sports Center for the Disabled
P.O. Box 1290
Winter Park, CO 80482
970-726-1540
info@nscd.org
www.nscd.org/nscd

National Wheelchair Basketball Association
c/o Charlotte Institute for Rehabilitation
1100 Blythe Blvd
Charlotte, NC 28203
704-355-1064

North American Riding for the Handicapped
Association
P.O. Box 33150
Denver, CO 80233
800-369-RIDE

United States Cerebral Palsy Athletic Association
200 Harrison Avenue
Newport, RI 02840
401-848-2460

Wheelchair Athletics of the USA (track & field)
30 Myano Lane
Stamford, CT 06902
203-967-2231

Wheelchair Sports USA
3595 East Fountain Blvd, Suite L-1
Colorado Springs, CO 80910
719-574-1150

14. ANESTHESIA

Fay Z. Safavi, M.B.B.S., F.F.A.R.C.S.

1. Why are anesthesiologists concerned about colds in children before surgery?

Upper respiratory infections (URIs) are the most common illnesses affecting children younger than 5 years of age. (Reported incidence of URI is 24% in this age group.) Children younger than 1 year of age have an average of 6.1 respiratory illnesses per year. Children between 1 and 5 years of age have an average of 4.7–5.7 respiratory illnesses per year. In children with a URI, there is an increased incidence of the following problems during and after surgery.
- Laryngospasm during induction of and emergence from anesthesia
- Bronchospasm. Viral URI will initiate wheezing more commonly in children than in adults, whether or not they have a history of asthma. Children younger than 5 years of age with pre-existing asthma or with respiratory syncytial virus are more prone to developing bronchospasm.
- Coughing due to increased airway secretion and hyperreactivity. Coughing can infrequently cause silent regurgitation and aspiration.

- Reduction in O^2 saturation intra- and postoperatively owing to above-mentioned factors and also owing to lung atelectasis and reduction of functional residual capacity (FRC).

2. Should routine surgery be canceled in all cases of runny nose?
No. Not every runny nose is due to a URI; it can be due to allergic rhinitis. Inquire if the child has allergies or if there is a family history of allergy.

3. How can I diagnose URI?
In general, two of the following criteria must exist.
- Sore or scratchy throat
- Sneezing
- Rhinitis
- Fever (mild)
- Congestion
- Malaise
- Nonproductive cough
- Laryngitis

Sneezing and runny nose do not necessarily indicate a URI, however. If in doubt, ask the mother if she feels that the patient has a URI.

4. Bottom line: in which group of children with URI should routine surgery definitely be canceled?
- Patients younger than 1 year of age
- Patients with *lower* respiratory infection
- Those with signs of overt viremia or bacteremia
- Patients awaiting operations of long duration that necessitate insertion of an endotracheal (ET) tube (because of increased incidence of intraoperative bronchospasm and postextubation croup)

5. How long must I wait before performing surgery on patients with a suspected respiratory tract infection?
Upper respiratory infection: One to 2 weeks after cessation of symptoms.
Lower respiratory infection: At least 4–6 weeks after cessation of symptoms.

6. How is perioperative fluid managed in children?
There are two types of fluids the body requires: maintenance and replacement. A balanced salt solution (BSS) such as lactated Ringer's or Plasma-Lyte is commonly used for fluid maintenance.

7. How is fluid requirement calculated?
- 4 ml/kg/h for the first 10 kg of body weight
- 2 ml/kg/h for the next 10 kg
- 1 ml/kg/h for any weight of more than 20 kg (i.e., a 30-kg child will receive 70 ml/hour)

8. What is the estimated blood volume (EBV) in children?

AGE	EBV (ml/kg)
Neonate (preterm)	100
Neonate (term)	90
Infant up to 1 year of age	80
Child 1 year or older	70

9. What criteria are used to assess the need for blood transfusion in children?
Healthy children can compensate for acute volume loss of 25–30% before any changes in blood pressure are observed. The most reliable early signs of hypovolemic shock in children are persistent tachycardia, poor capillary refill time (i.e., > 2 sec), and diminished pulse pressure.

Intraoperatively, I usually allow the hematocrit to drop to 21–25% before starting blood transfusion. If the patient is hemodynamically unstable despite what seems to be adequate hydration, however, I start blood transfusion earlier.

In patients with high thoracic spinal injury, such as meningomyelocele, I start blood transfusion much earlier than in other patient populations. In this group of patients, all efforts must be made not to challenge the cardiovascular system. Poor control of the autonomic nervous system in this group of patients increases the risk of life-threatening hemodynamic instability.

Postoperatively, if the patient does not exhibit clinical signs of anemia (such as postural hypotension and dizziness), the hematocrit can be allowed to drop to 18–20%.

10. How long should the nothing-by-mouth (NPO) period last?

Infants younger than 6 months of age can continue to have formula or breast milk up to 6 hours before surgery, followed by clear liquids (i.e., water, juice) until 3 hours before surgery.

Older infants and children are not given milk or food for 8 hours, but they can have clear liquids until 3 hours before surgery.

11. What are the different types of myopathies?

Myopathies (primary diseases of muscle fibers) are divided into three groups according to muscle biopsy examination.

1. Segmental necrosis of muscle fibers (e.g., muscular dystrophies such as Duchenne's muscular dystrophy [DMD] or Becker's muscular dystrophy).

2. Structural defects of muscle fibers (e.g., myotonic dystrophy or congenital myopathies).

3. Disorders of conduction function within muscle fibers or at the neuromuscular junction (e.g., myasthenia gravis).

12. What are the coexisting organ system dysfunctions in these groups of patients?

Cardiac abnormalities

- EKG abnormalities are seen in 90% of cases, as demonstrated by progressive decrease in R wave amplitude.
- Mitral valve prolapse and regurgitation have been documented in 20% of affected individuals and are due to papillary muscle dysfunction.

Cardiomyopathy

- Usually confined to the wall of the left ventricle, cardiomyopathy is responsible for the high incidence of cardiac arrhythmias.
- Ultimately, profound right ventricular dysfunction is also possible, leading to congestive cardiac failure.
- Cardiomyopathy is more common in DMD.

Cardiac conductive system abnormality

- More often seen in myotonic dystrophy, this results in dysrhythmias and atrioventricular block.
- The severity of cardiac lesions may not correlate with duration or severity of skeletal muscle disease. Also, restricted activity may mask compromised unstressed cardiac function.

Restrictive respiratory disease

- This is seen due to degeneration of inspiratory, expiratory, and diaphragmatic muscle fibers.
- Patients are more prone to aspiration of secretions owing to ineffective and weak cough and hence are more prone to pneumonia.

13. What preoperative investigations are necessary in patients with myopathy?

- EKG.
- Echocardiography and radionuclide studies, now indispensable in elucidating anatomic abnormalities (e.g., left ventricular wall thickness or mitral valve prolapse).
- Chest x-ray to detect cardiomegaly, diaphragmatic elevation, and pulmonary disease (e.g., infiltrates and mediastinal shifts secondary to scoliosis).
- Pulmonary function testing. Greatest reduction occurs in vital capacity. The reduction of vital capacity to 30–40% of predicted normal usually indicates the need for postoperative ventilatory support.

14. What are the anesthetic risks associated with these groups of patients?
- Malignant hyperthermia (MH) syndrome. This is an inherited myopathy characterized by a hypermetabolic state upon exposure to triggering agents. If untreated, it leads to death. Patients with myopathy (especially DMD) are susceptible to MH; this could be due to shared skeletal muscle disease or gene aberration. Triggering agents include all potent inhalational agents and succinylcholine.
- Cardiac rhythm disturbance.
- Postoperative ventilatory failure.

15. Why are anesthesiologists concerned about cervical spine disease?
- Cervical spine abnormality may result in neurologic dysfunction that significantly affects the anesthetic management.
- Airway management may be made more difficult because of limited range of motion.
- If spinal instability is present, the difficulty and importance of optimal airway management and patient positioning are dramatically increased.

16. What do anesthesiologists look for in their preoperative evaluation of cervical spine abnormality?
Cervical spine stability. If the cervical spine is unstable, movement (e.g., mask ventilation or intubation) may result in loss of normal alignment of the vertebrae, compression of the cord, and possibly permanent neurologic injury.

17. What radiologic examinations are important?
This depends in part on the disease process.

Patients with congenital diseases and those with chronically acquired disease (e.g., rheumatoid arthritis) require lateral spine films in neutral position and flexion and extensions views.

The acute trauma patient should have lateral, anteroposterior, and odontoid views in *neutral* position. If findings are equivocal, then CT scan or MRI may be necessary.

In preschool children, plain radiographs of the spine are difficult to interpret because of incomplete ossification of the spine. Hence, CT scan is the first-line investigation in this age group.

18. What is the best way to manage the airway in patients with cervical spine instability?
There is not one good method. There are many different approaches for intubation of the trachea. All have significant advantages and disadvantages. Whatever technique of intubation is used, the goal should be to eliminate neck and head movement during intubation and subsequent positioning.

19. What methods are used to immobilize the neck during intubation?
- Manual in-line stabilization, preferably by a neurosurgeon or an orthopaedic surgeon
- Halo traction or vest
- Cervical collars, which are least effective (they do not prevent neck movement during intubation) and must not be relied upon during intubation

20. What conditions are associated with cervical spine abnormality?
Congenital
- Down's syndrome (20% incidence of atlanto-occipital instability)
- Goldenhar's syndrome (craniovertebral abnormalities; may limit head extension)
- Klippel-Feil syndrome (fused cervical vertebrae, spinal cord compression)
- Achondroplasia (decreased head extension caused by abnormalities at the atlanto-occipital joint and the upper cervical spine, such as scoliosis, neurofibromatosis, and spondyloepiphyseal dysplasia)
- Mucopolysaccharidoses (Morquio, Hurler, Hunter's, Scheie's, and Sanfilippo's syndromes)

Acquired
- Rheumatoid arthritis
- Ankylosing spondylitis
- Still's disease

- Psoriatic arthritis
- Reiter's syndrome

Trauma

21. What is acute pain?

Acute pain refers to pain of short duration (usually 3–7 days) and is usually associated with surgery, trauma, or an acute illness.

22. Why should we as physicians strive for good management of acute pain?

Effective pain management has been shown to improve mortality and morbidity rates and immune function. Pain is a form of stress and causes release of stress hormones, which cause catabolism and impaired tissue healing.

The value of pre-emptive analgesia in certain conditions is well known. For example, patients who undergo amputation under a regional block have a decreased incidence of phantom pain.

23. Why has acute pain in children been undertreated?

- Lack of ability to assess pain in nonverbal children
- Our fear of respiratory depression and use of narcotic analgesia
- Wrong assumption that the pain pathways are not developed in babies, and therefore they do not feel pain

24. How is acute pain assessed in children?

Age-appropriate pain assessment is essential. Both subjective and objective assessment tools may be utilized depending on patient age and clinical status. Ideally, pain assessment tools *must* be introduced before surgery or before occurrence of pain.

In our institution (Texas Scottish Rite Hospital for Children), we use the Visual Analog Scale (VAS) for patients older than 7 years of age and the Objective Plan Scale for younger children and older, noncommunicative children (e.g., children with cerebral palsy).

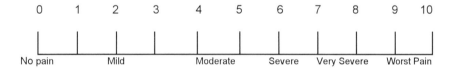

Visual Analog Scale

OBJECTIVE PAIN SCALE

OBSERVATION	CRITERIA	POINTS
Blood pressure	± 10% Preop	0
	> 20% Preop	1
	> 30% Preop	2
Crying	Not crying	0
	Crying; responds to TLC	1
	Crying; doesn't respond to TLC	2
Movement	None	0
	Restless	1
	Thrashing	2
Agitation	Asleep or calm	0
	Mild	1
	Hysterical	2
Verbal evaluation	Asleep or no pain	0
	Mild pain (cannot localize)	1
	Moderate pain (localize)	2

25. What methods are used in the management of pediatric acute pain?

Patient controlled analgesia (PCA). In hospitalized patients aged 5–6 years or older with postoperative acute pain, PCA is the most commonly used technique. Loading doses are necessary before initiation of PCA. I usually use morphine in a loading dose of 0.1–0.2 mg/kg. The PCA is then programmed as follows.

Dose:	0.02–0.03 mg/kg
Lock out:	5–10 minutes (usually 8 minutes)
Maximum hourly dose:	0.75–0.1 mg/kg

Continuous intravenous (IV) infusion. Used when PCA or regional anesthesia is not indicated. Preloading before continuous infusion is necessary. I usually use morphine in a loading dose of 0.1–0.2 mg/kg and then use continuous IV infusion of morphine at 0.01–0.03 mg/kg/hr. The infusion rate is slowly titrated to provide adequate pain relief. The infusion rate is then reduced by 10% every 12–24 hours if the patient is comfortable.

Oral route. Used when the patient is not under an NPO order.

Commonly Used Oral Opiates

MEDICATION	INGREDIENTS	USUAL DOSAGE
Acetaminophen + codeine elixir (Tylenol with codeine elixir)	Acetaminophen 120 + codeine 12 mg/5 ml	Acetaminophen 15 mg/kg Codeine 1 mg/kg/dose P.O. every 4–6 hr
Acetaminophen + codeine tablets (Tylenol No. 3)	Acetaminophen 300 mg + codeine 15 mg/tablet	1–2 tablets P.O. every 4–6 hr p.r.n.
Morphine sulfate oral solution	Morphine sulfate 2 mg/ml	0.3 mg/kg P.O. Every 4 hr p.r.n.
Acetaminophen + oxycodone (Percocet)	Acetaminophen 325 mg + oxycodone 5 mg	1–2 tablets P.O. Every 4–6 hr p.r.n.
Hydrocodone + acetaminophen (Vicodin)	Hydrocodone 5 mg + acetaminophen 500 mg per tablet	1–2 tablets P.O. Every 4– hr p.r.n.

Commonly Used Nonsteroidal Anti-inflammatory Drugs

Ketorolac—frequently used as an adjuvant for acute pain management	Bolus 0.5 mg/kg (max 30 mg) IV Then 0.5 mg/kg (max 30 mg) IV every 6 hr for 24–48 hr
Ibuprofen (Motrin)	8 mg/kg P.O. every 6 hr for 24–48 hr

Epidural analgesia. Extremely effective method of pain control in most postoperative patients. It provides good pain relief with smaller doses of narcotic and local anesthetic and less sedation than IV narcotics.

The most common insertion sites for epidural analgesia are caudal (for newborns to children 6 years of age), lumbar (for patients older than 6 years of age), and thoracic (for patients with specific indications, e.g., anterior spinal fusion).

In our institution, we use continuous-infusion epidural analgesia for all age groups. The three most commonly used epidural infusions are the following.

- Hydromorphone (Dilaudid, 20 μg/ml + 0.1% bupivacaine for postoperative pain management after posterior or anterior spine fusion.
- Fentanyl, 2 μg/ml + 0.1% bupivacaine after all lower periphery surgery in patients older than 6 months
- Fentanyl, 1 μg/ml + 0.05% bupivacaine in infants < 6 months

26. Does regional anesthesia mask compartment syndrome?

One of the complications of proximal tibial osteotomy is compartment syndrome, which is characterized by pain, neurologic dysfunction, decreased sensation, decreased motor function, and swelling.

When local anesthetics or narcotics are used in regional anesthesia, they interrupt the pain pathways. Local anesthetic alone also interrupts motor and sensory pathways. Therefore, the first two signs of compartment syndrome can be masked by regional technique. Marked increases in analgesic requirements may suggest the presence of compartment syndrome.

27. Are there any benefits to the use of nonpharmacologic methods of acute pain management?
Nonpharmacologic methods, such as relaxation, biofeedback, recreational therapy (methods such as distraction), hypnosis, and acupuncture, can improve the quality of pain control and should be utilized when appropriate.

28. What is the key to the success of an acute pain service?
- Must be a multidisciplinary team, which can include anesthesiologist, pediatrician, pediatric pain nurse, psychologist, physical therapist, and recreational therapist.
- Must implement appropriate assessment techniques.
- Must closely monitor the vital signs and pain scores every 2–4 hours.
- Must be able to recognize and treat the side effects of each modality, such as nausea and vomiting, itching, urinary retention, and, most importantly, respiratory depression.

29. What is latex allergy?
Latex allergy was first described by Nutter in 1979 as "contact dermatitis" following use of rubber gloves. Since then, many manifestations of latex allergy have been reported, such as urticaria, rhinitis, conjunctivitis, asthma, angioedema, anaphylaxis, and intraoperative cardiovascular collapse.

30. What is the pathophysiology of latex allergy?
Latex allergy is due to a type 1 reaction (hypersensitivity or anaphylactic reaction). Initial exposure to the antigen (i.e., latex) develops sensitization. Re-exposure to the antigen causes it to bind the IgE antibodies on the surfaces of mast cells and basophils. This causes release of mediators such as histamine, prostaglandins, eosinophilic chemotactic factor of anaphylaxis (ECF-A), leukotrienes, kinins, and platelet activating factor (PAF). The clinically observable signs of allergy are urticaria, bronchospasm, laryngeal edema, hypotension, and cardiovascular collapse.

31. Who are "high risk" patients for latex allergy?
- Patients with spina bifida (18–40%) and congenital urologic abnormality who have been in contact with latex through repeated urinary catheterizations, use of latex gloves during bowel evacuation, and repeated surgeries
- Physicians, nurses, and dental personnel, who are all chronically exposed to latex products
- Individuals who have a history of atopy (35–85% of those with latex allergy have a history of atopy)
- Patients with a history of allergy to balloons, rubber gloves, and bananas.

32. Are there any tests available to identify latex allergy?
- Skin-prick testing.
- Radioallergosorbent test (RAST), performed on the patient's serum. This test detects and quantifies IgE antibodies.

33. How do you manage the patient at high risk for latex allergy?
Preoperatively
- Have an increased index of suspicion.
- Obtain detailed medical history (family history of allergies, allergies to foods or drugs, previous problems).
- Do an allergy evaluation for high-risk patients (i.e., those with spina bifida).
Intraoperatively
- Avoid using latex surgical gloves and any latex-containing material that may come into contact with the patient.

- Most latex hypersensitivity reactions occur about 30 minutes after the induction of anesthesia (range is 10–290 min). Anaphylactic reactions vary in severity from mild bronchospasm and desaturation, which may be self limiting, to severe life-threatening episodes of bronchospasm and cardiovascular collapse.

34. How is an anaphylactic reaction managed?
1. Discontinue anesthetic agents, blood, or antibiotic infusion.
2. Administer 100% O_2 via positive-pressure ventilation.
3. Administer IV fluid (normal saline) to maintain blood pressure.
4. Administer epinephrine, 3–5 μg/kg bolus, followed by 1–4 μg/kg/min of epinephrine infusion as required.
5. Administer an antihistamine (diphenhydramine, 0.5–1.0 mg/kg IV).
6. Utilize β-agonist inhalers p.r.n.
7. Administer steroids (hydrocortisone, 1 g, or dexamethasone, 4–20 mg, IV).
8. Administer bicarbonate for severe persistent acidosis.
9. Do not extubate the patient, since there can be severe laryngeal edema. Allow time for edema to subside.
10. Obtain blood for RAST test.

BIBLIOGRAPHY

1. Berry FA, (ed): Anesthetic Management of Difficult and Routine Pediatric Patients, 2nd ed. New York, Churchill Livingstone, 1990.
2. Breucking E, Mortier W: Anesthesia in neuromuscular diseases [review]. Acta Anaesthesiol Belg 41(2):127–132, 1990.
3. Nguyen DH, Burus MW, Shapiro GG, et al.: Intraoperative cardiovascular collapse secondary to latex allergy. J Urol 146:571–574, 1991.
4. Nutter AF: Contact urticaria to rubber. Br J Dermatol 101:597–600, 1979.
5. Porter SS (ed): Anesthesia for Surgery of the Spine. New York, McGraw-Hill, 1995.
6. Ready L, Ashburn M, Caplain R, et al.: Practice guidelines for acute pain management in the peri-operative setting. Anesthesiology 82:1071–1081, 1995.
7. Schreiner MS, O'Hara I, Markakis DA, et al.: Do children who experience laryngospasm have an increased risk of upper respiratory tract infection? Anesthesiology 85:475–480, 1996.
8. Suderman VA, Crosby ET: Elective intubation in the unstable cervical spine patient. Can J Anaesth 37:S122, 1990.
9. Sullivan M, Thompson WK, Hill GD: Succinylcholine-induced cardiac arrest in children with undiagnosed myopathy. Can J Anaesth 41(6):497–501, 1994.

15. SURGERY

Kent Reinker, M.D.

1. What five prerequisites must be present before considering surgery on a child?
1. Parental and physician agreement on the need for surgery
2. Patient acquiescence with the surgery
3. Agreement regarding well-established outcome goals for surgery
4. Carefully defined pre-, peri-, and postoperative plans
5. Physician and family ability to carry out these plans

2. What are the indications for considering surgical treatment in a child?
Any of the following:
1. Failure of previous non-surgical management

2. Excessive patient or parental cost for nonsurgical management
3. Prophylaxis of expected deterioration in condition

3. How does surgical planning in a child differ from that in an adult?
The child is surrounded by one or more parents who are responsible for the child's welfare and who can be expected to be loving advocates for the child. The parents may not agree with each other, with other family members (e.g., grandparents), or with the child regarding surgical options. The surgeons must deal with these family conflicts.

4. What factors should be considered in determining parental and patient cost?
- Projected discomfort, anxiety, and pain
- Degree of temporary or permanent disability
- Separation from family
- Financial cost
- Time outlay
- Neglect of siblings

5. What time outlay costs must be considered in pediatric orthopaedic patients?
Because of the duration of healing following surgery for many orthopaedic conditions, the patient may lose considerable time from school. School makeup must be part of the surgical plan. The patient may need an attendant at home until he or she is ready to return to school. This may create a burden on the parents.

6. What caveat must be considered any time surgery is contemplated for a child?
Never sacrifice a happy childhood for nebulous or ill-defined gains in adulthood. Childhood can be one of the happiest periods of a person's life. It not only sets the stage for the rest of life—it is part of the play. Ideally, the surgery should yield a happier childhood as well as gains in adulthood.

7. Are there good and bad times for pediatric orthopaedic surgery?
Yes. Timing is important for most orthopaedic conditions and frequently is dictated by the medical situation. However, many surgical procedures can be deferred until it is most convenient for the family. Bad times for surgery include the following:
- During the first six months of life. Small tracheal size and the difficulty of finding venous access make anesthesia more difficult.
- During important holidays. Although parents frequently want surgery when school is not in session, children are very unhappy when they are in the hospital over the holidays or on their birthday.
- During junior or senior year in high school. Junior year is very important for college placement; senior year is a time of transition. Surgery should be deferred until after graduation, if possible.
- During summer vacations. School is certainly important, but most hospitals have tutoring available in-house or provided by the state while the child is unable to attend school. With good planning, schoolwork is usually not disrupted markedly by orthopaedic procedures. Some children with chronic conditions have every summer ruined by surgery and postoperative casting. This should be avoided.

8. What is the place of second opinions regarding surgical treatment?
They may be helpful in bringing to light aspects of the case that have not been previously considered. However, second opinions are encouraged by many medical plans in an attempt to save money by avoiding "unnecessary" surgery which may be very helpful for the patient. They are usually rendered by physicians who have seen the parents and patient only once and have not had the opportunity to get to know the family. Because few cities have more than a few pediatric orthopaedic surgeons, the second opinion may be rendered by a person with significantly less experience than the first surgeon. Under these circumstances, the second opinion is suspect.

In pediatric orthopaedics, issues are frequently complex and the problems unique. Therefore, complete agreement between two surgeons is unusual. Parents are frequently faced with a difficult decision when choosing between two surgeons with conflicting ideas. This may create a possibility for inappropriate treatment.

9. What should the surgeon do if the parents wish surgical treatment which is contrary to that recommended by the surgeon?
If the surgeon does not agree, he must explain his position to the parents. If the parents insist on the alternative option, the surgeon must determine whether he can, in good conscience, carry out that plan. If he cannot, he should indicate to the parents why he must decline to participate.

10. How is patient and family fear of surgery alleviated?
  • Frank and accurate communication regarding risks and discomfort
  • A friendly and trusting relationship with the patient and family
  • Preoperative introduction to the operating room setting and personnel

11. What errors are commonly made in preoperative communications?
  1. Talking only to the parents and leaving the patient out of the planning process. This accentuates patient fear and creates hostility. Adolescents in particular must be brought into the planning, and their own questions answered.
  2. Use of medical terminology in describing the surgery. Even the most simple concepts may be missed if the family's ignorance of medical terminology is not taken into account.
  3. Failure to adequately document counselling of parents and child.
  4. Failure to repeat counselling. Only about 30% of counselling information is absorbed in the first session.
  5. Failure to communicate risks quantitatively. Parents must be told not only that a risk exists but how great a risk it is.
  6. Lying to the patient. Telling the child that it will not hurt when it will creates distrust and fear.

12. What are the principles in managing perioperative pain in a child?
  1. Alleviate anxiety by repeated truthful reassurance.
  2. Avoid repeated intramuscular injections. Most children are frightened of shots. Even starting an IV line for surgery can be threatening. Needles should be avoided in favor of other techniques.
  3. Reassure parents that everything is being done to alleviate the patient's pain.
  4. Recognize that nurses and physicians frequently underestimate pain, particularly in the quiet, uncomplaining child.
  5. Children tolerate short-term pain reasonably well, but not long-term pain. Continued pain, even of low magnitude, must be avoided.

13. Are parents ever a handicap in accomplishing surgery?
Parents can occasionally become part of the problem instead of the solution. Communication can solve many of these problems. Difficult parents should not be avoided; a rule is that they should be seen twice as often as parents who are not difficult. The surgeon must recognize and overcome his own tendency to avoid awkward relationships in order to adequately deal with such parents.

14. What about the parent who is hostile to the surgeon?
The patient should not be operated upon until the hostility is overcome. If personality conflicts arise, the patient should be referred to another surgeon.

15. How does a surgeon gain the trust and cooperation of a parent?
By demonstrating that he or she cares greatly about their child.

16. What must the surgeon do immediately after surgery?
Find the parents and notify them of the patient's condition. This simple courtesy, so often neglected, is critical for good family relations. If the surgery lasts longer than expected, someone

on the surgical team should arrange to get word to the parents that surgery is progressing well and letting them know the expected completion time.

17. What must the surgeon do if surgery does not go as planned?
Parents must be immediately advised of any deviation from the surgical plan. The reasons for the deviation must be divulged, as should any changes from the expected surgical outcome. This parental counselling should be documented in the patient chart.

18. What if the surgery has an adverse outcome?
The surgeon must change the postoperative plan in order to make the best of the situation. This must be done in cooperation with parents. Maintaining communication is particularly important in this situation, and the surgeon must take the initiative in ensuring that the friendly and cooperative relationship continues.

19. Are anesthetic risks enhanced in the pediatric orthopaedic patient?
Yes. The incidence of cardiac arrest under anesthesia has been estimated at 4.7/10,000 for children and only 1.4/10,000 for adults. Death associated with anesthesia has been reported to be 1/40,000 anesthetics.

20. What additional risk factors are present in children?
Anesthetic risks are enhanced due to the following mechanisms:

1. Many orthopaedic patients have an increased risk of malignant hyperthermia. This is particularly true of those with muscle diseases, but patients with congenital deformities, such as club feet, are also at increased risk.

2. Congenital limb anomalies may have associated malformations of heart, lungs, kidneys, or other vital tissues. Radial aplasia, for example, may be associated with thrombocytopenia. Preaxial hand deformities may be associated with cardiac septal defects. Congenital scoliosis may be associated with renal or cardiac anomalies.

3. Many patients require surgical treatment during the first year of life, when the trachea is very small and easily occluded. Intubation and postoperative maintenance of airway may be difficult.

4. Reactive airway difficulties during anesthesia are greatly enhanced in severity and incidence if the child undergoes anesthesia during the two to three week period following an upper respiratory infection. The airway remains reactive for at least 7 weeks following upper respiratory infections. Unfortunately, the average child has 9 upper respiratory infections per year, making scheduling of surgery difficult.

5. Myelomeningocele patients have an increased risk of latex allergy, which can cause anaphylaxis under anesthesia, and acute shunt malfunction, which rarely can lead to catastrophic brain herniation during anesthesia.

21. What groups of children require preoperative clearance for cervical spine instability prior to surgery?
Arthritis, particularly juvenile rheumatoid arthritis
Bone dysplasias, many of which can lead to odontoid malformations
Congenital scoliosis, which may be associated with cervical spine anomalies
Down syndrome and other chromosomal anomalies

22. What is latex allergy, and how is it managed?
Many people are allergic to latex rubber of the type found in surgical gloves. Exposure of these people to even tiny amounts of latex can result in an anaphylactic reaction. As many standard items of surgical equipment contain latex, provision of a latex-free environment can be difficult. Latex allergy should be suspected if there is a history of swelling of the mouth after blowing up balloons, or allergy to cross-reactive food products such as bananas, potatoes, or tomatoes.

23. What other postoperative concerns are unique to the pediatric orthopaedic population?
Small children are little Houdinis, they are remarkably adept at slipping out of postoperative dressings and casts. Hand dressings, for example, are best protected by a long arm cast incorpo-

rating the entire hand. Following foot surgery, parents must be advised to notify the surgeon if toes disappear into the cast.

Children are also adept at dropping objects (money, suckers, small toys) into casts.

Children may be uncooperative with physical therapy or with activity restrictions. Crying is normal, and tantrums are not uncommon.

Infants and nonverbal patients may have difficulty communicating the presence of pain under a cast, as from a compartment syndrome or local pressure.

BIBLIOGRAPHY

1. Means LJ, Ferrari R, Fisher QA, et al: Evaluation and preparation of pediatric patients undergoing anesthesia. *Pediatrics* 98:502–507, 1996
2. Sussman GL, Tarlo S, Dolovich J: The spectrum of IGE-mediated responses to latex. *JAMA* 265:2844–2847, 1991.

16. POSTOPERATIVE MANAGEMENT

David D. Aronsson, M.D., and Marci D. Jones, M.D.

1. An 8-year-old boy with a closed femur fracture was treated with an immediate spica cast. The postoperative radiographs demonstrate satisfactory alignment. When should a follow-up appointment be scheduled?

The exact timing for a follow-up appointment varies considerably depending on whether you anticipate any problems or complications and whether it poses any particular problems for the patient or family. An 8-year-old boy treated with an immediate spica cast for a femur fracture is at risk of developing shortening or angulation at the fracture site. These potential problems are easily correctable if they are identified early; an appointment is recommended in 7–10 days to obtain a repeat radiograph in the cast to verify that the reduction remains satisfactory. Seven to 10 days after the injury, he should be relatively comfortable in the cast, and transportation to the office should not be painful.

2. A 13-year-old girl with cerebral palsy and spastic quadriplegia is recovering from a posterior spinal arthrodesis using allograft bone and segmental spinal fixation. How do you determine when to discharge the patient?

I recommend discharge as soon as medically possible. Hospitalization is a stressful event for anyone and can be even more stressful for a patient who has difficulty communicating with physicians, nurses, and caregivers. A posterior spinal arthrodesis is a major operation with risks for complications, and these risks are higher in children with cerebral palsy. It is documented that stress is reduced by returning the patient to a familiar comfortable environment. It is important that the patient be taking adequate fluids by mouth and be hemodynamically and nutritionally stable before discharge. Under these conditions, once the patient and family believe that the postoperative pain is satisfactorily controlled with oral medications, I recommend discharging the patient to a more familiar environment, usually 4–6 days after the operation. This helps reduce the incidence of complications such as gastritis or stress ulcers.

3. A 13-year-old girl with adolescent idiopathic scoliosis was treated with a posterior spinal arthrodesis using an iliac crest bone graft and segmental spinal fixation. Her postoperative course has been uncomplicated, and postoperative radiographs demonstrate satisfactory correction of the deformity. When should a follow-up appointment be scheduled?

A posterior spinal arthrodesis with an iliac crest bone graft is a painful operation, and patients often note just as much pain from the bone graft donor site as from the back itself. Since the patient is uncomfortable, I do not recommend an early appointment unless there are unusual circumstances, such as persistent drainage from the wound, that cause me to believe that the patient is at increased risk for development of complications. Under normal circumstances, I recommend an appointment in 3–4 weeks to obtain a posteroanterior and lateral radiograph to document that the internal fixation has not changed and that there has not been any loss of correction. By 3–4 weeks after the operation, the patient is usually experiencing minimal pain, so transportation to the office should not pose any particular problems for the patient and family.

4. A 13-year-old girl with cerebral palsy and spastic quadriplegia had a posterior spinal arthrodesis with allograft bone and segmental spinal fixation 3 days ago. The postoperative course has been complicated; she is still in the intensive care unit, and the family believes that she is having stomach pains. What do you recommend?
A posterior spinal arthrodesis with allograft bone and segmental spinal fixation is a painful operation that can be particularly stressful for the patient. The stress is even greater in patients who do not communicate because they may not understand why they are experiencing pain and are unable to ask questions. A prolonged stay in the intensive care unit (ICU) is known to be stressful; patients often become disoriented and confused, resulting in the development of ICU psychosis. This stress is associated with an increased risk of developing gastritis and gastric or duodenal ulcers, which can lead to a life-threatening upper gastrointestinal bleeding episode. I recommend prophylactic treatment with a histamine H_2-receptor antagonist to prevent this potentially devastating complication. The medication can usually be discontinued at the time of discharge, when the patient returns to a more familiar, less stressful environment.

5. At what rate should a child receive postoperative intravenous fluids?
The daily requirement for maintenance fluid can be calculated based on the weight of the child as follows: up to 10 kg, 100 ml/kg; 10–20 kg, 1000 ml for the first 10 kg then 50 ml/kg; and over 20 kg, 1500 ml for the first 20 kg, then 20 ml/kg. For example, a 25-kg child would have a 24-hour maintenance fluid requirement of 1600 ml/day or 67 ml/hour.

6. If a child requires a fluid bolus, what should be given?
A bolus of 20 ml/kg of Ringer's lactate or normal saline should be given. This may be repeated if there is no response. Use of hypotonic fluid (e.g., 5% dextrose in water) for a bolus replacement should be avoided because this may cause hyponatremia and a hypo-osmotic state that can result in seizures, especially in smaller children.

7. How does hypovolemia present in a child?
Hypovolemia can have subtle findings in children because they can maintain blood pressure by increasing heart rate and systemic vascular resistance. An increased heart rate, a weak peripheral pulse, and decreased urine output are signs of dehydration. Mild hypovolemia (< 25% volume loss) can present with thirst, restlessness or lethargy, postural hypotension, dry mucous membranes, and a sunken anterior fontanelle. More profound hypovolemia can cause combativeness, confusion, cool and clammy skin, decreased skin elasticity, hypotension, and shock.

8. If a child requires transfusion of packed red blood cells, what volume of replacement should be given?
A healthy child who has lost blood because of an operation can tolerate a low hematocrit much better than an adult. The risk of complications, including acute myocardial infarction, is also much lower than for an adult with a similar hematocrit. As a result, it is important to analyze the clinical setting to determine if a transfusion of packed red blood cells is merited. If required, the transfusion should be at a volume of 10 ml/kg, with a maximum of 15 ml/kg, to avoid volume overload. A transfusion of 10 ml/kg should raise the hematocrit by approximately 10%.

9. What are the risks of transfusion of packed red blood cells?

An immediate or delayed transfusion reaction, pulmonary edema, and bacterial or viral infections are all potential risks of blood product transfusion. An allergic or febrile transfusion reaction occurs immediately. Signs of a transfusion reaction include a fever up to 40°C, urticaria, edema, and, rarely, bronchospasm. One to two percent of patients given a transfusion will have an allergic reaction. The recommended treatment is to discontinue the transfusion and, if necessary, administer acetaminophen, diphenhydramine, diuretics, O_2, steroids, and epinephrine.

Hemolytic transfusion reactions can be either immediate or delayed. These are rare and are usually secondary to use of mismatched blood. Symptoms and signs include restlessness; anxiety; precordial, back, and abdominal pain; high fever; chills; dark urine; jaundice; and disseminated intravascular coagulation. The recommended treatment includes discontinuing the transfusion, intravenous hydration, osmotic diuretics, and laboratory evaluation of the transfused blood.

Bacterial infections fortunately are rare, but if they occur, they may cause overwhelming sepsis with a high mortality rate.

Viruses that can be transmitted in blood include cytomegalovirus (CMV), human immunodeficiency virus (HIV), human T-cell lymphotropic virus (HTLV), hepatitis B virus (HBV), and hepatitis C virus (HCV). CMV is ubiquitous, with 80% of healthy adults testing positive. An acute CMV infection can cause hepatitis and a syndrome similar to mononucleosis. In an immunocompromised host, CMV can cause serious interstitial pneumonia, so CMV-free blood should be used for these patients. Estimates of the incidence of infectious blood, based on blood donated during an infectious period prior to detectable infection, are 1 in 493,000 for HIV; 1 in 641,000 for HTLV; 1 in 63,000 for HBV; and 1 in 103,000 for HCV. The overall aggregate risk is 1 in 34,000, 88% of which is made up of HBV and HCV.

10. What is the recommended treatment for postoperative nausea and vomiting?

Nausea and vomiting are very common postoperatively and can occur in more than 40% of children. It is the most common cause of an unplanned admission following ambulatory surgery. Ondansetron, a serotonin receptor antagonist, can be effectively used both to prevent postoperative nausea and vomiting and to control established emesis. When administered preoperatively in an intravenous dose of 0.1 mg/kg (up to 4 mg) to children older than 2 years, ondansetron is effective in the prevention of nausea and vomiting in the first 4 postoperative hours. A single postoperative dose is effective for 24 hours in the treatment of established emesis as well and is less sedating than droperidol. Oral ondansetron has not been shown to be superior in controlling postoperative nausea and vomiting when compared with other oral agents. Ondansetron is preferable to promethazine because it can be given intravenously, whereas promethazine is usually given intramuscularly to avoid the possible serious side effects of skin necrosis and gangrene if extravasation occurs.

11. What is the significance of postoperative fever?

Postoperative fever is very common. There are multiple causes of fever, including atelectasis, infection, allergic reaction, thrombosis, trauma, anesthesia, transfusion, hematoma, drug reactions, and constipation. A recent study found that 73% of pediatric patients who had undergone open orthopaedic surgical procedures had a postoperative temperature of $> 38°C$ (100.4°F). The reliability and predictive value of fever is low, with a sensitivity of 67%, a specificity of 26%, and a positive predictive value of only 2%. If the definition of fever is changed to include only temperatures $> 39°C$ (102.2°F), it can be said that 10% of patients experience postoperative fever. The reliability of predicting complications increases specificity to 91%, but the positive predictive value is only 6%.

The utility of fever in predicting complications is low; clinical examination and judgment should be used to determine the need for a septic work-up.

BIBLIOGRAPHY

1. Angel JD, Blasier RD, Allison R: Postoperative fever in pediatric orthopaedic patients. J Pediat Orthop. 14(6):799–801, 1994.

2. Cooke CE, Mehra IV: Oral ondansetron for preventing nausea and vomiting. Am J Hosp Pharm. 51(6):762–771, 1994.
3. Holbrook PR: Textbook of Pediatric Critical Care. Philadelphia, W.B. Saunders Co., 1993.
4. Khalil S, Rodarte A, Weldon BC, et al. Intravenous ondansetron in established postoperative emesis in children. S3A-381 Study Group. Anesthesiology 85(2):270–276, 1996.
5. Rudolph AM, Hoffman JE, Rudolph CD: Rudolph's Pediatrics, 20th ed. Stamford, CT, Appleton and Lange, 1996.
6. Schreiber GB, Busch MP, Kleinman SH, et al. The risk of transfusion-transmitted viral infections. The Retrovirus Epidemiology Donor Study. N Engl J Med 334(26):1685–1690, 1996.
7. Ummenhofer W, Frei FJ, Urwyler A, et al.: Effects of ondansetron in the prevention of postoperative nausea and vomiting in children. Anesthesiology 81(4):804–810, 1994.
8. Yaster M, Sola JE, Pegoli W Jr, et al.: The night after surgery. Postoperative management of the pediatric outpatient—surgical and anesthetic aspects [review]. Pediatr Clin North Am 41(1):199–220, 1994.

17. PREVENTION OF COMPLICATIONS

J. Richard Bowen, M.D.

1. What is a complication?

Many physicians consider a complication to be an "unplanned negative event" occurring during evaluation and treatment of a patient. Patients expect to have their disease accurately diagnosed, their evaluation performed in a prompt and cost-conscious manner, and the goals of the treatment met. Often, patients may consider *anything less than the expected* as a complication.

2. What actions of a physician contribute to complications?

1. Perform poor history and physical examinations.

2. Estimate rather than calculate dosages in children (especially when ordering narcotics or fluids).

3. Work in a "bad hospital," one that routinely loses charts and radiographs, or one that has poorly trained staff with a bad work attitude.

4. Try to hide complications by destroying radiographs and changing charts.

5. Work with hostile physician peers who are overly competitive, critical, and envious.

6. Overwork and underpay your staff.

7. Promote or tolerate bad behavior such as lack of respect for patients, bad language, crude jokes, and sexual advances.

8. Have little weekend patient coverage.

9. Promote bad rapport with your patients by not taking the time to communicate, by never returning phone calls, or by flaunting your financial success.

10. Perform histories, physicals, or treatments without a chaperone.

11. Become an incompetent physician by never taking continuing education and training courses, by using alcohol or drugs, and by losing interest in medicine.

12. Fail to document important information on the chart.

13. Perform marginally indicated procedures.

3. What are the causes of complications?

Complications occur as a consequence of disease or as a consequence of health care (evaluation and treatment). Many diseases have associated complications. Generally, the more severe the injury or disease process, the greater the risk of complications. By altering the natural history of a disease, the incidence and severity of the associated complications may often be reduced.

Complications also occur as a consequence of health care (evaluation and treatment); Mercer Rang calls these complications "adverse events." He states, "An adverse event is an un-planned negative event that occurs during the evaluation or treatment of a patient." Examples are a spinal fusion for scoliosis complicated by paraplegia or an osteotomy complicated by in-fection.

4. How are complications classified?

I like Mercer Rang's classification of complications. He considers complications occurring during evaluation and treatment of a patient to be "adverse events." Adverse events are unplanned negative occurrences and come in three grades.

1. *An incident.* Occurrence of an event that does no harm. For example, the patient is given the wrong medicine but no harm occurs. (A tablet was given when the liquid form was ordered.) Incidences should be recorded and actions taken to reduce the probability of recurrence.

2. *Fault-free adverse event.* Occurrence of an event in which the patient is harmed but no one is obviously at fault. For example, the patient falls in the hallway or accidentally pulls out an intravenous line.

3. *Adverse event due to substandard or negligent care.* Occurrence of an event that is caused by actions below a reasonable standard of care. Examples are operating on the wrong hip, stiff-ness in a joint because of noncompliance, and transfusing the wrong blood.

Wagner believed problems and complications to be separate entities. *Problems* are adverse events that are expected and predictable and that if treated may not affect the outcome. An ex-ample is a pin tract infection during a leg lengthening that is treated with antibiotics and has no sequelae. *Complications* are adverse events that are not expected, cause severe injury, and affect the outcome. An example is thrombosis of the femoral artery during a leg lengthening that re-quires an amputation.

5. How common are complications?

There is no single answer to this question. The incidence of complications varies among procedures, physicians, patients, and hospitals. An overall complication rate is meaningless un-less each type of complication is considered within comparable groups. My personal experi-ence shows that limb lengthening in children is associated with almost a 100% incidence of skin infections from pin tracts, while I cannot remember a case of an infection due to a skin biopsy for collagen analysis. There are data available about the frequency of specific complications; however, before accepting and comparing complication rates as "gospel," I suggest a very care-ful evaluation of the original publications to determine the techniques of gathering and the methods of analyzing data. I am wary of suggesting that complication rates be the sole deter-minant of quality of care; however, high complication rates should not be ignored. For exam-ple, complications have been reported to be higher in teaching hospitals and adverse events caused by negligence have been reported to be higher in hospitals treating predominatly mi-nority groups.

Rates of common complications are reported frequently to evaluate trends. Examples are nosocomial infection rate, operative infection rate, mortality rate, length of hospital stay, and blood transfusion rate. Recently, disease severity scores have been applied to outcomes of treat-ment and incidences of complications as a determinate to calculate quality of care.

6. What is the course of a complication?

Complications have two different types of courses.

1. *Progressive warning signs that are followed by an adverse event or complication* Most complications develop after many warning signs. These warning signs may be minor or appear unimportant, may be overt and ignored, or may be overt and uncontrollable. Adverse events that occur after a "trail of warning" give us the greatest opportunity to correct minor problems before they become major complications.

2. *A sudden adverse event or complication* A few complications occur without warning, such as the patient falling and fracturing a leg. These sudden adverse events are often difficult to pre-dict and difficult to prevent.

7. How can a hospital prevent complications?

A hospital cannot prevent all complications; however, the prevalence of complications can be reduced. Hospitals can minimize complications by providing a quality staff, a good workplace, good equipment, and a chain of administrative responsibility that assures continued improvement of patient care. Some factors that should be considered include developing continuing educational programs, avoiding understaffing, encouraging an enthusiastic attitude, performing routine maintenance of equipment, providing good administrative support focusing on continued quality improvement, having the basic necessary equipment, keeping good patient records, handling radiographs and laboratory results accurately, and maintaining hospital accreditation.

8. How can an orthopaedist prevent complications?

An orthopaedist can minimize complications by being well educated and trained and by having a good attitude toward continued improvement of the quality of patient care. Other considerations in the prevention of complications include not being overworked or excessively fatigued, establishing a lifelong continuing medical education program, developing a positive attitude toward your profession, always looking for opportunities to improve patient care, and communicating well with your patients.

Common errors that lead to complications can be expressed in three stages.

- Pre-treatment stage. Errors in:
    Diagnosis. (Get a good history and physical.)
    Assessing severity.
    Choice of treatment. (Understand the indications.)
    Patient selection. (Noncooperative patient).
    Informed consent. (Make sure the patient understands reasonable complications and knows that many treatments do not restore the condition to normal.)
    Judgment of surgical skills (adequate training for the procedure).
- Treatment stage (operative treatment). Errors in:
    Operating on the wrong side.
    Operating on the wrong patient.
    Quantitative judgment (overcorrecting or undercorrecting, too long or too short).
    Equipment use (monitors, radiology).
    Judging skill of associated physicians (anesthesiologist, internist). A good rule of thumb is to trust everyone as long as you check on them.
- Posttreatment stage. Errors in:
    Establishing a good postoperative care plan.
    Explanation of the postoperative care plan to patient, family, and nurses.

9. How can patients and parents prevent complications?

Patients can minimize the prevalence and severity of many. Beware of patients who are noncompliant with treatment advice, who frequently miss scheduled appointments, and who are in such poverty that adequate medical resources are unavailable to them. Children are particularly susceptible, since they must rely on adults. Caution should be exercised when dealing with parents who are nearly incompetent, especially those who abuse alcohol and drugs. If a parent does not properly supervise a child, the risk of complications increases dramatically. For example, the cast may be allowed to get wet, coat hangers may be used to scratch under the cast, and the cast padding may be pulled out. Additionally, children will often not exercise without supervision, and joint stiffness may result. Parents may disagree about a choice of treatment. If agreement is not reached, family counseling may be necessary. I have also treated several children whose parents have different medical restrictions for religious reasons. Ethical questions of the parents' rights versus their children's rights arise when the parents' medical decisions increase the risk of complications for the children.

10. How do we manage complications?

All patients are candidates for complications, and most patients are very fearful of having one. When discussing complications, patients need to consider the physician as a down-to-earth, approachable, considerate, unpretentious professional who has their best interests at heart. The treatment of complications can be broken down into stages.

- Precomplication stage.
    Discuss reasonable complications with the patient and family.
    Discuss expected outcome of treatment, what a reasonable person would want to know.
    Obtain informed consent.
    Perform evaluation and treatment in a manner to minimize the risk of a complication.
- Complication stage.
    Recognize complications promptly and early. Pay attention to the nurses and to complaints of the patient.
    Explain the complication to the patient.
    Record the complication in the chart.
    Establish a rational treatment plan. "Spread the base," which means get consults and help as needed.
    "Never run from a complication," which means the patient and complication are your responsibility. You need to maintain a high standard of care even if intimidated by the process.
- Postcomplication stage.
    Be professional: Notice your choice of behavior.
    Maintain integrity.

11. What are the strategies to reduce complications?

Many strategies have been proposed to reduce the incidence of complications. Hippocrates suggested that the physician who commits faulty care should receive the same consequences as the patient. I do not believe the number of harmless incidents or fault-free adverse events would decline in this scenario; however, incompetent physicians who repetitively perform substandard or negligent care would rapidly disappear.

Codman published an annual "report card" with every patient's diagnosis, operation, complication, and result and suggested his colleagues do the same. To judge quality of care by this method seems inappropriate because the strategy does not account for variables that cause complications.

Today, many strategies are available to reduce complications, improve care, and assure quality. Examples are quality assurance programs, morbidity and mortality conferences, outcome analysis, utilization review, credentialing processes, accreditation reviews, risk management, board certification, licensing agencies, continued educational requirements and conferences, routine equipment evaluation, and patient care protocols. The "Zero Defect/Continuous Quality Improvement" strategies are most interesting to me. The goal is continuous improvement until all defects have been eliminated. With this strategy, every stage of care would be evaluated by a team and continuous efforts would be made to correct faults and improve performance.

12. What are the effects of complications?

There are many effects of complications. Patients and families often experience fear, depression, loss of confidence, pain, and disability. Physicians may become insecure or even stop performing certain procedures, develop a defensive attitude, form a thick-skinned approach to life, practice defensive medicine, and experience grief. Nurses may develop a defensive attitude. For society, complications significantly increase the cost of medicine and the number of malpractice suits.

13. What do you do when you are sued for malpractice because of a complication?

Remember that even with the best of care, complications will occur occasionally, and a poor outcome does not necessarily indicate negligence. As soon as you are notified of a suit, I would suggest that you have your office or the hospital personnel secure the records, radiographs, and any other item that may be useful. Never, never, never change or alter any record in any way. Ask for the pages to be counted and for a copy to be duplicated for yourself. Notify your insurance carrier, and hire a very good lawyer immediately. Do not discuss the case with anyone except your lawyer. I am aware of several physicians who thought they could solve the suit by "explaining the problem" to the patient or family, and that is a BIG mistake. Many conscientious physicians are devastated by a suit; however, remember, as a lawyer friend told me, "A suit is only about money." Select high-quality physicians as expert witnesses and avoid physicians who have become "legal prostitutes."

Always tell the truth! During deposition or trial answer the question by saying, "Yes, no, I don't know," or the exact answer. Smart or sarcastic answers are usually detrimental. Be professional and maintain integrity.

BIBLIOGRAPHY

1. Berwick DM: Continuous improvement as an ideal in healthcare. N Engl J Med 320:53–56, 1989.
2. Bowen JR, Angus PD, Huxster RR, MacEwen GD: Posterior spinal fusion without blood replacement in Jehohvah's Witnesses. Clin Orthop 198:284–288, 1985.
3. Brennan TA, Hebert LE, Laird NM, et al.: Hospital characteristics associated with adverse events and substandard care. JAMA 265:3264–3269, 1991.
4. Brennan TA, Leape LL, Laird NM, et al.: Incidence of adverse events and negligence in hospitalized patients—results of the Harvard Medical Practice Study. N Engl J Med 324:370–376, 1991.
5. Champion HR, Copes WS, Sacco WJ, et al.: The major trauma outcome study: establishing national norms for trauma care. J Trauma 30:1356–1365, 1990.
6. Codman EA: A study of hospital efficiency, as demonstrated by the case. Boston, T Todd, 1915.
7. Epps CH, Bowen JR (eds): Complications in Pediatric Orthopaedic Surgery, Philadelphia, J. B. Lippincott Co., 1995.
8. Karger C, Guille JT, Bowen JR: Lengthening for congenital deficiencies of the lower limp. Clin Orthop 291:236–245, 1993.
9. Rang M: Adverse events. In Epps CH, Bowen JR (eds): Complications in Pediatric Orthopaedic Surgery. Philadelphia, J. B. Lippincott Co., 1995.

18. CASTS

Alfred D. Grant, M.D.

1. What are casts used for?

Casts are most often used for **immobilization** when treating fractures and post-surgery to permit healing without unwanted motion.

Use for **positioning** is most often prescribed in paralytic states to position a part to enhance function. Similarly, casts can be used to rest a joint while allowing function, such as in inflammatory states.

One of the most common uses in children is for **corrective casting,** such as for clubfoot. Here, the casts are not the corrective device but are used to hold the position obtained during manipulation. Such casts can be applied serially, repeatedly reapplying the cast after manipulation until correction of the deformity is achieved.

Another use of casts in children is for tone reduction in cerebral palsy. These short leg casts, which position the toes in dorsiflexion, are controversial and without hard scientific evidence of benefit, yet are popular in some therapeutic circles.

2. How are casts applied?

Casts are applied either in a circular manner encompassing a part, or as splints.

Circular casts are more rigid, more easily contoured, less apt to change shape, more protective, and are thought to be more "permanent." Splints are applied as layers of casting material placed on one or more sides of a limb. They tend to be less secure and less "permanent." Splints are most often used either to allow for expansion—i.e., swelling, as can be seen in the acutely injured or operated limb—or where immobilization is desired, such as night splinting for positioning.

Casts and splints are rarely applied directly to the skin. Various types of padding are placed on the skin. They come in rolls which are applied either directly on the skin or over a layer of stocking-like material named "stockinet." The most common of these materials is "sheet cotton," or a non-woven batting named Webril. These both disintegrate when they are wet, making them undesirable when used with waterproof casting materials such as fiberglass. In such instances, synthetic material, which is stable when wet and dries easily, is advised. One manufacturer has recently produced a padding which does not absorb moisture but still permits the skin to "breathe" allowing for the evaporation of moisture. This material, Gortex, is more difficult to apply but has an advantage when treating children who may get casts wet with water or urine.

3. What is the composition of casting material?
The most commonly used material is plaster of Paris. It is imbedded in gauze rolls of different widths. Fiberglass casting material has become popular. Urethane material is embedded in knitted fiberglass rolls. Each of these materials is activated to harden by immersing in water.

4. What are the differences among various casting materials?
Plaster of Paris is easiest to work with, can be readily molded, but is much weaker than fiberglass. Plaster of Paris is the most forgiving of casting materials. It spreads apart easily in its hardened state when split longitudinally. Once it is spread, it tends to stay in the enlarged state since it does not have a "memory." Plaster is the most easily wedged of all materials. It is inexpensive and most readily available. One of the materials most commonly used in children is "Gypsona" plaster, a very quick-setting, fine-textured material. Other plasters, however, can serve the same purpose.

Fiberglass casts are difficult to apply due to stickiness, requiring gloves and a lubricant such as Vaseline to facilitate application. The most common types are Delta-Lite and Scotchcast. Some of the stickiness can be reduced by adding silicone to the fiberglass-knitted material. Examples are Delta-Lite S and Scotchcast Plus. Fiberglass is difficult to mold but is significantly harder, lighter, and waterproof. It is relatively radiolucent. If a circular fiberglass cast is split longitudinally and spread, it tends to return to its original state, having a "memory." Thus in order to expand a fiberglass cast it must be split on two sides and then spread on both sides.

There are other materials, such as Hexalite, which are thermoplastic. They are more difficult to use, weaker, and have little benefit when compared to the other materials. Theoretically, thermoplastic casts or splints can be heated and remolded to different positions. However, this is rarely done.

5. What occurs when casts harden?
The material changes its chemical composition. The reaction gives off heat. Thus, casts are hot when applied. The temperature can vary depending on the temperature of the water and room, and the cast thickness. The cast should not be covered until it is dry. Setting time depends on the material. Plaster casts set between 2 and 8 minutes, depending on type. However, thick casts can take up to 72 hours to completely dry. Fiberglass sets within 4 to 5 minutes and weight-bearing can begin after 20 minutes.

6. How are casts removed?
With special cast cutters. They look like rotating saws but are not! They vibrate. If the motion used to cut the cast is simply in and out, not pulling, it will cut the hard cast but not the underlying padding or skin (when pushed against the soft material). Strips of plastic or a tongue blade can be slipped under the cast to further protect the skin.

7. When casts are used to treat fractures, are there special guidelines?
1. Casts are used to immobilize a fracture or fractured part.
2. To immobilize a limb segment or part, the cast should extend across the joint above and below the fracture.

3. The cast is not used to reduce a fracture but to hold the position, either of an undisplaced fracture or that obtained by manipulation.

4. Failure to immobilize the joint above and below can result in displacement of the fracture.

5. Unstable fractures may displace in a cast:
   (a) as a result of muscle forces; (b) because the fracture has no intrinsic stability (i.e., comminution); because (c) room within a cast will permit displacement as swelling decreases.

6. Contouring and molding the cast enhance stability of the fracture.

7. Initial casting of fresh fractures is dangerous (see below). Therefore these casts must be split or the initial immobilization should be done with splints.

8. X-rays should be obtained before and after cast application to ensure and document proper treatment position.

9. The neurologic and vascular condition of the limb must be examined and documented before and after cast application.

10. Fractures that cannot be satisfactorily managed in a cast or splint are usually unstable. Stability may be achieved in such instances by introducing pins into the boney structures adjacent to the fractures and incorporating these pins into the cast. In other instances, surgical intervention may be necessary.

8. Can casts be applied over damaged skin, wounds, and surgical incisions?
Yes, if access to the involved skin is provided. This can be done with removable splits or by providing a window in the circular cast over the area needing inspection. If a window is used it should be replaced after observation and/or treatment of the skin to prevent swelling or window edema.

9. What major problem can occur in using a cast?
A cast that is too tight can cause serious neurovascular compromise.

10. What are the signs that a cast is too tight?
Pain—when moving the fingers/toes
Pallor—pale/white distal part due to lack of blood supply
Paresthesias—and possible numbness due to nerve compression and lack of circulation
Paralysis—due to loss of nerve function

11. How do you prevent a tight cast?
1. Use sufficient padding
2. Split the cast on both sides and spread the cast to allow for swelling (bivalving).
3. Split the padding—to the skin
4. Elevate the limb to prevent dependent edema and inflammatory swelling

12. Are there other problems in using the cast?
A cast that is too loose can result in displacement of a fracture. This occurs after initial swelling subsides in treating acute injuries. Casts must be replaced or adjusted to prevent this occurrence.

Pressure by the cast over boney prominences can lead to irritation and decubitus ulceration. This is prevented by extra padding over these areas, such as the head of the fibula, the anterior superior iliac spine and the malleoli.

A cast that is too tight across the abdomen, (e.g., in a hip spica) can cause superior mesenteric artery compression at the level of the third part of the duodenum. This can result in an acute abdominal crisis: gangrene of the bowel. Any suggestion of acute abdominal symptoms must be taken seriously!

Displacement of bones can occur from inadequate immobilization, when both adjacent joints are not immobilized. This may not always be practical. However, in such instances, frequent checking of the fracture position is necessary. Examples are when a hip joint or a shoulder joint is not immobilized in treating an injury to the thigh or arm. Obviously if the hip or shoulder were immobilized it would require that the casting material go across part of the trunk. If deciding not to do that, careful observation of the fracture is critical.

13. What should you remember at all times about a cast?

Pay attention to the patient's complaints!

A properly casted limb is comfortable, warm, has moving joints distally (e.g., digits) and proximally, and has normal color. Splints used to protect a joint or position a part should also be comfortable.

BIBLIOGRAPHY

1. Chapman DR, Bennett JB, Byran WJ, Tullos HS: Complications of distal radial fractures: pins and plaster treatment. J Hand Surg [Am] 7:509–512, 1982.
2. Cusick BD: Splints and casts: managing foot deformity in children with neuromotor disorders. Phys Ther; 68:1903–1912, 1988.
3. Gill JM, Bowker P: A comparative study of the properties of bandage-form splinting materials. Engineering in Medicine; 11:125–134, 1982.
4. Hinderer KA, Harris SR, Purdy AH, et al.: Effects of "tone-reducing" vs. standard plaster-casts on gait improvement of children with cerebral palsy. Dev Med Child Neurol; 30:370–377, 1988.
5. Hutchinson DT, Bassett GS: Superior mesenteric artery syndrome in pediatric orthopedic patients. Clin Orthop; 250:250–257, 1990.
6. Keenan WNW, Clegg J: Intraoperative wedging of casts: Correction of residual angulation after manipulation. J Pediatr Orthop; 15:826–829, 1995.
7. Martin PJ, Weimann DH, Orr JF, Bahrani AS: A comparative evaluation of modern fracture casting materials. Engineering in Medicine; 17:63–70, 1988.
8. Walker JL, Rang M: Forearm fractures in children: Cast treatment with the elbow extended. J Bone Joint Surg [Br]; 73:299–301, 1991.
9. Wolff CR, James P: The prevention of skin excoriation under children's hip spica casts using the Goretex Pantaloon. J Pediatr Orthop; 15:386–388, 1995.

19. ORTHOTICS, BRACES, AND SPLINTS

Peter F. Armstrong, M.D., FRCSC, FACS, FAAP, and Daniel D. Ramsey, M.A., C.P.O.

1. What is the history of splinting and bracing?

Splints of one type or another have been used, principally in the management of fractures, since prehistoric times. Hippocrates described in detail the closed reduction and splinting of fractures. Galen, in the second century, proposed the use of braces for scoliosis and kyphosis. In medieval times, armorers built various types of braces. Bracing was the key treatment for many deformities because surgery often resulted in the death of the patient. The advent of polio resulted in a tremendous increase in demand for braces to support weakened and unstable limbs. These braces were most commonly made of leather and iron. With the development of newer plastics, braces have become lighter, more versatile, and definitely more cosmetic.

2. What is an orthotic?

A support or brace for weak or ineffective muscles. An orthotic is a force system that acts on body segments. The amount of force that may be applied is limited by the tolerance of the tissue against which the force is applied, namely the skin and subcutaneous tissue.

Orthotics may be as simple as a soft arch support in a shoe or as complex as a reciprocating-gait orthosis, a brace that encompasses the pelvis and both hips, the knees, the ankles, and the feet.

3. What is the difference among the terms *brace*, *splint*, and *orthotic*?

In many respects, the terms are used interchangeably. *Orthotic* or *orthosis* is probably the broadest term. It includes leg braces, arm braces, spine braces, shoe inserts, shoe lifts, and other devices that are used in the treatment of orthopaedic problems. They are usually used for long periods of time. *Splint* most often refers to a supportive device that is used for shorter periods of time, often after injury or surgery.

4. What are the uses of orthotics?

Orthoses are used frequently in children with neuromuscular disorders. In these conditions, they may be needed **to replace the function of paralyzed or weak muscles**, such as with a drop-foot brace that allows dorsiflexion but not plantar flexion beyond the neutral position. Hinges may be needed to **stabilize unstable joints** in one plane while allowing motion in another. A parapodium or self-standing brace may allow a patient with high-level spina bifida or spinal cord injury to **be supported in the upright position** for periods of time. A specialized brace called a reciprocating-gait orthosis may help **simulate walking** in patients with intermediate-level spina bifida or spinal cord injury. In the case of cerebral palsy, the brace **may counteract the force of a spastic muscle**. An AFO (ankle-foot orthosis) may counteract the tendency toward equinus produced by a spastic calf muscle.

Protection of potentially fragile bones is often accomplished with orthotics. A total-contact or clamshell AFO or knee-ankle-foot orthosis (KAFO) may be used to try to prevent fracturing and subsequent development of congenital pseudarthrosis of the tibia. An orthosis may be used in an attempt **to prevent progression of a deformity**, possibly preventing the need for major surgery.

A brace may also be used to **prevent recurrence of a deformity**. Many surgeons use AFOs and KAFOs after clubfoot surgery for this purpose.

A brace may be used to **replace the function of a damaged or otherwise deficient anatomic structure** such as a cruciate ligament.

Restoration of normal anatomic relationships may be accomplished with orthoses.

There is not a clear consensus on whether a brace may be used to **correct deformity**. Some would argue that use of a Denis-Browne night splint actually corrects an inward torsional problem (intoeing) in the tibiae or that a KAFO can lead to correction of the genu varum associated with Blount disease. Others have designed braces and shoes that they feel gradually corrects a somewhat resistant metatarsus adductus. It is important to understand that a rigid type of deformity, such as clubfoot that has not responded to manipulation and casting, will not be corrected by orthotic use alone. In that instance, surgery is required. Similarly, an orthosis will not be able to correct permanently a deformity secondary to ligamentous laxity, such as flexible flatfoot.

5. How are braces described?

Orthotics are generally defined by the area of the body that they affect. Some are alternatively described by the function that they perform, such as a drop-foot splint. Some braces are given names that reflect the inventor or the place where the brace was first developed, such as the University of California Biomechanics Laboratory (UCBL) orthosis, a type of foot orthosis.

6. Describe the supporting devices for the lower limb.

An arch support or similar supporting device for the foot can be called a foot orthosis (FO). A brace that supports or stabilizes the ankle and foot is called an ankle-foot orthosis (AFO). KAFO refers to support extended to the knee, and HKAFO if extended to the hip. These braces may be further described as solid, articulating, or dynamic. A solid AFO would not allow any ankle motion. An articulating AFO would allow ankle motion in the sagittal plane. It could also be further limited to allow dorsiflexion but prevent plantar flexion (plantar flexion block). A KAFO may have a completely unconstrained joint at the knee. This could be modified to produce a temporarily fully constrained joint in extension with the addition of a drop-lock hinge. A dynamic AFO might allow active plantar flexion against elastic resistance of the material, but it returns the ankle to a neutral position as the material returns to its resting state.

7. Describe supporting devices for the upper limb.

A WHO is a wrist-hand orthosis. Usually this is further defined by the specific function it is to perform; for example, a cock-up WHO is used to stabilize the wrist and hand in dorsiflexion.

Above the forearm, there is no universally accepted description for orthoses. These are best described by the function they perform, such as a shoulder abduction splint.

8. Describe the supporting devices for the spine.

A support that stabilizes the lumbosacral spine is called a lumbar-sacral orthosis (LSO). Adjectives may supplement the description, such as rigid, bivalved, plastic LSO for symptomatic spondylolysis.

A spine support with a much higher trim level that encompasses part of the thoracic spine is described as a thoracic-lumbar-sacral orthosis (TLSO). One that also includes the cervical spine would be (CTLSO). Some of the TLSOs are known by other names, such as Boston brace or Charleston brace.

Neck braces most often have proper names associated with them, such as Lerman cervical brace or Guilford cervical orthosis, but some have a more anatomic designation, such as sternal-occipital-mandibular immobilizer (SOMI).

9. How are orthotics prescribed?

The ideal situation is to have the orthotist in the clinic or office with you. In some instances, an "off-the-shelf" item may be used with or without minor modifications. In many cases, a custom-designed orthosis must be made to fit the particular child. If the orthotist is not readily available, be as descriptive as possible concerning the function you want the device to achieve.

The next most important step in the process is to see the patient after the orthosis has been fit. You should be able to tell right away if the orthosis has been constructed to accomplish the goal for which it was prescribed. This allows adjustments to be made early, and the potential for success will be greater. A common mistake is to accommodate to a deformity rather than build in some correction for it.

10. What are the principles of orthotics?

Orthotics are generally force systems. Where and how the force is applied is determined by the construction of the device. The most common force principle used is that of three-point fixation. In the case of metatarsus adductus, there is a curved deformity with a convex and a concave surface. In order to correct the deformity, one has to place a fulcrum at the apex of the deformity on the convex side. Force in the opposite direction must be applied to the heel and the metatarsal heads on the concave side of the deformity. The amount of force will depend on the tolerance of the skin and subcutaneous tissues.

11. How are orthotics constructed?

When making a custom-molded orthosis, a plaster mold is made of the part to be braced. In the case of metatarsus adductus, the foot would be held in the corrected position while the plaster sets. The cast would then function as a mold to which more plaster is poured, creating a positive mold of the foot. Polypropylene is then vacuum molded to the plaster model. When hard, the mold is removed and finished. Using the same principles, bracing a knee with a weak quadriceps would involve application of pressure anteriorly at the patella and posteriorly above and below the knee on the thigh and calf. The longer the lever arms, the lower the force needed to maintain the correction or position. If both the hip and the knee needed to be stabilized in extension, four points of pressure would be needed: posterior calf, anterior knee, posterior upper thigh, and anterior abdomen. When any force is applied, it should be distributed over as large an area as possible to decrease the force per unit area. Care must also be taken to avoid friction over areas of bony prominence such as the malleoli or the base of the fifth metatarsal. This is of particular importance if sensation is diminished or absent in the part being braced, as is the case in children with spina bifida or spinal cord injury.

If the orthosis is to cross a joint, hinges of one type or another will need to be used. These hinges may be free, limited motion, or locked, depending on the need.

Every attempt is made to make the brace as strong as required while being as light and cosmetically acceptable as possible. The devices are finished with straps and padding where necessary.

12. What are some of the complications of wearing an orthosis?

Pressure areas can develop early if an orthosis is not fitted properly and later if adjustments are not made for growth of the child. As mentioned, the common sites for these are around the malleoli and the base of the fifth metatarsal. Another very common place is the medial longitudinal arch in a child or adolescent with marked flatfeet treated with a rigid arch support.

Muscle atrophy and, to a certain extent, **osteopenia** can also occur with long-time brace use. If the orthosis is not to be used for the rest of the child's life but has been used for an extended period of time, a period of weaning should be recommended with increasing periods of time out of the orthosis to allow the muscles and bones to recover their strength gradually.

13. What are the psychologic effects of wearing an orthotic device?

Children and adolescents do not like anything that suggests that they are different from their friends. Braces fashioned from steel and leather were very conspicuous. The steel uprights were fastened to unattractive shoes. This meant that those were the only shoes the child could wear. We will probably never know the magnitude of the psychologic trauma suffered by the children who had to wear these devices.

With the advent of the new plastic materials, it has been possible to achieve the desired function with orthoses that are much more cosmetically pleasing. Polypropylene AFOs now can be made to fit into almost any type of shoe. The spinal orthoses generally have a lower profile and are less obvious.

14. What is the role of part-time bracing?

Virtually no brace is worn 100% of the time. The Charleston brace was constructed so that an adolescent would be required to wear the brace only when at home and not while at school. It is quite different from the other spinal orthoses in that it was designed to correct completely or overcorrect a flexible curve. Some of the reports in the literature suggest that this approach is as successful as wearing the brace 23 or 24 hours. Many orthopaedic surgeons recommend that some of the other underarm spinal braces be used 16 hours a day in selected cases in which there is not an exceptionally high risk for progression. Patient compliance seems to be better with this plan. It is felt that the loss of a few degrees of final correction is an acceptable price to pay for a situation that is much better psychologically for the patient.

Some AFOs are worn only at night to try to prevent the development or recurrence of deformity. Quite frequently, after the spica cast is removed after closed or open reduction of the hips, a plastic flexion-abduction orthosis is used at night to promote development of the acetabulum.

BIBLIOGRAPHY

1. American Academy of Orthopaedic Surgeons: Atlas of Orthotics: Biomechanical Principles and Application. St. Louis, C.V. Mosby Co., 1985.
2. Alexander M, Nelson M, et al: Orthotics, adapted seating, and assistive devices. In Molnar G: Pediatric Rehabilitation. Baltimore, Williams & Wilkins, 1992, pp. 181–201.
3. Bowker P: Biomechanical Basis of Orthotic Management. Boston, Butterworth-Heinemann, 1993.
4. Heaver A, Kraft P, et al: Orthotics and Prosthetics Digest: Reference Manual. Ottawa, Edahl Productions, 1983.
5. Wenger D, Rang M: The Art and Practice of Children's Orthopaedics. New York, Raven Press, 1993.

20. PHYSICAL AND OCCUPATIONAL THERAPY

H. G. Watts, M.D., and S. K. DeMuth, D.P.T.

1. What is physical therapy?

Physical therapy (PT) developed from the need for rehabilitation of persons injured in World War I and grew rapidly during and after World War II. Involvement with children came from needs identified during the polio epidemics after World War II.

Physical therapy, as defined by the American Physical Therapy Association, means the evaluation and treatment of people by using therapeutic exercises and mobilization; rehabilitative procedures, including training in functional activities, with or without assistive devices; and the use of physical measures such as heat, cold, light, electricity, and water for the purpose of limiting or preventing disability and alleviating or correcting any physical or mental condition. It also includes the performance of tests and measurements that aid in diagnosis or evaluation of function.

2. What is occupational therapy?

Occupational therapy, which also developed out of the need to rehabilitate those injured by war, is defined by the American Occupational Therapy Association as the therapeutic use of self-care, work, and play activities to increase independent function, enhance development, and prevent disability. It may include the adaptation of tasks or the environment to achieve maximum independence and to enhance quality of life.

3. Is there a subspecialty of children's physical or occupational therapy?

How often have we been told, *"Children are NOT small adults"*? This truth is no less valid for physical or occupational therapy. While therapists used to dealing with adults are not incompetent with children, those dealing with children all the time are better able to understand what a child should be able to do at a given stage of development and what that child's needs are in the home or school.

4. What is the difference between occupational therapy and physical therapy?

Sometimes the margins between the two fields are blurred. This blurring is more common in working with children than with adults.

Over the decades, occupational therapy has focused on assisting people with the ability to succeed at school or work, adaptive behavior, rehabilitation of upper extremity injuries, and management of upper limb prosthetics. Physical therapy has tended to focus on walking and mobility with or without adaptive equipment such as braces and wheelchairs, the rehabilitation of trunk and lower extremity injuries, and lower limb prosthetics.

5. What does physical therapy have to do with children's orthopedics?

Physical therapists are knowledgeable in the assessment of children's problems with motor function. This involves not only the assessment of muscle strength by manual testing and range-of-motion evaluation, but also the assessment of a child's ability to manage age-appropriate activities of daily living (ADL). Physical therapists also are very involved in the care of children with movement disorders such as cerebral palsy and have an interest in the child's integration into the community.

6. What does occupational therapy have to do with children's orthopedics?

Occupational therapists have a strong background in assessing children's developmental difficulties. They usually make such assessments using standardized tests. In addition, occupational therapists have a strong interest in assuring that the child with developmental disabilities is able to manage age-appropriate activities of daily living (ADL). Obviously, children with upper extremity injuries and deformities are appropriate for occupational therapy (OT) assessment.

7. Is there only one category of worker in OT or PT?

No, there are also registered occupational therapists and certified occupational therapy assistants (COTAs). These assistants provide occupational therapy services under the supervision of a registered occupational therapist.

The same goes for physical therapy. There are licensed physical therapists and physical therapy assistants (PTAs). Assistants provide care under the supervision of a licensed physical therapist.

OTs, COTAs, PTs, and PTAs have all received their education at accredited colleges or universities.

Occupational and physical therapy aides are trained on the job and have not received any formal education in therapy.

8. Which children should be referred for physical therapy?

A child who had an injury or a recent operation would be greatly assisted by the physical therapist in learning how to use crutches or a walker, for example. He or she would be taught not only how to go from one point to another but how to go up and down stairs and how to transfer from a chair to a bed, toilet, and car. Children with cerebral palsy and other developmental disabilities frequently benefit from contact with physical therapists as well.

9. Kids are very agile. Do they really need to learn how to use crutches?

Yes. Kids can certainly learn to use crutches pretty easily, provided they get proper-fitting ones and have normal coordination.

10. You know of a child who could use a wheelchair. Who do you ask for advice?

The physical therapist is the one who usually helps with the decision and the fitting. For a small child whose parents want a convenient method of getting the child around while shopping, a stroller may be all that is needed. At other times, a *properly fitted* wheelchair may be the answer. For some children, a powered chair may be needed, but not if the home doesn't have the space to make it useful.

11. Which children should be referred for occupational therapy?

A child who had an injury or a recent operation would be greatly assisted by the occupational therapist in learning how to feed or dress, for example. He or she would be taught how to chew or swallow as well as how to use adapted utensils or how to use specific strategies to dress without assistance from an adult. Children with cerebral palsy and other developmental disabilities frequently benefit from contact with occupational therapists as well.

12. What role do the therapists play in splinting and bracing?

Occupational therapists have expertise in making splints to improve function or to prevent deformity. Physical therapists are knowledgeable about the use of braces to enhance function.

13. You look after a child with a new limb prosthesis. Who will help train the child in its use?

That depends. As a general rule, occupational therapists work with children with upper extremity prostheses, while physical therapists work with those with lower extremity prostheses. There may be some overlap, especially in children with multiple limb involvement.

14. Is the child the only one to benefit from PT or OT?

No. The family can get tremendous help from the therapist. The family can learn what to expect from the child, how to rearrange home furnishings to facilitate the care of the child and what equipment would be appropriate.

15. What kind of range-of-motion exercises are there for children?

In *passive range of motion*, the therapist or parent does the moving of the joint without the active involvement of the child. *Active exercises* are those in which the child is doing the motion himself, albeit usually with additional encouragement from the therapist or parents. *Active assisted exercises* are those in which the child moves the joint through a range of motion, but therapist or parent is assisting and supporting the child. Both the child and the therapist or parent have some control over the amount of motion. *Active resisted exercise* clearly involves the child doing the motion with the parent or therapist resisting the activity.

Because children are small and their muscles can be easily overpowered, *caution* has to be used so that a child does not get injured. With this in mind, there is very little place for passive exercise use in children except where there is no motor ability whatsoever.

16. What other kinds of exercises are there for children?

There are many therapeutic approaches to teaching children how to move or perform various tasks. You may see terms like Swiss Ball therapy, NDT (neurodevelopmental therapy), SI (sensory integration therapy), or PNF (proprioceptive neuromuscular facilitation). The important point is that there is no one approach that solves all the problems, and therapy approaches continue to change as new knowledge evolves.

17. Getting children to do exercises can be like having them clean their rooms. How would you suggest avoiding such turmoil?

With children, exercises should be modified into game playing. For example, ball kicking can be a means of strengthening the quadriceps muscle in the leg rather than going through the often frustrating activity of encouraging a child to straighten and bend the knee.

But these gamelike exercises must be appropriate for the stage of development that a child has reached. In addition, the therapist needs to know what activities are likely to sustain attention in a child at a given age.

18. Do these exercises need to be done in the presence of the therapist?

Certainly not. There are not enough therapists or days in the week to have the exercises limited to direct hands-on treatment. A major role of the therapist is to teach the parents how to do the appropriate exercises. This is usually done by demonstration and is reinforced by illustrations to take home as a reminder. The therapist may see a child fairly frequently to reinforce the teaching, but not necessarily to help the child with the exercises directly.

19. The role of therapy may be obvious in children with purely mechanical problems such as osteogenesis imperfecta. What can physical or occupational therapy do for a child with cerebral palsy?

A child with cerebral palsy may benefit by maintaining the range of motion of the extremities, but muscle strengthening where appropriate and particularly learning coping skills to manage ADL are also valuable.

20. What aspects of cerebral palsy are *unlikely* to benefit from physical or occupational therapy?

Fixed contractures of joints are not amenable to correction by exercises. In some places, physical therapists are mandated to apply plaster casts. In such situations, serial casting may be used to overcome fixed contractures.

Although there has been a great deal of interest in the subject, there is no scientific evidence that physical therapy is able to reduce spasticity.

21. Why do occupational and physical therapists work in school systems?

It is often in the school setting that evidence of a central nervous system disorder is first seen. Therapists are then asked by teachers to assess such children. This may be the child's introduction to the medical system. A therapist can help the teachers help the children in their daily activities, making sure that the activities are indeed possible and that equipment needed to help the child is available.

22. What are the indicators for occupational therapy referral of a school student?
The guidelines published by the California Department of Education are a good place to start. They suggest that students who demonstrate the following be referred to occupational therapy.
  1. Difficulty in learning new motor tasks.
  2. Poor organization and sequencing of tasks.
  3. Poor hand use (including writing and tool use).
  4. Difficulty in accomplishing tasks without the use of adaptive equipment, environmental modifications, or assistive technology.
  5. Unusual or limited play patterns.
  6. Deficits in adaptive self-help or feeding skills in the educational setting.
  7. Poor attention to tasks.
  8. Notable overreaction or underreaction to textures, touch, or movement.

23. What are the indicators for a referral for physical therapy?
The same guidelines suggest that students who demonstrate the following be referred to physical therapy.
  1. Delayed gross motor skills.
  2. Difficulty in learning new motor tasks.
  3. Unusual walking or movement patterns.
  4. Difficulty in moving or moving unsafely in the school environment.
  5. Difficulty in maintaining an appropriate sitting posture.
  6. Poor balance or falling frequently.
  7. Difficulty in accomplishing tasks without the use of adaptive equipment, environmental modifications, or assistive technology.
  8. Postural or orthopedic abnormalities.
  9. Reduced endurance or excessive fatigue.

24. What is the Individual with Disabilities Education Act (IDEA)?
This act defines which individuals are eligible for the special services in the school setting. IDEA is divided into parts A through I. Part A pertains to children from birth to 3 years of age. Part B pertains to children 3 through 21 years of age. Under part B, the federal government defines eligible disabilities as mental retardation; hearing impairments, including deafness; speech or language impairments; visual impairments, including blindness; serious emotional disturbance; orthopedic impairments; autism; traumatic brain injury; other health impairments; or specific learning disabilities.

25. What does this have to do with children's orthopedics?
Children with orthopedic problems often have problems in other systems as well and may need the services of therapists.

26. What is an IEP?
An IEP is an Individualized Education Program. This is a working document required by the IDEA for special education students 3–21 years of age that documents their eligibility for services; level of present functioning; appropriate goals, objectives, services, and services providers; and other specifics. When the IEP is signed and is accepted by the parent or legal guardian, it becomes the legal document insuring compliance with provision of service. The IEP team refers to all the members, including the parents, who provide services to special education students as part of a free and appropriate educational program.

27. What are some of the terms you are likely to see on a therapist's report?
When you get reports from therapists, they naturally employ their own jargon. For instance, ADL means activities of daily living. These are tasks that individuals engage in on a regular basis so that they can function and be sustained in the environments in which they operate.

Fine motor skills are the types of skills that require precise controlled movement of one's hands to perform an activity. This is contrasted with *gross motor skills,* an example of which is walking. *Motor planning* is the ability of the brain to conceive, organize, and carry out a sequence of unfamiliar actions. *Visual perception and integration* is the ability to use visual information to recognize, recall, and discriminate the meaning of what the child sees.

28. What is meant by "modalities"?

Therapists use the term *modalities* to mean externally applied physical agents such as hot packs, ice, diathermy, and ultrasound.

29. What is the role of these modalities in children?

You have to be a little cautious in using some of these agents with children. For example, there is experimental evidence that open epiphyses can be damaged by ultrasound. Therefore, ultrasound is generally not used in children.

Young children and those with developmental delays may not be able to communicate readily. In this instance, it is possible that excessive heat could be applied using a modality such as diathermy.

These same cautions are needed with manual therapy techniques (including mobilization and manipulation), which are generally not used with children.

30. What is meant by architectural barriers?

These are potential obstacles to wheelchairs. A good exercise is to spend a part of a day moving around and living your life in a wheelchair. You will find even thick rugs on the floor can be an impediment, let alone steps, the absence of ramps, or even the absence of elevators. While there are laws mandating the elimination of architectural barriers in public buildings, private homes and apartments can present enormous difficulties. For example, the doors into most bathrooms are too narrow for a wheelchair to be pushed through.

31. What is the role of electrical stimulation in children?

Electrical stimulation can mean a number of different things. Surface electrical stimulation has been used effectively for strengthening muscles. It has been tried and found wanting in the treatment of scoliosis, however. It has been used to maintain muscle bulk after a nerve injury while the nerve recuperates.

Outcomes are affected by variations in the stimulus—the *duration,* the *intensity,* the *frequency,* and even time of day during which the stimulus is applied. It is important to look at these specific qualities.

32. What is the role of biofeedback in children?

Biofeedback uses a physical end result of effort to signal to a child the outcome of the child's work. For example, EMG leads can be placed on an amputation stump and hooked up to the handset of a radio-controlled automobile. The child then learns to steer the car by using muscle contractions. This training can be used prior to fitting a child with a myoelectric prosthesis. Other biofeedback systems are used for less obvious outcomes, such as relaxation.

33. Does physical therapy have a role in teaching body mechanics?

The most important role may be to teach parents how to lift their child properly so the parents don't injure their backs as their child grows heavier.

34. What is the role of physical therapists in motion analysis laboratories?

The role of motion analysis laboratories ("gait labs") has grown as a means of documenting the pre- and postoperative status of children. This is particularly so with children with musculoskeletal problems secondary to cerebral palsy. They are also used in assessing children with other musculoskeletal problems such as myelodysplasia (spina bifida) and amputations. Such studies may include energy consumption assessments.

Many such gait laboratories are managed by physical therapists who have been specially trained in the field. As with all such laboratory tests, the findings need to be carefully integrated with results of the child's physical examination.

35. What is the role of aerobic conditioning exercises in children?
In the past, such activity has been confined to the treatment of adults. As our focus on the problems of obesity of adulthood sharpens, we recognize that patterns established by children, especially in their teenage years, are those continued into adulthood.

As a consequence, there is a greater interest in involving children in fitness programs such as "Fit Kids," established by the American Physical Therapy Association.

BIBLIOGRAPHY

1. American Physical Therapy Association: A guide to physical therapists' practice, volume I: A description of patient management. Phys Ther 75 (8,):707–756, 1995.
2. Guidelines for Occupational Therapy and Physical Therapy in California Public Schools: Sacramento, California Department of Education, Bureau of Publications, 1996.
3. Campbell SK, Gardner HG, Ramakrishnan V: Correlates of physicians' decisions to refer children with cerebral palsy for physical therapy. Dev Med Child Neurol 37(12):1062–1074, 1995.

21. SHOES FOR CHILDREN

Lynn Staheli, M.D.

1. Is going without shoes OK for infants and children?
Barefoot is a natural and healthy state for the foot at any age. Barefoot people have stronger feet with fewer deformities than those who wear shoes.

2. What are the benefits of wearing shoes?
Shoes, like other clothing, are worn for appearance and protection. Shoes protect the foot from cold, sharp objects, and from the eyes of those who don't like the appearance of the bare foot.

3. What are the harmful effects of wearing shoes?
This depends upon the shoe. Stiff shoes make the foot weaker and increase the frequency of flatfeet. Tight shoes can cause deformities of the toes.

4. Does the growing foot need support?
No. A *supportive* shoe limits movement, makes the foot weaker, and lowers the long arch. The foot should be free to move freely and to develop mobility and strength. We would think it ridiculous to place the hand in a rigid glove.

5. Are shoes "corrective"?
Shoes are not corrective and have never been shown to correct any deformity.

6. When should the infant be first fitted for shoes?
Usually parents fit shoes sometime during the first year. This is a clothing issue. The infant will do well in stockings around the house. Soft shoes may be fitted for appearance or to protect the foot when outside.

7. What shoes are best for the toddler?

Soft, flexible shoes are best. As the infant's foot is chubby, sometimes a hightop shoe is helpful just to keep the shoe on the foot.

8. What shoes are best for the teenager?

Shock-absorbing shoes reduce overuse injuries. Thick-cushioned soles make walking more comfortable.

9. What types of shoes should be avoided?

Most children's shoes are made better now than they were in the past. The major problems now are pointed toes with high heels for girls and cowboy boots for boys. Those with elevated heels force the foot forward and wedge the toes. This can cause discomfort, calluses, toe deformities, and can aggravate bunions.

10. What are the features (5 Fs) of a good shoe?

The best shoe is one that simulates barefootedness. The shoe should have the following features (Figure):

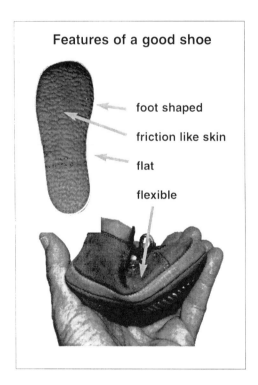

Flexible. The shoe should allow as much free motion as possible. As a test, make certain the shoe can be easily flexed in the parent's hand.

Flat. Avoid high heels that force the foot forward, cramping the toes.

Foot-shaped. Avoid pointed toes or other shapes which are different from the normal foot.

Fitted generously. Better to be too large than too short.

Friction like skin. The sole should have about the same friction as skin. Soles that are slippery or adherent can cause the child to fall. Slide the shoes across a flat surface and compare that with running the hand across the same surface. The resistance to sliding should be about the same.

11. How do we know if new shoes fit properly?
They should be comfortable and provide about a fingerbreadth of room for growth. It is preferable that the shoes be too large rather than too small. Sometimes shoes are sold without sufficient room for growth, shortening the useful life of the shoe.

12. How often should shoes be replaced?
In the growing child, shoes are nearly always outgrown before being worn out. Foot growth occurs earlier than that of the rest of the body and is completed before adolescence.

13. Can outgrown shoes be safely worn by younger sibs?
Hand-me-downs are OK. Minor alterations in shape of the shoe will not damage the younger sibling's foot. Fungal skin infections may be passed in the shoe.

14. Are expensive shoes best for the child's foot?
Provided that the shoe meets the criteria of a good shoe, the price is not important. It is often useful to emphasize this point to parents as some equate the quality of parenting to the quality of the shoes.

15. Does asymmetric shoe wear indicate a foot problem?
Not necessarily. If wear is asymmetric, examine the child's feet. Children with normal feet often will show asymmetric shoe wear.

16. Do stiff shoes, orthotics, or inserts prevent or correct flatfeet?
No. The belief that the foot needed support and that the arch would fall unless supported by inserts was once common. We now know that this concept is wrong. A stiff shoe actually increases the incidence of flatfeet. As one would expect, the stiff shoe, by limiting mobility, makes the foot weaker. This weakness results in a loss of the dynamic component of arch maintenance in a flatter foot.

17. Do shoe wedges or inserts help with intoeing or out-toeing?
No. In the past, countless children wore various wedges on their shoes to correct a rotational problem. When we studied this by applying various wedges to children's shoes and measuring the effect on the foot progression angle, we found that the wedges made no difference in how much the child toed in or out.

18. Are shoe wedges helpful in managing bowlegs or knockknees?
No. In the past, sole wedges were commonly prescribed for these conditions. Now we know that the improvement in these conditions was due simply to natural history.

19. Are orthotics useful in managing bunions in children?
No. This has been studied and found not to be useful.

20. Is there any harm in prescribing shoe modifications for children?
Yes. Shoe modifications are often uncomfortable, limit play, and are embarrassing. In addition, they can impart in the child a sense that they are defective. We found that adults who wore shoe modifications as children had a significantly lower self esteem than controls. They remembered the experience of wearing the devices as unpleasant.

21. Are inserts useful in reducing abnormal shoe wear?
Sometimes. Inserts such as heel cups may reduce the frequency of the shoe from breaking down. The cost, discomfort, and inconvenience for the child and possible effect on the child's self image makes this approaches to excessive shoe wear questionable. It is usually best for the parents to buy a sturdier shoe.

22. When are shoe inserts useful?
Shoe inserts and orthotics are useful to redistribute the load-bearing on the sole of the foot. Children with stiff, deformed feet may benefit from orthotics which are recessed under prominences.

This is most useful in children with clubfeet, who often have excessive loading under the base of the 5th metatarsal.

23. Are arch supports or orthotics useful in managing growing pains?
Controversial. Growing pains are common and resolve without treatment with time. The value of orthotics in changing the natural history has never been studied. I do not treat growing pains with shoe inserts because of possible long-term harmful effects on the child, cost for the family, and doubts regarding effectiveness.

24. What should I do if families insist on some treatment?
Prescribe a healthy lifestyle for the child (physical activity, limited TV time, healthy foods, etc.). Avoid mechanical interventions, as these can be both unpleasant for the child and risk possible long-term adverse psychological effects.

BIBLIOGRAPHY

1. Driano AN, Staheli LR, Staheli LT: Psychosocial Development and "Corrective" Shoewear Use in Child-hood. AAOS 1997.
2. Engle ET, Morton DJ: Notes on foot disorders among natives of the Belgian Congo. J Bone Joint Surg 13:311, 1931.
3. Kilmartin TE, Barrington RL, Wallace WA: A controlled prospective trial of a foot orthosis for juvenile hallux valgus. J Bone Joint Surg 76-B:210, 1994.
4. Knittle G, Staheli LT. The effectiveness of shoe modifications for intoeing. Orthop Clin North Am 7:1019, 1976.
5. Rao UB, Joseph B. The influence of footwear on the prevalence of flat foot: A survey of 2300 children. J Bone and Joint Surg 74B:525, 1992.
6. Sim-Fook L Hodgson A. A comparison of foot forms among the non-shoe and shoe-wearing Chinese population. J Bone Joint Surg 40A:1058, 1958.
7. Staheli LT, Chew DE, Corbett M. The longitudinal arch: a survey of eight hundred and eighty-two feet in normal children and adults. J Bone Joint Surg 69A:426, 1987.
8. Staheli LT, Griffin L. Corrective shoes for children: a survey of current practice. Pediatrics, 65:13, 1980.
9. Staheli LT. Shoes for children: A review. Pediatrics, 88:371, 1991.
10. Wenger DR, Mauldin D. Speck G, Morgan D. and Lieber RL. Corrective shoes as treatment for flexible flatfoot in infants and children. J Bone Joint Surg 71A:800, 1989.

22. JOINT ASPIRATION

Ken N. Kuo, M.D.

1. What is joint aspiration?
Joint aspiration is a procedure that introduces a syringe needle into a joint (arthrocentesis) and withdraws its content for diagnostic or therapeutic purposes.

2. What equipment is required for joint aspiration?
- Syringes: size will depend on the size of the joint to be aspirated.
- Needles: 18- to 22-gauge 1½-inch straight needle with short bevel. In the hip of a larger person, a 3½-inch spinal needle may be required. The gauge of the needle used partly depends on the viscosity of the fluid aspirated.
- 4x4 sponges
- Topical antiseptics: tincture of iodine or betadine stick, 70% alcohol wipes.
- Sterile barrier and sterile gloves.
- Local anesthetic (such as 1% plain lidocaine) and 3-ml syringe with 22-gauge needle.

- Plain or anticoagulated sterile fluid collection vials or test tubes.
- Culture tube as needed.

3. What are the indications for joint aspiration?
- For diagnostic purposes to rule out such diseases as septic arthritis, different types of inflammatory disorders and arthritis, or certain metabolic maladies.
- For decompression from acute traumatic hemarthrosis, septic arthritis, or a large effusion secondary to inflammatory disease.
- For therapeutic purposes such as intra-articular injection of therapeutic agents.

4. What are the absolute contraindications to joint aspiration?
- Soft tissue cellulitis or soft tissue abscess in the path of needle entrance, since one may introduce the pathogen into the joint.
- Pathologically uncontrolled bleeding tendency, such as hemarthrosis in a patient with hemophilia or in one receiving active anticoagulative therapy.
- The path of the needle going through tumorous tissue.

5. What are the precautions during joint aspiration?
- Avoid passing the needle through a vascular area.
- Avoid obvious nerve trunk structures.
- Do not wiggle the needle tip in the joint, because it may damage intra-articular structures such as articular cartilage. It may also cause unnecessary bleeding.
- It is a must to observe strict sterile techniques.

6. What is the best site for joint aspiration?
So long as one observes the above-mentioned indications, contraindications, and precautions, it is generally acceptable to perform the aspiration where the fluid can be most easily seen and felt. The location for entrance to each joint is different dependent on its specific anatomic structure.

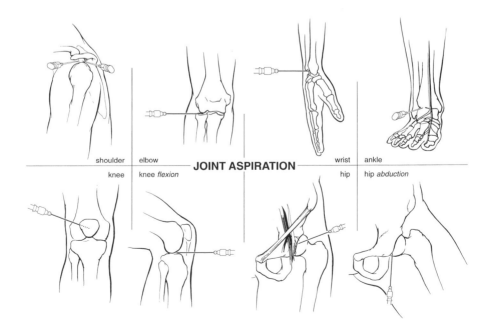

| shoulder | elbow | **JOINT ASPIRATION** | wrist | ankle |
| knee | knee *flexion* | | hip | hip *abduction* |

7. What is the approach for shoulder joint aspiration?
The shoulder joint can be approached through either the anterior or the lateral aspect just below the acromial process. The needle should enter the joint directly. Avoid sticking the needle directly into the convexity contour of the humeral head.

8. What is the approach for elbow joint aspiration?
The elbow joint can be easily entered from the posterolateral aspect to avoid the medial neurovascular structure. The needle should enter the space between the lateral humeral condyle and the radial head. The structure can be palpated with the forearm in supinated position. At the time of aspiration, the elbow can be placed in flexion and the forearm in pronation.

9. What is the approach for wrist joint aspiration?
The easiest one is the dorsal radial approach. The needle can be inserted distal to Lister's tubercle at the joint line. The wrist should be kept in pronated position and slight ulnar deviation. Other approaches are radial entrance at the tip of the radial styloid and ulnar entrance at the tip of the ulnar styloid.

10. What is the approach for finger joint aspiration?
With the finger or thumb slightly flexed and distracted (by pulling the finger or thumb distally), the needle can enter from either the dorsal ulnar or the dorsal radial angle.

11. What is the approach for hip joint aspiration?
 The hip joint is the most difficult joint to aspirate. The patient should be placed under general anesthesia or heavy sedation with local anesthesia. Unless the patient is very thin and in the hands of a very experienced physicians, fluoroscopic guidance is often required. The approach can be medial, anterior, or lateral.

 The *medial approach* enters just below the adductor longus in the groin and advances in the cephalad direction. The needle tip enters the joint through the anterior inferior joint capsule.

 The *anterior approach* enters anteriorly about one fingerwidth lateral to the femoral artery pulse and distal to the inguinal ligament. The needle advances posteriorly and enters the joint through the anterior joint capsule.

 The *lateral approach* enters the area proximal to the tip of the greater trochanter. The needle advances medially and in a slightly cephalad direction. It enters the joint through the lateral joint capsule. This approach travels the longest distance and is not practical in larger patients.

12. How can you be sure the needle is in the hip joint?
 * Rotate the hip joint gently. One should feel the needle scratching on the femoral head. If it is fixed, the needle may have penetrated the articular cartilage of the acetabulum or the femoral head.
 * Use fluoroscopic observation to ensure that the tip of needle is between the femoral head and the acetabulum.
 * Use an obturator during needle insertion to avoid soft tissue plugging the needle lumen.
 * If there is no fluid aspirated, inject 0.5–1 ml of normal saline, then disconnect the syringe. The saline will backflow quickly when the needle tip is in the joint.
 * Confirm negative hip aspiration by injecting arthrographic dye.

13. What is the approach for knee joint aspiration?
 Commonly, the joint can be approached in two ways, superolateral or anterior medial. In the *superolateral approach,* one inserts the needle just under the superolateral corner of the patella with knee in full extension. The needle is advanced medially into the suprapatellar pouch or slightly distally into the patellofemoral junction.

 In an *anterior approach,* with the knee in 90° of flexion, one inserts the needle into the triangle formed by the patellar tendon, medial femoral condyle, and medial tibial plateau. The needle will go straight into the medial knee joint.

14. What is the approach for ankle joint aspiration?
The ankle joint can be easily and safely entered anterolateral to the pedis dorsalis pulse. The needle enters proximal to the talus in a straight posterior direction into the ankle joint. In a smaller child, precautions should be taken not to enter the distal tibial epiphyseal plate, which is only a short distance from the joint line.

15. What is the approach for toe joint aspiration?
With the toe in slight flexion and distracted by being pulled distally, the small needle can enter dorso medially or dorso laterally.

16. What should one observe and test once the joint fluid has been aspirated?
One should describe the general characteristics of the gross appearance. The aspirated fluid is inspected for viscosity by the "string test," clarity, color, and the presence of blood. The aspirated fluid is then placed in different containers and sent for laboratory tests depending on the differential diagnosis. In general, testing often includes a cell count with differential, an immunologic test for arthritis, and analysis of glucose and protein. A smear for gram stain and a bacterial culture are ordered when infection is suspected.

BIBLIOGRAPHY

 1. Crenshaw AH (ed): Campbell's Operative Orthopaedics, 8th ed. St. Louis, C.V. Mosby Co., 1992.
 2. Hughes WT, Buescher I: Pediatric Procedures. Philadelphia, W.B. Saunders Co., 1980.
 3. Leversee JH: Aspiration of joints and soft tissue injections. Prim care 13:579, 1986.
 4. Pfenninger JL: Infection of joints and soft tissue: Part I. General guidelines. Am Fam Physician 44:1196, 1991.
 5. Pfenninger JL: Infection of joints and soft tissue: Part II. Guidelines for specific joints. Am Fam Physician, 44:1690, 1991.
 6. Sholkoff SD, Eyring EJ: Arthropuncture technique. Clin Orthop 72:393, 1970.
 7. Staheli LT: Fundamentals of Pediatric Orthopedics. New York, Raven Press, 1992.
 8. Tachdjian MO: Clinical Pediatric Orthopedics: Art of Diagnosis and Principles of Management. East Norwalk, CT, Appleton & Lange, 1977.
 9. Tachdjian MO: Pediatric Orthopedics, 2nd ed. Philadelphia, W.B. Saunders Co., 1990.
10. Wenger DR, Rang M: The Art and Practice of Children's Orthopaedics. New York, Raven Press, 1993.

23. PREVENTION OF INJURY

Merv Letts, M.D., and Darin Davidson

1. What is the most common cause of death in the first two decades of life?
Trauma is the major cause of death in children over one year of age and it is the major cause of morbidity among children of all ages in the United States and Canada. Approximately 22,000 children die secondary to trauma in the United States each year, representing a mortality rate of 30.3 per 100,000 children. Farm injuries alone were responsible for an estimated 23,500 injuries to children, 300 of whom died as a result of their injuries. Injuries kill more children than all other causes of death combined. Seventy-percent of the deaths among teenagers are due to injury. For every injury-related death, there are 45 hospital admissions, and 13,000 visits to emergency departments for trauma-related injury.

2. Are injuries the result of accidents?
Accidents are unpredictable acts of fate, over which we have no control. More than 90% of injuries are both predictable and preventable in children.

3. What are the most common causes of farm injuries to children?

Approximately 40% of farm-related injuries in children occur as a result of tractor-induced injury followed by auger injuries, power take-offs, conveyor belts, and wagons. Extremity fractures are the most common injuries, with the upper extremity being more frequently involved than the lower. Amputations are the most common cause of long-term morbidity, sometimes reaching as high as 40% of farm injuries. (see Figure).

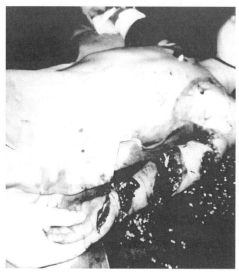 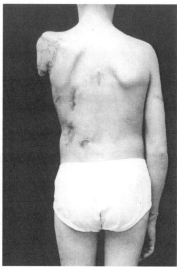

Child whose arm became entangled in an auger. Amputation was required at a high level.

4. How can farm injuries be prevented and minimized?

By encouraging the compilation of data concerning farm trauma in children to increase awareness of the problem. We can encourage the use of safety devices on augers and power take-offs and support public awareness campaigns to discourage children from sitting on the fenders of tractors and riding dangerous equipment.

5. In children presenting with a mangled limb, how can amputation be prevented or minimized?

The mangled limb in a child should not be subjected to the same criteria for amputation as in adults. Do not apply the mangled limb extremity score developed for adults in the same manner to children, since their regenerative capacity is much greater. Nerve and vascular repair are more successful in maintaining limb viability in children.

6. What is the epidemiology of bicycle trauma in North America?

In bicycle trauma, factors relating to the environment, the vector or vehicle, and the operator's behavior must all be considered when examining the causes of bicycle accidents. The accident rate in the United States for bicycle injuries is 200 minor injuries per 100,000 bicyclists; 85 severe injuries per 100,000 bicyclists each year; and two fatal bicycle accidents per 100,000 bicyclists each year.

7. What age group is most vulnerable to death and injury from bicycle riding?

Children under 10 years of age. Young children have difficulty interpreting road signs and understanding rules of the road and are more likely to carelessly ride out into busy traffic.

8. What is the most common risk factor responsible for bicycle injuries in children under 10 years of age?
Children under 10 are most frequently injured in mid-block rideouts. This occurs when the child rides out of the end of a driveway in the middle of a block into oncoming traffic. This type of trauma is preventable, perhaps by temporary barriers at the end of driveways where young children are cycling.

9. In the age group of 11 to 19, what is the most common cause of bicycle accidents?
In this age group errors in operating the bicycle are common. Training courses would seem to be a logical way to reduce bicycle trauma in teenagers, as well as encouraging city planners to incorporate dedicated bicycle paths and lanes into their traffic plans.

10. What is the most common cause of death in the bicyclist?
Ninety percent of all deaths involving bicycles are secondary to collision with a motor vehicle. Head injuries are the most common cause of death and the most common reason for hospitalization. Bicyclists actually have a higher incidence of severe head injuries than motorcyclists.

11. What is the most common musculoskeletal injury resulting from a bicycle accident and how can it be prevented?
Eighty-five percent of all bicycle injuries involve the shoulder or upper extremity. "Bicycle shoulder" may occur when the bicycle is suddenly stopped and the rider is thrown over the handle bars. Bicyclists can try to prevent this by keeping a tight grip on the handle bars and being taught to roll with the bike, allowing it to absorb some force of the fall.

12. Does the use of helmets by motorcyclists and bicyclists decrease the mortality rate in accidents?
Emphatically yes! The death rate for motorcycle accidents was 15 per 10,000 in the 1960s and has now fallen to six per 10,000 in areas enforcing universal helmet laws.

13. What has been the effect of restraint systems on morbidity and mortality in children?
Infant car seats properly restrained and placed in the rear seat facing the rear will protect an infant from a force of 60 g. In Michigan, following the implementation of the child restraint law, there was a reduction in injury in infants 0–1 year of age by 50% and in children 1–3 years of age by 17%.

14. Can seat belts cause trauma in children?
The lap belt, when worn without the shoulder harness, does predispose to so-called Chance fracture, a hyperflexion injury which in children may not only cause a typical transverse fracture through the body and spinous process, but also may result in an atypical fracture line running through the disk or the vertebral apophysis. Occasionally the shoulder lap belt, when not applied properly, may produce similar forces across the cervical spine resulting in cervical spine fracture.

15. How efficient are seatbelts in preventing injury in infants and young children?
In the United States, motor vehicle accidents account for over 600 deaths per year in children under the age of five. They are the leading cause of childhood death in this age group. The design of seatbelts is optimized for the fiftieth percentile male and this is the size used in federal safety standard testing in both Canada and the United States. For young children, properly installed safety seats and booster seats are the most effective restraint system and have reduced fatal injury by as much as 69% in some studies.

16. Are air bags effective in preventing injury in children?
The air bag has been very effective in reducing trauma in adults and teenagers. In young children, however, the force of the explosion of the bag has the potential to cause sudden hyperextension of the cervical spine and in younger children the bag may obstruct breathing. It is best to have in-

fants and young children positioned in the back seat and strapped into infant seats or car seats. This will prevent any possible trauma from the sudden explosion of the bag.

17. How can blood loss be minimized or prevented during surgery for trauma victims?
Blood loss during surgery and postoperatively is always a major concern to surgeons operating on acute trauma patients. A good history is mandatory for any traumatized children, as many bleeding problems can be recognized and corrected prior to surgery. Identifying children with bleeding disorders may allow the appropriate preoperative treatment of the condition, such as AHG for hemophiliacs, or DDAVP for von Willebrand's disease. A history of pharmaceuticals and drugs being taken by the child is absolutely essential. Many drugs (salicylates, non-steroid anti-inflamatories or anticoagulants) may increase bleeding, and appropriate management to decrease hemorrhage during the procedure and eliminate a major cause of blood loss can be undertaken.

18. What is the role of falls in causing injury?
Falls on the outstretched arm are the most common cause of fractures of the upper extremity in children. Although fracture of the hip typically occurs as a result of a fall in the elderly, it is uncommon in children except in falls from heights. Although children are at high risk of fall injury, their death rate is low. Falls on stairs account for one-eighth of the childhood falls treated in the emergency room. This has been substantially reduced with the ban on infant walkers, which were a common cause of infant falls.

19. What preventive measures can be taken to minimize falls for children?
It is difficult to modify children's behavior, hence the environment needs to be adapted. Playground modification, including guidelines for playground equipment, has contributed to a decrease in falls at playgrounds. The use of wood chips or sand around playground equipment, rather than cement or asphalt, assists in cushioning falls. In high-rise apartment buildings, potential falls out of windows can be minimized by window guards and window modifications. Falls down stairs have been reduced by discouraging the use of infant walkers.

20. What is the leading cause of injury in the 12–17 year age group?
A comprehensive survey of injured children admitted to Massachusetts emergency rooms and hospitals revealed that sports were the leading cause of injury from age 12–17 years. Each year one child in 27 sustained a sports injury severe enough to warrant hospital treatment. Almost two-thirds of these sports injuries resulted from team contact sports, such as football, basketball or soccer.

21. What is the best way to prevent confusion or concern regarding the type of surgery being performed on a child?
The most important aspect of signing a consent form prior to surgery is the discussion that centers on consent. The form itself is not the "consent." The explanation given by the surgeon and the dialogue between the surgeon and parents about the proposed treatment are the all-important element of the consent process. The form is simply written confirmation that explanations were given and that the family agreed to what was proposed. A signed consent form will be of little value later if the family can convince a court that the explanations were inadequate, or worse, not given at all.

22. What areas of prevention must take top priority in preventing spinal cord injuries in children?
Prevention programs must address the most common causes of spinal cord injury in children: motor vehicle accidents, gun shot injuries, and contact sports such as hockey and football. Improvement in motor vehicle child restraints have been helpful but more are needed. Modification of athletic rules, such as abolishing checking from behind in hockey and spearing a football, is an example of how spinal cord trauma has been minimized in sports, but continued enforcement is necessary.

23. Is it possible to prevent atlanto axial spinal cord injury in children with marked ligamentous laxity?

Atlanto-axial instability is a common accompaniment of a number of syndromes characterized by marked ligamentous laxity. Down syndrome is one of the more common, and these children are at higher risk in sports where there may be hyperflexion of the cervical spine. The American Academy of Pediatrics has suggested these guidelines for minimizing trauma to the atlanto-axial region: (1) all children with Down's syndrome who desire to train or compete in at-risk sports should first obtain flexion-extension radiographs of the lateral cervical spine to determine the atlanto dens interval; (2) if the atlanto dens interval is greater than 4.5 mm or if odontoid dysplasia is present then at-risk sports should be avoided and regular follow up begun; (3) if the ADI is greater than 4.5 mm and abnormal neurologic signs are present, it is recommended that the child be evaluated for C1–C2 fusion.

24. What pharmaceutical method can be used to prevent or minimize loss of spinal cord function?

The standard treatment for acute spinal cord injury is intravenous steroids. Other compounds of GM-1 gangliocide are being investigated as are techniques for spinal cord regeneration.

25. How is it possible to prevent further cervical trauma in the transport of infants with cervical spine injuries?

Upper cervical spine injuries are more common in infants due to the larger size of the head and increased forces this exerts on the upper aspect of the cervical spine. When transporting these infants it was pointed out by Herzenberg and Hensinger et al. that by using a transport board with a cut-out in order to accommodate the occiput, flexion of the head is prevented. When transporting the traumatized child, there would be less flexion force on the cervical spine, and further injury to the spinal cord is minimized.

26. What is one of the major problems that prevents the spinal cord injured from regaining their full potential?

One of the greatest barriers to regaining a full and productive life is the development of impairments and disabilities secondary to the spinal cord injury, such as severe scoliosis, chronic renal infection, or pressure sores. These can be prevented through a good orthopaedic rehabilitation program and improved understanding of stable seating.

27. How can we prevent or minimize the high costs associated with spinal cord injury?

With the longer life expectancy of children with spinal cord injury, together with improved medical technology, the costs associated with modern rehabilitation of the spinal cord-injured patient is enormous. It is cost-effective to reduce the incidence of rehospitalizations because of complications from the spinal cord injury, such as pressure sores, contracture, and urinary tract infection. Returning the spinal-cord–injured young person to gainful employment and schooling is also an excellent way to maximize rehabilitation.

28. What are the best methods to prevent pressure ulceration in spinal-cord–injured children?

Any bony prominence is susceptible to pressure ulceration in the spinal-cord–injured child. The older and heavier the child, the more susceptible they are to developing pressure ulceration, hence proper sitting in the wheelchair is essential. As the child grows in height and weight, a total education on maintaining skin integrity is essential. They must be taught to (a) regularly inspect their insensate skin, especially over pressure areas; (b) develop skin tolerance through the gradual use of an orthosis or gradual pressure release such as push ups or side-to-side motion; (c) develop proper positioning techniques, especially when sitting in the wheelchair, and maintain proper hygiene to keep the skin dry and clean.

29. What is now the second most common cause of spinal cord injury in children in the United States?
In the United States, many spinal cord injury centers are experiencing a dramatic increase in gunshot trauma as a cause of spinal cord injury. In most major centers this form of spinal cord injury is now the second most common in children.

30. Why are all-terrain vehicles such a major hazard to inexperienced childhood riders?
The three-wheeled all-terrain vehicle is very unstable, and easily tipped over by the inexperienced. As a result of their involvement in thousands of deaths and severe injuries, this vehicle was banned in 1987 in North America. There have been recommendations to ban the four-wheel all-terrain vehicle due to its propensity to flip backwards. This is an example of the first of Haddon's ten basic strategies in the prevention of injury, that is, to prevent the creation of the hazard in the first place. Another illustration of this strategy is the American Academy of Pediatrics recommendation in 1977 that the use of school trampolines be banned. Following this, there was a decrease of more than 60% in the number of trampoline head and neck injuries. A final illustration of this strategy is a creation of a ban on high-risk activities such as human pyramids, which result in major injuries to cheerleaders each year.

31. In most major trauma centers in North America what is the most common cause of amputation and how can it be prevented?
Most recent studies on amputations have revealed that the power lawn mower now accounts for the majority of amputations to children less than ten years of age. Prevention is mostly common sense and is based on the concept that familiarity breeds contempt. Young children should never be allowed to ride on lawn mowers, either alone or accompanied by an adult. Children under 14 should not be allowed to operate riding mowers, which are one of the most common causes of amputations in children. Young children should also not be present in a yard in which a power mower is being used.

32. What is the major cause of skiing accidents in children and adolescents?
Most catastrophic pediatric skiing injuries result from collisions with stationary objects, with two predominate risk groups, being beginners and experienced male skiers. The main reasons for such injury are excessive speed and loss of control. Lower extremity injuries have decreased over the past decade with improved equipment, but upper extremity injuries have not. Most injuries result from impact with the snow surface or a bending or twisting motion of the lower extremities during falls. The injury rate is highest in beginners, with 20 to 40% of total injuries occurring in children under 16 years of age.

33. Why has there been an increase in the incidence of stress fractures of the pars interarticularis in adolescent athletes?
Over the past decade there has been an increased interest by North American adolescent athletes in highly competitive sports such as gymnastics, weightlifting, and figure skating, as well as traditional team sports such as hockey and football. This has resulted in increased training and competition time. Participation to an extreme (hours of practice daily with frequent stressful competition) may be required of the adolescent athlete to excel at a national level. Any of these training exercises, as well as the actual sport, involves frequent flexion and extension of the lumbar spine. The L5 pars interarticularis experiences considerable stress over a small area. The cross-sectional area of the pars at L5 measures 0.75 cm^2, for a total cross-sectional area of 1.5 cm^2 for each neural arch. It has been demonstrated by Hutton and coworkers that in vitro cyclical stress loading will produce fractures of the pars after as few as 1,536 cycles at a force of 570 + 190 Newtons in a vertebral column taken from a 14-year-old child. The tensile and sheer forces across the pars interarticularis in normal flexion and extension have been calculated to be on the order of 400–630 N. Thus it is quite conceivable that with numerous flexion-extension movements such as in training of a gymnast, this area of the vertebrae is indeed exposed to the dangers of fatigue fracturing.

34. How can this injury be prevented in high-level adolescent athletes?

Since abnormal stress such as vigorous training involving multiple flexion-extension of the lumbar spine does increase the incidence of micro-fractures, coaches should be taught to avoid extensive exercising involving these training methods. Persistent back pain in athletes involved in high-level competitive sports such as gymnastics should never be dismissed, since identification of the fatigue fracture at an early stage greatly facilitates its healing using a lumbosacral orthosis. It should be emphasized that oblique radiographs may not show the lesion and a bone scan is often necessary to demonstrate the increased uptake in the region of the stress fracture in the pars interarticularis.

35. The application and maintenance of a halo for a small child has a complication rate as high as 40 percent. How can this high incidence be minimized in young children?

Because skull thickness varies considerably up to 6 years of age, the use of CT bone windows may be very helpful in choosing the best pin sites. This is of greater importance when there are congenital skull abnormalities or generalized bone disease which may alter cortical thickness. The use of multiple insertions using 6 or 8 pins rather than the usual 4 will give improved fixation. This reduces the need for any one pin to be inserted deeply, and thus the chances of either penetration or loosening are reduced.

36. Is it possible to allay anxiety and fears in children prior to major orthopaedic procedures?

Where there is to be a loss of a body segment of tissue, such as an amputation, or the application of casts, traction or fixation devices, it has been shown in children under 6 or 7 years of age that puppetry and doll play can be used to prepare children for this type of surgery and minimize guilt feelings and hostility. Children between 1 and 3 years of age establish a certain representation of their bodies separate from the rest of the world. We must help these children heal the body as well as the psychic damage created by amputations of extremities. The portion of the body to be operated on is explained together with any defect that will be left, the casting, and in some cases of amputation, the artificial leg. Acceptance in the home and school can also be dealt with. Children, although physically recovering well, may be left emotionally distressed, perhaps even furious, because they feel their bodies were wantonly invaded and injured. Doll play and puppetry by nursing staff and child life specialists can provide an opportunity to work out these feelings for the child and prevent ongoing emotional distress for both the child and the family.

37. How is it possible to reduce and prevent the incidence of recurrent fractures of the lower extremities in children with severe osteogenesis imperfecta or in children with osteoporosis secondary to paraplegia?

Severe osteogenesis imperfecta and disuse osteoporosis may result in frequent fracturing of lower extremity bones when the child assumes upright weight-bearing. To prevent such breaking and to provide simple comfortable standing, specialized orthosis, such as "vacuum pants" can be used. This can be augmented by standing devices, such as the standing frame and parapodium in young children to allow the child to safely bear weight. Bone densitomitry studies of the tibia have revealed an increase in both mineral content and bone density above that expected for growth alone in patients with osteogenesis imperfecta who can safely bear weight with these devices. In older children this can be facilitated by intramedullary rodding of the femur and tibia in order to provide more intrinsic support and again facilitate weight-bearing and the stimulation of new bone formation through Wolfs' law.

38. In the assessment of children with physeal injury, how can permanent growth plate arrest be minimized or avoided?

It is not always possible to prevent a growth plate arrest secondary to a physeal injury since the growth plate may have been damaged at the moment of impact, the so-called type 5 injury of Salter and Harris, which may accompany more innocuous looking type 1 or type 2 injuries. However, by ensuring a good anatomic reduction, especially of the type 3 and 4 injuries, growth plate arrests secondary to bony bars created by displacement of the growth plate can certainly be minimized. Approximately 15% of injuries to the long bones involve the epiphyseal plate in childhood. Injuries involving the growth plate should be dealt with early, since they tend to heal more rapidly, and trying to obtain a reduction a week after the injury may result in damage to the growth plate during the reduction itself. The displaced type 3 epiphyseal injury, which is intra-articular and extends from the joint surface to the weak zone of the epiphyseal plate then along the plate periphery, requires an accurate reduction often involving an open reduction with internal fixation with smooth K wires. Similarly a type 4 epiphyseal injury, which is intra-articular extending from the joint surface through the epiphysis across the full thickness of the epiphyseal plate and through a portion of the metaphyses, also is often displaced and requires an open reduction and internal fixation.

39. What is the role of the physician in the prevention of child abuse?
Often the first indication of abuse is the presentation of a child in the Emergency Department with an extremity fracture and a history that does not fit the fracture. The so-called corner fracture with periosteal elevation is pathognomonic of child abuse in children under 2 years of age until proven otherwise. A high degree of suspicion must be maintained in any child under 3 years of age who has a fracture. It is essential that the physician act as an advocate for the child. If there are any other signs of neglect, such as skin burns, inappropriate history of injury, or evidence of other healing fractures, such children should be admitted for their own protection and the appropriate children's aid or child abuse team informed so that the home situation can be assessed thoroughly.

40. How can the increasing epidemic of gunshot trauma in children be minimized and prevented?
This requires input not only from the pediatric care teams, but also from public health officials, social workers, and child protection teams. All children with these injuries should be admitted to a hospital for appropriate social service and child protection team intervention. The majority of such injuries are due to children obtaining handguns in the home. Education of the whole family is required, including children, whenever there is a gun in the home. Areas of the country characterized by high rates of firearm ownership have the highest rate of unintentional firearm injury to children. Some type of firearm control is needed to minimize gunshot injuries in children which is directly related to a lack of gun control legislation.

41. What is the most common cause of serious injury and amputations in children in countries following an armed conflict?
In countries that have experienced recent wars such as Cambodia, Afghanistan, Vietnam, Mozambique, and Bosnia, death and limb loss from landmines and unexploded ordnance are a major public health problem. A significant proportion of landmine injuries involve children since they are usually responsible for gathering wood, tending cattle and sheep or playing in areas uncleared of mines. It is estimated that there are over 110 million buried landmines in some 60 countries that will continue to maim or kill 26,000 people a year. Most of the survivors will have an amputation of one or more extremities. As physicians we should support the United Nations General Assembly resolution calling for a permanent world-wide moratorium on the exports of any land mines and assist in efforts to de-mine countries affected.

BIBLIOGRAPHY

1. Cushman R: Injury prevention: A time has come. Can Med Assoc J. 21:152, 1995.
2. Rowe BH, Rowe AM, Bota GW: Bicyclists and environmental factors associated with bicycle related trauma in Ontario. Can Med Assoc J. 45–51:152, 1995.
3. Baker SP, O'Neill B, Ginsburg MJ, Li G: The Injury Fact Book, 2nd Ed. New York, Oxford University Press, 1992.
4. Friede AM, Azzara CV, Gallager SS, et al: The epidemiology of injuries to bicycle riders. Pediatr Clin North Am. 32:141–151, 1985.
5. Letts M, Kaylor D, Gouw G: A biomechanical analysis of halo fixation in children. J Bone Joint Surg 708:277–279, 1988.
6. Letts M, Monson R, Weber K: The prevention of recurrent fractures of the lower extremities in several osteogenesis imperfecta using vacuum pants. J Pediatr Orthop 8:454–458, 1988.
7. Letts M, Smallman T, Afanasiev R, Gouw G: Fractures of the pars interarticularis in adolescent athletes: A clinical-biomechanical analysis. J Pediatr Orthop 6:40–46, 1986.

8. Letts M, Stevens L, Coleman J, Kettner R: Puppetry and doll play—an adjunct of pediatric orthopaedics. J Pediatr Orthop. 3:605–609, 1983.
9. Letts RM, Gammon W: Auger injuries in children. Can Med Assoc J 118:519–522, 1978.
10. Spence LJ, Dykes EH, Bohn DJ, et al: Fatal bicycle accidents in children: A plea for prevention. J Pediatr Surg. 28:214–216, 1993.
11. Stucky W, and Loder RT: Extremity gunshot wounds in children. J Pediatr Orthop. 11:64, 1991.
12. Stover E, Keller AS, Cobey J, Sopheap S: The medical and social consequences of landmines in Cambodia. JAMA 272:57, 1994.
13. Trautwein LC, Smith DG, Rivara FP: Pediatric amputation injuries: Etiology, cost, and outcome. J Trauma. 41:831–838, 1996.

24. EVALUATION OF THE INJURED CHILD

Marc F. Swiontkowski, M.D.

1. What are the anatomic features of the growing child that must be considered in evaluation?
Features unique to the growing child include the presence of preosseous cartilage, thicker and stronger periosteum, the presence of multiple physes, and, depending on the unique features of growth and age, a smaller size.

2. How is the injury produced by falls affected by the age of the child?
Growing children have body proportions that are unique. The younger the child, the greater the head size relative to the torso. In this situation, the head and neck are more likely to be injured during a fall.

3. What are the key features in the history of the mechanism of injury that should be obtained from the parents or emergency rescue personnel?
The size of the child and the orientation of the force are the key elements. Depending on the size and position of the child, different injuries may be produced. The treating physician should

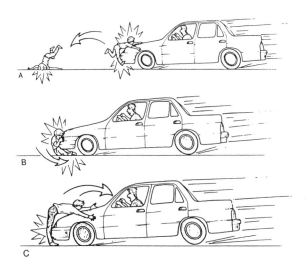

Injury patterns are different depending on the size of the child and his or her position to the injuring force. A, Ipsilateral femur fracture and chest injury followed by head injury in a child 6–10 years old (Waddell's triad). B, A smaller child receiving a direct blow to the head and chest followed by a crush injury of the pelvis and lower extremity. C, Taller adolescent with trauma to the proximal tibia and knee region.

note whether the child was on a bicycle, walking, or running and whether the child was wearing a helmet at the time he or she was struck. Other important features would be an estimation of the height of the fall and the type of surface that the child struck.

4. Which key elements of the history must be noted to avoid missing a case of child abuse?
A history of previous trauma is important. Similarly, the mechanism of injury should make sense when considered in relation to the child's injury. A careful social history should also be obtained, focusing on the presence of new individuals in the house, history of substance abuse among the caretakers, and other socioeconomic stresses.

5. How common is serious life-threatening trauma in children?
Trauma is the leading cause of death in children 14 years of age and younger, accounting for 50% of all deaths. Fifteen thousand children in this age group die from accidental injuries each year in the United States, and an additional 19 million are injured seriously enough to seek medical care or to restrict their activities. Approximately 13% of the children seen in the busy emergency department of an urban teaching hospital had serious injuries.

6. What are common mechanisms of injury in children?
The most common mechanism of serious injury in a child is by being struck by a car while a pedestrian or on a bicycle. This mechanism accounts for approximately 80% of significant injury in children. The next most common mechanism is being an unrestrained passenger in a motor vehicle accident. Finally, falls, collisions with trains or other heavy equipment, injuries from lawnmowers, and injuries sustained as passengers on motorcycles make up the remaining most common mechanisms.

7. Is there justification for pediatric trauma centers?
The improved outcome for children injured by trauma who are treated at pediatric trauma centers is well documented in the literature. The American College of Surgeons has set standards for the level of trauma care that an institution should provide to be categorized as a pediatric trauma center. These guidelines are used in verification visits conducted for statewide trauma systems. Guidelines detailing which children should be transported to these centers have been published.

*Guidelines for Referral to Pediatric Trauma Center
from the American College of Surgeons Committee on Trauma*

More than one body system injury
Injuries that require pediatric ICU care
Shock that requires more than one blood transfusion
Fractures with neurovascular injuries
Fractures of the axial skeleton
Two or more major long bone fractures
Potential replantation of an amputated extremity
Suspected or actual spinal cord injury
Head injuries with any of the following:
    Orbital or facial bone fractures
    Altered state of consciousness
    Cerebrospinal fluid leaks
    Changing neurologic status
    Open head injuries
    Depressed skull fractures
    Requirements of intracranial pressure monitoring
Ventilatory support required

8. What are the key aspects of the physical exam?
The physical exam should be directed by the history obtained from the caregiver or emergency personnel. If the injury is of high degree, the basic ABC evaluation (airway, breathing, circulation)

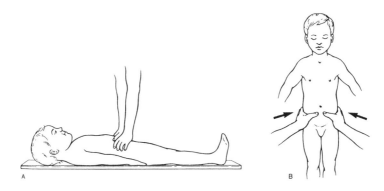

The basic examination for pelvic stability. A, Anterior/posterior instability. B, Rotational (external) stability.

should be conducted. Once the child is determined to have an adequate airway, functional breathing exchange, palpable pulse, and adequate blood pressure, the secondary survey should begin. This should include a careful abdominal examination to detect injuries to the liver, spleen, pancreas, or kidney. Surface bruising from externally directed trauma or a seatbelt should be evaluated. Sites of potential external bleeding are assessed. Extremity swelling, deformity, or crepitus is noted. These basic observations should be followed by an evaluation of pelvic stability.

9. What details are important in the evaluation of the upper extremity?
In addition to the examination for swelling, discoloration, open wounds, deformity, and crepitus, careful observation of motor function in the fingers of the younger child is appropriate. The older child should be asked to flex and extend the individual wrist, interphalangeal, metacarpophalangeal, and elbow joints. This should be followed by a sensory examination of light touch and two-point discrimination in the older, more cooperative child.

10. What details are important in the evaluation of the lower extremity?
In addition to the screening examination for swelling, contusion, open wounds, deformity, and crepitus, the specifics of the examination should include palpation of the thigh and lower leg compartments. Careful evaluation of the child's expression and demeanor on passive stretching of the toe dorsiflexors and plantar flexors should be noted to rule out compartment syndrome. Motor strength should be assessed in the cooperative child; in the younger child, an assessment of the ability to move the ankle, foot, and knee should be performed. The sensory examination for light touch and sharp touch should be completed in the older, cooperative child.

11. What are the key components of the spinal exam?
The child who has a history of significant trauma and presents on a backboard should be carefully logrolled at the end of the secondary survey. The back should be evaluated for a palpable increase in the interspinous space, the location of flank contusions, the existence of a kyphotic or an excess lordotic deformity, and the presence of wounds. The extremity neurologic examination for sensory changes in nerve root distributions, motor strength, and reflexes at the knee, ankle, triceps, and brachioradialis then follows. A digital rectal examination for tone should be performed in the most seriously injured children.

12. How should unsplinted fractures be managed?
Immediately after completion of the initial ABC's and secondary survey, limbs with deformity and crepitus should be aligned and appropriately splinted. Most emergency rooms have simple cardboard or air splints available for use until appropriate radiographic examination can be completed and early treatment undertaken. Ultimately, these will be switched to well-padded plaster splints in most instances.

13. Should the parents be present for the evaluation?

No one correct answer is apparent. A cooperative calm parent can often be helpful in managing the injured awake child. For the most seriously injured children, parents are generally best served by being escorting from the room, particularly when invasive procedures are necessary. Parents are extremely helpful in explaining the history, particularly of the injury and of past medical events, current medications, allergies, and past surgical procedures.

14. Are orthopaedic surgeons always required for evaluation of injured children?

The definitive diagnosis of a growth plate injury, dislocated joint, spinal fracture, open fracture, or fracture of the pelvis or femur requires evaluation by an orthopaedic surgeon or transfer to a pediatric trauma center. Simple fractures of the forearm or minimally displaced or nondisplaced fractures of the lower extremity (i.e., tibia) may be managed by the well-trained pediatrician, family physician, or emergency room specialist.

15. Are there any scoring systems that are useful in the evaluation of injured children?

The Modified Injury Severity Score, Glasgow Coma Scale, and Pediatric Trauma Score are all useful for individual patient management and for trauma systems research.

16. What are the prerequisites for sedation prior to conclusion of the evaluation?

One of the prerequisites before sedation of the injured child to manage fracture or dislocation reduction and splinting is a completed evaluation, including the primary survey (ABCs), secondary survey, and directed evaluation of extremity injuries.

17. Should ketamine be used?

Although ketamine has been extensively used for sedation in emergency patients, careful monitoring is required. Ketamine is generally best avoided in emergency patients without a protected airway. The patients may become deeply sedated and therefore must be carefully monitored. This is not considered the optimum method for sedation of the injured child.

18. Is nitrous oxide an appropriate sedative agent for injured children?

Children who are too young to cooperate with self-administration of nitrous oxide are generally inappropriate candidates for this form of sedation. Generally speaking, an equilibration period of 3 minutes should be allowed prior to instituting a painful procedure. Nitrous oxide administration may need to be supplemented with use of a local fracture block for improved success.

19. What are the risks of the use of the pediatric cocktail (DPT)?

The mixture of meperidine (Demerol), promethazine (Phenergan), and chlorpromazine (Thorazine) still remains widely popular for the sedation of children. The sedation can be prolonged and profound, however. Additionally, hypotension is possible along with severe respiratory depression. Most authors feel that this combination of medications should NEVER be used.

20. What are the signs and symptoms of local anesthetic toxicity?

Maximum Recommended Doses of Commonly Used Local Anesthetics in Children

	INJECTION DOSE (MG/KG)	
AGENT	PLAIN	WITH EPINEPHRINE*
Lidocaine† (Xylocaine)	5	7
Bupivacaine‡ (Marcaine, Sensorcaine)	2.5	3
Mepivacaine (Carbocaine)	4	7
Prilocaine§	5.5	8.5

*The addition of epinephrine (vascoconstrictor) reduces the rate of local anesthetic absorption into the bloodstream, permitting use of a higher dose.
†For IV regional anesthesia (Bier blocks), the maximum lidocaine dose is 3 mg/kg. Preservative-free lidocaine without epinephrine should be used for either Bier blocks or hematoma blocks.
‡Due to its cardiotoxicity, bupivacaine should never be used for IV regional anesthesia or for hematoma blocks.
§Of the amide local anesthetics, prilocaine is the least likely to produce CNS and cardiovascular toxicity. However, a by-product of prilocaine metabolism may lead to severe methemoglobinemia in young children. Prilocaine is, therefore, contraindicated in children < 6 mo old.

Although seizures and cardiac arrest may be the initial manifestations of systemic toxicity in patients who rapidly obtain a high serum level of medication, other symptoms generally predominate. These include numbness of the lips and tongue, lightheadedness, visual and auditory disturbances, shivering, muscle twitching, tremors, and unconsciousness. Seizures, coma, respiratory arrest, and cardiovascular depression and collapse can follow.

21. What is the normal blood pressure in an injured child?

Normal Values for Blood Pressure by Age

AGE	BLOOD PRESSURE (MM HG)	
	SYSTOLIC	DIASTOLIC
Full-term infant	60 (45)*	35
3–10 d	70–75 (50)	40
6 mo	95 (55)	45
4 yr	98	57
6 yr	110	60
8 yr	112	60
12 yr	115	65
16 yr	120	65

*The numbers in parentheses refer to mean arterial blood pressure.
(Steward, D.J.: Manual of Pediatric Anesthesia. New York, Churchill-Livingstone, 1990, p. 24, and Rasch, D.K., and Webster, D.E.: Clinical Manual of Pediatric Anesthesia. New York, McGraw-Hill, 1994, p. 17)

Calculation of Normal Blood Pressure by Age

80 + (2 × age in years) = normal systolic BP for age
70 + (2 × age in years) = lower limit of normal systolic BP for age

(Rasch, D.K., and Webster, D.E.: Clinical Manual of Pediatric Anesthesia. New York, McGraw-Hill, 1994, p. 197)

22. What are the normal values for pulse in an injured child?

Normal values for heart rate by age are provided in this Table. In an agitated child, heart rate may increase 20–30 points above the normal range.

Normal Values for Heart Rate by Age

AGE	RANGE (BEATS/MIN)
Newborn	110–150
1–11 months	80–150
2 years	85–125
4	75–115
6	65–110
8	60–110

(Rasch, D.K., and Webster, D.E.: Clinical Manual of Pediatric Anesthesia. New York, McGraw-Hill, 1994, p. 16)

23. What is the best environment for assessment of an injured child?

For all but the most seriously injured unconscious children, the evaluation should take place in the most comfortable environment. The child should be supine on a comfortable stretcher or bed. The area should be as quiet as possible. The parents should be present at least for the initial part of the evaluation. Appropriate wall coverings for children are often comforting, as are stuffed animals, a warm and caring nursing staff, and a comfortable room temperature.

24. What about "style issues" in evaluating children?

The most important part of evaluating children is speaking directly to them and giving them age-appropriate information about what you are going to do next. If a procedure will incur some pain, you should give them a truthful and calm explanation of when, how, and why this will occur. The details of the screening examination of the extremities should be explained while it is being conducted. Gentleness and calmness are the critical aspects of this section of the evaluation.

BIBLIOGRAPHY

1. Mann DC, Rajmaira S: Distribution of physeal and nonphyseal fractures in 2,650 long-bone fractures in children aged 0–16 years. J Pediatr Orthop (10(6):713–716, 1990.
2. Mizuta T, Benson WM, Foster BK, Paterson DC, Morris LL: Statistical analysis of the incidence of physeal injuries. J Pediatr Orthop 7:518–523, 1987.
3. Ogden JA: Injury to the growth mechanisms of the immature skeleton. Skeletal Radiol 6:237–253, 1981.
4. Peterson CA, Peterson HA: Analysis of the incidence of injuries to the epiphyseal growth plate. J Trauma 12(4):275–281, 1972.

25. CHILD VERSUS ADULT TRAUMA: MANAGEMENT PRINCIPLES

R. Jay Cummings, M.D.

1. What challenges exist in the care of childhood trauma victims that generally do not exist in the care of adult trauma victims?

If the trauma was not witnessed by an adult, details about how the injury occurred may not be available or may not be complete because of the child's inability or unwillingness to provide them. Children frequently resist examination, making detection and localization of injuries difficult. Finally, the physicians caring for the child must develop a rapport not only with the child, but also with the parents.

2. Does trauma lead to death and disability more commonly in children or in adults?

In children. Moreover, trauma is five times more common a cause of death in children than the next most common cause.

3. Is the type of trauma seen in children the same as that seen in adults?

Penetrating injury is more common in adults than in children. Children are more likely to present with injuries caused by blunt trauma.

4. What is the most common cause of death in pediatric trauma victims?

Between 30–70% of trauma deaths in children are due to head injury. In the pediatric age group, the head is larger in proportion to the body than in adults. Furthermore, children's neck muscles are weaker, skulls are thinner, and scalps are more vascular than those of adults. Children, however, recover more often and more completely from head trauma than do their adult counterparts.

5. What is the second most common cause of death in pediatric trauma victims?

Hemorrhage due to intra-abdominal injury. Children are at increased risk because their liver and spleen are larger relative to their overall size than in adults and their ribs are more flexible than in adults.

6. Do clinical signs mirror hypovolemia in the same way in children as in adults?

No, in children hypotension is a late manifestation of hypovolemia. Tachycardia and poor skin perfusion are the early signs of hypovolemia in a child.

7. Are there differences in the ability of children and of adults to maintain body temperature?

Children have a higher body surface-to-mass ratio than adults. In addition, their skin is thinner, and they have smaller fat stores than adults. These factors make the child more prone to hypothermia than the adult. This hypothermia can prolong acidosis, increase coagulation time, and affect nervous system function.

8. Are there any special precautions that need to be taken in the transport of pediatric trauma patients?

In children, the cervical spine is especially susceptible to injury because of the child's large head size relative to body size and because of the relatively weak neck muscles. The use of adult trauma boards places the neck in flexion in children less than 6 years old. Since children are more prone to upper spine (C1, C2) injuries than adults, use of special trauma boards with accommodations for the child's relatively larger head size is advised.

9. In children, multiple trauma is more common than in adults. Does this increase the risk for pulmonary problems?

No. Fat embolism is uncommon in the pediatric age group, and deep vein thrombosis and pulmonary embolism are also uncommon.

10. What differences exist between the child's bone structure and an adult's? How do these differences affect the way children's bones fail?

Children's bones are less dense and more porous than adult bones. In addition, the child's bone has more vascular channels. Because of these differences, children's bone may deform without actually macroscopically fracturing (see Figure). Children's bones may also fracture incompletely. When this occurs in compression, a torus or buckle fracture is produced. When this occurs in distraction, a greenstick fracture is produced. Finally, the differences between the child's and the adult's bone make comminuted fractures less common in children than in adults.

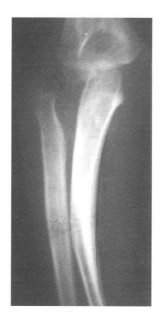

Anteroposterior x-ray of an elbow. Note the plastic deformation of the ulna leading to dislocation of the radial head.

11. Are there any other structural differences between children's and adults' bones that are clinically significant?
The periosteum in children is thicker and more vascular than it is in adults. Because of their more biologically active periosteum, children are usually able to reconstitute segmental bone defects that would persist in adults.

12. Does bone healing in children differ in any other ways from bone healing in adults?
Children's bones can remodel during and after fracture healing much more than adult bones can. Because of this, children can correct offsets and to some degree angulation, especially when it is in the plane of the adjacent joint's motion. Adults do not have this ability. Children's fractures also heal more rapidly than adults'. For example, a femur fracture that takes months to heal in an adult will heal in younger children in weeks. Finally, delayed union and nonunion are much less common in children than in adults.

13. Children's bones have growth centers that are separated from the rest of the bone by growth plates or physes. Does the presence of these structures affect the way the child's bone fails?
Because the physis is made of cartilage and because cartilage is weaker than bone, fractures in children frequently involve the physis. In addition, the ligaments that are attached to growth centers are also stronger than the physis. As a result of this, forces that in the adult would lead to ligament rupture usually cause failure of the physis instead in children.

14. Does the presence of growth centers and growth plates in children have any effect on the ability to diagnose injury in a child?
They make evaluation and diagnosis more difficult. Some fractures are not visible on x-ray examination because they pass completely through the physis without extension into the epiphysis or metaphysis. Other fractures extend through unossified growth centers and are also invisible on radiography. Therefore, when children have pain well localized to their growth centers, one must assume that a fracture exists until proven otherwise.

15. Can the way in which growth centers ossify and growth plates fuse affect the ability to diagnose injury in children?
Children's epiphyses may ossify from multiple locations or may be associated with accessory growth centers. These accessory growth centers and multiple ossific nuclei may be mistaken for fractures.

16. Do fractures that involve the physis affect bone growth?
If all goes well, they have no effect at all. When the fracture results in significant damage to the physis, growth may be impaired. If the damaged area is small and the remainder of the physis continues to grow, angular deformity will be produced. If the area of damage is large, growth may cease altogether, leading to shortening of the involved bone.

17. Do fractures in children that do not involve the growth centers and their physes have any effect on growth?
They may. In fractures involving the child's femur, so-called "overgrowth" may occur. This refers to an increase in the growth rate of the fractured femur that occurs during healing. Because of overgrowth, if the bone is reduced end-to-end, the fractured femur may grow to be longer than the normal femur. To avoid this, children 2–12 years old are often placed in a cast with the ends of the femur overlapped 1–1.5 cm.

18. Are there any problems that may arise in the care of children that are not usually present in the care of adults during fracture healing?
Adults can usually be relied upon to restrict activity, maintain immobilization devices, and use ambulatory assist devices during recovery. Children, on the other hand, frequently tend to resume their normal activity after pain subsides and, if left unattended, may go without splints they have been advised to use.

19. After fracture healing and discontinuance of immobilization, do children rehabilitate in much the same way as their adult counterparts?

Children tend to recover range of motion and strength more readily and more rapidly than adults. Extensive physical therapy is frequently unnecessary in children after bone healing.

BIBLIOGRAPHY

1. Barkin RM (ed): Pediatric Emergency Medicine Concepts and Clinical Practice. St. Louis, C.V. Mosby Co., 1992.
2. Fuhrman BP, Zimmerman JJ: Pediatric Critical Care. St. Louis, C.V. Mosby Co., 1992.
3. Levin DL, Morriss FC: Essentials of Pediatric Intensive Care. St. Louis, Quality Medical Publishing, Inc., 1990.
4. Ogden JA: Skeletal Injury in the Child. Philadelphia, W.B. Saunders Co., 1990.
5. Rockwell CA Jr, Wilkins KE, Beaty J (eds): Philadelphia, J.B. Lippincott Co., 1996.

26. PHYSEAL INJURIES

Hamlet A. Peterson, M.D.

1. Describe the epiphysis.

The epiphysis is the secondary center of ossification located at the end of the long bone in a child. The cartilage between the epiphysis and the diaphysis is termed the epiphyseal growth plate, or the physis. This is the area from which longitudinal growth of the bone occurs. Damage to the physis is referred to as an epiphyseal growth plate injury or, more commonly, a physeal injury.

2. What are the most common causes of physeal injury?

The vast majority of injuries to the physis are due to fracture. Other sources of damage to the physis include infection, radiation, tumors, disuse, heat (burns), cold (frostbite), electrical and laser burns, arterial damage, and iatrogenic causes (placement of pins, screws, staples, etc., across the physis).

3. What is the incidence of physeal fracture?

Injury to the growth plate occurs in 18–30% of all fractures in children.

4. What is the rate of physeal fracture?

The overall rate of physeal fracture is 365.8 fractures per 100,000 person years for males and 181.4 fracture per 100,000 person years for females. In a community with an average child/adult ratio, this is approximately 100 fractures in 100,000 total population per year.

5. Is the incidence of physeal fracture equal in boys and girls?

The boy-to-girl ratio of physeal fracture is 2:1, primarily because the physes of boys remain open longer.

6. At what ages are physeal fractures most common?

Boys have the highest rate of physeal fractures at age 14; girls at ages 11–12. Since girls stop growing sooner than boys due to growth plate closure, it is uncommon for a growth plate fracture to occur after age 15 in girls and after age 17 in boys.

7. Which bones are most often involved in a physeal fracture?

The phalanges of the fingers have by far the greatest incidence of physeal fracture, followed by the distal radius. This is not surprising, as each upper extremity has fourteen phalanges and only one distal radius.

8. What are the different types of physeal fractures?

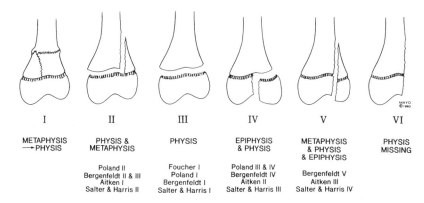

I	II	III	IV	V	VI
METAPHYSIS →PHYSIS	PHYSIS & METAPHYSIS	PHYSIS	EPIPHYSIS & PHYSIS	METAPHYSIS & PHYSIS & EPIPHYSIS	PHYSIS MISSING
	Poland II	Foucher I	Poland III & IV		
	Bergenfeldt II & III	Poland I	Bergenfeldt IV	Bergenfeldt V	
	Aitken I	Bergenfeldt I	Aitken II	Aitken III	
	Salter & Harris II	Salter & Harris I	Salter & Harris III	Salter & Harris IV	

The anatomic pattern of fracture of a growth plate can vary, with implications as to both the mechanism of injury and the outcome. Several classifications of physeal fractures have been developed, and there is great overlap of fracture type among the various classifications. The most recent and statistically verified classification contains six types (see Figure).

9. What is the anatomic basis of this classification?
There is a progressive increase in the amount of physeal cartilage damage from type I to type VI fracture.

10. What is the epidemiologic significance of this classification?
So far, type II has been found to be the most common physeal fracture, followed by types I, III, IV, V, and VI. Type I fracture was only recently described and often can be found only on oblique or three-quarter radiographs. It may prove to be the most common physeal fracture.

11. What is the prognostic value of this classification?
The rates of both initial surgery to treat the fracture and late surgery to treat complications gradually progress from type I fractures (surgery rarely necessary) to type VI fractures (surgery always necessary).

12. What is the etiology of physeal fractures?
Statistically, falls from all sorts of activities account for 20% of physeal fractures in children. This is followed by football and bicycle accidents. Physeal fractures are recorded in many childhood sports, both organized and unorganized. Automobiles, motorcycles and all-terrain vehicles account for only 5% of physeal fractures.

13. How are physeal fractures evaluated?
History and physical examination determine the appropriate body site for which to obtain radiographs. Good-quality radiographs in at least two planes, usually anterior–posterior and lateral, are required. If questions arise, additional planes, usually three-quarter views will help delineate the fracture. When questions persist, comparison views of the opposite uninjured extremity, as well as stress views, tomograms, arthrograms, ultrasound, CT scans, and MRI, can be helpful in defining the fracture.

14. How are these fractures treated?
In general, physeal fractures are treated by anatomic reduction and maintenance of reduction until they heal. Often this can be accomplished by closed reduction and immobilization.

15. What factors determine the prognosis?

The prognosis depends on these factors, in descending order of importance:

1. The severity of the injury, including displacement, comminution, and open versus closed injury
2. The age of the patient
3. The specific physis injured
4. The type of fracture

The treatment is dependent on these factors and in itself also has an important bearing on the prognosis.

16. What percentage of patients require surgery?

All physeal injuries involving an open wound require surgical debridement and irrigation. Adding these few to those injuries that require surgery to obtain adequate reduction and stabilization brings the total to 7% of all physeal fractures. The decision about whether to operate depends on the ability to obtain and maintain anatomical alignment of the growth plate to enhance the possibility of continuing normal growth.

17. Do fractures of the physis heal in the same manner as fractures elsewhere?

Because the fracture is through growing cartilage, physeal fractures heal much more rapidly than fractures involving only bone. Most of these fractures are stable in 3–4 weeks; earlier in younger patients and later in older patients.

18. What are the major complications of physeal growth plate fractures?

By far the most common and serious complication is damage to the growth plate resulting in premature complete or partial growth plate closure. Complete growth plate closure ensures that the injured bone will not grow as long as the contralateral uninjured bone. Partial growth plate closure tethers growth in the damaged area while allowing the remaining uninjured portion of the physis to grow, thus producing an angular deformity. Other complications include delayed union, nonunion, infection, and avascular necrosis, all of which are infrequent.

19. How early can growth plate closure be detected after surgery?

It is difficult to document a premature growth plate closure prior to 3 months post-injury, even in cases in which there is a high suspicion that it will occur. Often the growth plate closure only becomes manifest several months or even years after the traumatic incident.

20. How are growth rate closures treated?

There is no way to reestablish growth following complete growth plate closure. Its treatment requires arresting the physis of the contiguous bone (as in the case of the radius/ulna and tibia/fibula), as well as either surgical arrest of the contralateral physis, surgical lengthening of the injured shorter bone, or surgical shortening of the normal longer uninjured bone. In the case of partial arrest, these same modalities can be used. However, growth can sometimes be reestablished by surgically excising the bony bar and preventing bar reformation by insertion of an interposition material.

21. Which physeal bars respond most successfully to excision?

Bar excision in an attempt to reestablish growth is most successful when the bar comprises less than 50% of the total area of the physis in children who have significant growth remaining (girls aged 12 years and under, and boys aged 14 years and under).

BIBLIOGRAPHY

1. Mann DC, Rajmaira S: Distribution of physeal and nonphyseal fractures in 2,650 long-bone fractures in children aged 0–16 years. J Pediatr Orthop (10(6):713–716, 1990.

2. Mizuta T, Benson WM, Foster BK, Paterson DC, Morris LL: Statistical analysis of the incidence of physeal injuries. J Pediatr Orthop 7:518–523, 1987.
3. Ogden JA: Injury to the growth mechanisms of the immature skeleton. Skeletal Radiol 6:237–253, 1981.
4. Peterson CA, Peterson HA: Analysis of the incidence of injuries to the epiphyseal growth plate. J Trauma
   12(4):275–281, 1972.
5. Peterson HA: Partial growth plate arrest and its treatment. J Pediatr Orthop 4:246–258, 1984.
6. Peterson HA, Madhok R, Benson JT, Ilstrup DM, Melton LJ: Physeal fractures: Part 1. Epidemiology in
   Olmsted County, Minnesota, 1979–1988. J Pediatr Orthop 14:423–430, 1994.
7. Peterson HA: Physeal fractures: Part 3. Classification. J Pediatr Orthop 14:439–448, 1994.
8. Peterson HA: Physeal and apophyseal injuries. In Rockwood CA Jr, Wilkins KE, Beatty JH (eds): Fractures in Children, 4th ed. Philadelphia, J.B. Lippincott, 1996, pp 103–165.
9. Peterson HA: Physeal fractures: Part 2. Two previously unclassified types. J Pediatr Orthop 14:431–438,
   1994.

27. PITFALLS IN TRAUMA

Randall T. Loder, M.D.

1. In spite of appropriate analgesic doses, a child with a fracture of the supracondylar humerus is still experiencing severe pain. Why?

A compartment syndrome with impending Volkmann's ischemic contracture is highly likely. It may be associated with a traumatic lesion in the brachial artery at the level of the fracture site. Immediate orthopaedic consultation is needed to (1) reduce and stabilize the fracture, (2) assess the function of and measure the compartment pressures in the volar compartment, and (3) assess the vascular supply and viability of the hand. Following these actions, further intervention such as release of the affected compartment(s) and/or brachial arterial exploration/repair may be urgently needed.

2. How should a minimally displaced midshaft ulnar fracture be managed?

The pitfall here is the elbow joint. Innocuous-looking ulnar fractures can be associated with radial head dislocations at the elbow (Monteggia lesion). These dislocations require, at a minimum, closed reduction and application of a long-arm cast in a position as dictated by the type of radial head dislocation. Older children and adolescents often require open reduction and internal fixation. For this reason, all ulnar fractures necessitate adequate radiographs of both the elbow and wrist.

3. A child who sustains a nondisplaced lateral condylar fracture of the humerus is placed in a long-arm cast. What follow-up care is required?

Fractures of the lateral condyle must be watched closely. They may displace in the first 2 weeks after injury, and repeat radiographs are needed approximately every 5 days. These radiographs should be obtained out of the cast as a subtle displacement or shift is easily obscured by overlying shadows from the cast material. Another pitfall with lateral condylar fractures is the risk of nonunion, even when nondisplaced. They must be followed for several months to ensure union and then for a few years at infrequent intervals to ensure that angular or growth deformities do not occur.

4. What are the physical findings in a compartment syndrome?

Classically the five P's have been described: **p**ain, **p**aresthesias, **p**allor, **p**ulselessness, and **p**aralysis. The most important finding is severe pain or restlessness. Once pallor, pulselessness, and paralysis are present, permanent damage may have already resulted. All efforts should be made to not reach this point. A low threshold should be maintained at all times, as children often will not communicate the early sign of paresthesias. If the physician has any concern, appropriate compartment pressure measurements should be taken, even if a general anesthesia is necessary. A frightened child with a fresh fracture often cannot cooperate sufficiently during the physical examination to ensure that the examiner obtains an accurate clinical assessment of the compartment's condition.

5. A 7-month-old child presents to the emergency room with a history of falling off a couch, and radiographs are interpreted as indicating a dislocation of the elbow. What treatment is required?

The pitfall here is the diagnosis. Elbow dislocations in young children are essentially nonexistent. Instead, this child has sustained a displaced distal humeral physeal fracture. The distal humeral epiphysis is still cartilaginous and not yet ossified; therefore, it cannot be seen radiographically. Thus, its displacement mimics the appearance of an elbow dislocation. To help differentiate the two, the physician should remember that a fracture of the distal humeral epiphysis is usually displaced posteromedially, whereas an elbow dislocation is usually displaced posterolaterally. My preferred method of treatment is closed reduction and percutaneous pinning in the operating room. **Caution:** This fracture has a high association with child abuse, and the circumstances of the accident should be explored.

6. A 3-year-old child is injured in a motor vehicle crash. Lateral radiographs of the cervical spine obtained in the emergency room are interpreted as demonstrating a ligamentous injury at the C2–3 level. Is this an expected finding?

No. True ligamentous instability at the C2–3 level in young children is extremely rare, whereas pseudosubluxation is quite common. Pseudosubluxation can be differentiated from pathologic (true) instability by using the posterior line of Swischuk (see figure).

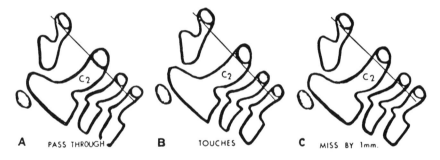

| A | PASS THROUGH | B | TOUCHES | C | MISS BY 1mm. |

The posterior cervical line of Swischuk is drawn from the anterior cortex of the posterior arch of C1 to the anterior cortex of the posterior arch of C3. In pseudosubluxation (or physiologic displacement) of C2 on C3, the posterior cervical line may pass through the cortex of the posterior arch of C2, touch the anterior aspect of the cortex of the posterior arch of C2, or come within 1 mm of the anterior cortex of the posterior arch of C2. In pathologic subluxation of C2 on C3, the posterior cervical line misses the posterior arch of C2 by 2 mm or more. (From Swischuk LE: Anterior displacement of C2 in children: Physiologic or pathologic? A helpful differentiating line. Radiology 122:759–763, 1977, with permission.)

7. An 8-year-old boy sustains a "minimally displaced" fracture of the medial malleolus. What type of treatment should he receive?

The pitfalls here are both the amount of displacement and the possibility of nonunion. Fractures of the medial malleolus are rare in children, yet they must be aggressively treated. As perfect a reduction as possible should be achieved, and the threshold for performing an open reduction and internal fixation should be very low. The risk of physeal growth arrest is much higher if an anatomic reduction is not obtained. If the fracture is truly nondisplaced, it needs to be monitored carefully to ensure that it does not displace in the first few weeks after injury and also that it proceeds to union.

8. A 12-year-old girl presents with a displaced midshaft fracture of both bones of the forearm. After closed reduction and application of a short-arm cast, when should the child be rechecked?

Short-arm casts have no role in the immobilization of midshaft forearm fractures of both bones. Rather, a long-arm cast is mandatory. Because this girl, at age 12 years, is nearing skeletal maturity, only minimal angulation and displacement can be permitted. Frequent checks are needed after the reduction to ensure that the fracture position remains acceptable. I typically recheck these fractures on a weekly basis for the first 3 weeks after reduction. If any shifting has occurred, I perform either a repeat closed reduction with intramedullary stabilization or an open reduction–internal fixation.

9. A 6-year-old boy, restrained and seat-belted, is involved in a motor vehicle crash. He is admitted to the hospital for abdominal pain and also complains of some mild discomfort of the lumbar spine, even though the abdominal CT scan shows only a small hepatic hematoma. What is the cause of his back pain?
The classic injury in a restrained lap-belted passenger is Chance's fracture, which results from forward flexion over the seatbelt, distracting the posterior vertebral elements. In adults, this type of trauma usually results in a bony fracture. In children, however, it usually results in a ligamentous injury, disrupting the interspinous ligaments, facet capsules, posterior longitudinal ligaments, and intervertebral disc. Ecchymosis in the lap belt distribution is frequently seen on physical examination, and the presence of lumbar ligamentous disruption is strongly associated with abdominal visceral injury. CT scans are usually not diagnostic, since the axial CT cuts are in the same plane as the horizontal fracture/dislocation. Lateral radiographs of the spine are needed to make the diagnosis. For this reason, every child who has sustained abdominal trauma from a lap belt injury should have radiographs of the thoracolumbar spine.

10. A 14-year-old boy injures his left knee in a football game. Swelling rapidly ensues. Physical examination reveals tenderness of the medial femoral condyle and instability to valgus stress, yet the radiographs are negative. Why?
In children with open epiphyseal plates, athletic injuries to the knee frequently result in physeal fracture rather than ligamentous injury. This boy likely has sustained a Salter I fracture of the distal femoral physis which is nondisplaced, thus giving a "negative" radiographic appearance. Stress radiographs under controlled circumstances should be performed to determine the anatomic location of the instability and subsequent appropriate treatment.

11. While playing basketball, a 10-year-old boy jumps up for a rebound, and his knee suddenly gives way. Physical examination reveals a markedly swollen knee. Radiographs demonstrate a "chip" fracture at the distal pole of the patella. What is the appropriate treatment for this fracture?
This child has sustained a sleeve fracture of the patella. This fracture is an avulsion of a large portion of the patellar articular cartilage along with a small bony fragment. This avulsion can result in an extensor lag with considerable long-term morbidity. If the "chip" is truly nondisplaced, then cast immobilization is all that is required. If there is an extensor lag or if the avulsed fragment remains separated from the remainder of the patella, then surgical repair is required.

12. A 6-year-old boy steps on a nail while wearing tennis shoes and sustains a puncture wound to the plantar aspect of the foot. Ten days later he presents to the emergency room with a complaint of increasing pain and warmth over the plantar aspect of the metatarsal heads during the last 48 hours. There is slight drainage from the wound. How should this condition be managed?
These signs and symptoms most likely indicate infection due to *Pseudomonas*—both a septic arthritis of the metatarsophalangeal joint and osteomyelitis of the metatarsal. The rubber soles of tennis shoes harbor *Pseudomonas,* which is then introduced into the foot from the puncture wound. Appropriate therapy consists of surgical debridement and intravenous antibiotics appropriate for *Pseudomonas* until the surgical culture results are available.

13. An obese 14-year-old boy sustains a fall during a football game. Over the next few weeks he complains of increasing knee pain and a limp. Knee radiographs are normal. What should the next step be in the work-up?

Obese adolescent children are prone to develop a slipped capital femoral epiphysis, with the initial symptoms often related to a mild episode of trauma. Hip pain is often referred to the knee, and thus radiographs of the hips should be obtained. Both AP and lateral pelvis radiographs are needed, since early on the slip is seen only on the lateral radiograph. Up to 35% of these injuries are bilateral, with the opposite hip being asymptomatic or "silent."

14. While playing football, a 15-year-old boy sustains a patellar dislocation with spontaneous reduction. He has a swollen knee and radiographs demonstrate an "osseous chip fracture" near the patella. What does this mean?

During patellar dislocation, the patella rapidly impacts on the lateral femoral condyle. This may result in an osteochondral fracture of the patella. An arthroscopic examination of the knee is usually necessary to determine the extent of the injury to the patellar articular surface and the appropriate treatment (e.g., removal of the fragment, if small, or fixation of a large fragment).

15. A 10-year-old boy falls and injures his ring finger while playing soccer. Radiographs demonstrate a fracture of the distal metaphyseal portion of the middle phalanx with "slight angulation and translation." How long should the finger be splinted?

A simple finger splint is not adequate for this fracture! The pitfall here is the fracture location. It is far removed from the epiphyseal plate; thus, the potential for remodeling of any malunion is minimal, especially at 10 years of age. These fractures need an anatomic reduction; this may require either a closed reduction or open reduction. Often internal fixation after the reduction is needed to ensure that the fracture does not shift while healing.

BIBLIOGRAPHY

1. Letts RM (ed): Management of Pediatric Fractures. New York, Churchill Livingstone, 1994.
2. Morrissy RT, Weinstein SL (eds): Lovell and Winter's Pediatric Orthopaedics, 4th ed. Philadelphia, Lippincott-Raven, 1996.
3. Ogden JA: Skeletal Injury in the Child, 2nd ed. Philadelphia, W.B. Saunders, 1990.
4. Rockwood CA Jr, Wilkins KE, Beaty JH (eds): Fractures in Children, 4th ed. Philadelphia, Lippincott-Raven, 1996.

28. CHILD ABUSE

William L. Oppenheim, M.D.

1. What is child abuse?

Child abuse is any form of maltreatment deleterious to a child's welfare by an adult responsible for nurturing and caring for that child. It involves much more than the simplistic "three fractures in different stages of healing," which at one time constituted the traditional orthopaedic definition. Today, the term encompasses emotional neglect, starvation, sexual abuse, as well as physical abuse. Specifically, the term *battered child syndrome* refers to cases of abuse in which a child presents with fractures and other overt physical injuries. *Shaken infant syndrome* describes brain injuries sustained by forceful shaking of the cranial contents without overt skull fracturing.

Because fractures occur rather late in the course of physical abuse, the physicians' role is to recognize nonaccidental trauma and the social milieu surrounding it, and to intervene early so that further injury or neglect is prevented. The Federal Child Abuse Prevention and Treatment Act of

1974 established a National Center on Child Abuse and Neglect, but specific legal mandates are formulated and carried out on a state-by-state basis.

2. How common is child abuse?

More than 1.5 million cases are reported across the United States each year. But many cases go unreported. Some health professionals are reluctant to report information gathered in an otherwise confidential manner, many do not want to become involved with the legal system, and some simply refuse to believe that otherwise normally appearing parents would purposely injure their children.

3. What happens to abused children eventually?

If unrecognized, a child returned to an abusive environment faces a 50% chance of further battering and perhaps as high as a 15% chance of death. Death is most often caused by intracranial injury, followed by ruptured abdominal viscus injuries. Undetected survivors may become the next generation of child abusers, [or grow up to pay their parents back with elder abuse.] When the diagnosis is recognized, and appropriate intervention deployed, the vast majority of children can remain in or eventually be reunited within their families. Only in extreme cases are the children remanded to foster care.

4. What is the physician's role in diagnosing child abuse?

It is usually not possible for a physician to come to a definitive conclusion regarding any one episode of trauma. However, it is not necessary to come to a definitive conclusion. Only a reasonable *suspicion* of abuse is necessary to trigger mandatory reporting of potential abuse or nonaccidential injury, according to most state laws.

Since abuse most often takes place in the private confines of a home, and since small nonvocal children are frequently involved, any legal action will of necessity involve circumstantial evidence. This requires involvement of many other professionals beyond the physician, so that actual proof by the physician is neither expected nor required. In fact, physicians should not be accusatory in their approach, or their ability to elicit useful information and thus protect the child will be quickly compromised.

Failure to report one's suspicions is usually punishable simply by fines, but children returned to an abusive environment frequently sustain additional injuries, and when these children are eventually sent to foster care, the new parents may sue the physician who missed or ignored the diagnosis. Settlements can be substantial and threaten continued insurance coverage.

All states grant legal immunity to reporting physicians. Society has deemed it more important to protect innocent children than to enforce patient–physician confidentiality in this instance.

5. What background circumstances might raise the suspicion of abuse?

Although abuse cuts across all socioeconomic levels, there are some associations worth looking for in the history. These include:

- Parents who themselves were abused as children (intergenerational abuse)
- Drug and alcohol abuse
- Social isolation of the family
- A history of family crises
- Prior intervention
- A history of an abused sibling
- Acute severe financial pressures

Most parents know exactly when their children are injured and under what circumstances. Vagueness as to how the injury took place is suspicious. The history must be consistent both with the developmental milestones and with the injury. A delay in seeking care demands an explanation. It is hard to imagine how an attentive parent could miss a fracture event, although there is a chance that a parent might not seek immediate care for a swollen limb based on financial considerations, or that a minor fracture might initially be misinterpreted as a "sprain." A lack of appropriate concern on the caretaker's behalf even when the diagnosis becomes clear should be noted in the record. Finally, small children look to their custodians for protection. A vacant, listless child who runs from a caretaker or who fails to make eye contact with him or her is quite unusual and should raise a red flag in the physician's mind.

6. What physical findings point toward abuse?

An old aphorism of child abuse holds that the injuries speak for the child who cannot. Most physically abused children are less than 5 years of age. (Sexual abuse is more common after the age of 6, and most frequent in the teenage group.) Repetitive trauma, frequent bruising beyond normal play expectations, the failure to thrive syndrome, or multiple fractures with no clear etiology all raise the issue of nonaccidental trauma or neglect.

Some aspects of abuse are obvious upon reflection. For example, fractures of long bones prior to the age of walking are sufficiently rare to raise concern. Even after the age of walking, rib fractures, vertebral body fractures, and skull fractures are rarely seen in healthy children without an obvious explanation. The finding of traumatic brain injury along with other unexplained manifestations of trauma (e.g., long bone fractures), in the absence of a significant historical traumatic event is strong evidence for abuse. Children who present with *two* black eyes, a torn frenulum (from a fisted uppercut), bite marks, cigarette burns, or bilateral long bone shaft fractures reportedly sustained during normal play activities are difficult to accept as cases of accidental injury. Natural injuries tend to be irregular in character.

Multiple injuries with *linear* edges are characteristic of whipping with belts, extension cords, broomsticks, and other slender objects. Similarly, circumferential marks about a limb indicate binding or restraining with ropes, chains, belts, or other cord-like objects. Examination of the genitalia can reveal evidence of sexual abuse or venereal disease.

7. Where do burns fit into the picture of abuse?

Soft tissue injury is much more common than fractures, and about 20% of such injuries in abused children are caused by burns. Burns caused by cigarettes are relatively easy to spot with their irregular concentric imprints and resultant scarring. Children who are forced to stand in a scalding hot bath for punishment demonstrate clearly delineated "stocking glove" burn patterns on their feet and legs. Flat iron or curling iron branding injuries yield similar linear-edged burns, as do injuries caused when children are forced to stand on or touch a hot radiator. In contrast, when a child pulls over a hot water kettle or bowl, the resulting injury is scattered and variable. Similarly, when young infants are dipped into scalding water, reflex flexing of the hips and knees results in popliteal sparing, a pattern quite different from that seen when children fall in and attempt to extricate themselves.

8. How should physical findings of abuse be documented?

Physicians should use special forms available to document suspected cases of abuse for later use in legal precedings. Photographs can be helpful, but only if they clearly depict the actual injuries. Some states prefer that evidence technicians from the local law enforcement organization obtain such photographs, rather than the physician or hospital.

9. What laboratory and diagnostic tests should be obtained?

A bone survey remains the standard diagnostic test. Bone scans may show occult fractures earlier and may highlight rib and spine fractures, which are otherwise easy to overlook. However, these scans should not, in my estimation be a routine part of the work-up. Ultrasound imaging and MRI likewise may also have their place in selected circumstances, but are not routinely performed. Intra-abdominal injury calls for its own evaluation, including testing for hematuria, melena, and amylase and liver enzymes. A chronically low hematocrit suggests malnourishment or excessive blood loss due to fracturing. PT/PTT results will be necessary in court as the defense will raise the issue of a bleeding diathesis with easy bruisability. Levels of calcium, phosphorus, alkaline phosphatase, BUN, and creatinine, along with a bone density scan may be helpful at times in ruling out metabolic or genetic diseases that may be confused with abuse. Cultures to rule out venereal disease can also be obtained, as warranted.

10. What confirmation should be sought on x-rays?

Okay, "three fractures in different stages of healing" works. But the goal should be to recognize the problem *before* there are multiple fractures. While any single long bone injury could be nonaccidental, bilaterality is suggestive of abuse. An important aspect of fracture evaluation is a closer look at the fracture itself. Corner metaphyseal fractures result from pulling on a limb with stretching of the periosteum/perichondrium over the growth plates. This yields a classic picture of abuse as far as the bones are concerned, with either a "bucket handle" appearance of the physis, or a "bone within a bone" appearance as the elevated periosteum lays down excessive new bone. (See Figures.) These findings, sometimes referred to as metaphyseal fragility, are still considered pathopneumonic for battering 40 years after their initial association with the syndrome. Unfortunately, such fractures are present in only one-quarter of child abuse cases. Excessive callous formation is often a sign of lack of fracture immobilization. When such x-ray findings are combined with the history or lack thereof, physical findings, and a careful social services evaluation, most abuse can be recognized at this point.

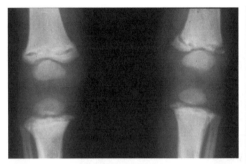

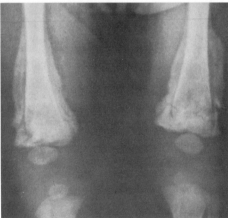

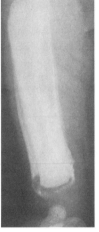

These x-rays illustrate the bilaterality and metaphyseal fragility characteristic of an abused child in the absence of underlying metabolic or genetic disease. Other findings include the "bone within a bone" appearance caused by excessive periosteal stripping, and the "bucket handle" appearance of a healing physis.

11. What should be considered in the differential diagnosis?

Metabolic or genetic diseases such as rickets, malnourishment, and hypervitaminosis A; chronic disease processes such as renal osteodystrophy or liver disease; and complications post-transplant steroid administration must all be considered. Osteogenesis imperfecta (OI) is a special consideration in cases of suspected abuse. Most parents of children with this syndrome, unless diagnosis is prompt, will have unfounded allegations lodged against them. This can be devastating for a family that is doing the correct thing and seeking care for a sick and frail child. Osteogenesis imperfecta can be recognized in 90% of cases based on the family history, and findings of a helmet shaped skull, blue sclera, prenatal fractures, thin fragile skin, joint hypermobility, excessive sweating, discolored breakable teeth, minimal soft tissue swelling associated with the fractures, and the gracile appearance of the bones on x-ray. Blood tests or skin biopsy with subsequent tissue culture and collagen analysis raise the diagnostic accuracy to 95% or better.

Other confounding issues include physiological periostitis, scurvy, copper deficiency, and Caffey's disease. The spiral distal tibial fracture (or toddler's fracture) is common in children after walking age and should not be misconstrued as abuse. Although some texts suggest a high probability of abuse based on the location and character of the fracture (e.g., a spiral humeral fracture), I have not found a single isolated long bone fracture, either transverse or spiral, to be suggestive of abuse unless accompanied by the ancillary factors mentioned in questions 7 and 8, earlier.

12. How can you confront the parents with your suspicions and still maintain a trusting relationship with the family?
Reporting is mandatory under the law. This should be explained to the family. At the UCLA Medical Center only half of the children referred to the Suspected Child Abuse and Neglect (SCAN) team are eventually confirmed as cases of abuse. The fact that half of these children need to be screened to protect the other half is a price most rational parents accept. Finally, if the physician is simply not comfortable enough to handle the situation, the patient can be referred for further evaluation to a larger facility where a SCAN team or its equivalent can be allowed to pursue the diagnosis. This removes the physician from direct confrontation with the parents, but does not relieve the physician of his or her reporting obligation under the law. Frequently, for the sake of a thorough evaluation, suspiciously injured children are admitted for their protection while investigations are carried out. If the parents do not voluntarily accept this, a legal "hold" can be readily obtained, but at that point the case is headed for a court hearing rather than simple decision making by the local social services or law enforcement organization.

13. The lawyers say you can never be sure the child does not have osteogenesis imperfecta, instead.
First of all, child abuse cases are rarely prosecuted, though often supervision is required of the family. When such cases are prosecuted, defending lawyers will often use this ploy, but by that time additional information is usually substantial. As noted, over 95% of osteogenesis imperfecta can be diagnosed definitively through collagen analysis in combination with the clinical findings, history, and x-ray results described in question 12. Although the magnitude of precipitating trauma is small, the fractures are noted immediately. This scenario, combined with additional physical evidence and the social services reports, will usually differentiate cases of OI from child abuse. In extreme cases of abuse, removal from the home for 6 months, often by placing the child in the care of a grandparent, results in complete cessation of fractures during this period, also clarifying the diagnosis. It has been said that carrots, gravy, and meat by themselves do not make stew, but when you put them all together, you have the requisite meal. Likewise in child abuse, no one finding is definitive, but putting it all together usually tells the story.

BIBLIOGRAPHY

1. Carty HM: Fractures caused by child abuse. J Bone Joint Surg 75B:849–857, 1993.
2. Dent JA, Paterson CR: Fractures in early childhood: Osteogenesis imperfecta or child abuse? J Pediatr Orthop 11:184–186, 1991.
3. Galleno H, Oppenheim WL: The battered child syndrome revisited. Clin Ortho Rel Res 150:8–15, January 1982.
4. Loder R, Bookout C: Fracture patterns in battered children. J Orthop Trauma 5:428–433, 1991.
5. Thomas SA, Rosenfeld NS, Leventhal JM, et al: Long bone fractures in young children: Distinguishing accidental injuries from child abuse. Pediatrics 88:471–476, 1991.

29. POLYTRAUMA

Walter W. Huurman, M.D.

1. Is childhood polytrauma a significant problem in North America?

Approximately 10% of hospital admissions due to trauma in this age group are due to multiple injury. For every fatality, four are permanently disabled; the U.S. Department of Health estimates the cost of these injuries to exceed $7.5 billion annually.

2. What are the major differences between the child and the adult when dealing with issues related to polytrauma?

The patterns of injury differ because the child is smaller, resulting in a greater application of force per unit area. The absence of significant amounts of subcutaneous fat with greater proximity of internal organs to the surface results in a higher incidence of multisystem injury. This vulnerability extends to the brain; 80% of severely injured children have head injuries. The thinner skull simply is less protective of its contents.

3. How does the child respond to the assault of multiple injuries?

A child has greater physiologic reserve than the adult, is most often free of complicating organ system disease, and possesses a central nervous system with greater ability to recover from severe damage. This can be a two-edged sword, however. The tremendous reserve capacity may mask very severe cardiovascular compromise right up to the point where the system suddenly collapses into irreversible shock. Many of the prodromes seen in the adult, such as falling blood pressure, are not present in the child until hypovolemia has led to a life-threatening state.

4. How does one initiate care of the polytraumatized child?

- **A**irway. The child's tongue and pharynx tend to be lax. The shorter length and narrower diameter of the trachea present a risk of obstruction due to foreign bodies, emesis, or direct tracheal injury.
- **B**reathing. Because of greater elasticity of the chest wall and underdevelopment of the associated musculature combined with an increase in metabolic demand, it is imperative to note the character of the chest wall movement, the respiratory rate, and the breath sounds. Pneumothorax, tension pneumothorax, hemothorax, or pulmonary contusion are diagnosable at this stage.
- **C**irculation. The child will maintain a normal blood pressure until 20–30% of blood volume is lost, developing a variable tachycardia as a response to hypovolemia. Normal blood volume is 80 ml/kg, or about 2.5 liters for a 72-pound child. Assessment of the circulatory system includes observation of the child's color, peripheral pulse (a palpable peripheral pulse indicates a systolic pressure of 80, a palpable central pulse, 50–60 mm), skin temperature, capillary refill, and blood pressure.
- **D**isability. The nervous system is not as well developed in the less mature individual, and assessment should be age based. Intracranial shear forces may result in contusion or subdural or epidural bleeding. Notation of pupillary response and extremity motion should be made.
- **E**xposure. Children have a larger surface/area volume ratio and infants shiver less; hence they may lose body temperature at a greater rate. Body surfaces should be evaluated for evidence of hypothermia. The necessity of undressing the patient for an adequate exam should not overlook the need to preserve body heat.

5. What are the first steps in managing an airway problem?

Immobilize the cervical spine to avoid further neurologic damage; clear the throat of foreign material and tongue obstruction; and pull the jaw forward to open the posterior pharynx.

6. What about treatment of breathing problems?

Cover open chest wounds. Initiate advanced airway management with assisted ventilation as necessary.

7. Circulation difficulties demand what initial approach?

After airway and breathing problems have been stabilized, hemorrhage can be controlled with direct pressure. Then obtain intravenous access and administer 20 ml/kg of balanced salt solution. If veins are not accessible in a small child, emergent intraosseous administration of fluids is acceptable.

8. How do you initially treat head or spinal injuries?

Immobilize the child on a spinal board. Remember that the child's head is proportionately larger than that of the adult. If the back of the head is lying on the same surface as the shoulders, the cervical spine is pushed into flexion. Allowing the head to drop back moderately avoids this. Mildly elevate the head and hyperventilate the child.

9. If exposure has been a problem, what are the appropriate steps to take?

Externally warm the patient, then transport the child to radiology, the operating suite, or the ICU with appropriate warmed blankets. If necessary, consider warming IV solutions.

10. Mentioning a primary survey implies the existence of a secondary review. What does this include?

The secondary survey is a systematic assessment of organ systems after an adequate airway, effective respiratory efforts, and the circulation have been insured.

11. What type of musculoskeletal physical examination should be performed on the polytraumatized patient?

The cervical spine should be first cleared; in a cooperative child, normal pain-free motion combined with normal anteroposterior, lateral, and odontoid x-rays is sufficient to accomplish this. The extremities should be visually examined for areas of swelling, evidence of lacerations, abrasions, and neurocirculatory competence. Palpation of the long bones for tenderness, crepitance, and instability will identify areas requiring x-ray studies.

12. What are the key orthopaedic x-rays to obtain? What special views are recommended?

Anteroposterior (AP), lateral, and odontoid views of the cervical spine are the basic studies. If they are negative but significant pain is present or the mechanism of injury suggests a high risk for problems, controlled flexion-extension views are required. An AP view of the pelvis to include the hips is required in the case of pelvic/abdominal trauma. An AP and lateral view of the thoracolumbar spine is indicated if there is tenderness, an abnormal neurologic exam, or a suggestive mechanism for spine injury present. Two views taken at 90 opposing degrees are the accepted standard in any suspicious extremity area. If the Glasgow coma scale score is less than 14, a CT of the head should be performed.

13. What are some of the commonly missed injuries encountered later in this patient population? How do you increase the risk of late identification?

The incidence of missed fractures in patients with polytrauma is actually quite low, 2–12% in seven different studies. Initially undisplaced growth plate injuries lead the list. Some people recommend a technetium bone scan several days after admission to avoid the late sequelae of missed fractures.

14. Are the same classifications of injury severity used in children as in adults, and what purpose do they serve?

The various scoring systems used in cases of multiple trauma provide a mechanism for identifying patients at major risk for morbidity or mortality, performing outcome studies, and comparing results between trauma centers. The Glasgow Coma Scale has been modified for infants. The Pediatric Trauma Score, Revised Trauma Scale (which omits parameters difficult to assess at night), and Modified Injury Severity Scale serve these purposes as well.

Glasgow Coma Scale (GCS)			GCS Modified for Infants	
ACTIVITY	BEST RESPONSE	SCORE	BEST RESPONSE	SCORE
Eye opening	Spontaneous	4	Spontaneous	4
	To verbal stimuli	3	To speech	3
	To pain	2	To pain	2
	None	1	None	1
Verbal	Oriented	5	Coos, babbles	5
	Confused	4	Irritable crying	4
	Inappropriate words	3	Cries to pain	3
	Nonspecific sounds	2	Moans to pain	2
	None	1	None	1
Motor function	Follows commands	6	Normal, spontaneous movement	6
	Localizes pain	5	Withdraws to touch	5
	Withdraws to pain	4	Withdraws to pain	4
	Flexion to pain	3	Abnormal flexion	3
	Extension to pain	2	Extension to pain	2
	None	1	None	1

Pediatric Trauma Score

	SEVERITY POINTS		
COMPONENT	2+	1+	−
Size	20+ kg (40 lb)	10–20 kg	−10 kg
Airway	Normal	Maintainable	Unmaintainable
Systolic blood pressure	90+ mm Hg	50–90 mm Hg	−50 mm Hg
Central nervous system	Awake	Obtunded/loss of consciousness	Coma/decerebrate
Skeletal	None	Closed fracture	Open/multiple fractures
Cutaneous	None	Minor	Major/penetrating

Sum _____

From Tepas JJ III, Ramenofsky ML, Molitt DL, et al.: The Pediatric Trauma Patient Score as a predictor of injury severity: an objective assessment. J Trauma 28:425–429, 1988.

Trauma Score		Revised Trauma Score	
ATTRIBUTE	CODED VALUE	ATTRIBUTE	CODED VALUE
Respiratory rate		Respiratory rate	
10–24	4	10–29	4
25–35	3	29+	3
35+	2	6–9	2
0–9	1	1–5	1
		0	0
Respiratory effort			
Normal	1		
Shallow, retractive	0		
Systolic blood pressure		Systolic blood pressure	
90+	4	89+	4
70–89	3	76–89	3
50–69	2	50–75	2
0–49	1	1–49	1
		0	0
Capillary refill			
Normal	2		
Delayed	1		
Absent	0		
Glasgow Coma Scale		Glasgow Coma Scale	
14–15	5	13–15	4
11–13	4	9–12	3
8–10	3	6–8	2
5–7	2	4–5	1
3–4	1	3	0
Total Trauma Score		Unweighted Revised Trauma Score	

15. Which of these may be applied early to facilitate the ability to make treatment decisions and provide accurate information to parents regarding the magnitude of the problem?
The Modified Injury Severity Score (MISS) has been accepted and recognized as fulfilling this role.

16. What is the mechanism of determining the Modified Injury Severity Score, and upon what is it based?
The body is divided into five areas. Each area is assigned a score from one to five depending on the magnitude of injury to that region. The three areas receiving the highest scores are noted, their scores are squared, and the sum of these three determinants is designated as the MISS.

Modified Injury Severity Score (MISS) for Children with Multiple Injury

BODY AREA	1—MINOR	2—MODERATE	3—SEVERE, NOT LIFE-THREATENING	4—SEVERE, LIFE-THREATENING	5—CRITICAL, SURVIVAL UNCERTAIN
Neural Face/ neck	GCS 13–14 Vitreous or conjunctival hemorrhage; fractured teeth	GCS 9–12 Laceration of eye, disfiguring laceration	GCS 9–12 Displaced facial fracture, blow-out fracture of orbit	GCS 5–8	GCS 4
Chest	Muscle ache or chest wall stiffness	Simple rib sternal fracture	Multiple rib fractures, hemo- or pneumothorax diaphragmatic rupture	Open chest wounds, pneumomedi-astinum, myocardial contusion	Lacerations of trachea, mediastinum, myocardium
Abdomen	Muscle ache, seat belt abrasion	Major abdominal wall contusion	Contusion of abdominal organs, retroperitoneal hematoma, extraperitoneal bladder rupture, thoracic or lumbar spine fractures	Major laceration of abdominal organs, intraperitoneal bladder rupture; spine fractures with paraplegia	Rupture, severe laceration of abdominal vessels or organs
Extremities and pelvic girdle	Minor sprain, simple fractures and dislo-cations	Open fractures of digits, nondisplaced long bone or pelvic fractures	Displaced long bone or multiple hand or foot fractures, single open fracture	Multiple closed long bone fractures, amputation of limb fracture	Multiple open long bone fractures

Adapted from Mayer T, Matlak ME, Johnson DG, Walker ML: The Modified Injury Severity Scale in pediatric multiple trauma patients. J Pediatr Surg 15:719–726, 1980.

17. After the MISS has been obtained, what does the specific score imply?
Review of a large series of polytrauma victims has demonstrated the following relationship to the score.

	MISS 40+	*MISS 25+*	*MISS 25−*
Mortality	100%	60%	0%
Morbidity			2.5%
Dependency (disability)		16.7%	0%

18. What do the other scores imply?
Any patient with a Glasgow Coma Scale Score of 12 or less, a Trauma Score of 12 or less, a Revised Trauma Score of 9 or less, or a Pediatric Trauma Score of 8 or less should be admitted to a trauma center.

19. What are the orthopaedic considerations for definitive treatment in children with polytrauma?

The size of the patient must be considered. Studies show that these children have fewer complications when fractures are stabilized operatively at the time of surgery for other injuries. Although closed treatment is normally preferred for most pediatric fractures, open reduction and fixation are often recommended for skeletal fractures accompanying other serious injuries.

20. What are the types of treatment?

Nonsurgical treatment with traditional casting, splinting, and various types of traction must be considered first. Surgical stabilization, either internally with plates, pins, rods, or screws or externally with a fixator, must be performed with full cognizance of and adjustment to the vagaries of the immature skeleton.

21. What type of spinal cord injury is unique to children?

Spinal cord injury without radiologic abnormality (SCIWORA) is occasionally noted secondary to severe trauma. Hence, all child victims of severe trauma must be placed under appropriate precautions until acute and delayed spinal cord injuries are ruled out.

22. Should the child with spinal cord injury be treated with steroids to decrease cord edema?

Use of corticosteroids has not been shown to be of benefit but has been noted to increase the risk of pulmonary complications.

23. Are cervical spine injuries common in children? How about neurologic deficits?

No, cervical spine injuries represent only 2% of all vertebral fractures. This may be an underestimate due to the difficulty in interpreting the x-ray of a spine composed of much cartilage. Neurologic deficits are less frequently seen than in adults, and the prognosis is better.

24. What kinds of injuries do occur, and what part of the cervical spine is most subject to trauma?

The upper cervical area (C1–C3) is most prone to injury owing to the relatively large cranium and the young child's natural hypermobility. The vertebral epiphyses may be traumatically separated, and facet joint subluxation or dislocation may occur, often fatally. As the age approaches adolescence, injury patterns become adultlike, and the lower cervical spine is more often involved.

25. Is the polytraumatized child exposed to unique thoracic or lumbar spine injuries?

Lap-type seat belts, which cross the lower abdomen rather than the pelvis, are the source of flexion/distraction injuries concentrated at the thoracolumbar junction. Ligamentous attachments are avulsed posteriorly, and the facet joints are disengaged. Anterior ligamentous or physeal disruption allows the spine to hinge on the anterior longitudinal ligament, stretching the cord and causing complete or incomplete neurologic compromise. Symptoms may be delayed, calling for a strong index of suspicion and ongoing reassessment.

26. What must the physician be aware of when faced with trauma to the child's pelvis?

The child's pelvis is very elastic, has great capacity for remodeling, and is rarely the site of long-term morbidity. In adults, hemorrhage from pelvic fracture can be the cause of mortality. In the child with pelvic fracture, death more often results from associated head or abdominal trauma. Hence, pelvic fracture in the child should stimulate a thorough search for injury to other organ systems.

27. When is operative treatment for the child's pelvic fracture required?

Faced with an unstable pelvic fracture in a hemodynamically unstable child, the treating orthopaedist must be prepared to stabilize the pelvis emergently with an external factor. Open reduction of a significantly displaced sacroiliac dislocation or acetabular fracture may be appropriate, but these are not urgent problems in the polytraumatized youngster.

28. What are the advantages of operative stabilization of long bone fractures in the polytraumatized child?
Traction is poorly tolerated by the patient with multiple injuries. Patients with head injuries may be agitated. Those with chest injuries need upright posturing. Access to the abdomen may be required, and frequent imaging studies may require repeated transport to the radiology department.

29. If long bone fractures are best treated with fixation, what considerations are important?
The open physis must be respected and not crossed with screws, rods, or plates. This may make the external fixator the best choice when choosing operative treatment for the closed or open fracture.

30. What about an intramedullary rod for femur fractures?
In children younger than 12 years of age, a small but troublesome incidence of capital femoral epiphyseal avascular necrosis has been associated with the use of intramedullary rods for femoral shaft fractures. Recovery from the polytrauma is probable; hence, another choice for the femur that avoids iatrogenic morbidity should be considered.

31. What alternatives to the intramedullary rod exist?
External fixation or bone plates can be used. Flexible intramedullary nails may be introduced proximally through the trochanter or distally above the distal femoral physis, avoiding the complications associated with avascular necrosis and growth plate compromise.

32. Must upper extremity injuries also be as frequently treated operatively?
Many upper extremity fractures can be successfully and appropriately treated with closed methods without interfering with the care of other injuries. Open fractures, articular fractures, displaced epiphyseal injuries, and injuries to the arm and forearm resulting in a "floating elbow" are best treated with operative stabilization.

BIBLIOGRAPHY

1. Armstrong PF: Management of the multiply injured child: The ABC's. Am Acad Orthop Surg Instructional Course Lectures 41:347–350, 1992.
2. Buckley SL, Gotschall C, Robertson WR, Sturm P, Tosi L, Thomas M, Eichelberger M: The relationship of skeletal injuries with trauma score, injury severity score, length of hospital stay, hospital charges and mortality in children admitted to a regional pediatric trauma center. J Pediatr Orthop 14:449–453, 1994.
3. Cramer KE: The pediatric polytrauma patient. Clin Orthop 318:125–135, 1995.
4. Heinrich SD, Gallagher D, Harris M, Nadell JM: Undiagnosed fractures in severely injured children and young adults. J Bone Joint Surg 76A:551–572, 1994.
5. Tepas JJ, Ramenofsky MI, Mollett DL, et al.: The Pediatric Trauma Score as a predictor of injury severity: an objective assessment. J Trauma 28:425–429, 1988.
6. Ziegler MM, Templeton JM: Major Trauma. In Fleisher GR, Ludwig S (eds): Textbook of Pediatric Emergency Medicine, 3rd ed. Baltimore, Williams & Wilkins, 1993, pp 1089–1101.

30. FOOT AND ANKLE TRAUMA IN CHILDREN

Andrew Sullivan, M.D.

1. How do fractures about the foot and ankle occur in children?

In children, the physes are still open, and this is the weakest part of the bone ligament interface. When a force is applied against the foot or ankle, it can cause either a sprain or, if enough force is exerted, a fracture. While serious ankle sprains can occur in children, more often the ligament remains intact and pulls off a piece of bone. On the lateral side, this pulls off the entire fibular epiphysis with an intact physis and sometimes a very small fragment of the metaphysis. On the medial side in a very young child, usually the entire tibial epiphysis comes off with the physis and a portion of the metaphysis. Since the entire physis is usually intact in these injuries, in most instances normal growth will resume.

2. What classification system is used to describe children's epiphyseal fractures?

All systems consider the position of the foot, the force applied, and the resulting pathoanatomy, but the Salter-Harris classification is the most useful for planning treatment and predicting outcomes in the skeletally immature patient. The Salter-Harris I–IV types are most frequently seen/presented; type V is a crush injury and is rarely, if ever, demonstrated.

3. Is there a fracture pattern that corresponds with age?

In the very young child, the injury most often occurs so that the entire epiphysis and physis are disrupted from the metaphysis. If the physis and epiphysis is intact, so is the articular surface. As skeletal maturity nears, the physis of the distal tibia begins to close, first medially and then laterally. A fracture may occur through the articular surface, epiphysis, and physis toward the lateral side remaining open. This results in Salter-Harris III and IV injures as opposed to I and II types, which are more common in a younger child.

4. Which factors help predict the outcome of ankle fractures in children?

- Salter-Harris classification
- How well the fracture is reduced
- The level of skeletal maturity
- The degree of displacement
- Any modifier (an open fracture, a vascular injury, a systemic illness, or an infection)

Salter-Harris I and II are the most predictable, and the incidence of complications remains approximately the same for both regardless of the amount of displacement. However, some type II injuries of the distal tibia which have been reduced and appear benign may develop premature growth closure; these must be followed for several years.

Salter-Harris III and IV injuries have higher complication rates. Because they involve the articular surface and cross the growth plate, anatomic or near anatomic reduction is required in addition to internal fixation to maintain the alignment. Premature closure, angular deformity, and leg length discrepancy are more likely to result from these injuries. Particular attention must be paid to the medial malleolus, in which there is a high incidence of premature physeal closure.

5. How are fractures about the ankle managed?

In the young child, fractures about the ankle are most often Salter-Harris II of the distal tibial physis with a fracture of the fibula. Most can be reduced, closed, and satisfactorily maintained with a long leg walking cast which can then be converted to a short leg walking cast after two weeks. **Salter-Harris I** injuries occur in the distal tibia, and more commonly, in the distal fibula. These must be differentiated from an ankle sprain. Their diagnosis is based on a history of inversion injury combined with swelling and tenderness directly over the physis as opposed to the lig-

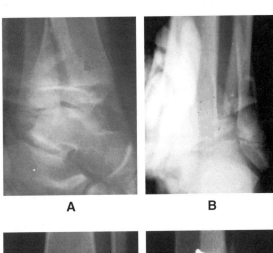

(A) AP radiograph and (B) lateral radiograph of a triplane ankle fracture. The fracture lines extend all 3 planes (triplane).

A   **B**

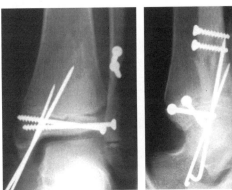

Postoperative radiographs. Note that fixation devices extend into the sagital, frontal, and coronal planes.

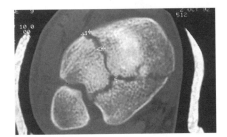

CT scan showing multiple fragments.

ament complex. The x-ray may appear normal or the physis slightly widened. If there is any question, the extremity should be immobilized for three weeks in a short leg walking cast.

Salter-Harris II injuries of the distal tibial epiphysis can be treated with a long leg weight-bearing cast for four weeks. Walking casts promote early healing, a rapid return to full activity, and have a low complication rate.

Salter-Harris III fractures occur in the distal tibial epiphysis (fracture of Tillaux). A fragment of the lateral epiphysis remains attached to the anterior talofibular ligament. These will often require open reduction and internal fixation of the fragment with a pin or screw. Fractures of the medial malleolus can be either Salter-Harris III or IV. If they are undisplaced, they can be treated closed in a long leg nonweightbearing cast for three weeks, followed by a short leg walking cast for three weeks. These are among the most unpredictable of ankle epiphyseal injuries. Near anatomic reduction must be achieved, even if it requires open reduction or internal fixation.

Salter-Harris IV fractures include those of the medial malleolus and the so-called triplane fracture, in which the fracture lines extend into the transverse, sagittal, and coronal planes (see Figure). This is best diagnosed by looking carefully at both the AP and lateral x-ray. CT scan will accurately diagnose and identify the pathoanatomy prior to open reduction and internal fixation. In the past, these have been associated with a high complication rate but if reduced well surgically, the results should be good. Because these patients are approaching skeletal maturity, physeal arrest is less likely to cause angular deformity or leg length discrepancy. The articular surface must be reduced. These injuries should be treated for six weeks in a cast.

6. What are the most common fractures of the foot?

Fractures due to direct trauma. The metatarsals are frequently fractured. Most fractures of the shafts of the metatarsals can be satisfactorily treated in a short leg walking cast for 4–6 weeks. A more serious fracture is that of the base of the fifth metatarsal, the point of attachment of the peroneus brevis tendon on the apophysis of the base of the fifth metatarsal. An inversion injury may avulse this apophysis. Findings include tenderness at the base of the fifth metatarsal, pain with attempted eversion against resistance, and swelling. X-ray may show widening of the apophysis. These fractures will heal uneventfully. Immobilization with crutches and an elastic bandage until pain subsides is usually satisfactory. Two to three weeks in a short leg walking cast can also produce favorable results.

The so-called Jones fracture is one of the proximal diaphyses of the fifth metatarsal and is less common in the skeletally immature patient. Initially each patient needs to be managed conservatively; immobilization in a short leg walking cast should be the first form of treatment. If this results in delayed union or nonunion, operative intervention with screw fixation and bone grafting should be done. Established nonunion requires a reopening of the medullary canal.

Fractures of the toes can be treated by taping to the adjacent toe. Perhaps the only operative indication in children would be a Salter-Harris III or IV type of the proximal phalanx of the great toe (while I have seen several of these, none have been sufficiently displaced to require operative treatment).

7. What causes stress fractures and how are they managed?

Stress fractures may result from a sudden increase in training or a change in training surface or in shoe type. While these are most frequent in the metatarsals, they can occur in the navicular and the medial sesamoid. Diagnosis requires vigilance and a high index of suspicion. Bone scan is not necessary unless you are dealing with an elite athlete who must return to competition. In most cases, immobilization in a short leg walking cast for 2–3 weeks and repeat x-ray will show periosteal new bone confirming the diagnosis. Be aware that the initial radiograph may appear normal in more than half the cases.

8. How frequent are fractures of the calcaneus, and how are they treated?

They occur much less frequently than in the adult. Most occur as children approach skeletal maturity. As in the adult, these are often associated with other injuries such as fractures of the lumbar spine or pelvic injuries. Many of these involve the tuberosity of the posterior portion and will heal uneventfully with either nonweightbearing or weightbearing as tolerated. It is less common for them to involve the articular surface. Fractures that are intra-articular often require surgical management and reconstitution of the articular surface. Those that are minimally displaced or nondisplaced can be treated with nonweightbearing until they heal in about 6 weeks.

9. How frequent are fractures of the talus, and how are they managed in children?

Fortunately, these are rare in children, and are somewhat different from the equivalent adult injury. They usually result from forced dorsiflexion and can involve the body or the neck. If they are nondisplaced, use a long-leg, nonweightbearing cast. Weightbearing is commenced when there is some sign of healing. Displaced fractures require open reduction and internal fixation. This should be done as soon as possible, as there may be embarrassment of the blood supply to the talus which can result in avascular necrosis (AVN). Placement of a cannulated screw allows good control and compression of the fracture site. They are then treated in a nonweightbearing cast until signs of healing appear, followed by weightbearing. These must be followed for AVN, which is the most significant complication that occurs with them. AVN can occur in either displaced or nondisplaced fractures, indicating that children may be at greater risk than adults for developing this problem. One must look for the subchondral lucency signifying loss of circulation and viability of the talus. The question of whether these should be treated with weightbearing has not been resolved, but most are treated with nonweightbearing.

The dome of the talus can also be injured from significant trauma. I have seen complete AVN and disruption of the talus as a result of an ankle injury that was associated with a Salter-Harris type III injury of the distal tibial physis, indicating that the talus was probably compressed against the articular surface of the tibia as a result of a motor vehicle accident.

Osteochondral fractures occur in children particularly as they approach skeletal maturity, requiring anatomic reduction and internal fixation which can be difficult in youths.

10. Do injuries to Lisfranc's joint occur in children?
Yes. Previously unrecognized, it is now known that this tarsal metatarsal disruption does occur and requires a precise diagnosis and anatomic reduction. Some can be reduced closed but must be maintained with some type of internal fixation, such as pins or wires. The second metatarsal that keys into the tarsals must be reduced and stabilized. Pins may be necessary in the other metatarsals to maintain their reduction.

11. What are the disease processes and normal variants that can be confused with fractures in children?
Children have a variety of osteochondroses that may be confused with injury. These include osteochondroses of the second metatarsal head (Freiberg's disease) and the navicular joint (Kohler's disease), and irregular ossification of the calcaneal apophysis (Sever's disease). In addition, there are a variety of sesamoids in the foot that can be mistaken for fractures. For instance, it is not unusual for the sesamoid associated with the first metatarsal to be bipartite and mistaken for a fracture of the sesamoid. The os trigonum located immediately behind the talus may either be an integral part of the talus or separate. There are also often irregularities in ossification of the epiphyses of the medial malleolus and fibular malleolus which can be confused with fractures. All of these are distinguishable from a fracture in that they are more rounded, sclerotic, and do not have the appearance of acute fracture. When in doubt, radiographs of the opposite foot or ankle should be obtained for comparison.

BIBLIOGRAPHY

1. Ashworth A, Hedden D: Fractures of the Ankle. In Letts RM (ed): Management of Pediatric Fractures, 1st ed. New York: Churchill Livingstone, 1994; pp 713–734.
2. Jarvis JG: Tibial Triplane Fractures. In Letts RM (ed): The Management of Pediatric Fractures, 1st ed. New York: Churchill Livingstone, 1994; pp 735:–750.
3. Carrol N: Fractures and Dislocations of the Tarsal Bones. In Letts RM (ed): The Management of Pediatric Fractures. 1 ed. New York: Churchill Livingstone, 1994; pp 751–766.
4. Baxter MP: Fractures and Dislocations of the Metatarsals and Phalanges. In Letts RM (ed): The Management of Pediatric Fractures, 1st ed. New York: Churchill Livingstone, 1994; pp 767–788.
5. Sullivan JA: Ankle and Foot Fractures in the Pediatric Athlete. In Stanitski CL, DeLee JC, Drez DD, Jr. (eds): The Management of Pediatric Fractures, 1st ed. Philadelphia: W.B. Saunders, 1994; pp 441–455.
6. Crawford AH: Fractures and Dislocations of the Ankle: In Green NE, Swiontkowski MF (eds): Skeletal Trauma in Children, 1st ed. Philadelphia: W.B. Saunders, 1994; pp 449–516.
7. Ertl JP, Barrack RL, Alexander AH, VanBuecken K: Triplane fractures of the distal tibial epiphysis: Long-term follow-up. J Bone Joint Surg Am 70:967, 1988.

31. KNEE INJURIES

Kit M. Song, M.D.

1. What are important anatomic and mechanical considerations in knee injuries in children?

All knee ligament origins and insertions and capsular attachments are to the epiphyses, except for the medial collateral ligament and the tibial collateral insertions, which have attachments to the tibial epiphysis, the tibial metaphysis, and the fibular head. This arrangement makes the proximal tibial physis more resistant to injury than the distal femoral physis. Both are physeal growth plates and the ligaments have viscoelastic properties, and their strength is determined by the total force applied and the rate of loading. Pure ligamentous injuries are secondary to low-energy rapid-loading events, and injuries to the physis or tendon-bone junctions occur with high-energy slow-loading events.

2. Describe important points of the clinical evaluation of knee injuries in children.

- A careful history. This will be more vague than for adults. Information regarding mechanism of injury, timing of the onset of effusion, a "pop" felt at the time of injury, mechanical blocking symptoms, and feelings of true instability will often be lacking.
- A detailed physical examination. Always examine the uninjured knee first. If possible, examine the patient walking. Children will seldom tolerate ligamentous laxity testing or provocative maneuvers following an acute injury. In the absence of an obvious fracture, immobilization and repeat examination 1–2 weeks later are appropriate. The physical examination findings in the preadolescent will be less accurate than in adults or adolescents. A careful neurovascular examination should be performed. Always examine the hips of children presenting with knee pain. **Remember that hip problems in children can cause referred pain to the knee.**
- Selective imaging of the knee.

3. What imaging modalities are helpful in evaluating knee injuries in children?

Plain radiographs remain important in evaluating knee injuries in children and can demonstrate physeal injuries and lesions that mimic meniscus injuries. Double contrast arthrography remains useful in evaluating the pediatric knee owing to the large amount of cartilage present prior to maturity. It has an accuracy rate of greater than 90% in experienced hands but has the great disadvantage of being invasive. Magnetic resonance imaging (MRI) has been increasingly applied to the evaluation of knee injuries. MRI is very sensitive and specific for the detection of acute injuries to the anterior cruciate ligament (ACL). The sensitivity of MRI is 95% for medial meniscus injuries and 90% for lateral meniscus injuries.

4. What is the differential diagnosis for an acute hemarthrosis of the knee in a child?

For preadolescents, meniscal tears (47%), ACL injuries (47%), and osteochondral fractures (13%) account for the majority of injuries with hemarthrosis. For adolescents, ACL tears (65%), meniscus tears (45%), and osteochondral fractures (5%) account for the majority of hemarthroses.

5. How can you differentiate a true ligament injury from a physeal injury in a child?

Both injuries present with swelling and pain within and about the knee. Age younger than 14 years, prepubertal status, and the mechanism of injury will be the most helpful clues to suspecting a physeal injury. A nondisplaced fracture through the physis may be difficult to visualize radiographically. Oblique, comparison, and stress views may be helpful. It must be remembered that physeal fracture and ligament disruption can occur simultaneously. Evaluation of ligamentous stability after fracture management is advised.

6. How common are knee ligament injuries in children?

The incidence of ACL injuries is 0.3–0.38 per 1000 per year. The majority of injuries are related to the sports of football, soccer, skiing, and basketball. The incidence of avulsion of the tibial spine is estimated to be 3 in 100,000 children per year. Skeletally immature patients account for 3–4% of all ACL tears. Isolated lateral collateral ligament (LCL) injuries in children are rare and are associated with polytrauma in younger children. Isolated medial collateral ligament (MCL) injuries in children are not uncommon, but the incidence is not known. Isolated posterior cruciate ligament (PCL) injuries are rare in children.

7. How does failure of the anterior cruciate ligament occur in children?

Bony avulsion of the tibial insertion of the anterior cruciate ligaments occurs in preadolescent children. Intrasubstance tears are more common in adolescents. The mechanism of injury is generally hyperextension, sudden deceleration, or a valgus rotational force with a stationary foot.

8. What is the natural history of the ACL-deficient knee in a skeletally immature patient?

The natural history of ACL deficiencies in preadolescent children is not well defined owing to the small number of such injuries. For adolescents, the natural history appears to be similar to that in young adults. Episodes of "giving way" are reported in 33–86% of subjects with ACL tears treated nonoperatively. Activity level, not age, is the primary risk factor for recurrent instability. Because adolescents are very active, conservative treatment will fail in a greater number of these patients. A relatively inactive adolescent, however, may have a very satisfactory outcome without ligament reconstruction.

9. How are bony avulsions of the ACL insertion on the anterior tibial spine classified?

Avulsion injuries of the ACL are classified on the basis of displacement.

Type I fractures are minimally displaced and are best managed with cast immobilization in slight flexion.

Type II fractures have a posterior hinge but are still attached to the tibial epiphysis. These fractures should undergo closed reduction and cast immobilization.

Type III fractures are displaced and require open reduction and suture or screw fixation, avoiding crossing the physis.

10. What are the management options for an isolated intrasubstance tear of the ACL in a skeletally immature child? In a skeletally mature child?

In the absence of a torn meniscus, ACL injuries in preadolescent children are best managed with activity modification and observation. Repair of the ligament is at best controversial and will have a high rate of failure. Children with more than 1 year of growth remaining should not undergo ligament reconstruction with bone tunnels that cross the epiphyseal growth plate. For the rare situation of a prepubertal child with an intrasubstance tear and significant instability, an extra-articular reconstruction can be done (in a very young child) or a hamstring reconstruction using a tibial tunnel and placement "over the top" of the femoral condyle can be performed (in an older child).

The adolescent with an ACL disruption should be managed as an adult. It must be established that the ACL injury is an isolated one. If there is an associated meniscus tear that is repairable, an aggressive approach to reconstruction of the ACL is justified.

11. What are the clinical findings and mechanism of injury associated with a torn posterior cruciate ligament in a child?

The mechanism of injury to the PCL is a direct blow to the tibia, hyperflexion of the knee, or hyperextension of the knee. Hyperflexion injuries are associated with avulsion of the PCL origin from the femur. The posterior drawer test is usually positive, but it may be negative if Wrisberg's and Humphry's ligaments are intact.

12. What are the treatment options for a torn PCL in a child?

Intrasubstance tears of the PCL in a skeletally immature child are best managed with activity modification and observation. An avulsion of the PCL origin from the femur or insertion onto the tibia is best treated with open reduction and internal fixation. Intrasubstance PCL disruptions in the skeletally mature patient should be managed as in an adult, with reconstruction if the patient is symptomatic.

13. What is the clinical presentation of meniscal injuries in children?
The primary symptoms of meniscus injuries in children are pain (95%), effusion (71%), snapping (63%), giving way of the knee (63%), intermittent locking of the knee (54%), and a locked knee (7%). The symptoms may change over time. Joint-line tenderness and McMurray's test are not as reliable in children as in adults.

14. What is the outcome of meniscectomies for a torn meniscus in children?
The outcome of complete meniscectomies in children is very poor, with a 60% unsatisfactory outcome at 7-year follow-up examination. Preservation of the meniscus is important, and whenever possible operative repair should be done. Peripheral tears are more common in children than in adults; the repair of peripheral tears in children has a favorable outcome in 80–90% of cases. Tears of the meniscus in the avascular zone should be treated with a partial meniscectomy.

15. What is a discoid meniscus? Where does it occur?
Early reports had suggested that a discoid meniscus was caused by an arrest in embryologic development with a failure of resorption of the central portion of the meniscus. Subsequent studies did not find a meniscus with a discoid morphology at any stage of fetal development. It is believed that this condition is acquired when an initially normal meniscus has abnormal peripheral attachments that lead to meniscal hypermobility and hypertrophy. The meniscus may be stable or unstable (Wrisberg) with or without meniscotibial attachments. The stable meniscus may be either complete or incomplete depending on how much of the tibial plateau it covers. The clinical finding is a disc of meniscal cartilage covering the lateral tibial plateau. There are no reports of a medial discoid meniscus.

16. What is the incidence of discoid meniscus?
There is considerable cultural variation in the incidence of discoid menisci. The reported ranges are 3–20%, with the highest incidence in the Japanese.

17. What are the presenting symptoms and findings with a discoid meniscus?
Symptoms include lateral knee pain, snapping or popping within the knee, decreased extension of the knee, and episodes of giving way, with slight swelling that rapidly resolves. An asymptomatic or unstable meniscus that is popping back and forth within the knee but is not causing pain is best left untreated until it does become symptomatic. As children reach puberty, tears of the meniscus become more common. Most discoid menisci remain asymptomatic.

18. What are the options for treatment of a symptomatic discoid meniscus?
Excision of the torn portion of the meniscus, sculpting of the meniscus by excision of the torn central portion, or complete meniscectomy.

19. What is the outcome of complete meniscectomy for symptomatic discoid meniscus?
At 20-year follow-up, 75% of patients will show degenerative changes of the lateral condyle radiographically. Despite this, the majority of patients will have clinically acceptable function.

20. What is osteochondritis dissecans?
Osteochondritis dissecans is a lesion of bone and cartilage that results in bone necrosis and loss of continuity of the subchondral bone. This may or may not lead to loss of articular cartilage continuity. The cause of this lesion is unknown. Theories have ranged from abnormal vascular anatomy, leading to ischemic injury to bone, to existence of a normal accessory ossification center that fails to fuse with the surrounding bone.

21. What are the most common sites for osteochondritis dissecans in the knee?
The most common site is the lateral middle to posterior portion of the medial femoral condyle (57–83%). Other sites are the lateral femoral condyle (20%) and the patella (15%).

22. What is the initial management of osteochondritis dissecans in a skeletally immature child?

In children with open growth plates, there is a much higher potential for healing with immobilization than in adults. If the subchondral bone is intact, immobilization in a cast for 2–3 months may produce healing. This is especially true in girls younger than the age of 11 and boys younger than the age of 13. If the subchondral bone is disrupted or there is a loose fragment, immobilization is unlikely to succeed, and surgical treatment should be offered.

23. What are the principles of surgical treatment of osteochondritis dissecans of the knee?

The optimal treatment is controversial. The basic concepts are 1) fragmented displaced lesions are best excised, 2) painful lesions in continuity with the surrounding bone should be drilled, 3) displaced small lesions should be excised and curetted, and 4) displaced large lesions with subchondral bone attached to cartilage should be fixed with or without bone grafing. A wide variety of fixation devices, bone grafting techniques, and surgical approaches exist.

24. What is Osgood-Schlatter disease?

Osgood-Schlatter disease is an alteration in the development of the tibial tuberosity due to repeated application of tensile forces. It is generally a self-limited condition and will respond to rest. It is bilateral in 20–30% of cases. A small number of children will develop painful ossicles within the patellar tendon that will require surgical removal.

25. How common are fractures of the tibial tubercle relative to all growth plate injuries?

The reported incidence is 0.4–2.7% of all growth plate injuries.

26. What is the average age at which fractures of the tibial tubercle occur?

The average age in most series is 14 years, and most of the patients are boys.

27. What factors guide the management of tibial tubercle fractures?

The degree of displacement and the size of the fragment involved. Minimally displaced small fragments can be treated nonoperatively. Displaced fragments are treated operatively with reduction and internal fixation.

BIBLIOGRAPHY

1. Beaty JH: Intra-articular and ligamentous injuries about the knee. In Rockwood CA, Wilkins KE, Beaty JH (eds): Fractures in Children, 4th ed. Vol. 3. Philadelphia, Lippincott-Raven, 1996.
2. Beaty JH, Kumar A: Fractures about the knee in children. J Bone Joint Surg 76A:1870, 1994.
3. Meyers MH, McDeever FM: Fracture of the intercondylar eminence of the tibia. J Bone Joint Surg 52A:209, 1959.
4. Smith AD, Tao SS: Knee injuries in young athletes. Clin Sports Med 14:629, 1995.
5. Stanitski CL, DeLee JC, Drez D (eds): Pediatric and Adolescent Sports Medicine. Philadelphia, W.B. Saunders Co., 1994.
6. Stanitski CL, Harvell JC, Fu F: Observations on acute knee hemarthrosis in children and adolescents. J Pediatr Orthop 13:506, 1993
7. Vahassarja V, Kinnuen P, Serlo W: Arthroscopy of the acute traumatic knee in children. Prospective study of 138 cases. Acta Orthop Scand 64:580, 1993.
8. Vahvanaen V, Aalto K: Meniscectomy in children. Acta Orthop Scand 50:791, 1979.
9. Wojtys EM (ed): The ACL Deficient Knee. Rosemont, IL, American Academy of Orthopedic Surgeons, 1994.

32. TIBIAL INJURIES

Kit M. Song, M.D.

1. Describe the anatomic and developmental features of the tibia and the fibula in the growing child.

The tibia develops from three ossification centers, one in the diaphysis and two in the epiphyses. The proximal epiphysis appears shortly after birth and closes at approximately 16 years of age. A secondary ossification center forms for the tibial tuberosity and appears at age 7–9 years, fusing with the remaining epiphysis in adolescence. The distal epiphysis appears in the second year of life and closes at approximately 16–18 years. There may be a secondary ossification center in the medial malleolus that appears at age 7–9 years and fuses with the remaining distal tibia by age 14–15 years. Accessory malleolar ossification centers can also be present in the medial malleolus, which can be confused with fractures. Closure of the distal tibial epiphysis is in a posteromedial to anterolateral direction over 1½ years. This pattern of closure creates characteristic fracture patterns.

The distal and proximal fibular epiphyses begin to ossify at age 2 and 4 years, respectively. Distal epiphyseal closure is at age 16, and proximal closure is 1–2 years later. The distal fibular epiphyseal growth plate is at the same level as the tibial growth plate at birth and descends to the ankle joint by the age of 7 years.

2. How often do fractures and injuries of the tibia and fibula occur in children?

The tibia and fibula are the third most commonly injured long bones in children, after the radius and ulna. Tibial fractures are the most common lower limb fractures in children, accounting for approximately 15% of pediatric long bone fractures.

3. In what location and by what mechanism do most fractures and injuries of the tibia and fibula occur in children?

Fifty percent of fractures occur in the distal tibia. These are most common in the older child and are usually due to indirect trauma. Thirty-five percent of fractures are in the middle third. Fifteen percent involve the proximal tibia and are most common in children 3–6 years of age. Thirty percent of tibial fractures will also involve the fibula. The most common mechanism of injury is direct force from pedestrian motor vehicle injury (50%), followed by indirect twisting injuries (22%), falls from a height (17%), and motor vehicle injuries (11%). The tibia is fractured in 26% of children who are victims of child abuse.

Fracture of the proximal fibula is uncommon and can be displaced owing to the pull of the biceps. Open reduction and internal fixation are often needed. Subluxation or dislocation of the proximal tibiofibular joint is also uncommon, but early recognition within the first week can lead to a successful closed reduction. Isolated fibular diaphyseal fractures are rare and are generally due to direct blows.

4. What is a common deformity after treatment of proximal tibial fractures in children? What are its causes?

Valgus deformity after union of proximal tibial fractures is common and occurs in the first 6 months after injury. The deformity is not progressive. The cause of this can be poor reduction, but it is seen even in children with an anatomically correct reduction. Other theories to explain this are injury to the pes anserinus tendon, with loss of its normal tethering effect upon medial growth of the tibia; enchondral bone overgrowth due to increased vascularity of the medial tibia; relative overgrowth of the tibia to the fibula, leading to a lateral tethering; and valgus angulation. Spontaneous correction of the deformity has been reported. The deformity can recur after osteotomy of the tibia, and early correction is not recommended.

5. What vascular and neurologic complications can be seen with tibial fractures in children?

Vascular and neurologic injuries are uncommon in children, but the anterior tibial artery may be injured proximally as it passes through the interosseous membrane or distally if there is posterior displacement of the distal fragment. Displaced metaphyseal tibial fractures will require closed reduction, usually under general anesthesia. If there is clinical evidence of a dysvascular foot after reduction, arteriography should be considered. The peroneal nerve can be injured with proximal fibular injuries.

Compartment syndrome can and does occur in children with tibial injuries. The exact incidence is unknown. The assessment of pain and clinical detection of muscle compartment swelling in young children can be very difficult, making early detection of compartment syndrome difficult. Distal swelling may be an early finding.

6. Does overgrowth of tibial fractures occur in children?

Overgrowth of the tibia does occur in children younger than the age of 10 years but is not as predictable or as well documented as for fractures of the femur. Shortening greater than 1 cm is not likely to resolve. Tibial overgrowth can be observed following femur fractures even in the absence of a tibial fracture.

7. How much spontaneous correction of angular deformity will occur following tibial shaft fractures?

The cumulative experience of several large series suggests that angular correction can occur up to 18 months after fracture, with the range of improvement being 13–100%. Deformities greater than 10° should not be expected to correct fully. Children under the age of 10 years have the best chance of some correction. Varus malalignment will generally correct better than valgus malalignment. Rotational deformities do not spontaneously correct. The degree of malunion that can be accepted without long-term morbidity has not been defined.

8. What factors affect fracture healing in children with tibia fractures?

The age of the child, the degree of soft tissue injury, and the presence of deep infection have the greatest impact on healing of tibial fractures in children. The time required for osseous union of a closed diaphyseal fracture is 2–3 weeks in a neonate, 4–6 weeks for a toddler and younger child, and approaches the average 16 weeks seen in adults by the age of 14 years. The time required for osseous union increases for open fractures and parallels the grade of injury, with average healing times of 6 months for adolescents and 5 months for preadolescents with Gustillo grade III injuries. Nonunions and delayed unions are rare in children under the age of 11 years, but in adolescents these complications approach the incidence seen in adults. The presence of infection also greatly delays healing but is uncommon in younger children, even with open fractures, if adequate soft tissue débridement is done. The use of external fixation is associated with longer healing times. Location and fracture pattern will also affect healing times. Metaphyseal and spiral or long oblique fractures will heal more quickly than transverse diaphyseal fractures. Loss of periosteum (as in penetrating trauma with segmental bone loss) can also lead to delayed union or nonunion.

9. What are the operative stabilization options that can be used in children with tibial fractures?

Monolateral external fixators with pins more than 1 cm from the growth plates, plate fixation with open reduction, limited internal fixation with wires or screws, and flexible intramedullary nails can be used in a child of any age and are preferred for children with more than 1 year of growth remaining if surgical stabilization is needed. Children who are within 1 year of skeletal maturity can be treated with reamed or unreamed tibial nails.

10. When is operative stabilization of tibial fractures indicated for children?

Open fractures require operative débridement and aggressive soft tissue management, just as in adults. Only 9% of tibial fractures in children are open, and many Gustillo grade I or II injuries can be managed with a cast or splint. Severe soft tissue injuries, complex or unstable fractures, fractures involving the articular surface, polytrauma in which fracture stabilization facilitates care, and vascular injury needing repair require bone stabilization with internal or external fixation.

11. What is a toddler's fracture?

A toddler's fracture is a fracture of the tibia in a child 9 months to 3 years of age due to low-energy forces, which may lead to a limp and fracture of the tibia. This injury may be a stress fracture of the tibia. There is generally not an associated fracture of the fibula. The fracture, if visible, is a spiral fracture of the distal diaphysis and metaphysis.

12. What are the clinical and radiographic findings for a toddler's fracture?

The child suddenly refuses to bear weight with no observable trauma. There may be localized redness, warmth, and tenderness. The child will usually crawl but not walk, which is important in differentiating this from problems at the hip.

The initial evaluation should include a complete blood count with differential and analysis of the erythrocyte sedimentation rate and C-reactive protein. Oblique radiographs can help visualize the fracture line. Technetium bone scanning can be helpful if x-ray findings are normal. Immobilization and repeat radiographs in 10 days to 2 weeks will show periosteal reaction and sclerosis.

13. What is the most common location of a stress fracture in an older child? What is the management of this problem?

The proximal third of the tibia is the most common site of stress fractures in children. The peak incidence is 10–15 years of age. Fibular stress fractures are less common and occur from 2–8 years of age. The management of tibial stress fractures is rest and immobilization for 4–6 weeks. Fibular stress fractures may be managed with activity modification and immobilization as needed for comfort.

14. What is a "floating knee"? How is it treated?

A floating knee is characterized by both a distal femoral and an ipsilateral tibial fracture. These are high-energy injuries and will be seen primarily in adolescents. Coincidental ligamentous injury of the knee is seen in 10% of cases. Operative stabilization of at least one of the bones is recommended because closed management of both injuries is associated with at least a 30% incidence of postfracture complications.

BIBLIOGRAPHY

1. Buckley SL, Smith G, Sponseller PD, Thompson JD, Griffin PP: Open fractures of the tibia in children. J Bone Joint Surg 72A:1462, 1990.
2. Buckley SL, Smith GR, Sponseller PD, Thompson JD, Robertson WW, Griffin PP: Severe (type III) open fractures of the tibia in children. J Pediatr Orthop 16:627, 1996.
3. Hansen BA, Greiff J, Bergmann F: Fractures of the tibia in children. Acta Orthop Scand 47:448, 1976.
4. Heinrich SD: Fractures of the shaft of the tibia and fibula. In Rockwood CA, Wilkins KE, Beaty JH (eds): Fractures in Children, 4th ed. Vol. 3. Philadelphia, Lippincott-Raven, 1996.
5. King J, Defendorf D, Apthorp J, Negrette VF, Carlson M: Analysis of 429 fractures in 1889 battered children. J Pediatr Orthop 8:585, 1988.
6. Letts M, Vincent M: The "floating knee" in children. J Bone Joint Surg 68B:442, 1986.
7. Ogden JA: Subluxation and dislocation of the proximal tibiofibular joint. J Bone Joint Surg 56A:145, 1974.
8. Oujhane K, Newman B, Oh KS, Young LW, Girdany BR: Occult fractures in preschool children. Trauma 28:858, 1988.
9. Salter RB, Best TN: Pathogenesis of progressive valgus deformity following fractures of the proximal metaphyseal region of the tibia in young children. Instr Course Lect 41:409, 1992.
10. Shannak AO: Tibial fractures in children: follow-up study. J Pediatr Orthop 8:306, 1988.
11. Song KM, Sangorzan B, Benirschke S, Browne R: Open fractures of the tibia in children. J Pediatr Orthop 16:635 1996.
12. Zionts LE, MacEwen GD: Spontaneous improvement of post-traumatic tibia valga. J Bone Joint Surg 68A:680, 1986.

33. FEMUR FRACTURES

Deborah Stanitski, M.D.

1. How common are fractures of the femoral shaft in children?
Various studies have estimated the incidence of femoral shaft fracture at approximately 1% of children under the age of 12

2. In children between the onset of walking and 3 years of age, what is the most common mechanism of injury?
A fall.

3. What age range experiences the maximum incidence?
Children Aged 2–5 years.

4. What is the most common location for femoral shaft fracture?
Approximately 70% of these fractures occur in the middle third, 22% in the proximal third, and 8% in the distal third of the diaphysis.

5. What is Waddell's triad of injury when a child is struck by a car while crossing the street?
Fractured femur, head injury, and thoracic injury.

6. How are femoral fractures classified?
Like other fractures, femoral fractures are classified according to:
- Position
- Fracture pattern
- Whether open or closed

7. What is the most important etiology to exclude in children less <1 year of age who sustain a femoral fracture?
Child abuse is the most common cause of femoral fractures in children who have not yet begun walking.

8. What is the first consideration in treatment of a femoral fracture?
A femoral fracture is very painful because it produces strong muscle spasms in the thigh, which has the largest muscle mass in the body. Splinting or skin traction (max. 5 lbs) is recommended to improve patient comfort.

9. What general treatment methods can be used for femoral shaft fractures?
- **Operative,** including external or internal fixation
- **Nonoperative,** including immediate cast application or traction followed by cast immobilization

10. Identify the two basic types of traction.
Skin traction and skeletal traction. The latter involves drilling a traction pin through the distal femur from which the patient's limb is suspended.

11. When can Bryant's overhead skin traction be used?
Patients less than 20 lb or 2 years of age can be treated with overhead traction. Heavier patients risk neurovascular complications.

12. When is skeletal traction necessary?
Skeletal traction is only necessary for those fractures for which alignment cannot be controlled by skin treatment. This may include subtrochanteric fractures, which tend to flex and abduct excessively unless treated in 90°–90° skeletal traction.

13. Where should the traction pin be placed for skeletal traction?
The distal femur, proximal to the physis.

14. How long is traction required prior to cast application in those patients treated with traction?
The answer is dependent on age and fracture pattern. There must be adequate provisional callus to avoid excessive shortening once traction is removed. This varies from 7–10 days in the young child to as much as 3–4 weeks in the adolescent.

15. What are the relative indications for external fixation?
Again, this is a controversial area. Open fractures clearly can be treated with external fixators. Multiple injuries, a floating knee, or vascular injury are also good indications for external fixation.

16. What kind of cast must be used to treat femoral fractures?
Children with reliable families, <50 lbs, with fractures that are shortened <2 cm on initial radiographs.

17. In what position should the broken leg be placed?
The leg needs to be positioned in the optimum position to best reduce the fracture. This usually involves 30–45° of hip and knee flexion. The leg should be abducted or adducted to align the fracture. The anterior superior iliac spine, patella, and foot should be aligned to prevent rotational malunion.

18. What is the best treatment for closed femoral shaft fractures in children between the age of 5 years (or >50 lbs) and adolescence?
This area is controversial. Operative treatment with external fixation, in some authors' reports, has resulted in the lower total treatment cost, fewer x-rays, and far shorter hospitalization than traction followed by spica cast application.

19. What are the two basic types of intramedullary implants?
Reamed intramedullary rods or flexible intramedullary pins.

20. What are the candidates for reamed intramedullary nailing?
This is controversial. Good results have been described in patients as young as 5 years. Most surgeons reserve this treatment for the adolescent or older patient, however.

21. What is the most serious complication recently reported of reamed intramedullary nail use?
Avascular necrosis of the femoral head.

22. When are flexible intramedullary nails contraindicated?
In unstable comminuted or, possibly segmental fractures in which rotation and shortening will be difficult to control.

23. What are current operative methods for treatment of femoral shaft fractures?
Intramedullary rod (flexible or reamed), plate, or external fixation.

24. How should a femoral fracture with a coexisting severe closed head injury be treated?
With operative stabilization followed by either internal or external fixation. This approach facilitates nursing care (e.g., head position, moving patient), accommodates CT or MRI scans with ease, and promotes early rehabilitation.

25. List other indications for operative treatment of femoral fractures.
Associated vascular injury, compartment syndrome, and ipsilateral tibial shaft fracture.

26. Who are the best candidates for immediate spica treatment?
Patients less than 40–50 lbs. with a stable fracture pattern, less than 2 cm of initial shortening, and no associated injuries.

27. What is the most common complication following a femoral fracture?
Leg length discrepancy. Longitudinal growth may be accelerated in patients 2–11 years old, but is most commonly in those under age 8. This phenomenon, when it occurs, is limited to the first 18 months postinjury. Many authors have documented that this growth most often accounts for no more than 1 cm difference and is therefore insignificant.

28. What is the acceptable amount of angulation during healing?
This is somewhat controversial and is age- and direction-dependent. Anterior and posterior angulation in the plane of the knee joint will remodel more readily than varus and valgus angulation. Generally, guidelines should be <20 of anterior angulation and <10° of varus/valgus angulation in the preadolescent child.

29. How much shortening or overriding can be accepted?
Ideally, no more than 1–2 cm should be accepted. The principle of "overgrowth" in children between 2 and 11 years of age is hotly contested. Thus, one should not assume that initial shortening of 2 cm will ultimately resolve.

BIBLIOGRAPHY

1. Aronson DD, Singer RM, Higgins RF: Skeletal traction for fractures of the femoral shaft in children: A long-term study. J Bone Joint Surg 69A:1435–1439, 1987.
2. Aronson J, Tursky EA: External fixation of femur fractures in children. J Pediatr Orthop 12:157–163, 1992.
3. Bohn WW, Durbin RA: Ipsilateral fractures of the femur and tibia in children and adolescents. J Bone Joint Surg 73A:429–439, 1991.
4. Canale ST, Tolo VT: Fractures of the femur in children. J Bone Joint Surg 77A:294–315, 1995.
5. Herndon WA, Mahnken RF, Yngve DA, et al: Management of femoral shaft fractures in the adolescent. J Pediatr Orthop 9:29–32, 1989.
6. Martinez AG, Carrol NC, Sarwark JF, et al: Femoral shaft fractures in children treated with early spica cast. J Pediatr Orthop 11:712–716, 1991.
7. McCartney D, Hinton A, Heinrich SD: Operative stabilization of pediatric femur fractures. Orthop Clin North Am 25:635–650, 1994.
8. Reeves RD, Ballard RI, Hughes JL: Internal fixation versus traction and casting of adolescent femoral shaft fractures. J Pediatr Orthop 10:592–595, 1990.
9. Shapiro F: Fractures of the femoral shaft in children: The overgrowth phenomenon. Acta Orthop Scand 52:649–655, 1981.

34. HIP AND PELVIC FRACTURES

James H. Beaty, M.D.

1. Are hip fractures as common in children as in adults?
No. Fractures about the hip account for fewer than 1% of all pediatric fractures, and the prevalence of fractures of the hip in children is less than 1% of that in adults.

2. Why are fractures of the hip in children different from those in adults?

The anatomy of the proximal femur. In children, injuries can occur through the proximal femoral physis. Because the orientation of the trabeculae and femoral neck in children is not along stress lines, fracture surfaces are smooth with very little interlocking impaction, making closed reduction less stable in children.

3. How are hip fractures in children classified?

The most widely accepted classification is that proposed by Delbet. Type I fractures are transepiphyseal with or without dislocation from the acetabulum, type II are transcervical, type III are cervicotrochanteric, and type IV are intertrochanteric.

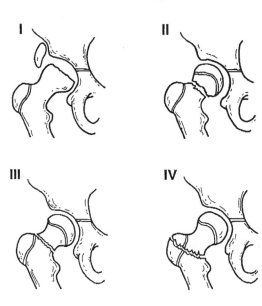

Classification of hip fractures in children. Type I, transepiphyseal with or without dislocation from the acetabulum. Type II, transcervical. Type III, cervicotrochanteric. Type IV, intertrochanteric. (From Canale ST, Beaty JH: Pelvic and hip fractures. In Rockwood CA Jr, Wilkins KE, Beaty JH (eds): Fractures in Children, 4th ed. Philadelphia, Lippincott-Raven, 1996, p 1151.)

4. What is the mechanism of injury?

Most hip fractures in children (75%) are caused by severe trauma and high-velocity forces, including motor vehicle accidents and falls. Other fractures can occur through pathologic bone, such as unicameral bone cysts, aneurysmal bone cysts, and fibrous dysplasia. In toddlers and infants, hip fractures can occur owing to child abuse.

5. How are hip fractures in children treated?

Treatment is based on fracture classification and degree of displacement. Occasionally in infants, closed reduction and spica casting can be used for minimally displaced type I injuries. For type I injuries in most children, however, closed or open reduction should be followed by internal fixation. Smooth pins can be used in children younger than the age of 6–8 years, and cannulated screw fixation can be used in children older than the age of 8 years. If the femoral head is dislocated from the acetabulum, closed reduction may be attempted once, but usually open reduction will be required. If open reduction is performed, the surgical approach should be in the direction of the dislocated femoral head (i.e., posterior approach for posterior dislocation of the femoral head and anterior approach for anterior dislocation). For type II transcervical fractures, closed or open reduction and pin or screw fixation are indicated.

Type III cervicotrochanteric fractures should be treated by reduction and internal fixation. Occasionally, with a completely nondisplaced fracture in a child younger than 8 years, spica cast immobilization is adequate; however, late displacement or coxa vara can occur, and close supervision and observation of the fracture are necessary during the initial week after injury. Any question of fracture stability should be an indication for reduction and internal fixation.

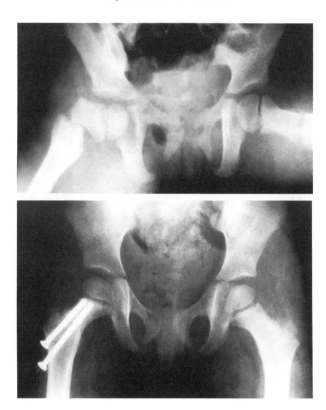

A, Type II (transcervical) displaced femoral neck fracture. *B*, After open reduction and internal fixation with 4.0-mm cannulated screws. (From Hughes LO, Beaty JH: Current concepts review. Fractures of the head and neck of the femur in children. J Bone Joint Surg 76A:283–292, 1994.)

Type IV intertrochanteric fractures can be treated by traction and casting in young children or by open reduction and internal fixation with a pediatric hip compression screw, especially in an older adolescent with multiple injuries.

6. What operative treatment is of benefit in hip fractures in children?

Surgery is most frequently indicated for placement of smooth pins or cannulated screw fixation after closed reduction of type II and III fractures. Open reduction through an anterolateral Watson-Jones approach frequently is required in children in whom adequate closed reduction cannot be obtained.

7. What surgical technique tips are helpful in the management of hip fractures in children?

The most important consideration is the choice of internal fixation, which is based on the child's age and the injury. In general, for types II and III fractures, I prefer smooth pins in children younger than 3 years of age, cannulated 4.0-mm screws in children aged 3–8 years, and 6.5-mm cannulated screws in children older than 8 years. I use a pediatric hip compression screw in the young child and an adult hip compression screw in older adolescents. The femoral neck in children is of harder consistency than the osteoporotic bone in elderly patients, so predrilling and pretapping may be necessary before the insertion of all screws. Spica casting after internal fixation of hip fractures frequently is required to support the internal fixation in children younger than 10 years. *The most important surgical goal is stable fixation of the fracture. Preservation of the physis of the proximal femur is a secondary goal!*

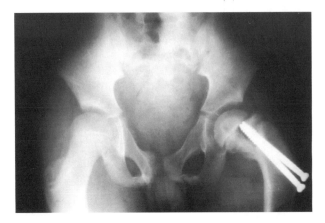

Unstable fixation of type II (transcervical) fracture with loss of reduction and nonunion. If fracture stability is questionable, fixation should extend into the femoral head, regardless of the type of fracture of age of the child. (From Canale ST, Beaty JH: Pelvic and hip fractures. In Rockwood CA Jr, Wilkins KE, Beaty JH (eds): Fractures in Children, 4th ed. Philadelphia, Lippincott-Raven, 1996, p 1163.)

The physis of the proximal femur only grows 3–4 mm a year, so fear of limb-length discrepancy should not compromise fracture fixation. If stability is questionable, the internal fixation device should extend into the femoral head for rigid stable fixation, regardless of the type of fracture or the child's age.

8. What are the major complications after hip fractures in children?

The most frequent complication is avascular necrosis of the femoral head, with an incidence of approximately 40%. I believe that avascular necrosis is related to the initial displacement of the fracture. About half of all displaced types II and III fractures and almost all type I fractures with dislocation of the femoral head will result in avascular necrosis.

Coxa vara deformity occurs after hip fractures in children owing to growth arrest of the proximal femoral physis or the fracture healing in a varus position. If the femoral neck–shaft angle decreases to 110° or less, subtrochanteric valgus osteotomy and fixation yield satisfactory results.

Nonunion after femoral neck fractures occurs in approximately 5% and can occur after the injury itself or if loss of reduction occurs after closed management or internal fixation. Treatment is early subtrochanteric valgus osteotomy, fixation, and bone grafting.

9. What is the prognosis for hip fractures in children?

Unfortunately, because of the high complication rate, the prognosis may be fair or guarded, especially if complications have occurred. If the fracture heals without avascular necrosis, coxa vara, or nonunion, the child should be followed to skeletal maturity to evaluate growth of the hip and extremity.

10. How are pelvic fractures in children different from those in adults?

Pelvic fractures can occur in children (as in adults) owing to high-velocity trauma. In children, however, because of the uniqueness of the skeletally immature pelvis, pelvic avulsion from muscle origins and insertions also can occur owing to less severe trauma and sports injuries. The other difference is the triradiate cartilage of the acetabulum, which when injured can cause acetabular dysplasia or growth disturbance in children. A child's pelvis is more flexible than an adult's, so single breaks in the pelvic ring are more common. Because significant pelvic-ring disruption is less frequent in children than in adults, the mortality rate in children with pelvic fractures is much lower than that in adults.

11. What are the clinical signs of pelvic fracture?

(1) A large hematoma superficially beneath the inguinal ligament or in the sacrum, (2) a decrease in

the distance from the greater trochanter to the pubic spine on the affected side in lateral compression fractures (Roux's sign), and (3) a bony prominence or large hematoma and tenderness on rectal examination, indicative of a severe pelvic fracture (Earle's sign). Posterior pressure on the iliac crest will cause pain at the fracture site as the pelvic ring is opened, and compression of the pelvic ring at the iliac crease from lateral to medial will cause pain and possibly crepitation. Downward pressure on the symphysis pubis and posteriorly on the sacroiliac joints will cause pain and motion if there is a break in the pelvic ring. Flexion and extension of the hips may cause pain in the inguinal area.

12. What type of imaging is useful?
In addition to anteroposterior and inlet and outlet roentgenograms of the pelvis, computed tomography is useful in complex injuries to assess possible articular surface involvement of the acetabulum and to evaluate injuries of the sacrum or sacroiliac joint.

13. What classification system is used to describe pelvic fractures in children?
In young children, Key and Conwell's classification, which describes single or multiple injuries of the pelvic ring and fractures of the acetabulum, can be used. In adolescents approaching skeletal maturity, the classifications of Letournel and Tile are more widely used.

14. What other injuries occur with pelvic fractures in children?
In a polytrauma setting, I frequently see children who have head, neck, chest, and abdominal injuries. Related or local injuries include vascular, urologic, and neurologic injuries. The greatest morbidity and mortality occur in children with more severe Malgaigne-type injuries. Hemorrhage is treated as in adults, including use of antishock trousers and arterial embolization. Frequently, simple placement of an external fixator in an unstable pelvis will decrease the number of raw bony surfaces and will help control hemorrhage. Urethral or bladder lacerations occur in about 5% of children with pelvic fractures and can be diagnosed by insertion of a Foley catheter followed by examination of the urine for gross or occult blood. With any signs of urinary tract disruption, a cystoureterogram should be performed followed by an intravenous pyelogram. Neuologic injury of the lower extremity is uncommon after pelvic fractures in children, occurring in about 1.5%.

15. Are pelvic fractures in children treated differently from those in adults?
Compared with pelvic fractures in adults, many of which are severe injuries that require surgical intervention, most pelvic fractures in children involve a single injury of the pelvis and can be treated nonoperatively with bed rest with or without traction and protected ambulation. For unstable Malgaigne-type injuries, either reduction with external fixation or a combination of external and internal fixation, especially of the sacroiliac joint, can be used. Malgaigne fractures in children younger than 4–5 years may remodel with conservative treatment, but in juvenile and adolescent children, treatment should be similar to that in adults.

16. How are avulsion fractures of the pelvis treated in children?
Conservative treatment (bed rest and protected ambulation) is sufficient for these injuries, and almost all patients return to their previous level of sports participation. Most pelvic avulsion fractures occur as a result of overpull of muscles in those participating in sports activities, especially gymnastics, football, and track.

17. What complications should be anticipated after pelvic fractures in children?
Complications are rare but can include nonunion, triradiate cartilage closure, avascular necrosis, sciatic nerve palsy, or myositis ossificans.

BIBLIOGRAPHY

1. Canale ST: Fractures of the hip in children and adolescents. Orthop Clin North Am 21:341–351, 1990.
2. Davison BL, Weinstein SL: Hip fractures in children: a long-term follow-up study. J Pediatr Orthop 12:355–388, 1992.

3. Forlin E, Guille JT, Kumar SJ, Rhee KJ: Complications associated with fracture of the neck of the femur in children. J Pediatr Orthop 12:503–509, 1992.
4. Garvin KL, McCarthy RE, Barnes CL, Dodge BM: Pediatric pelvic ring fractures. J Pediatr Orthop 10:577–582, 1990.
5. Hughes LO, Beaty JH: Current concepts review. Fractures of the head and neck of the femur in children. J Bone Joint Surg 76A:283–292, 1994.
6. Ismail N, Bellemare JF, Mollitt DL, et al: Death from pelvic fracture: children are different. J Pediatr Surg 31:82–85, 1996.
7. Oveson O, Arreskov J, Bellstrom T: Hip fractures in children: a long-term follow-up of 17 cases. Orthopedics 12:361–367, 1989.
8. Sundar M, Carty H: Avulsion fractures of the pelvis in children: a report of 32 fractures and their outcome. Skeletal Radiol 23:85–90, 1994.
9. Waters PM, Millis MB: Hip and pelvic injuries in the young athlete. Clin Sports Med 7:513–526, 1988.

35. FRACTURES OF THE NECK AND SPINE

Thomas S. Renshaw, M.D.

1. How common are fractures of the neck and spine in children?

Not very. Most large children's hospitals and trauma centers admit only 2–3 cases per year, and in published series of spinal injuries, children < 16 years old seldom comprise more than 10% of cases. About half the fractures occur in the cervical spine, and 40% of these are associated with neurologic injuries. Because considerable force is usually necessary to produce a fracture of the lower spine, it is not surprising that 50% of these fractures are associated with other injuries and 20% are accompanied by neurologic damage.

2. What are the most common causes of these injuries?

Motor vehicle accidents involving occupants of automobiles, pedestrians, bicyclists, motorcyclists, and riders of all-terrain vehicles are responsible for about 50% of these fractures. Other common causes are diving and other sports injuries, firearms, falls from a height, child abuse, and birth trauma.

3. How should suspected neck and spine injuries be handled at the trauma scene?

- All unconscious children should be assumed to have a spinal injury.
- Use sandbags and tape or, as a second choice, apply a cervical collar after gently placing the child on a rigid spine board while manually supporting the neck and spine in a neutral position (ear canal level with the center of the shoulder). *Do not apply traction. In an unstable spine, this can be catastrophic!*
- **In children < 8 years of age:** Because the head is disproportionately larger than the chest, a board with an occipital recess should be used or folded blankets placed under the chest to prevent cervical kyphosis. A small lumbar support will maintain normal lordosis when thoracolumbar or lumbar trauma is suspected.

4. What about neck injuries from football?

The helmet should be left in place, but the face mask cut away to facilitate airway management. At the hospital the neck is manually supported while the helmet is spread and then carefully removed without flexing the neck.

5. What steps should be taken in the emergency department when a child presents with possible fracture of the neck or spine?

ATLS principles are applied. Next, the spine is examined by looking for evidence of trauma to the head, neck, chest, abdomen, or extremities; palpating the spinous processes and paraspinal muscles; and performing a complete neurologic examination (repeated at intervals to detect progression or the late development of a lesion). A calm, gentle, thorough approach is essential when evaluating an uncooperative child.

6. Which imaging studies should be obtained?

To start, plain radiographs, which are taken without changing the protected alignment of the spine. The entire spine should be imaged in AP and lateral projections, as injuries at multiple spinal levels may occur in up to 15% of patients. However, obtaining an open-mouth odontoid view will be difficult at best and is often impossible.

An awake, cooperative child may be able to actively flex and extend his or her neck to permit assessment of cervical spine stability on the lateral views, but such flexion/extension should never be done passively in a less than completely responsive child. When neurologic abnormalities are present, an MRI may be necessary to define the pathology and assess for soft tissue lesions, such as disc or ligament disruption or spinal cord compression.

Remember that the anatomy of the young child's spine is different than the adult's and a knowledgeable expert in interpreting these imaging studies is essential, particularly at the atlanto-occipital and other cervical levels. Finally, the physician should not forget about SCIWORA (spinal cord injury without radiographic abnormality).

7. What are the normal radiographic variations in the child's cervical spine?

Myriad. For starters: synchondroses with variable closure times; multiple ossification centers; angulation of the dens; horizontal articular facets; absence of cervical lordosis; anterior vertebral body wedging; hypermobility from ligamentous laxity; psuedosubluxation at C1-C2, C2-C3, or C3-C4; congenital anomalies; prevertebral swelling from crying; etc.

8. What is SCIWORA?

This stands for spinal cord injury without radiographic abnormality. It represents from 10–30% of all spinal cord injuries in children and may present as delayed paralysis after transient symptoms at the time of the injury. SCIWORA is most likely caused by a subluxation or even a dislocation of the spine that has spontaneously reduced. It is more common in the cervical region and in younger, more elastic spines. An MRI may not reveal an identifiable myelopathic lesion, and dynamic films or fluoroscopy may or may not show an unstable spinal lesion. Somatosensory and/or motor-evoked potentials usually document abnormalities. Although patients with incomplete neurologic injuries often recover function, those with complete lesions almost never do. Treatment consists of immobilization of the spine for 3 months and then dynamic studies to confirm stability.

9. Should children with spinal cord injuries be given the steroid protocol?

Yes, although little data is available for children. Treatment with methylprednisolone in the first 8 hours postinjury may improve neurologic recovery. The dose is 30 mg per kg in a 15-minute bolus infusion, followed by a 45-minute pause, then a 23-hour maintenance infusion of 5.4 mg per kg per hour.

10. Explain the diagnosis and treatment of altanto-occipital disruption.

This lesion is rarely seen because most patients do not survive it. It is more common in young children than in adults because the cervical fulcrum is more cephalad and the facets more horizontal. Neurologic findings vary greatly and may include cranial nerve, brainstem, or more caudal signs.

The radiographic diagnosis can be a real bear. Films are often of poor quality. A pediatric orthopaedist and a pediatric orthopaedic radiologist should be called in. They will draw all sorts of strange lines on the films and use words like *basion, dens, opisthion, Power's ratio,* and *many eponymous lines.* Application of traction is absolutely contraindicated as it may cause fatal neurologic or vascular damage. Treatment is halo-cast or halo-brace immobilization, usually followed by a difficult posterior occipitocervical fusion when the child is stable.

11. Describe the cause and treatment of fracture of the atlas (the Jefferson fracture).
These are usually burst fractures that result from axial compression. They are very rare in children, because the synchondroses of the ring of C1 are flexible. CT imaging is most helpful and will distinguish fractures from normal synchondroses. Most fractures of the atlas are treated with halo immobilization for 2–4 months.

12. How do you put a halo on a small child?
Very carefully. In children under 7 years of age, a CT scan is recommended because the thickness of the skull is variable. The physician should use 8 or 10 pins, with 2 inch-pounds of torque, in children under 2 years of age; consult the CT image; and keep all pins below the greatest circumference of the cranium. Caution must be taken to avoid the supraorbital and supratrochlear nerves, and pins should not be put in the temporalis fossa. In children from 2–7 years of age, 6 or 8 pins with 4 or 5 inch-pounds of torque are used.

In children aged 7 or older, the skull may be considered as "adult." If a halo brace cannot be used, an experienced orthopaedist should be enlisted to help put on a Minerva cast, but care must be taken. Minerva casts can slide up or down and may fail to provide adequate immobilization.

13. Do odontoid fractures occur in children?
Yes. In young children these are usually separations through the physis (epiphysiolysis) at the base of the dens. Most are displaced and angulated, which makes diagnosis possible by plain radiography. Fractures through a more cephalad level of the odontoid are much less common.

14. How are these fractures treated?
Treatment consists of positional reduction and halo or Minerva cast immobilization for 2–3 months, followed by dynamic films to document stability and healing. Failure to diagnose this fracture may lead to development of a nonunion, the os odontoideum, which requires surgical C1-C2 fusion if unstable or painful, and sometimes even if not. The physis at the base of the dens closes by about age 8 years, so in older children odontoid fractures occur in adult patterns; however, these fractures are very rare until chronologic adulthood.

15. How often does traumatic atlantoaxial instability without fracture occur? How is it treated?
Not often. Usually the odontoid physis separates. However, the transverse ligament complex *can* rupture; this is detectable by noting an atlantodens interval of more than 5 mm on the neutral or flexion lateral radiograph. Treatment consists of positional reduction, usually by slight extension, and immobilization by halo cast or vest for 2–3 months, followed by dynamic films to assess stability. Posterior C1-C2 fusion is necessary if instability persists.

16. What about hangman's fracture (C2 pedicles)?
These fractures occur in children, even in infancy, but are rarely accompanied by neurologic deficit. The diagnosis can be confused by the normal, apparent anterior wedging of C3 and physiologic hypermobility at C2-C3 that are common in younger children. Treatment is nonsurgical, using halo immobilization after positional reduction of displaced fractures and a less complex orthosis for those with no or minimal displacement. Bony union is the rule in 3 months, and slight anterior displacement of the body of C2 is not uncommon. Surgery is reserved for nonunion (virtually unheard of).

17. Explain how birth injuries of the spine occur.
Fortunately, these injuries are becoming less common. Intrauterine trauma is usually the result of a hyperextended neck position; when this is detected, a caesarian section delivery should be considered. Neurologic injury has been reported in up to 25% of infants with this positioning. The other major cause of obstetrical trauma to the spine is traction on the head during a difficult delivery. Overstretching of the very elastic cervical spinal column can produce spinal cord damage

and must be avoided. Although an infant's vertebral column may stretch up to 2 inches and recover, the infantile spinal cord can rupture at greater than ¼ inch of stretch.

18. How do fractures in the mid and lower cervical spine in children differ from those fractures in adults?

Although cervical spine injuries in children younger than 8 years occur most often in the region from the occiput to C3, in older children and adolescents the most common injuries occur from C3 to C7. These injuries, which include compression fractures, burst fractures, and facet dislocations, are treated as one would manage an adult-type lesion. Two caveats to be kept in mind:

1. Use of allograft bone should be avoided in pediatric cervical fusions; it often does not heal well.

2. Anterior fusion, alone, is not appropriate in the young child; this can tether anterior growth and the unopposed posterior growth may produce a substantial kyphosis.

19. Are fractures in the thoracic, thoracolumbar, and lumbar regions also different in children?

Not as much as are fractures in the cervical spine. As in adults, compression fractures, fracture-dislocations, burst fractures, limbus fractures, and seat belt fractures may be seen. Compression fractures are common, but greater segmental elasticity plus increased disc and end-plate strength tend to spread forces over more levels. This results in more vertebral bodies being compressed, but to a lesser degree at each body. Superior end plates are injured more often than inferior, and the posterior column is more often spared. Although burst fractures are not as common in children, CT imaging will avoid mistaking a potentially unstable burst lesion for an uncomplicated compression fracture.

20. Is their treatment different?

Not very much. Fractures with some kyphotic deformity, especially if multiple vertebrae are involved, should be followed during growth so that appropriate intervention can prevent insidious progression of kyphosis. Without going into great detail, fractures with no significant malalignment, instability, or canal compromise can be treated by observation, an orthosis, or a cast. Those that do not meet these criteria should be considered for surgical treatment, which may include realignment, stabilization, decompression, and fusion.

21. What are the concerns when seat belt fractures occur in children?

These injuries occur in the lumbar and thoracolumbar regions with lap belts and in the cervical spine with shoulder restraints. Usually they are flexion-distraction injuries, and often sentinel contusions from the belt are present across the abdomen or chest. Children with seat belt fractures have a higher likelihood of spinal cord injury (up to 30%) than do adults. A high index of suspicion must be maintained for associated internal injuries.

Many of these fractures are reducible and stable in extension and can be maintained by an appropriate cast or orthosis. Those that do not reduce may require surgical realignment and posterior tension band fixation. It must be emphasized that use of car seats, seat belts, and air bags has saved many, many more lives than would have been the case had these children been unrestrained in automobile collisions. To be effective, these devices must be applied properly and used diligently. This requires adult responsibility, the lack of which should not be an indictment of the restraint system. Furthermore, in any collisions involving extreme forces, severe injuries and fatalities will still occur.

22. What is a limbus (vertebral end plate) injury?

It is a displaced transverse fracture involving all or part of the vertebral apophyseal end plate, with or without a small bony fragment attached to the apophysis. This makes it difficult or impossible to detect on a standard plain radiograph. The most accurate means of diagnosis is by CT imaging.

23. Is this something new?

No, just newly recognized and emphasized, thanks in large part to imaging techniques such as MRI and particularly CT scans, especially with contrast and/or 3-D reconstruction.

24. How is this lesion diagnosed and treated?

An end plate fracture is most often seen in the lumbar spine and may mimic a herniated disc, with low back pain, myospasm, weakness, numbness, and other signs and symptoms. The diagnosis is frequently delayed and undoubtedly some of these fractures have been misdiagnosed as SCI-WORA. Depending upon the alignment, stability, canal compromise, or neurologic deficit, these fractures may require operative decompression and fusion or may simply need a cast or an orthosis and monitoring.

25. What are the concerns when fractures of the transverse process and spinous process occur?

By themselves, these are innocuous injuries that are painful for a few weeks and require analgesics, but do not need reduction or immobilization. However, most are caused by substantial blunt trauma. Consequently, these fractures are often accompanied by other spinal injuries and major, perhaps life-threatening problems such as pelvic fractures, intra-abdominal trauma, or chest injuries. Diligent evaluation of the entire patient is therefore essential when these seemingly trivial fractures are encountered.

26. Are there common patterns of spinal fracture in child abuse?

Yes. The thoracolumbar and lumbar vertebrae are most often involved and multiple fractures are common. The lesion that most often results is anterior wedging from compression. Spinous and transverse process and end-plate fractures are sometimes encountered, and SCIWORA should be considered when neurologic deficit is present.

27. Any last take-home messages?

You bet. Physicians should always suspect spinal trauma when a child is badly injured. In addition, all health care providers who work with children should:

- Know the presenting signs and symptoms of spinal fractures (see table) and appropriate emergency care.
- Initiate and support efforts to increase the proper use of child restraint systems in automobiles.
- Learn about and advocate methods for reducing child pedestrian accidents.

Clinical Findings in Children's Spinal Fractures

Neck pain	Palpable spinal tenderness
Occipital pain	History of transient neurologic symptoms
Torticollis	Physical signs of trauma to the head, neck, or trunk
Limited active range of motion	A positive neurologic finding
Paraspinal muscle spasm	Any unconscious patient
A palpable spinous process gap	

BIBLIOGRAPHY

1. Bracken MB, Shepard MJ, Collins WF, et al. A randomized, controlled trial of methylprednisolone or naloxone in the treatment of acute spinal cord injury: Results of the Second National Acute Spinal Cord Injury Study. N Engl J Med 322:1405–1411, 1990.
2. Cattell HS, Filtzer DL. Pseudosubluxation and other normal variations of the cervical spine in children: A study of one hundred and sixty children. J Bone Joint Surg 47A:1295–1309, 1965.
3. Letts RM, ed: Management of Pediatric Fractures. New York, Churchill Livingstone, 1994.
4. McGrory BS, Klassen RA, Chao EYS, et al: Acute fractures of the cervical spine in children and adolescents. J Bone Joint Surg 75A:988–995, 1993.
5. Mubarak S, Camp J, Vuletich W, et al: Halo application in the infant. J Pediatr Orthop 9:612–614, 1989.
6. Pang D, Pollack IF: Spinal cord injury without radiographic abnormality in children: The SCIWORA syndrome. J Trauma 29:654–664, 1989.
7. Rumball K, Jarvis J: Seat belt injuries of the spine in young children. J Bone Joint Surg 74B:571–574, 1992.
8. Swischuk LE: The cervical spine in childhood. Curr Probl Diagn Radiol 13:1–26, 1986.
9. Weinstein SL, ed: The Pediatric Spine—Principles and Practice. New York, Raven Press, 1994.

36. SHOULDER INJURIES

Kathryn E. Cramer, M.D.

1. What is the most commonly fractured long bone in a child?
The clavicle.

2. Which portion of the clavicle is most commonly fractured in children?
Fractures involving the shaft account for approximately 85% of clavicle fractures in children.

3. What is the standard treatment for a clavicle shaft fracture in a child?
Clavicle shaft fractures in children heal rapidly, and treatment is symptomatic. While a figure-of-eight harness may be used, a sling is simpler and easier for children (and parents!) to manage.

4. Which long bone is the first to ossify?
The clavicle develops from two primary ossification centers that appear during the fifth or sixth week of fetal life.

5. Which epiphyseal center is the last to fuse?
The medial clavicle epiphysis forms a center of ossification at 18 years of age, and fusion with the metaphysis occurs between 22 and 25 years of age.

6. A 16-year-old football player is evaluated in the emergency room for complaints of shoulder pain after a block. Physical exam confirms local tenderness and swelling about the medial aspect of the clavicle. What injury is suspected?
Local swelling and tenderness about the medial clavicle should lead one to suspect a medial clavicle physeal injury or a medial clavicle shaft fracture.

7. What radiographic studies should be ordered?
A clavicle series should confirm the presence or absence of a shaft fracture, and a serendipity view (cephalic tilt) allows evaluation of the sternoclavicular joint. Computed tomography will delineate the direction and extent of displacement, if present.

8. Medial clavicular fractures can displace either anteriorly or posteriorly. Which occurs more commonly?
Because the posterior sternoclavicular ligament is stronger, anterior displacement is more common.

9. When reduced, which fracture is usually stable?
Posteriorly displaced fractures are generally stable when reduced, while anteriorly displaced fractures are notoriously less stable. Because these are physeal injuries in children, remodeling can be expected.

10. Posterior displacement of a medial clavicular physeal injury may compromise which vital structures?
The trachea, esophagus, and great vessels lie behind the medial clavicle and may be compressed if it is posteriorly displaced.

11. Which fracture occurs most commonly during birth?
The clavicle is most commonly fractured at birth. The incidence of clavicle fracture ranges from 2.8–7.2 per 1000 live births.

12. What factors are associated with neonatal clavicle fractures?
Newborn weight, gestational age, and shoulder dystocia.

13. Distal clavicle fractures in children have been described as "peeled bananas." What does this mean?
    In children, the ligamentous attachments to the distal clavicle are very strong. When the weaker bone or physis is fractured, the shaft portion of the clavicle may be displaced superiorly; however, the periosteal tube remains intact, held in position by the ligaments. The displaced shaft fragment comes out of the periosteal sleeve like a "banana from its skin." Because the periosteal tube is intact, remodeling occurs, and functional disability is rare.

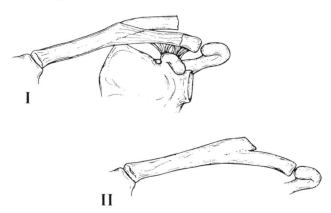

I, Distal clavicle fracture in a child. A banana "peeled" from its skin. II, Healing within the intact periosteal tube. (Reproduced with permission from Webb LX: Fractures and dislocations about the shoulder. In Green NE, Swiontkowski MF (eds): Skeletal Trauma in Children. Philadelphia, W.B. Saunders Co., 1993.)

14. What does "pseudodislocation" of the acromioclavicular joint in children mean?
The secondary ossification center of the distal end of the clavicle remains unossified until it unites with the shaft at approximately 19 years of age. The inherent weakness of the physeal-metaphyseal region during growth relative to the ligamentous structures makes fracture of the physis much more common than acromial-clavicular separation. While the injury may appear radiographically to be an acromial-clavicular separation, the unossified physis is the site of injury.

15. What treatment is appropriate?
Conservative treatment (sling or figure-of-eight harness) allows heating without functional disability.

16. What should the parents be told about the outcome?
A cosmetic "bump" over the injured area may result; however, function will be normal.

17. When does the proximal humeral physis close?
The proximal humeral physis generally closes between the ages of 14–17 years in girls and between the ages of 16–18 years in boys.

18. The Salter-Harris classification is widely used in describing physeal injuries in children. Using this classification system, what injury predominates in proximal humeral physeal fractures in children under the age of 5 years?
Salter-Harris I or transepiphyseal fractures predominate in very young children and are treated conservatively.

19. A 10-year-old boy is seen in the emergency room following a fall during a soccer game, complaining of shoulder pain. Although there is no gross deformity, his shoulder is swollen and tender to palpation over the proximal humerus. What radiographic studies are appropriate?
Appropriate radiographic studies include an anteroposterior (AP) and lateral view in the plane of the scapula and an axillary lateral view.

20. A moderately displaced proximal humeral physeal injury is discovered. What treatment should be prescribed?
Symptomatic treatment (sling or shoulder immobilizer) is adequate.

21. What is the prognosis?
The fracture will heal rapidly, and, because of the rapid growth of the proximal humeral physis, remodeling of the displacement will occur with time.

22. How are scapular fractures in children classified?
Scapular fractures in children are classified according to the anatomic areas involved. These include the body, glenoid, acromion, and coracoid.

23. What is an os acromiale?
The os acromiale is an acromial epiphysis that may be mistaken for a fracture. Careful clinical examination and comparison films may be helpful.

24. Which is correct? Anterior dislocation of the shoulder in children
  A. is associated with a high incidence of neurovascular injury
  B. is associated with a high recurrence rate
  C. results in permanent loss of range motion
  D. is extremely common.
Answer: **B.** Anterior dislocation of the shoulder in children is unusual, and associated neurovascular injury is rare. Full range of motion is usually regained quickly; however, the risk of recurrent dislocation is great.

25. Why are glenohumeral dislocations rare in children younger than 10 years of age?
During childhood, because the proximal humeral physis is open and there is rapid growth of the remodeling metaphysis, these areas are the weakest points in the glenohumeral articulation. During adolescence, as the bone in the metaphysis becomes stronger and the physis begins to close, dislocations occur more frequently.

26. Atraumatic voluntary dislocation of the shoulder is more common in which group of patients, children or adults?
Atraumatic voluntary dislocation of the shoulder is more commonly seen in children and may be seen in association with psychological problems. Patient education and physical therapy designed to strengthen the muscles about the shoulder are the mainstays of treatment.

27. A 6-month-old child is evaluated in the emergency room. A history obtained from the parents reveals that the child has not been moving the arm normally for several days. A nondisplaced spiral fracture of the humeral shaft is diagnosed based on radiographs. In addition to immobilizing the fracture, what else should be done?
A humeral shaft fracture in a very young child without a history of violent trauma should prompt the physician to investigate the possibility of child abuse.

BIBLIOGRAPHY

1. Black GB, McPherson JA, Reed MH: Traumatic pseudodislocation of the acromioclavicular joint in children. A fifteen year review. Am J Sports Med 19(6):644–646, 1991.

2. Chez RA, Carlan S, Greenberg SL, Spellacy WN: Fractured clavicle is an unavoidable event. Am J Obstet Gynecol 171(3):797–798, 1994.
3. Havranek P: Injuries of distal clavicular physis in children. J Pediatr Orthop 9(2):213–215, 1989.
4. Kohler R, Trillaud JM: Fracture and fracture separation of the proximal humerus in children: report of 136 cases. J Pediatr Orthop 3(3):326–332, 1983.
5. Larsen CF, Kiaer T, Lindequist S: Fractures of the proximal humerus in children. Nine-year follow-up of 64 unoperated on cases. Acta Orthop Scand 61(3):255–257, 1990.
6. Lewonowski K, Bassett GS: Complete posterior epiphyseal separation. A case report and review of the literature. Clin Orthop 281:84–88, 1992.
7. Marans HJ, Angel KR, Schemitsch EH, Wedge JH: The fate of traumatic anterior dislocation of the shoulder in children. J Bone Joint Surg [Am] 74(8):1242–1244, 1992.
8. Oppenheim WL, Davis A, Growdon WA, Dorey FJ, Davlin LB: Clavicle fractures in the newborn. Clin Orthop 250:176–180, 1990.
9. Thomas SA, Rosenfield NS, Leventhal JM, Markowitz RI: Long-bone fractures in young children: distinguishing accidental injuries from child abuse. Pediatrics 88(3)471–476, 1991.
10. Webb LX: Fractures and dislocations about the shoulder. In Green NE, Swiontkowski MF: Skeletal Trauma in Children. Philadelphia, W.B. Saunders Co., 1993, pp 257–282.

37. ELBOW INJURIES

K. *Wilkins*, M.D.

1. What are the bones most commonly injured around the elbow in children?

Around 86% of fractures in the elbow region occur in the distal humerus. Of these, 79.8% are supracondylar fractures, 16.9% involve the lateral condyle, and 12.5% involve the medial epicondyle. Medial condyle, T-condylar, and lateral epicondyle fractures combined occur less than 1% of the time.

2. What is a supracondylar fracture of the humerus?

It is a fracture through the distal metaphysis, proximal to the distal physis (growth plate). The fracture is usually transverse in the coronal plane (medial to lateral). In the sagittal (anterior to posterior) plane, the fracture line is often oblique, from anterior distal to posterior proximal.

3. Why are extension supracondylar fractures commonly seen in the last half of the first decade (i.e., 6–7 years)?

Around the age of 6–7 years, the child achieves maximum ligamentous laxity. Thus, when the child falls on the outstretched upper extremity, the elbow is directed into a hyperextension position. This forces the tip of the olecranon into its fossa. As a result, all the linear force originally directed proximally up the upper extremity when the hand hit the ground is converted to a bending force in the supracondylar area of the distal humerus. Since this is new and relatively immature metaphyseal bone, it fails quite easily. The degree of completeness of the fracture depends on the combination of the bending moment and the severity of the force applied.

4. What are the major displacement patterns of extension supracondylar fractures and how is this classification used in determining the method of treatment?

Type I displaced fractures are essentially undisplaced and can be treated with simple immobilization using either a long-arm cast or a posterior splint.

Type II fractures usually have enough intrinsic stability, because of the intact posterior cortex, that when the elbow is flexed up to the safe limit of 120°, the distal fragment does not rotate when the upper extremity is fully internally or externally rotated. Thus, this type of fracture pattern can be treated with long-arm cast in which the elbow is flexed up to around 120°. If there is so much swelling about the elbow that there is evidence of vascular compromise distal to the extremity at 120° of elbow flexion, then this *type II* fracture must be stabilized as for *type III* fractures so that the elbow can be placed in less flexion.

Type III fractures are completely displaced, and thus there is no intrinsic stability. In addition, because of the more severe nature of this injury, there is usually a much greater degree of swelling of the soft tissues around the elbow. As a result, once a closed reduction is achieved, it is usually stabilized by pins placed percutaneously across the fracture fragments. Once stabilized by these pins, the elbow is then protected with a splint or cast. Because the fragments are stabilized internally, the elbow can then be immobilized at the safer angle of 90° of flexion.

5. What are the two major types of supracondylar fractures?

The *extension type* is most common, observed in 90–95% of all supracondylar fractures. This type is caused by a hyperextension mechanism in which the distal fragment (distal metaphysis and humeral condyles) is displaced posterior to the proximal fragment.

The *flexion type* usually occurs when the child falls directly on the flexed elbow. In this type, the distal fragment is hyperflexed and lies anterior to the distal fragments. It is less common, accounting for only 5–10% of all supracondylar fractures.

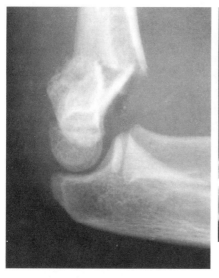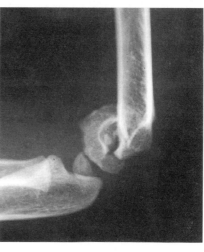

Left, Extension-type supracondylar fracture in which the distal fragment is extended and posterior to the proximal fragment. Right, Flexion-type pattern in which the distal fragment is flexed and anterior to the proximal fragment.

6. What are the associated injuries occurring with extension supracondylar fractures?

Nerve injuries. Any of the three major nerves (median, radial, ulnar) can be injured with supracondylar fractures. Originally it was shown that the *radial nerve* was the most commonly injured in extension supracondylar fractures. Recent studies by Cramer and associates have shown, however, that if a very careful neurologic examination is performed, one will find that the *anterior interosseous nerve* is probably the most commonly injured. This branch of the median nerve stimulates the muscles that flex the interphalangeal joints of the index finger and thumb. There is no sensory deficit. Fortunately, at least 95% of the nerve injuries resolve spontaneously. The *ulnar nerve* is most commonly injured with flexion supracondylar fractures.

Vascular injuries. The brachial artery can be injured by the sharp edge of the distal portion of the proximal fragment. This more commonly occurs if the distal fragment is displaced both posteriorly and laterally. The range of injuries varies from temporary compression to partial or complete obstruction due to interval tears to complete rupture of the artery. Fortunately, in most cases, there is sufficient collateral circulation to maintain the viability of the extremity.

Compartment syndrome. In some cases, injury to the brachial artery produces vasospasm at the meta-arteriole level, producing ischemia of the forearm muscles, especially the flexors. This ischemia causes a dysfunction of the muscle cell, resulting in severe swelling of the compartment, which in turn produces more ischemia. If not recognized early, the muscle cells become fibrotic, producing the characteristic *Volkmann's ischemic contracture.* Fortunately, this complication occurs in less than 1% of cases.

7. What are the classic clinical findings for an impending forearm compartment syndrome associated with a supracondylar fracture?

Remember the 5 Ps. The extremity is usually **pulseless.** (In some cases, however, the pulse may be present.) There is usually severe **pain** in the forearm due to ischemia of the muscles. There is dysfunction of the muscles manifest by **paralysis.** The compromise of the arterial supply produces **pallor.** Compression of the nerves produces **paresthesias** and in some cases even anesthesia.

8. What is the most common iatrogenic complication?

The most common problem associated with inadequate treatment of extension supracondylar fractures is a deformity termed *cubitus varus.* This occurs because the distal fragment can tilt into a varus alignment in relationship to the shaft if the fragment is neither adequately reduced nor stabilized (see Figure).

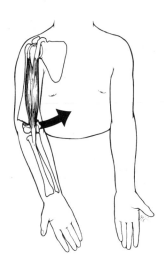

Cubitus varus deformity. The eccentric pull of the biceps tilts the distal fragment into varus position (*arrow*), producing the gunstock deformity of cubitus varus.

9. What are the effects of a cubitus varus deformity?

Usually, this results primarily in a strictly cosmetic deformity in which there is an unsightly prominence of the lateral condyle and the forearm is angulated in a varus direction in relation to the arm. There is rarely significant functional deficit associated with this malalignment of the distal fragment.

10. How long does it take for this fracture to heal?

Since this is an area of active growing bone, healing is rapid. There is usually adequate fracture callus to remove all forms of stability (pins, casts) at 3 weeks to allow *active* motion.

11. What is the usual long-term outcome of these fractures?

If an adequate reduction is achieved and stabilization is appropriate, a full return of motion can usually be expected in almost all cases. Because of the magnitude of soft tissue injury, it may be 2–3 months after case removal before full elbow motion has been accomplished. Postfracture physical therapy usually is not indicated. In fact, it may lead to a delay in resumption of motion.

12. What is the most common iatrogenic complication of a flexion supracondylar fracture?
Flexion injuries, if not adequately reduced, may result in loss of elbow extension. The cosmetic deformity associated with this fracture pattern is most commonly a cubitus valgus deformity.

13. What is a fracture of the lateral condyle?
Characteristically, this is an injury in which instead of being completely transverse, the fracture line goes obliquely from the articular surface of the distal humerus and exits laterally in the lateral distal humeral metaphysis. The fracture can originate in either the radiocapitellar groove (Milch type I) or the trochlea (Milch type II).

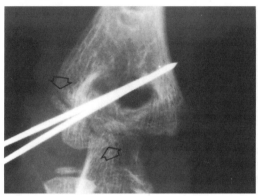 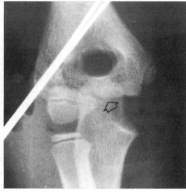

A   B

Lateral condyle fractures. The fracture line (*arrows*) can originate in either the radial capitellar grove (A) or the trochlea (B). The fracture line exits in the lateral metaphysis.

14. How does the mechanism of injury in this fracture differ from that of a supracondylar fracture?
The injury is created when the elbow is forced into varus. The fragment is either pulled off by the extensor muscles or pushed off by the radial head or semilunar notch of the olecranon.

15. What are the possible long-term effects of this injury?
Since this is an exact-fitting joint, if the articular surface is not reduced to an anatomic alignment, incongruity may result, producing loss of motion with subsequent degenerative arthritis. In addition, since the fracture line traverses the physeal plate, growth abnormalities can occur, which also can create functional difficulties. Rarely does this type of fracture produce any type of injury to the neurovascular structures.

16. How are the types of lateral condylar fractures differentiated?
Stage I. The fracture fragment is essentially undisplaced. The fracture gap is < 2 mm.
Stage II. There is greater than 2 mm of gap between the fragments, but the condylar fragment is still in close proximity to the distal humerus and is usually laterally rotated only minimally.
Stage III. There is wide displacement, and the condylar fragment is markedly rotated, in some cases as much as 180°, so that the articular surface may be facing the fracture surface of the distal humerus.

17. How does the clinical appearance of lateral condylar fractures differ from that of supracondylar fractures?
With lateral condylar fractures, usually there is little displacement in the sagittal plane so that the elbow does not appear hyperextended. Since the fracture line involves only the lateral articular surface, hematoma formation is usually localized laterally over the condyle. Because of the lesser displacement, the degree of pain is often less with lateral condyle fractures.

18. How does the stage of displacement affect the usual treatment of these injuries?

Stage I injuries usually require only immobilization with a cast or splint until there is sufficient fracture callus seen on the follow-up x-rays.

Stage II injuries require reduction of the condylar fragment and stabilization with smooth pins
placed across the fracture site. In some cases, if the fracture hematoma is still fresh and the displacement is minimal, the reduction can be achieved by closed manipulation and the pins placed
across the fracture site by percutaneous techniques using an image intensifier.

In many stage II fractures and almost all stage III fractures, the fracture fragment cannot be
reduced adequately by closed manipulative techniques. In these cases, the fracture site must be
approached surgically first to achieve a reduction. Then the fracture fragments are stabilized with
two pins, usually placed laterally across the fracture site.

19. What is the most common complication of the treatment of stage I fractures?

In these fractures, the lateral condylar fragment contains the origin of the forearm extensor muscles. Even if immobilized in a cast, these muscles can still contract and cause a late displacement
of the condyle fragments. Thus, if this type of lateral condyle fracture is immobilized only with
a cast or splint, it needs to be followed and x-rays must be taken again at 5 to 7 days to be sure
there is no late displacement. Fractures stabilized with pins do not, as a rule, displace late.

20. How long do these fractures require immobilization?

The cast or pins can be removed in 3 weeks to allow early active motion.

**21. What is the more common injury involving the distal humerus in infants and small chil-
dren?**

The entire distal humeral physis becomes separated from the distal humeral metaphysis. The distal fragment involves both the lateral and the medial condyles.

22. How is a fracture of the distal humeral physis recognized?

In some patients, especially very young infants, the secondary centers have not ossified. The
diagnosis is correlated with the clinical finding of severe elbow swelling and so-called muffled
crepitus (named because the raw fracture edge of the distal metaphysis is rubbing against the
softer physeal cartilage of the distal fragment). On radiographs, the proximal forearm ossification
centers lie posterior and medial to the ossification of the distal humeral metaphysis. The exact lo-

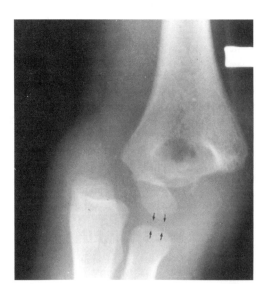

A fracture of the distal humeral physis in which
the ossification center of the lateral condyle remains aligned with the proximal radius (*arrows*). The proximal portion of the distal fragment is displaced posteriorly and medially.

cation of the unossified epiphyseal fragment must be confirmed with either an elbow arthrogram or ultrasound.

In the older child in whom the lateral condyle has ossified, this secondary ossification is always directly opposite the proximal radial metaphysis. The distal epiphyseal fragment is almost always posterior and medial to the distal humeral metaphysis.

23. What is the most common mechanism for fractures of the entire distal humeral physis?
In the small infant, this is usually the result of a twisting force. Children of this age do not run and thus don't fall on their outstretched extremities. As a result, many of these injuries in this age group are the result of child abuse.

24. How are fractures of the entire distal humeral physis usually treated?
Usually, these fractures are easily reduced with manipulative closed reduction. Because in a small child the extremity is short and fat, however, cast immobilization is usually inadequate. These fractures almost all require stabilization with pins placed percutaneously. At the time of the reduction, an arthrogram is usually required to confirm the adequacy of the reduction.

25. What are the most common complications associated with fractures of the entire distal humeral physis?
Often these are unrecognized or neglected, especially if the injury is the result of child abuse. Fortunately, these fractures heal quite rapidly with considerable remodeling. If the distal epiphyseal fragment remains tilted, however, some degree of cubitus varus may remain. Rarely is cubitus varus following this injury of significant magnitude to require surgical correction.

In some cases, the vessels supplying the secondary ossification centers of the trochlea (medial condyle) can be injured. Avascular necrosis develops, resulting in a secondary disruption of the articular surface with loss of elbow motion.

26. Do fractures of the medial condyle occur in children?
Yes, but they are very rare, accounting for less than 0.5% of fractures of the distal humerus.

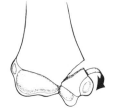

Fracture of the medial condyle. This includes the medial epicondyle and the ossification center of the medial aspect of the trochlea. This fragment may be displaced anteriorly and medially by the origin of the forearm flexor muscles (*arrow*).

27. What is an epicondyle?
An epicondyle is an apophysis; i.e., it is a secondary ossification center for a bony prominence that serves as the origin of muscles. The medial epicondyle is a separate prominence that serves as the origin of the forearm muscles. In the distal humerus, the medial epicondyle ossifies at about 5–7 years of age. The lateral epicondyle serves as the origin of the muscles for the forearm extensors. This secondary ossification center ossifies around the age of 9–11 years.

28. What is the most common humeral epicondyle injury?
Avulsion of the medial humeral epicondyle accounts for about 14% of all injuries involving the distal humerus in the child. Isolated fractures of the lateral humeral epicondyle are extremely rare.

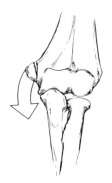

The medial epicondyle is often avulsed by the ulnar collateral ligaments or flexor muscles of the forearm (*arrow*).

29. With what other elbow injury is a fracture of the medial epicondyle often associated?

The medial (ulnar) collateral ligaments all arise from the medial epicondyle. When the elbow sustains a traumatic dislocation in the adult patient, the collateral ligaments are often ruptured. In the pediatric patient, however, the collateral ligaments are stronger than the physeal plate of the medial epicondyle. Thus, failure occurs through the relatively weaker physeal plate of the epicondyle. In more than 50% of acute traumatic elbow dislocations in pediatric patients, the medial epicondyle may be avulsed from its attachment to the distal humerus.

Other mechanisms of injury, such as direct blows to the epicondyle, sudden forceful flexure muscle forces as seen with arm wrestling or throwing, or simply a severe valgus stress to the elbow, can also cause the epicondyle to become avulsed from the distal humerus.

30. What is the most severe complication associated with avulsions of the medial epicondyle?

When the elbow is dislocated, the epicondylar fragment can become interposed between the articular surface of the distal humerus and the olecranon. When the elbow is reduced, this epicondylar fragment usually is extruded to return to close to its original attachment to the distal humerus. It may remain within the joint, however. If unrecognized, this interposed epicondyle can produce severe damage to the articular surface of the elbow. In addition, the incarcerated epicondyle and adjacent flexor mass may become wrapped around the ulnar nerve to produce compression neuropathy.

Thus, after reducing a traumatic elbow dislocation, it is very important to be sure that the medial epicondyle has not become incarcerated within the joint and that the ulnar nerve is functioning fully.

31. How are avulsion fractures of the medial epicondyle usually treated?

Treatment usually is by nonoperative methods. The key is to re-establish elbow motion with encouragement of early active motion exercises. Even if the epicondylar fragment remains displaced and forms a fibrous nonunion, rarely is there any significant disability in elbow function.

32. What are the indications for surgical fixation of the medial epicondyle?

First and foremost, if the epicondylar fragment is incarcerated within the joint, it must be removed surgically.

The other indications for surgical intervention remain controversial. Some believe that in high-performance athletes who use their upper extremities extensively, the elbow must be extremely stable. There is some evidence that an ununited medial epicondyle may produce sufficient elbow instability to interfere with high performance. Thus, in these individuals, open reduction with internal fixation of the fragment may be indicated.

The presence of ulnar nerve dysfunction is relative. Certainly, if both motor and sensory functions are lacking, the epicondyle and nerve should be explored. If there is only mild paresthesia or motor weakness, then simple observation may be appropriate.

33. What is the most common complication associated with avulsion of the medial epicondyle?

Although incarceration of the epicondyle within the elbow joint can produce severe elbow dysfunction, it is a relatively rare complication. The most common sequela following this injury is loss of elbow motion. This is especially true if it is associated with an elbow dislocation.

34. In the pediatric patient, what portion of the proximal radius is especially vulnerable to injury and why?

The *radial neck* is the area of the proximal radius most commonly injured. This is because it is a metaphyseal structure, composed of a high percentage of weak cancellous bone.

35. Where may the pain associated with a fracture of the radial neck manifest?

Often in the child, pain associated with a fracture of the radial neck is referred to the area of the wrist. The key to differentiating an injury of the radial neck from an injury of the distal radius is that there is usually no swelling or local tenderness over the distal radius with a fracture of the radial neck. The tenderness and swelling are localized distally at the elbow over the proximal radius. In addition, the pain of a fracture of the radial neck is accentuated when the forearm is supinated and pronated.

36. What are the major mechanisms of injury for fractures of the radial neck in children?

The most common mechanism is a *valgus force* applied to the elbow. A compressive force is applied against the radial head by the lateral condyle. Failure occurs at the weaker area of the radial neck. In this type of fracture, the radial head is forced into varying degrees of lateral angulation and translocation in relationship to the distal shaft.

A second, but rarer, mechanism occurs *during an elbow dislocation*. The lateral condyle can force the radial head off during either dislocation or reduction. In this rarer mechanism, the radial head is usually completely dislocated from the radial shaft.

The radial neck can also undergo stress fractures, which are very rare. Torsional injuries can force the neck and shaft away from the head. The shaft is primarily displaced, and the head remains within the confines of the orbicular ligament.

37. What warning should the parents of a child with a fracture of the radial neck be given prior to initiating treatment?

In this injury, the bone is small, and to the uneducated eye of the parents, the fracture displacement often appears minimal. The parents need to understand that in addition to the fracture there is often a considerable amount of soft tissue injury, especially if the head fragment is displaced. Because of this soft tissue injury, there may be postreduction stiffness, especially with loss of supination and pronation, even if an anatomic reduction is achieved. This is especially true if the reduction has to be achieved by open operative techniques.

38. In fractures of the radial neck, what are the usually accepted methods of treatment?

In the more common *valgus injuries*, the treatment is usually dictated by the degree of angulation with the radial neck. Angulation of 30° probably does not need manipulation. Greater than 30° but less than 60° of angulation can usually be reduced to an acceptable limit of less than 30° by one of the closed manipulative techniques. Greater than 60° of angulation usually requires some type of operative technique to obtain an adequate reduction.

In completely displaced *fractures associated with the elbow dislocations*, an open operative procedure is almost always required.

39. What other injuries are commonly associated with fractures of the radial neck?

Since this fracture is most commonly the result of a valgus stress to the elbow, the medial epicondyle may be avulsed. This valgus stress can also produce a greenstick fracture of the olecranon.

40. What are the common complications associated with fractures of the radial neck?
The most common complication is a loss of range of forearm motion, usually pronation. Other complications such as radial head overgrowth, nonunion, avascular necrosis of the radial head, or proximal radioulnar synostosis can also result in a loss of elbow or forearm motion.

41. What is unique about the ossification process of the olecranon?
The olecranon is structurally an apophysis that serves primarily as the insertion for the triceps tendon. This apophysis contributes very little to the length of the ulna. The apophysis may have more than one ossification center. Initially, the unossified portion of the olecranon apophysis supports greater than 50% of the articular surface of the olecranon. As it matures, the ossification front of the proximal metaphysis of the olecranon migrates proximally so that it supports only 25% or less of the articular surface.

42. What are the common mechanisms responsible for fractures of the olecranon in children?
The most common mechanism is probably an injury that occurs with the elbow locked in extension (*extension injury*). In this position, the forearm is subjected to varus or valgus forces, causing the metaphyseal portion of the olecranon to undergo a greenstick type of failure. If a valgus force is applied, there is usually an associated fracture of the radial neck laterally or avulsion of the medial epicondyle medially. If a varus force is applied, the radial head may dislocate (Monteggia type III lesion).

If the elbow is forced into hyperextension, a type of failure may occur in which the posterior cortex or periosteum of the olecranon is intact, but the anterior articular surface is disrupted.

If the elbow is stressed while it is flexed (*flexion injury*), failure of the olecranon metaphysis occurs posteriorly, and there is a resultant separation of the fragments with a loss of the extension mechanism of the elbow.

43. How are extension fractures of the olecranon commonly treated in children?
In varus and valgus injuries, the elbow is manipulated into extension and the deformity is corrected by applying the reverse force (i.e., a varus force applied to a valgus deformity).

In hyperextension injuries, if the posterior extension mechanism remains intact, the fracture can be reduced by simply hyperflexing the elbow.

44. How are flexion injuries of the olecranon treated?
With these injuries, the posterior extensor mechanism of the olecranon is usually completely disrupted. If there is only a slight displacement (i.e., 2 mm or less), the elbow can be forced into extension and immobilized in this position until adequate callus is produced. Usually, there is greater than 2 mm of disruption, and thus the fracture fragments need to be reduced by operative methods. Because of the deforming effect of the extensor forces on the muscles, this reduction needs to be secured with some type of internal fixation device.

45. How are Monteggia's lesions classified?
The four basic types are based on the direction of displacement of the radial head and the fracture pattern of the proximal ulna.

Type I. In this type, the radial head is displaced *anteriorly*, and there is an oblique fracture of the proximal shaft of the ulna. This type usually occurs as the result of a hyperextension force to the forearm and elbow.

Type II. This type is extremely rare in children. The fracture pattern is a flexion type of injury to the proximal ulnar metaphysis. The radial head dislocates *posteriorly*. The mechanism is usually the same as for traumatic dislocation of the elbow in which a linear force is applied proximally up the forearm to a semiflexed elbow.

Type III. This is the result of application of a varus force to the extended elbow. There is a greenstick varus fracture of the proximal ulna or olecranon and a lateral dislocation of the radial head.

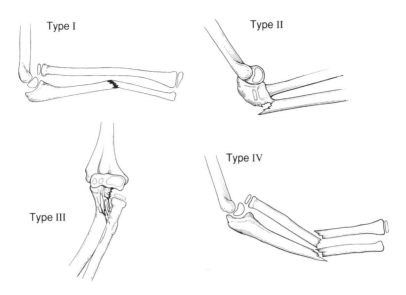

The four types of Monteggia's lesions.

Type IV. This is a fracture involving the shafts of both the radius and the ulna (usually at different levels) and an associated dislocation of the radial head, which is usually either anteriorly or laterally.

46. What are Monteggia's equivalents?

These are injuries involving the proximal radius or ulna for which Bado believed that the mechanism of injury was similar to that of a classic Monteggia's lesion. With the exception of the type IV lesion, equivalents have been described for each of the major types of lesions. For example, an isolated traumatic dislocation of the radial head is classified as a type I equivalent.

47. What frequent iatrogenic complications are associated with Monteggia's fracture?

Often, the fracture of the ulna is quite obvious both clinically and radiographically. The dislocation of the radial head may be subtle and may not be appreciated. If left untreated, this chronically dislocated radial head can produce a significant disability in elbow function.

Thus, it is extremely important in all cases in which the ulnar shaft is fractured to inspect the relationship of the radial head to the ossification center of the lateral condyle carefully to be sure that there is not a coexistent disruption of this joint. A line drawn proximally up the long axis of the proximal radius through the radial head should always pass proximally through the center of the ossification center of the lateral condyle.

48. How are type I Monteggia's lesion usually treated?

Treatment of the type I lesion requires two steps. First, the length of the ulnar shaft must be re-established by reducing the fracture, which is usually angulated anteriorly. Once the ulnar length has been re-established, the second step is to reduce the radial head. This is usually easily performed by applying a force directly over it in a posterior direction while hyperflexing the elbow. If the ulnar fracture is unstable, it may need to be stabilized with an intramedullary pin. After reduction, the elbow is immobilized in some degree of hyperflexion to decrease the potential of the deforming force on the biceps muscle.

On rare occasions, the orbicular ligaments may become interposed, preventing closed reduction of the radial head. In this case, open reduction may be necessary.

49. How are type II Monteggia's lesions usually treated?

The olecranon fracture and radial head can usually both be reduced by extending the elbow and immobilizing it in extension.

50. How are type III Monteggia's lesions usually treated?

These are essentially extension varus greenstick fractures of the olecranon. The olecranon fracture is first reduced by extending and applying a valgus force to the elbow. This usually simultaneously reduces the radial head. Occasionally, as with type I lesions, the orbicular ligament becomes interposed and may require surgical extraction.

51. How are type IV Monteggia's lesions usually managed?

The type IV lesion is converted to a type I lesion by surgically stabilizing the shafts of both the radius and the ulna with either intramedullary fixation or plates and screws. Once the shafts have been stabilized, the radial head is then reduced by manipulation in the same manner as for a type I lesion.

52. What is the common injury associated with type III lesions?

The anterolateral displacement of the radial head may produce compression of the posterior interosseous branch of the radial nerve. This results in a loss of wrist and finger extension. Almost all these disorders resolve following reduction of the radial head.

53. How does the incidence per age group of elbow dislocations differ from that of supracondylar fractures?

The peak age incidence for supracondylar fractures is 7 years, which is the period of maximum ligamentous laxity. Elbow dislocations tend to be more of a second decade injury, with the peak occurring around 12–13 years of age.

54. In what direction do most elbow dislocations occur?

In most traumatic elbow dislocations, the proximal radioulnar complex displaces in a posterolateral direction.

55. What is a nursemaid's elbow?

A so-called "nursemaid's elbow" usually occurs before the age of 5 years. It occurs when the forearm is pulled into hyperpronation as the elbow is forced simultaneously into extension. Because of the weakness of its distal portion, the orbicular ligament slips proximally over the radial head to become interposed between the lateral condyle and the radial head. With the orbicular ligament interposed between the articular surfaces, the child becomes reluctant to flex the elbow and holds it in an extended position at the side of the body.

Reduction is easily achieved by reversing the inciting mechanism; i.e., the forearm is supinated and the elbow is forced into hyperflexion. If the surgeon's thumb is placed over the lateral edge of the radial head as this is performed, the orbicular ligament can be felt as it is extruded out of the elbow joint. Elbow pain is soon relieved, and the patient promptly resumes active elbow flexion.

BIBLIOGRAPHY

1. Bado, JL: The Monteggia lesion. Clin Orthop 50:71–86, 1967.
2. Bernstein SM, King JD, Sanderson RA: Fractures of the medial epicondyle of the humerus. Contemp Orthop 637–641, 1981.
3. Cramer KE, Green NE, Devito DP: Incidence of anterior interosseous nerve palsy in supracondylar humerus fractures in children. J Pediatr Orthop 13:502–505, 1993.
4. DeLee JC, Wilkins KE, Rogers LF, Rockwood CA Jr: Fracture separation of the distal humerus epiphysis. J Bone Joint Surg 62A:46–51, 1980.
5. Flynn JC, Zink WP: Fractures and dislocations of the elbow. In MacEwen GD, Kasser JR, Heinrich SD (eds): Pediatric Fractures, A Practical Approach to Assessment and Treatment. Baltimore, Williams & Wilkins, 1993.

6. Foster DE, Sullivan JA, Gross RH: Lateral humeral condylar fractures in children. J Pediatr Orthop 5:16–22, 1985.
7. Fowles JV, Kassab MT: Displaced fractures in the medial humeral condyle in children. J Bone Joint Surg 62A:1159–1163, 1980.
8. Green NE: Fractures and dislocations about the elbow. In Green NE, Swiontkowski MF (eds): Skeletal Trauma in Children. Philadelphia, W.B. Saunders Co., 1994.
9. Jakob R, Fowles JV: Observations concerning fractures of the lateral humeral condyle in children. J Bone Joint Surg 57B:430–436, 1975.
10. Josefsson PO, Danielsson LG: Epicondylar elbow cases: 35 years follow-up of 56 unreduced cases. Acta Orthop Scand 57:313–315, 1986.
11. Letts J, Locht R, Wiens J: Monteggia fracture dislocations in children. J Bone Joint Surg 65B:724–727, 1985.
12. McIntyre W: Supracondylar fractures of the humerus. In Letts RM (ed): Management of Pediatric Fractures. New York, Churchill Livingstone, 1994.
13. Ogden JA: Elbow. In Skeletal Injury in the Child, 2nd ed. Philadelphia, W.B. Saunders Co., 1990.
14. Pirone AM, Graham HK, Krajbich JL: Management of displaced extension-type supracondylar fractures of the humerus in children. J Bone Joint Surg 70A:641–650, 1988.
15. Rang M: Elbow. In Children's Fractures, 2nd ed. Philadelphia, J.B. Lippincott Co., 1983.
16. Salter RB, Zaltz C: Anatomic investigations of the mechanism of injury and pathologic anatomy of "pulled elbow" in young children. Clin Orthop 77:134–143, 1971.
17. Wilkins KE: The operative management of supracondylar fractures. Orthop Clin North Am 21:269–289, 1990.
18. Woods GM, Tullos HG: Elbow instability and medical epicondyle fracture. Am J Sports Med 5:23–30, 1977.
19. Yoo CI, Kim YJ, Suh JT, Kim HT, Suh KT, Kim YH: Orthopedic surgery in Korea. Avascular necrosis after fracture separation of the distal end of the humerus in children. Orthopaedics 15:959–963, 1992.

38. FOREARM FRACTURES

Richard M. Kirby, M.D.

1. How do you differentiate between a wrist sprain and a fracture?
Wrist sprains are rare in children; if a sprain is being considered, the most likely diagnosis is a distal radius fracture. The differential diagnosis is really between a **contusion** and a fracture. The best finding on clinical examination (unless there is obvious deformity) is **point tenderness**. When in doubt, immobilize the wrist in a splint or cast for a couple of weeks, and then repeat x-rays.

2. If a forearm fracture is suspected, what x-rays should be ordered?
Most fractures are visible with standard anteroposterior (AP) and lateral radiographs of the forearm. It is essential to include the entire forearm, including the wrist and elbow joints. True AP and lateral x-rays require proper positioning for both views. A common error is to obtain the second view by rotating the forearm, thereby obtaining only one view of the elbow.

3. If the x-rays are equivocal, what next?
Obtain comparison views of the uninjured side. This can help if there is a subtle torus fracture or if the patient has plastic bowing of one bone or both bones. In a patient older than 10 years of age with tenderness over the snuff box, a carpal scaphoid view is indicated. If a fracture is suspected on clinical exam and the x-rays are not diagnostic, it is always reasonable to immobilize the area for a couple of weeks and then repeat x-rays.

4. How are forearm fractures classified?
The fractures are classified as compression (buckle or torus), greenstick (incomplete), or complete. Note the location in the forearm (proximal, middle, or distal third) and whether the radius

or ulna (or both) is fractured. Fractures through the growth plate of the distal radius are usually described using the Salter-Harris classification scheme.

5. How is the direction of angulation described?
This is an area of ongoing confusion. Fracture angulation in orthopedics is described based on the direction of **apex** of the angle. This applies as much to distal radius fractures as to any others. Thus, the typical distal radius fracture with the distal fragment pointing dorsally (similar to the adult Colles' fracture) is *not* "dorsally angulated." It has volar angulation.

This confusion can be eliminated by adding the word "apex" when describing fracture angulation. The distal radius fracture in this example is therefore best described as "apex volar angulation."

6. What about rotation in forearm fractures?
Rotational deformity is one of the biggest concerns with fractures of the forearm. The bones are less capable of remodeling rotation than angulation. The most common residual impairment after a forearm fracture is loss of pronation or supination.

7. How are angulation and rotation linked in forearm fractures?
There is tight association between angulation and rotation. Fractures with apex volar angulation also include supination of the distal fragment with respect to the proximal fragment. Fractures with apex dorsal angulation also include pronation through the fracture site. This is important to consider when reducing the deformity. The reduction maneuver must correct the angulation as well as the rotation (see Figure).

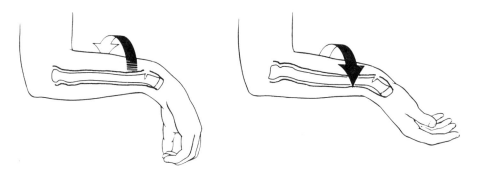

Left, Distal radius fracture with apex dorsal angulation and associated pronation deformity. Note the intact volar periosteal hinge. *Right,* Distal radius fracture with apex volar angulation and associated supination deformity. The intact periosteal hinge is dorsal with this fracture pattern.

8. What happens to the periosteum in forearm fractures?
The periosteum is a well-developed structure in growing bones and very important in forearm fractures. In angulated fractures, the periosteum is disrupted on the outer side of the angle and intact on the inner side. It is helpful to think about the "hinge side" of a fracture when reducing it. The periosteal "hinge" (intact portion) provides stability to the reduction and needs to be preserved as the fracture is reduced.

9. Which fractures need to be reduced?
Compression (buckle or torus) fractures are almost never unstable or displaced enough to need reduction.

Greenstick (incomplete) fractures tend to develop increased angulation, even in a cast. Most authorities recommend gently reducing these enough to feel or hear a "pop" in the intact cortex.

Care should be taken not to overreduce these fractures. This might disrupt the periosteum on the hinge side of the deformity and render the reduction unstable.

Most complete fractures should be reduced, particularly if there is rotation with angulation.

10. How, and under what circumstances, should the reduction be performed?

Greenstick fractures can be reduced in the Emergency Department or clinic, and no anesthesia is required. They lend themselves to reduction as a cast or splint is applied. The parents need to be cautioned that the child will experience pain for a minute or so following the reduction and then will typically be comfortable after immobilization.

11. How are complete fractures treated?

For complete fractures that require reduction, good analgesia or anesthesia as well as sedation for the reduction is indicated. The traditional approach has been to take the patient to the operating room for general or regional anesthesia and to perform the reduction with the aid of an image intensifier.

In this age of cost awareness, almost all complete forearm fractures at our facility are now reduced in the Emergency Department, and the patients are treated as outpatients. The patient is sedated with midazolam (Versed), 0.02–0.5 mg/kg (maximum 5 mg) and morphine, 0.05–0.1 mg/kg. The FluoroScan unit is used to check the reduction. Occasionally, a hematoma block can be added. Blood pressure, heart and respiration rate, and O_2 saturation are routinely monitored.

12. What is the best position of rotation of the forearm during immobilization?

This is another area of controversy, with experts advising a range of options from full pronation to full supination for the same fractures! There are some theoretical advantages to immobilization in supination due to relaxation of the brachioradialis and possibly gravity effects. In most fractures, however, a *neutral* rotation of the forearm is probably the best. The intact portion of the periosteum provides enough natural support that most fractures are well aligned in neutral position. In addition, if there is some rotational stiffness following a fracture, it is best tolerated if the forearm is close to the neutral position.

A notable exception is the Monteggia fracture, in which there is a fracture of the ulna and anterior dislocation of the radial head. This is a hyperpronation injury that needs to be supinated for reduction. In most cases, immobilization is best with the elbow flexed 90° and the forearm fully supinated. Without full supination, the radial head tends to redislocate.

13. Which fractures require pin fixation, and which require open reduction with internal fixation?

Most forearm fractures in children do not require open reduction or pin fixation. Open fractures, even grade 1 (puncture wounds), should be treated with formal irrigation and débridement in the operating room. In some instances, fractures cannot be adequately reduced, or a stable reduction cannot be maintained, and percutaneous longitudinal pinning can be helpful.

In adolescent patients with midshaft fractures, open reduction with plate fixation is frequently needed for a satisfactory result.

14. How much angulation is acceptable?

Most experts agree that forearm fractures angulated up to 30° in children 8 years of age or younger will remodel with minimal to no residual deformity or limitation of rotation. Other than that, guidelines are rather vague. In general, distal fractures in the area of the metaphysis or growth plate remodel sooner and more completely than midshaft fractures. If a child's forearm looks significantly deformed, it is usually easier to reduce the deformity than to explain to the parent why you are not reducing it.

15. How does one decide between above-elbow and below-elbow casts?

Fractures that need reduction and fractures that may be unstable should be immobilized in above-elbow casts. These limit forearm rotation and help maintain the reduction. Patients who have stable fractures but who experience pain with pronation and supination are also happier in an above-elbow cast. Children younger than 2 years of age, even with undisplaced torus fractures, should be in above-elbow casts because the below-elbow casts will slip off their conical forearms.

16. Are there any tricks to aid reduction?
The need to correct both the angulation and the rotation has already been emphasized. I find it very helpful to keep in mind that the *periosteum is intact* on the hinge side of the deformity. This is an ally in maintaining a stable reduction and needs to be considered in obtaining the reduction. Because of the intact periosteum, the reduction is best achieved by reproducing the original deformity and "walking" the bone ends out until the cortices hook on the hinge side of the fracture. The angulation and rotation can then be corrected without excessive force and without disrupting the intact portion of the periosteum (see Figure).

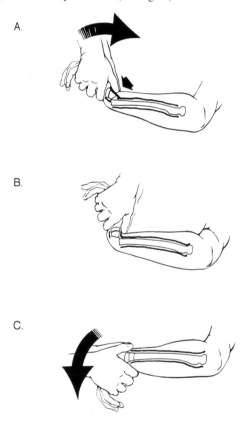

Use the intact periosteal hinge to assist in reduction of a displaced fracture of the distal radius. *A,* Increase the angulation to take tension off the intact dorsal periosteum. *B,* Walk the bone ends out until the dorsal cortices are aligned. *C,* Flex (and pronate) to complete the reduction.

17. When is a splint applied, and when can a patient's limb be placed directly into a cast?
Splinting is safer and is best for most fractures, particularly if reduction is required. A handy approach is to apply dorsal and volar plaster slabs on the forearm and circumferential cast material from midforearm to above the elbow. This provides good fracture stability and avoids excessive bulk at the elbow. The splint can be converted to a cast 4 to 7 days later when the child comes

in for repeat x-rays. By this time, the swelling has decreased, and the splint can be tightened a bit as it is overwrapped with fiberglass cast material.

Others favor applying a full cast at the time of fracture reduction and splitting it on the dorsal side of the forearm. Studies have shown, however, that this technique does not decrease the risk of neurovascular compromise due to casting. Also, this does not allow for the cast to be tightened when the swelling decreases in 4 to 7 days.

18. How long do forearm fractures need to be immobilized?

Torus fractures and fractures through the distal growth plates are well healed in 3 to 4 weeks. The casts can be removed at that time, even in older children. Fractures that require reduction, particularly in the diaphyseal portion of the bones, require protection for 6 to 7 weeks. Children do not develop stiffness due to prolonged immobilization. When in doubt, it is safer to err on the side of longer immobilization.

19. How frequently must x-rays be taken to monitor fracture healing?

This is another area of concern in this era of cost consciousness. We have recently seen problems in our clinic related to inadequate x-ray follow-up by "gatekeepers" who were trying to limit costs.

Patients with stable fractures (e.g., torus fractures) do not need x-rays during casting, and it is debatable whether they need x-rays when the casts are removed.

X-rays should be obtained in 4 to 7 days for fractures that require reduction and again at 10 to 14 days in order to confirm satisfactory alignment. If the fracture has drifted between the first and second weeks, but not enough to require remanipulation, then x-rays at 3 weeks are necessary. X-rays should be obtained for these fractures at the time the cast is removed.

For fractures involving the growth plate, repeat x-rays should be obtained 4 to 6 months postinjury to assess the status of the growth plate.

20. What physical therapy is needed after a forearm fracture?

None. Children recover at the optimal rate without specific therapy.

21. What is the risk of refracture?

Fractures through the growth plate and well-reduced metaphyseal fractures rarely refracture. One study of 500 consecutive displaced forearm fractures found a 7% incidence of refracture at the same site of the original fracture. The average time from the original fracture to refracture was 6.5 months. Risk factors for refracture included increased age (average 12.9 years in boys and 11.75 years in girls), presence of a transverse fracture line, and fracture of a dominant extremity.

22. Parents want to know when their children can resume sports after cast removal. Are there guidelines for this?

Not really. Factors to consider include the age of the child, the location of the fracture, and the position of the fracture at the time of healing. As a rule of thumb, it is advisable for children to avoid contact sports for as many additional weeks as their arm had been immobilized. Even then, refracture remains a concern. (See Question 21.) Fortunately, the refractures seem to heal as well as the initial fractures.

BIBLIOGRAPHY

1. Dicke TE, Nunley JA: Distal forearm fractures in children, complications and surgical indications. Orthop Clin North Am 24:333–340, 1993.
2. Evans EM: Fractures of the radius and ulna. J Bone Joint Surg [Br] 33:548–561, 1951.
3. Friberg KSI: Remodelling after distal forearm fractures in children. Acta Orthop Scand 50:731–749, 1979.
4. King RE: Fractures of the shafts of the radius and ulna. In Rockwood CA, Wilkins KE, King RE (eds): Fractures in Children. Philadelphia, J.B. Lippincott Co., 1984, pp 301–362.

5. O'Brien ET: Fractures and dislocations of the wrist region. In Rockwood CA, Wilkins KE, King RE (eds): Fractures in Children. Philadelphia, J.B. Lippincott Co., 1984, pp 273–299.
6. Rang M: Children's Fractures. Philadelphia, J.B. Lippincott Co., 1974, pp 124–140.
7. Tredwell SJ, Van Peteghem K, Clough M: Patterns of forearm fractures in children. J Pediat Orthop 4:604–608, 1984.

39. PEDIATRIC HAND INJURIES

Peter M. Waters, M.D.

1. What is the most common pediatric hand fracture?

A physeal (growth cartilage) fracture of the proximal phalanx is the most common injury in children, and most often occurs in preadolescents. In toddlers and young children, a distal phalanx fracture associated with a nailbed laceration due to a crush injury occurs most commonly.

2. Are mallet fingers different in children than in adults?

In young children, the physis will separate rather than the terminal tendon, creating the mallet posture. The terminal tendon is still intact in this situation because it inserts on the more proximal epiphysis. Adolescent injuries will be similar to adult injuries, with either a tendon disruption or an avulsion fracture.

3. Do all pediatric finger fractures do well?

The vast majority (75–80%) heal without problems. The potential problem areas are phalangeal neck, phalangeal shaft with malrotation (see Figure), and intra-articular fractures.

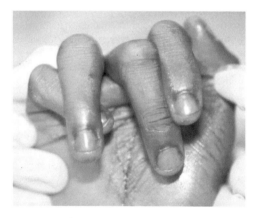

Wrist tenodesis reveals significant malrotation of this ring finger with a proximal phalanx fracture.

4. What is the controversy regarding the treatment of late-presenting phalangeal neck fractures?

The problem with late open reduction of the malunited fracture is the risk of avascular necrosis (AVN). Most authors advocate allowing for complete healing and maximal motion before performing a subchondral fossa reconstruction several months postfracture. Recently, percutaneous osteoclasis with a C-wire has been proposed to realign the fracture and lessen the risk of AVN. For this to be appropriate, the healing must be incomplete.

5. What is the main complication of phalangeal neck fractures?
These fractures are often considered a benign injury when seen in the emergency setting. Follow-up is often delayed, and the fracture frequently heals in a malunited position upon presentation to the orthopedist. The loss of the subchondral fossa due to the malunion leads to a loss of flexion (see Figure).

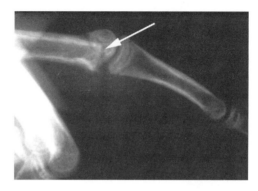

Lateral radiograph reveals a malaligned, nearly united phalangeal neck fracture. Too often, patients with this fracture present late with a malunion resulting in significant loss of proximal interphalangeal joint flexion.

6. What is the pediatric equivalent of an adult gamekeeper's thumb?
A Salter-Harris III physeal fracture of the proximal phalanx. This requires open reduction with internal fixation to align anatomically and to stabilize the joint and physis. The ulnar collateral ligament is intact in this situation; operative exposure needs to avoid injury to this ligament.

7. What is the difference between scaphoid fractures in adults and in children?
They often are distal pole avulsions that heal with cast immobilization. Waist fractures do occur in the skeletally immature, however, and carry the same risks of fracture nonunion and proximal pole avascular necrosis as in the adult.

8. What is an irreducible metacarpophalangeal (MCP) joint dislocation?
This is a complex dislocation in which the volar plate becomes entrapped between the proximal phalanx and the metacarpal head, preventing closed reduction. An open reduction of the dislocation is necessary to extract the entrapped volar plate and reduce the dorsally displaced proximal phalanx.

9. Is there a controversy regarding operative exposure for an irreducible MCP dislocation?
The issue is whether a volar or a dorsal approach is more appropriate. A volar approach allows for full visualization of the pathoanatomy, including the subcutaneous metacarpal head lassoed by the flexor tendons. Extreme care must be taken to avoid iatrogenic laceration of the displaced radial neurovascular bundle, however. A dorsal approach is thought to be safer. It requires a longitudinal incision in the volar plate to allow for reduction of the metacarpal head into the joint.

10. How can you diagnose flexor tendon or digital nerve laceration in an uncooperative child?
- Check the cascade of the fingers. A finger with a flexor tendon laceration will be more extended as the hand rests on a table.

- Move the wrist passively and observe the movement of the fingers by tenodesis. Again, a finger with a flexor tendon laceration will remain more extended.
- A "wrinkle test" will help in diagnosing a nerve laceration. Normally, innervated skin will wrinkle when immersed in saline for a prolonged period of time. A finger with a nerve laceration will fail to wrinkle after prolonged immersion.

11. What is the best postoperative program after a flexor tendon repair in a child?
Cast immobilization for 4 weeks in a protected position yields results equal to or better than Klienert or Duran programs of splinting and mobilization in children younger than 15 years of age.

12. When is two-point discrimination a reliable test for a nerve laceration in a child?
Discriminatory sensibility does not develop until approximately 5 years of age. In addition, the examiner needs to be meticulous in testing young school-aged children so as not to be fooled by their guessing.

13. What are the indications for replantation in a child?
An amputation at any level, including single-digit amputations in zones I and II, should be replanted in a child.

14. What factors favor digital survival in a pediatric replantation?
- Sharp amputation
- Body weight > 11 kilograms
- More than one vein repaired
- Bone shortening
- Interosseous wire fixation
- Vein grafting of arteries and veins
- Prompt reperfusion after arterial repair

BIBLIOGRAPHY

1. Hastings H, Simmons BP: Hand fractures in children: A statistical analysis. Clin Orthop 188:120, 1984.
2. Fischer MD, McElfresh EC: Physeal and periphyseal injuries of the hand: Patterns of injury and results of treatment. Hand Clin 10:287–301, 1994.
3. Campbell RM: Operative treatment of fractures and dislocations of the hand and wrist region in children. Orthop Clin North Am 21:217, 1990.
4. Dixon GL Jr, Moon NF: Rotational supracondylar fractures of the proximal phalanx in children. Clin Orthop 83:151–156, 1972.
5. Simmons BP, Peters TT: Subcondylar fossa reconstruction for malunion of fractures of the proximal phalanx in children. J Hand Surg 12:1078, 1987.
6. Green DP: Hand injuries in children. Pediatr Clin North Am 21:903, 1977.
7. Bohart PG, Gelberman RH, Vandell RF, Salamar PB: Complex dislocations of the metacarpal phalangeal joint. Clin Orthop 164:208, 1982.
8. Baker G, Kleinert J: Digit replantation in infants and young children: Determinants of survival. Plast Reconstr Surg 94:139–145, 1994.

40. YOUTH SPORTS AND RELATED INJURIES

Michael T. Busch, M.D.

1. What portion of youth sports injuries occur in organized sports?
Approximately one third. The remainder occur during physical education classes and nonorganized sports.

2. In the United States, what sports produce the highest rates of injuries?
When injury data are adjusted for a number of participant hours, the trend is for American football to be the highest-risk sport, followed by basketball, gymnastics, soccer, and baseball. Approximately one third of these injuries occur in youths between the ages of 5 and 14, with two thirds occurring in those 15 years or older. American football produces the highest rate of injury, with varsity high school athletes having an injury rate between 20% and 40%; however, 75% of these injuries are minor, resulting in minimal loss of participation. Up to 10% can require hospitalization, and 2% need reconstructive procedures.

3. In the United States, fatal injuries occur most often in which sport?
Baseball. Fatal injuries are usually related to bat or ball blows to the chest or head. Proper equipment, good supervision, and appropriate rules are important in reducing these injuries.

4. In preparticipation screening evaluations, what component is the most sensitive for identifying individuals at significant risk for injury from sports participation?
The medical history is the most cost-effective component of the screening evaluation. Episodes of prior musculoskeletal injury, neurologic injury, and cardiopulmonary problems should be noted. Questions related to general health, immunizations, hospitalizations, and limitations of function are helpful as well. Specifically, athletes should be asked about prior history of concussion, unconsciousness, paresthesias, heat-related illness, and previous musculoskeletal treatments or problems. Syncope is an important clue to undetected heart disease. Unfortunately, even with conscientious screening, identifying all individuals at high risk for sudden death (usually cardiac in origin) is not possible. Athletes and parents should always be informed that screening cannot insure protection from and prevention of all injuries.

5. What specific factors significantly increase risk for heat illness during sports participation?

Obesity	Lack of recent conditioning in the heat
Recent viral illness (especially gastroenteritis)	Failure to replenish previous day's water
History of previous heat illness	loss
Prepubescence	Chronic illness such as cystic fibrosis and
Mental retardation	inflammatory bowel disease

6. What situational factors place all participating youths at increased risk of heat illness?

High heat	First practice of the season
High humidity	Artificial turf
Direct sunlight	Long event
No breeze	Multiple competitions in a day or on
Dark or heavy clothing (e.g., football	consecutive days
pads, helmets, and uniforms)	Recent fluid restrictions.

7. What guidelines can be used to reduce the incidence of heat illness?
- Athletes should be acclimatized prior to the start of a sports season.
- Weather conditons should be evaluated for the combination of temperature, humidity, sunlight, and wind.
- Rest breaks in the shade should be scheduled and followed.
- Individuals at risk should be identified.
- Chilled fluids should be readily available.
- Enforced periodic drinking breaks should occur.
- Water restrictions should never be used as discipline.
- Deliberate dehydration for weight loss must be discouraged.
- Clothing should be lightweight and of light color.
- Events should not be scheduled during peak hours of heat and sun.
- Players, parents, and coaches all need to be educated about the potential risks of heat illness and how they are avoided.

- Athletes at significant risk should have daily weights recorded to assure adequate rehydration after the previous day's practice.

8. How much salt replacement is needed in fluids?

Sweat is hypotonic to body fluids, containing 40–80 mEq/L of sodium and less than 5 mEq/L of potassium. Initially, plain water adequately replaces these losses. Electrolyte solutions are needed only after 1–2 hours of continuous rigorous activity. Salt tablets and hypertonic solutions are dangerous because they can produce intracellular dehydration owing to their osmotic effect in the serum.

Ideally, water should be cooled to stimulate thirst. While sugar added to the solution may improve palatability, a high sugar concentration slows gastrointestinal motility and can cause bloated feelings and nausea.

9. What is the difference between weight lifting and weight training?

Weight training refers to the use of free weights or weight and resistance machines to enhance strength and endurance. Submaximal weights are lifted repeated until the muscles fatigue. The object is to enhance performance for other sporting activities. In weight lifting, the object is to perform a one-repetition maximal lift.

10. Before puberty, can children gain strength from weight training?

Prepubescent children can increase strength by 20–40% in a well-supervised program. While these children lack the higher level of androgens that facilitates hypertrophy of muscles, strength gains do occur owing to a combination of enhanced recruitment of motor units, synchronization, and some degree of muscle hypertrophy.

11. For children, does the risk of using weights outweigh any potential benefits?

With proper instruction and supervision, weight-training programs can be relatively safe, even for children. A proper strength conditioning program should be a prerequisite for youths participating in contact sports. Strength, particularly of the cervical spine, can reduce the incidence of injuries. For a program to be safe, proper technique needs to be emphasized. The equipment must be in good repair. An attentive partner is important whenever free weights are used. Strengthening should be balanced with a consistent stretching program. Most authorities recommend avoiding maximal weight lifting in children.

12. What are the two most common anatomic sites of injury for high school basketball players?

Injuries of the ankle are by far the most common, followed by injuries of the knee. Up to 70% of all high school varsity basketball players will sustain an ankle sprain during their career. Up to a third of these are recurrent. The occurrence rate of ankle sprains is similar in both boys and girls. Girls, however, are at an increased risk for knee injuries, particularly rupture of the anterior cruciate ligament.

13. Do high-top shoes (with or without inflatable air chambers) prevent ankle sprains in basketball players?

Probably not. Most data suggest no statistical reduction in ankle injury rates with use of high-top shoes. Taping and the use of lace-up braces do support the ankle and reduce injuries, compared with shoes alone.

14. How effective are modern American football helmets in preventing cervical spine injury?

Since their introduction, helmets (and face guards) have significantly reduced the incidence of closed head injuries and facial injuries. The cervical spine, however, remains at risk, with quadriplegia now being more common than fatal head injuries. Among high school participants in American football, the rate of quadriplegia is approximately 0.7 per 100,000 players (compared with 2.7 per 100,000 players at the collegiate level).

15. What is the most common scenario associated with catastrophic head or neck injury in American football players?

Defensive players sustain 70% or more of all catastrophic injuries, with 75% occurring while tackling. A direct axial load to the straight or flexed cervical spine (spearing) is the most common mechanism.

16. What can be done to minimize the risk of these catastrophic injuries in American football?

In 1976, the NCAA and the National Federation of State High School Associations made rule changes to prohibit using the head (like a battering ram) as the initial point of contact when blocking or tackling. This has greatly reduced the incidence of quadriplegia but has not eliminated it. Players must be repeatedly instructed about the dangers (and therefore, illegal nature) of spearing. Parents, coaches, and health professionals must be sure proper techniques are being taught and used. Rules must be enforced. Helmets and pads should fit properly. A weight training program to strengthen the neck muscles should be a requirement for all athletes involved in contact sports, particularly American football.

17. What two sports have the highest rate of quadriceps contusion? What are its causes and complications?

Soccer and American football. This injury usually results from a direct blow to the anterior aspect of the thigh. Although pads have been developed for American football to try to prevent this injury, contact from an opponent's knee, shoulder pad, or helmet can occur on the margins of the pad and produce this injury. Untreated, this injury can easily be exacerbated with recurrent bleeding leading to prolonged loss of time from sports. Occasionally, myositis ossificans can result as well. This injury should not be overlooked.

18. How do hip pointers occur?

Commonly occurring in contact or collision sports like American football and soccer, this injury results from a direct blow to the iliac crest apophysis. These heal with rest and time but are notoriously painful, debilitating in the short run, and slow to resolve (up to 8–10 weeks). American football waist pads are designed to reduce the occurrence of this injury but must be fitted properly.

19. How do stingers and burners occur?

These terms refer to an injury of the brachial plexus that is typically transient. It usually results from a stretching mechanism, often occurring in American football from a direct blow that depresses the shoulder and simultaneously bends the neck in the opposite direction. The result is paresthesias and paralysis that can take moments to weeks to resolve. Recurrent injury often results from premature return to contact sports. This can lead to progressive fibrosis of the brachial plexus and occasionally results in persistent symptoms or permanent disability. Recurrent stingers or burners can be related to relative stenosis of the cervical canal as measured by the Pavlov ratio. Unless this is accompanied by other changes in the radiographic appearance of the cervical spine, these individuals do not seem to be at significantly increased risk for development of subsequent cervical spinal cord injury.

20. What are the most common causes of wrist pain in gymnasts?

An overuse syndrome of the distal radial physis is a fairly common cause of gradual-onset wrist pain in a gymnast. The process is termed a physiolysis and appears to be analogous to a stress fracture involving the physeal (growth) plate. With rest, this usually resolves without complication; however, occasionally premature closure of the distal radial physis can occur with subsequent relative overgrowth of the ulna. This "positive ulnar variance" can result in excessive pressure on the lateral carpus and ongoing wrist pain.

Other considerations include Kienböck's disease (osteonecrosis of the lunate), impingement of the dorsal interosseous nerve at the wrist, synovial or capsular impingement of the wrist joint, and tears or inflammation of the triangulofibrocartilage complex.

21. What tests should be obtained in the evaluation of a prepubescent female gymnast with an injury to the proximal hamstring area following a stretching-type maneuver?
AP radiograph of the pelvis. While the mechanism described is consistent with the common hamstring strain, most of these injuries occur at the musculotendinous junction and are usually at the midportion of the distal thigh. In the skeletally immature gymnast, proximal injuries are often due to ischial avulsion fractures, resulting from a "pike position" stretch. After appropriate history and physical examination, a single AP pelvic radiograph will most often demonstrate widening of the affected apophysis. Typically, the other ischium provides a normal study for comparison.

22. What should be considered in the differential diagnosis of low back pain in a gymnast?
One of the most common problems is spondylolysis, which is most likely induced by recurrent hypertension stresses, which are very common to many gymnastic positions and stunts. While typically associated with very minimal grades of slippage, a substantial amount of spondylolisthesis can result. Initially, spondylolysis may be radiographically normal and only detectable by bone scan.

Many times the cause of back pain in gymnasts cannot be specifically identified. Impingement of the posterior elements and facets is often suspected. Disk injury or herniation should be considered. Significant trauma, fracture, and displacement of the ring apophysis can occur as well.

Night pain and subtle neurologic findings should suggest the possibility of a more serious source of the back pain such as tumor, infection, tethered cored, intradural lipoma, or other spinal anomaly. Occasionally, osteoid osteoma occurs in the lumbar spine of youths as well.

23. What are the most common injuries in the immature skeleton in young runners?
Most young runners participate, at least initially, with relatively few injuries. With time, they can develop overuse syndromes similar to their adult counterparts. Apophyseal problems such as Sever's disease (calcaneal apophysitis), Osgood-Schlatter disease, and avulsion fractures of the apophyses about the hip and pelvis are common in young runners. Stress fractures of the metatarsals, tibia, fibula, and femoral neck can occur as well.

24. What is the most common source of injuries in young runners?
Like adults, training errors are by far the most common cause of injury. A sudden increase in training distance and intensity is the most common error. Excessive mileage, lack of rest, running on hard surfaces, inadequate shoe wear, and lack of a concurrent stretching program are other mistakes.

BIBLIOGRAPHY

1. Busch M: Sports medicine. In Morrissy RT (ed): Lovell and Winter's Pediatric Orthopaedics, 4th ed. Philadelphia, J. B. Lippincott Co., 1996, p 1181.
2. Caine D, Roy S, Singer K, Broekhoff J: Stress changes of the distal radial growth plate. Am J Sports Med 20(3):290, 1992.
3. Cantu R, Mueller F: Catastrophic football injuries in the U.S.A.:1977–1990. Clin J Sport Med 2(3):180, 1992.
4. Lysholm J, Wiklander J: Injuries in runners. Am J Sports Med 15(2):168, 1987.
5. Maffulli N: Intensive training in young athletes. Sports Med 9(4):229, 1990.
6. Smith N: Is that child ready for competitive sports? Contemp Pediatr 3:30, 1986.
7. Smith N, Stanitski C, Dyment P, Smith R, Strong W: The prevention of heat disorders in sports. Am J Dis Child 138:786, 1984.
8. Zillmer D, Powell J. Albright J: Gender-specific injury patterns in high school varsity basketball. J Women's Health 1(1):69, 1992.

41. STRESS FRACTURES

Neil E. Green, M.D.

1. What is the cause and natural history of stress fractures?
Stress fractures are the result of repetitive stress to bones that do not have the ability to recover. Repetitive activities produce nonpainful microfractures of bone trabeculi. If the trauma is minimal or if the child rests between episodes of trauma, the microfractures will heal. On the other hand, if the child continues with the offending activity, such as running and playing, the microfractures will increase to the point that pain will occur with activity. This is the first symptom of a stress fracture in most, although some young children may limp without complaining of pain. If the child heeds the pain and reduces the stress at this point, the fracture should heal without other treatment. If the child continues with the activity, the stress fracture will become more evident clinically and radiographically.

2. What are the symptoms of a stress fracture?
Children with a stress fracture will complain of pain with activity but will not have pain when they are sedentary. Young children may not complain of pain, but their parents will notice that they limp during activity. Because children will usually continue to be active in spite of pain, the child's limp will worsen with increasing activity. Older children will be able to pinpoint the site of the pain; however, young children will usually not be able to tell their parents or the physician where they have pain.

3. How does one make the diagnosis of a stress fracture?
In children whose symptoms suggest a stress fracture, the clinical examination will reveal point tenderness of the bone at the point of the stress fracture. Adults or teenagers with stress fractures may present for diagnosis and treatment before the radiographs are abnormal, because radiographic changes frequently lag behind clinical symptoms by weeks. In individuals with symptoms of a stress fracture with normal radiographs, a bone scan may be helpful. Since young children complain about pain less frequently than the older individual however, radiographic changes are usually present by the time they present for diagnosis and treatment.

4. What are the radiographic findings with a stress fracture?
Stress fractures of a long bone are usually cortical. There will be periosteal reactive bone proximal and distal to the lesion. The cortex of the bone is thickened as a result of the increased bone density resulting from the healing of the fracture. If the fracture persists, the fracture line may become evident beginning at the cortex and progressing centrally. The longer the patient is symptomatic, the more evident the fracture becomes.

5. What is the differential diagnosis of a stress fracture?
The most common lesion that one will mistake for a stress fracture is an osteoid osteoma. The pain of an osteoid osteoma usually does not increase with activity, however. It will cause pain at times of both activity and inactivity, especially at night. Both lesions will produce periosteal reactive bone and cortical thickening. The nidus of the osteoid osteoma can usually be identified on a computed tomography (CT) scan if the differential diagnosis is difficult. In addition, osteoid osteoma will produce a more intense and widespread reaction on a bone scan, as opposed to the more localized reaction seen with a stress fracture.

A malignancy such as Ewing's sarcoma can be differentiated by its more widespread periosteal reaction and bone destruction. Very occasionally, an area of subacute or chronic bone infection may simulate a stress fracture.

6. Do stress fractures occur only in high-performance athletes?

Stress fractures can and do occur in anyone. Children in particular are very prone to the development of stress fractures because of their high energy level and the relative lower density of their bones. Most children with a stress fracture seen in an orthopaedic practice will be those who are very involved in play or in many sports and activities. Even relatively sedentary children may develop a stress fracture so long as the involved level of activity produces stress greater than the bone's ability to resist it.

7. Are some people more prone to the development of a stress fracture than others?

Since stress fractures are the result of excessive stress, if one has an abnormally angulated bone or portion of an extremity, increased stress will be delivered to a bone, increasing the chance of development of a stress fracture. For example, a child with a varus deformity of the hindfoot will place more stress than normal on the base of the fifth metatarsal, which may result in the development of a stress fracture of the proximal diaphysis of the fifth metatarsal (Jones fracture). Another example is stress fracture of the anterior cortex of the middle third of the tibia, which is the result of an anterior bow of the tibia. This anterior bow increases the tension stress on the tibia, which may result in a stress fracture.

Stress fractures can also be seen in children who have been immobilized. For example, the child who has sustained a traumatic fracture of the lower extremity requiring immobilization will develop osteopenia in the entire immobilized extremity. If the child returns to any activity too vigorously and too soon, he or she is prone to develop a stress fracture. Simple walking may even be sufficient to produce a stress fracture of a metatarsal.

8. What are the most common locations of stress fractures in children?

Stress fractures occur most commonly in the bones of the lower leg and foot. Their most common location is in the posterior medial aspect of the proximal tibia. One will see increased bone density with some evidence of periosteal healing. The child will have point tenderness over the stress fracture in the tibia.

The medial aspect of the distal tibia is another common location of a stress fracture, as is the distal third of the fibula and the calcaneus. The calcaneal stress fracture is frequently not seen on the initial radiograph, but if the diagnosis is made on a clinical basis and the foot is immobilized, the stress fracture will be seen after the cast is removed. Metatarsal stress fractures are also frequently seen in children, not only in those children involved in sports, but also in children who have been immobilized.

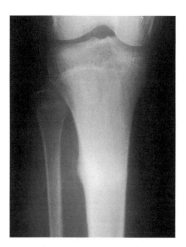

Anteroposterior radiograph of the tibia of an 11-year-old female who had pain in her leg with activity. She played basketball during the winter and softball in the spring. Throughout the softball season, she complained of pain; however, she continued to play. She finally sought medical attention because of her inability to continue to participate in her sport. The radiograph demonstrates an area of increased bone density on the anteromedial aspect of the proximal tibia. The periosteum is thickened, and there is also endosteal callus (the transverse line of internal callus). Simple reduction of her activity level allowed the fracture to heal completely.

9. What is the treatment of a stress fracture?

The stress fracture is treated by elimination of the offending activity. In the high-performance athlete, one may simply eliminate the activity that is the cause, such as running. In children, however, elimination of the stress is important, but immobilization of the extremity is equally important. Young children whose stress fractures are the result of normal activities must be immobilized to rest the bone adequately and to allow healing of the stress fracture. Immobilization is continued for 4–6 weeks or until there is no tenderness of the bone and radiographs show periosteal healing. The child is then allowed to walk, but with activity modification.

In the adolescent or teen who is able to comply with a more complicated regimen, one may use immobilization for a shorter period of time or may simply reduce stress with crutch ambulation. Conditioning may be maintained by changing activities, e.g., by swimming or bike riding instead of running.

10. Do stress fractures occur in the spine? What are some causes?

Spondylolysis or fracture of the pars interarticularis is in most cases a stress fracture. The pars is part of the posterior elements of the vertebrae. Stress may be concentrated in the pars interarticularis, resulting in a stress fracture. It has been shown that certain activities will increase the risk of developing spondylolysis. Axial loading of the extended spine with the lumbar spine in lordosis increases the stress on the pars interarticularis of the lower two lumbar vertebrae, especially L5. Gymnasts are especially prone to the development of spondylolysis because they axially load their spines in extension. (Picture the gymnast's landing posture at the ending of her routine.) Interior football linemen are also uniquely susceptable to a stress fracture of the pars interarticularis. They come up from their three-point stance to block defensive linemen with their spines in lordosis.

11. How does one make the diagnosis of spondylolysis?

Clinically, children with spondylolysis will complain of back pain with activity. On examination, these children will have pain with spinal motion, especially extension. They frequently have hamstring tightness, as demonstrated by limited forward bending. The lesion may be seen on a lateral radiograph of the lumbosacral spine if the fractures are bilateral and have been present for a sufficient period of time to become evident radiographically. The oblique radiograph of the lumbosacral spine will best show the stress fracture of the pars interarticularis. If the radiographs do not demonstrate the lesion, a bone scan will usually reveal increased uptake of the nucleotide in the region of the pars. Single-photon emission computed tomographic images should also be obtained to see and localize the lesion better. Finally, a CT scan of this area of the spine will demonstrate the fractures.

12. How should one treat spondylolysis?

Patients with spondylolysis will have back pain with activity. As the lesion progresses, pain may persist, even when the patient is sedentary. The pain will be more severe during periods of activity, however. Once the diagnosis has been made, reduction of stress is the main treatment, as it is for any stress fracture. The stress fracture of the pars is unlikely to heal, however. The lesion that may heal is the stress fracture that has recently occurred and is not complete. A bone scan should be performed; if there is significantly increased activity in the region of the pars interarticularis, one may assume that the stress fracture is attempting to repair itself.

Immobilization of these patients may result in complete healing of the fracture. In most patients, immobilization of the spine with a thoracolumbosacral orthosis (TLSO) allows the inflammation to subside. Most of the time, the fracture heals with a fibrous nonunion that is stable. Once the patient is comfortable, he or she is begun on an exercise program that will allow progressive return to sports.

13. What is spondylolisthesis? How is it classified?

If a stress fracture does not heal or does not develop stable fibrous nonunion, the fracture fragments may separate. This allows the vertebral body to slide anteriorly while the posterior elements of the vertebra remain in their normal position. Once the vertebral body has slipped forward far enough that it is identifiable radiographically, spondylolysis has become spondylolisthesis.

The severity of spondylolisthesis is graded according the amount of forward slippage. If the slippage is 25% or less as measured against the next caudal vertebra or sacrum, the spondylolisthesis is classified as grade I. In grade II spondylolisthesis, the slipped vertebra has moved 25–50% forward. In grades III and IV, the slippage is 75% and 100%, respectively. In grade V spondylolisthesis, or spondyloptosis, not only has the body of L5 slipped 100% in front of the sacrum, but it has also actually slipped far enough forward that it has begun to descend caudally in front of the sacrum.

14. Do stress fractures occur in growth plates?

Stress fractures of growth plates are uncommon, but they do occur. Children with open physes may experience stress applied mainly to a growth plate. The physeal stress fracture will have the same symptoms as the stress fracture of the ossified portion of the bone, namely, pain with activity. Gymnasts may develop stress fractures of their distal radius physis. Stress fractures of the olecrenon apophysis can be seen in skeletally immature weightlifters. Another apophyseal stress injury is the stress reaction of the tibial tubercle called Osgood-Schlatter disease. This lesion may occasionally lead to a complete fracture of the tibial tubercle if a very forceful contraction of the quadriceps muscle pulls loose an already weakened tibial tubercle.

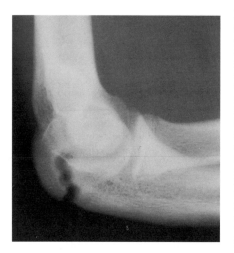

Lateral radiograph of the right elbow of a 14-year-old male who had pain in both elbows for more than 5 months. He played football, and to increase his upper body strength, he had been lifting weights for more than a year. In addition, he did more than 100 push-ups every day. In spite of the pain in both elbows, he continued with football and with the weightlifting and the other exercises. He had no pain at rest but did have pain over the olecrenon with all activities that required the use of his arms. This radiograph demonstrates a very wide olecranon apophysis. The apophysis should be nearly closed in a male of this bone age, since all the physes of the elbow are closed on this radiograph. He had point tenderness directly over the apophysis of both elbows. Immobilization resolved the pain in the left elbow, but the right elbow pain persisted. Because there was no improvement with immobilization, the fracture was operated on. The fracture was mobile at exploration. It was internally fixed with an intramedullary screw, and the fracture defect was bone grafted.

15. What are the two types of stress fractures?

Stress fractures on the compression side of a bone are the most common type. They are the result of axial loading of an extremity. For example, a stress fracture of a metatarsal is the result of increased axial bone stress. Stress fracture of the posterior medial cortex of the proximal tibia is also the result of increased axial stress.

The second type of stress fracture occurs on the tension side of a bone. This is the result of a combination of bending forces and muscle forces acting to increase bending of a bone. As mentioned, if the tibia has an increase in its anterior bow, excessive stress will result in a stress fracture of the anterior cortex of the tibia (tension side of the bone).

16. What type of stress fractures occur in the femoral neck? What is their management?

Although less common than stress fractures in the lower leg and foot, stress fractures do occur in the neck of the femur in children. If the fracture is not adequately treated, a complete fracture with displacement may occur, which risks the blood supply of the femoral head.

There are two sites of femoral neck stress fractures: the compression side and the tension side of the bone. The compression-side stress fracture will usually heal with reduction of the stress, i.e., crutch ambulation with lack of weightbearing on the injured extremity. On the other hand, a stress fracture that occurs on the tension side of the femoral neck heals with more difficulty, and it may not heal with simple crutch ambulation. These types are the most likely to result in a complete fracture. Therefore, if this fracture does not heal with conservative measures, internal fixation with screws in the femoral neck may be required.

17. Can stress fractures occur in the upper extremity?
Stress fractures can occur in almost any bone if excessive stress is applied to a bone that does not have the ability to recover. I have seen stress fractures in the upper extremity develop when a certain activity produces sufficient repetitive force.

18. Will all stress fractures heal with reduction of stress or immobilization?
Most stress fractures will heal with reduction of the stress, which usually requires immobilization in children. Stress fractures on the tension of a bone, as mentioned previously, are more prone to nonunion. The two most common locations for tension-side stress fractures are the superior cortex of the femoral neck and the anterior cortex of the midtibia if there is an associated anterior bow of the tibia. Both these fractures frequently require surgical treatment. In the femoral neck, if the tension-side stress fracture does not heal with avoidance of weightbearing, then internal fixation of the femoral neck will be required.

BIBLIOGRAPHY

1. Devas MB: Stress fractures in children. J Bone Joint Surg 45B:528–541, 1963.
2. Green NE, Rogers RA, Lipscomb AB: Nonunion of stress fractures of the tibia. Am J Sports Med 13:171–176, 1985.
3. Walker RN, Green NE, Spindler KP: Stress fractures in skeletally immature patients. J Pediatr Orthop 16:578–584, 1996.

---

42. UPPER EXTREMITY SPORTS INJURIES

Christopher K. Kim, M.D., and Henry G. Chambers, M.D.

1. What is acromioclavicular (AC) joint injury?
Fractures of the distal clavicle represent approximately 10–12% of all clavicular fractures. A fall on the point of the shoulder that drives the scapula downward usually causes an acromioclavicular dislocation in the older adolescent and adult, but fractures of the distal clavicle are much more common in children with the same mechanism. These fractures represent "pseudodislocations" because the distal shaft is herniated upward through a rupture of the thick periosteal tube that surrounds the distal clavicle. The coracoclavicular and acromioclavicular ligaments remain intact to the periosteal tube along with the usually apparent distal clavicular physis.

2. What diagnostic views are necessary in an AC joint injury?
Adequate radiographic views need to be taken to evaluate AC joint injuries. Routine radiographs of the shoulder are often well centered on the glenohumeral joint and therefore allow too much penetration to visualize the distal clavicle and acromioclavicular joint adequately. An axillary view and a 20° cephalic tilt view can further demonstrate the displacement in the AC region. When injuries to the region of the distal clavicle are suspected but not well defined on routine views, stress radiographs can be requested. Radiographs of both acromioclavicular joint regions are taken simultaneously on the same x-ray cassette. The first view is taken without weights, and the second stress view is taken with weights suspended from the wrists.

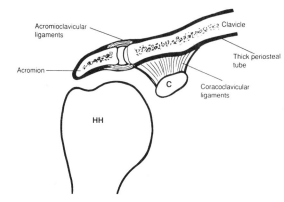

Anatomy of the distal clavicle and acromio-clavicular joint in children. Note the thick-ened periosteal tube surrounding the distal clavicle that is continuous with the acromio-clavicular and coracoclavicular ligaments.

3. How are AC injuries treated?

Most authors agree that distal clavicular injuries in children and adolescents represent frac-tures through the distal physis or pseudodislocations rather than true adultlike acromioclavicular separations. Most agree that so long as there is no gross deformity or instability, this injury can be treated conservatively. Therefore, types I–III can usually be treated with a short period of im-mobilization followed by progressive range-of-motion and strengthening exercises. Most frac-tures will heal, and function will be regained within 4–6 weeks. Return to sports is delayed until full shoulder motion and strength are obtained. Residual bony prominence is not a contraindica-tion to return to sports.

Types IV–VI injuries that show fixed deformity or gross displacement will generally require open reduction and internal fixation. Surgically, the joint will need to be reduced and the peri-osteal tube repaired. In the older patient, supplemental temporary fixation is performed with a coracoclavicular screw. This screw is removed in 6–8 weeks when rehabilitation is begun.

4. How are AC joint injuries classified?

Rockwood's classification is similar to that used in adults for acromioclavicular dislocation. The classification in children is based on the position of the distal clavicle and the accompanying injury to the periosteal tube rather than on injury of the ligaments, as occurs in true dislocation.

Type I Mild ligamentous sprain of the acromioclavicular ligaments without disruption of the periosteal tube. The distal clavicle is stable on examination, and x-ray findings are normal com-pared with the opposite shoulder.

Type II There is partial disruption of the dorsal periosteal tube with some instability at the distal clavicle on examination. Radiographically, there is a slight widening of the acromioclavic-ular joint but no change in the coracoclavicular interval.

Type III There is a large dorsal longitudinal split in the periosteal tube with gross instability of the distal clavicle. Radiographs reveal superior displacement of the clavicle in relation to the cora-coid and acromion. The coracoclavicular interval is 25–100% greater than on the normal shoulder.

Type IV This injury is similar to type III, but the clavicle is displaced posteriorly and is but-tonholed through the trapezius muscle fibers, with the distal end completely buried in muscle. On anteroposterior (AP) radiographs, there is little superior migration. The axillary radiographs show posterior displacement of the distal clavicle in relation to the acromion.

Type V There is a complete dorsal periosteal split with superior subcutaneous displacement of the clavicle. This is often associated with a split of the deltoid and trapezius attachments. On ra-diographs, the coracoclavicular distance is greater than 100% compared with the normal shoulder.

Type VI An inferior dislocation of the distal clavicle occurs, with the distal clavicle lodged beneath the coracoid process.

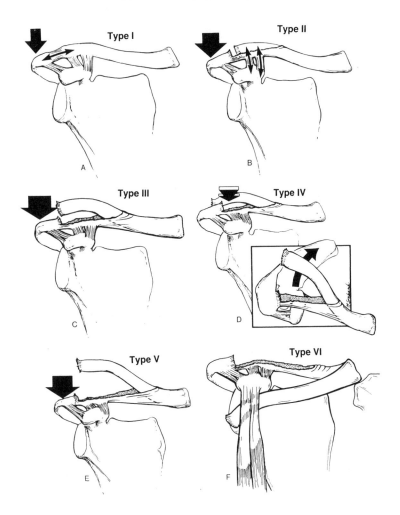

The Rockwood classification for distal clavicle injuries in children. Refer to the text for a complete description of this classification system. (Reproduced with permission from Rockwood CA Jr. Green DP (eds) *Fractures,* 2nd ed. Philadelphia, J. B. Lippincott, Co. 1984.)

5. What is sternoclavicular (SC) joint injury?

The sternoclavicular joint in children is much less commonly affected by injuries than the physis or medial metaphysis. True dislocations of the sternoclavicular joint in children are reported but are extremely rare. Most injuries about the medial end of the clavicle involve the medial physeal plate and occur as Salter-Harris type I or II fractures. Injuries to the medial clavicle can occur in athletic events, predominantly in contact or collision sports. The most common mechanism of injury is an indirect blow to the lateral aspect of the shoulder that transmits force along the clavicle, resulting in a fracture of the physis medially. If the shoulder is compressed and rolled forward, a posterior displacement at the medial end will occur. If the shoulder is compressed and forced posteriorly, anterior displacement will occur. These injuries are best described using the Salter-Harris classification of fractures and also the direction of the displacement of the shaft fragment.

6. How is shoulder instability classified?

By degree of instability, direction of instability, and cause of the dislocation. The etiologic classification is the most important when formulating treatment options and predicting prognosis. The degree of instability can be broken down into subluxation versus dislocation. The directions of instability are anterior, posterior, inferior, and multidirectional. Anterior dislocations of the glenohumeral joint in children are the most common, constituting greater than 90% of injuries. Isolated cases of posterior dislocations in children and adolescents have been reported, but true traumatic posterior instability of the shoulder is rare. Inferior dislocations are very rare. Instability can be traumatic or atraumatic, which can be further broken down into voluntary versus involuntary, and recurrent. To be classified as a case of traumatic instability, a history of significant high-energy trauma and an appropriate mechanism should exist. Atraumatic instability of the glenohumeral joint only exists in the presence of multidirectional laxity of the shoulder. Recurrent instability can exist after either traumatic or atraumatic instability.

7. What are the causes of traumatic instability?

Anterior instability of the glenohumeral joint is the most common form of traumatic injury. A fall onto an outstretched hand that forces the arm into excessive abduction and external rotation is the primary mechanism of injury. The humeral head is levered anteriorly, tearing the anterior glenohumeral ligament complex and eventually dislocating, with the humeral head lodging against the anterior neck of the glenoid. Commonly, this results in a Bankart-type injury, in which the inferior glenohumeral ligament attachment is stripped off the anterior neck of the glenoid. Posterior dislocations are not commonly reported in children.

With traumatic anterior glenohumeral dislocations, patients present with obvious deformity, swelling, and (always) pain. The arm is held slightly abducted, externally rotated, and supported by the other arm. The neurologic and vascular status must be assessed. The axillary nerve is the most common nerve to be injured with anterior dislocation, but the entire brachial plexus can be involved. The sensory distribution of the axillary nerve is along the upper lateral arm and can be tested by light touch or pinprick. The motor innervation to the deltoid can be tested by having the patient voluntarily contract the deltoid in an attempt to abduct the elbow lightly.

Traumatic posterior dislocation is less apparent on clinical examination. Looking at the shoulder from above, flattening of the anterior aspect of the shoulder is noted with the hand across the abdomen. The hallmark of posterior dislocation is the lack of external rotation and an inability to supinate the forearm.

AP of the glenohumeral joint, axillary lateral view, and scapular lateral view should be obtained. In the AP view, there will be an empty glenoid sign in which the articular surface of the humeral head does not fit into the glenoid. In the other two views, the head will be seen either anterior to or posterior to the glenoid.

In acute situations, we have performed a closed reduction by one of the standard and accepted techniques. Light sedation with either intravenous or intramuscular techniques is adequate for reduction. Any maneuver that gently and carefully reduces the joint is acceptable. X-rays should be obtained after the reduction maneuver. Postreduction care is somewhat controversial. In the limited literature available on anterior dislocation in the child, it is inconclusive whether immobilization after reduction truly alters the prognosis. After a period of immobilization, an aggressive rehabilitation program should be instituted that focuses on strengthening the rotator cuff and deltoid. The most common problem with anterior dislocation of the shoulder is recurrent instability. For posterior dislocations, a gentle reduction maneuver should be performed. After reduction, the arm is immobilized in neutral position or slight external rotation with the arm at the side. This may require a modified spica cast or a custom brace.

8. What are the causes of atraumatic instability?

This is the most common type of instability in children and adolescents. A shoulder dislocation in a child without a clear-cut significant history of trauma should arouse suspicion that this may be an instance of atraumatic instability. These patients have inherent joint laxity, and the glenohumeral joint can be dislocated either voluntarily or involuntarily as a result of minimal trauma. Voluntary instability is accomplished by consciously firing certain muscles while inhibiting their antagonists. Voluntary instability can be associated with psychologic instability.

The most notable finding is the lack of pain associated with subluxation or dislocation. In most cases, reduction is not required because spontaneous reduction occurs. Clinical exam shows multiple-joint laxity, which may include hyperextensibility of the elbows, knees, and metacarpophalangeal joints. Skin hyperelasticity and striae may be present. In cases of acute trauma, the opposite shoulder should be examined for findings of multidirectional laxity because the affected shoulder may be too painful to undergo a complete examination. These signs of multidirectional laxity at the glenohumeral joint include a positive sulcus sign and significant humeral head translation on anterior and posterior drawer tests. The sulcus sign, a dimpling of the skin below the acromion when manual longitudinal traction is applied to the arm, is due to inferior subluxation of the humeral head within the glenohumeral joint. The drawer test is performed with the examiner seated at the side of the patient. The scapula is stabilized with one hand while the opposite hand manually translates the humeral head anteriorly and posteriorly. In patients with atraumatic instability, all are painless. The radiographic exam results in these patients are usually normal.

In treating the patient with atraumatic instability, a nonoperative approach emphasizing a vigorous rehabilitation program involving strengthening of the rotator cuff will be used. Most patients without significant emotional or psychiatric problems successfully improve shoulder stability with this program. For patients with multidirectional instability who fail to improve after a thorough rehabilitation program, capsular-type reconstruction has been recommended.

9. How frequent are recurrent dislocations? How should they be treated?

The literature on the natural history of glenohumeral dislocation in adolescents and young adults demonstrates recurrence rates of 25 to 90%. The true incidence of recurrent dislocations of the glenohumeral joint in a child is difficult to assess because of both the rarity of the injury and the variations in reports in the literature. In 1963, Rowe reported a 100% incidence of recurrence in children younger than the age of 10 who sustained anterior dislocation. He reported a 94% incidence of recurrence in adolescents and young adults between the ages of 11 and 20 years. In 1975, Rockwood reported a recurrence rate of 50% in a series of patients between 13.8 and 15.8 years of age. Recently, Marans and associates reported on the fate of 21 children between the ages of 4 and 15 years with open physes at the time of initial dislocation. They found a 100% recurrence rate no matter what postreduction treatment program was used.

Treatment of the patient with recurrent anterior dislocation of the shoulder should begin with an attempt to confirm the cause of the dislocation. If the cause is atraumatic, then continued nonoperative treatment is recommended. If it is determined that recurrent dislocation has a true traumatic cause, treatment is surgical.

10. What is impingement syndrome?

Impingement is much less common than in adults, but can be a cause of symptoms in the pediatric athlete. Classically, impingement occurs as the structures (greater tuberosity, supraspinatus tendon, long head of the biceps, and subacromial bursa) pass beneath the anterior and inferior surfaces of the coracoacromial arch, which is composed of the coracoid, acromion, and coracoacromial ligament. This mechanical contact on a repetitive basis leads to acute and chronic inflammation and to the changes and clinical symptoms that we describe as impingement syndrome. Neer described impingement as a continuum; if left untreated, the process can progress from stage I (which includes acute inflammation and swelling) to stage II (a more chronic phase of inflammation, chronic scarring, and tendinitis) through to stage III (which is defined as a rotator cuff tear).

Most athletes in sports that require overhead repetitive shoulder function such as swimming, baseball, and tennis perform at a high level just below maximum stress. This repetitive microtrauma can lead to structural changes in the tendon, ligaments, and capsule. An intrinsic overload in the rotator cuff tendons can lead to tendinitis, secondary muscle weakness, and biomechanical imbalance.

Younger patients, both pediatric and adolescent, have a higher incidence of inherent multidirectional instability. In sports activities requiring repetitive stress on the shoulder, these patients require greater dynamic stability by the rotator cuff musculature. As the rate of stress increases and the rotator cuff becomes fatigued, impingement results secondary to the multidirectional instability. Treatment is therefore directed at improving joint stability rather than primarily correcting impingement phenomenon.

11. What are the symptoms of impingement syndrome?
The presenting symptom in all patients is pain. In mild cases, pain occurs only with certain activities, but as severity increases, the pain can become constant. Night pain is the hallmark symptom of rotator cuff disease. The pain is usually described as anterior or deep and can radiate down the lateral aspect of the arm to the area of the deltoid insertion. As the process becomes more severe, range of motion and strength can be diminished. Deficits in elevation and internal rotation are usually the first signs noted by the patient. The gross appearance of the shoulder is normal. In advanced cases, atrophy of the deltoid and the supraspinatus can appear. Range of motion is often normal. Strength can be affected by pain. The impingement sign is always positive in patients with pure impingement. It is elicited by stabilizing the scapula while forcing the arm into internal rotation and forward flexion. This maneuver compresses the subacromial space and causes pain in patients with impingement. The impingement test is done to confirm the diagnosis in the absence of instability. Substantial relief of symptoms occurring after injection of 10 ml of 1% Xylocaine (lidocaine) into the subacromial space indicates a positive test result. Great care should be taken to elicit signs of instability and generalized laxity on examination to confirm a diagnosis of secondary impingement.

12. How should impingement be treated?
Most young athletes present with mild symptoms only during specific activities. These patients may continue to participate while beginning treatment with oral nonsteroidal anti-inflammatory medications and rehabilitation. They should use moist heat-to-ice contrast treatment, along with a program of flexibility and rotator cuff strengthening exercises on a daily basis. In moderately severe cases in which the patient has pain at rest after athletic events, the athlete is removed from the activity. Nonsteroidal anti-inflammatory medications and modality treatments such as ultrasound are initiated. When the pain at rest subsides, the athlete should begin the usual rehabilitation program, to include flexibility and strengthening. In severe cases that have persisted more than 3 months despite a supervised treatment program, further work-up with shoulder MRI is performed. If the diagnosis of impingement is confirmed, the athlete continues with the rehabilitation process. Rarely, in older adolescents, surgical treatment may be necessary.

The young athlete with impingement should be made to realize that overuse is the common denominator in this problem. The overhand athlete should be painfree and actively involved in a rehabilitation program before returning to specific sports.

13. What are the stresses on the throwing elbow? What disorders can occur?
In both the young throwing athlete and the mature thrower, four distinct areas are vulnerable to throwing stress: (1) tension overload of the medial elbow restraints, (2) compression overload on the lateral articular surface, (3) posterior medial shear forces on the posterior articular surfaces, and (4) extension overload on the lateral restraints.

During early cocking and especially during late cocking, a significant distraction force is applied to the medial aspect of the elbow. The resultant force presents as tension on the medial epicondylar attachments, including the flexor muscle origin and the ulnar collateral ligaments. With overuse, the weakest link in the medial complex can be injured. In the young athlete, subsequent injury or avulsion of the medial epicondylar ossification center is often encountered. The ulnar collateral ligaments may be stretched, resulting in traction spurs on the coronoid process. Traction injury to the ulnar nerve and flexor muscle strain may also ensue.

Compression of the lateral articulation, in which the radial head abuts the capitellum, occurs mainly during early and late cocking. Sequelae include growth disturbances, chondral or osteochondral fractures of the capitellum, and growth disturbances and deformation of the radial head.

Posterior articular surface damage develops in two phases of throwing. During late cocking, a posterior medial shear force develops about the olecranon fossa. Throughout follow-through, hyperextension of the elbow is prominent, placing stress on the olecranon and anterior capsule. These stresses commonly produce disease at three sites: (1)posterior medial spur, (2) true posterior olecranon spurs, and (3) traction spurs of the coronoid process.

Lateral extension overload occurs during acceleration when extreme pronation of the forearm results in a tension force applied to the lateral ligaments and lateral epicondyle. Consequently, lateral epicondylitis may develop.

14. What are the biomechanics of the throwing elbow in baseball?

The pitch is divided into five stages: Phase 1 is the wind-up or preparation phase, ending when the ball leaves the glove hand; phase 2, termed early cocking, is a period of shoulder abduction and external rotation that begins as the ball is released from the nondominant hand and terminates with contact of the forward foot on the ground; phase 3, the late cocking phase, continues until maximum external rotation is obtained; phase 4 is the short propulsive phase of acceleration that starts with internal rotation of the humerus and ends with ball release; and phase 5 is the follow-through phase, which starts with ball release and ends when all motion is complete.

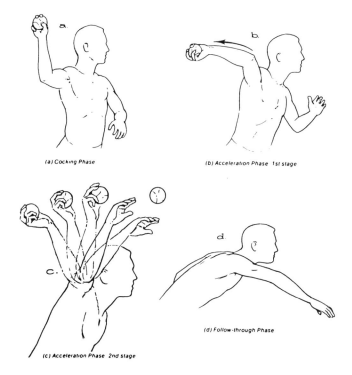

(a) Cocking Phase

(b) Acceleration Phase 1st stage

(c) Acceleration Phase 2nd stage

(d) Follow-through Phase

The three phases of pitching, *A*, Cocking phase *B–C*, Acceleration phase, *D*, Follow-through phase. (Reprinted with permission from Woods GW, Tullos HS, King JW: The throwing arm: Elbow joint injuries. J Sports Med [supp 4]45, 1973.)

15. What is little leaguer's elbow?

This is a group of pathologic entities in and about the elbow joint in young developing throwers. The injury includes (1) medial epicondylar fragmentation and avulsion, (2) delayed or accelerated apophyseal growth of the medial epicondyle, (3) delayed closure of the medial epicondylar growth plate, (4) osteochondrosis and osteochondritis of the capitellum, (5) deformation and osteochondritis of the radial head, (6) hypertrophy of the ulna, and (7) olecranon apophysitis with or without delayed closure of the olecranon apophysis. These abnormalities are secondary to the biomechanical throwing stresses placed on the young developing elbow.

16. What factors should be considered in the evaluation of the elbow of a young athlete?

A timely and accurate diagnosis is the keystone to successful treatment of the many conditions associated with little leaguer's elbow.

Age, position, handedness, activity level, location of pain, duration of pain, radiation, trauma, mechanism of injury, nature of onset, and past medical history are all salient factors in the history. The age of young throwers can be divided into three groups: (1) childhood, which terminates with the appearance of secondary centers of ossification; (2) adolescence, which terminates with the fusion of all secondary centers of ossification to their respective long bones; and (3) young adulthood, which terminates with completion of all bone growth and the achievement of final muscular form. During childhood, the most frequent complaints are sensitivity about the medial epicondyle, which is usually secondary to microinjuries at the apophysis and ossification center. When the athlete enters adolescence, the athlete increases the valgus stresses on the elbow, and the result can be an avulsion fracture of the entire medial epicondyle. Some adolescents develop enough chronic stresses to cause delayed union or possibly nonunion of the medial epicondyle. By young adulthood, the medial epicondyle has fused, and injuries of the muscular attachments and ligaments of the epicondyle become more prevalent.

The position played by the thrower provides insight into the magnitude of stresses placed on the elbow and the relative incidence of elbow complaints. The usual order of prevalence of elbow complaints among players is in pitchers, infielders, catchers, and outfielders.

Most throwers present with elbow problems in the dominant extremity unless direct trauma is the cause of the problem. Pain is the most common complaint. Localization, duration, character, temporal sequence, activity level, and nature of onset are all clues to the underlying problem. Although pain is the most frequent complaint, related but less frequent problems include decreased elbow motion, mild flexion contracture, swelling-decreased performance, and local sensitivity of the elbow. It is also helpful to remember that the elbow may be the site of referred pain. Therefore, associated neck, shoulder, and wrist pain or restricted motion must be appraised.

Young throwers often have unilateral hypertrophy of the muscle and bone of the dominant extremity. Therefore, the presence of hypertrophy, valgus deformity, and flexion contracture should not be considered uncommon in young throwers.

17. What are the types and symptoms of medial complex injuries? How should they be treated?

Most children with little leaguer's elbow present with medial elbow complaints. Medial complex injuries can be divided into three entities: (1) medial tension injuries, (2) medial epicondylar fractures, and (3) medial ligament rupture.

Medial tension injuries will present with a triad of symptoms including progressive medial pain, diminished throwing effectiveness, and decreased throwing distance. Repetitive valgus stresses and flexor forearm pull usually produce a subtle apophysitis or stress fracture through the medial epicondylar epiphyses. Physical manifestations include tenderness, swelling over the medial epicondyle, and an elbow flexion contracture of more than 15°. Radiographs show fragmentation and widening of the epiphyseal lines compared to the contralateral elbow. In most cases, a 4–6 week course of rest from throwing along with ice and nonsteroidal anti-inflammatory medications will result in cessation of symptoms. After 6 weeks, when the patient has no symptoms and a pain-free range of motion, strengthening exercises are begun. A progressive throwing program is initiated at 8 weeks. Occasionally, symptoms may reappear when throwing is resumed; in these cases, throwing should be delayed until next season.

When more substantial acute valgus stress is applied through violent muscle contraction during throwing, an avulsion fracture of the medial epicondyle may ensue. There may be a painful elbow with point tenderness over the medial epicondyle and an elbow flexion contracture that may exceed 15°. Radiographs most often show only a minimally displaced epicondylar fragment or significant displacement with or without displacement into the joint. Woods and Tullos have divided these lesions into two types. Type 1 occurs in younger children and produces a large fragment that involves the entire medial epicondyle and often displaces and rotates. Type 2 occurs in adolescents and produces a small fracture fragment. Most treatment protocols center on how much displacement is present. In minimally displaced (less than 2 mm) or nondisplaced fractures, simple posterior splint immobilization is initiated. After the acute symptoms have subsided, the patient's arm may be removed from the splint, and active motion exercises may be started. Radiographic evidence of healing should be apparent by 6 weeks, and aggressive active range-of-motion exercises as well as a progressive strengthening program should be begun. Competitive throwing may be resumed when the patient has normal painless range of motion, strength, and endurance while on the throwing program. In moderately displaced (more than 2 mm) fractures with a large fragment, open reduction and internal fixation are appropriate. Two small cancellous screws may be necessary to prevent rotation. Early motion after the surgery is extremely advantageous in the adolescent. Depending on the quality of the fixation, range-of-motion exercises begin 1 to 2 weeks after surgery while the patient is wearing a functional orthosis.

Injuries to the ulnar collateral ligaments are not common in young throwing athletes. Most patients have tenderness about the medial aspect of the elbow for months to years before the ligament is injured. Commonly, a rupture occurs as a catastrophic event. Clinically, there will be subtle medial elbow instability, which can be demonstrated by flexing the elbow to 25° to unlock the olecranon from its fossa and gently stressing the medial side of the elbow. Treatment of complete tear of the ulnar collateral ligament in young throwers who wish to resume their activity is surgical. This can be accomplished by direct repair or reconstruction using a tendon graft.

18. What is Panner's disease (osteochondrosis)? How is it treated?

This entity is a disease of the growth or ossification centers in children that begins as degeneration or necrosis of the capitellum and is followed by regeneration and recalcification. Panner's disease is a focal localized lesion of the subchondral bone of the capitellum and its overlying articular cartilage. The lesion is usually noted in the anterior central capitellum where it is in maximal contact with the articulation of the head of the radius. Radiographs show that the capitellar ossification center is fragmented owing to irregular patches of relative sclerosis alternating with areas of rarefaction. The natural history of Panner's disease is that as growth progresses, the capitellar epiphysis eventually assumes a normal appearance in size, contour, and subchondral architecture. Initial treatment should consist of rest, avoidance of throwing, and sometimes splinting until the pain and tenderness subside.

19. How is osteochondritis dissecans evaluated, classified, and treated?

Osteochondritis dissecans (OCD) is presently looked upon as a singular entity within the multiple entities encompassed by the term "little leaguer's elbow." OCD of the capitellum appears to be secondary to compressive forces occurring between the capitellum and the radial head during throwing. Osteochondritis is a focal lesion of the capitellum occurring in the 13 to 16-year-old age group, usually characterized by elbow pain and a flexion contracture of 15° or more. Onset is insidious, with a focal island of subchondral bone demarcated by a rarefied zone on radiographs. Sequalae include loose bodies, residual deformity of the capitellum, and often residual elbow disability. OCD must be differentiated from Panner's disease. Age, onset, loose body formation, radiographic findings, and deformity of the capitellum all aid in the differentiation. Panner's disease usually affects a younger population, and the onset is acute with fragmentation of the entire ossific nucleus.

Etiology of OCD of the elbow has not been determined. Three popular theories include ischemia, trauma, or genetic factors. Typically, the patient with OCD presents with a dull, poorly localized pain that is aggravated by use, especially throwing, and relieved by rest. These patients commonly complain of limitation of motion. Later in the course of the disease, locking and catching with severe pain may supervene. Radiographs will usually show the typical rarefaction, irregular ossification, and a crater adjacent to the articular surface of the capitellum. Arthroscopy is an excellent method of determining the size of the lesion, its fixation, and the condition of the articular cartilage of the capitellum and radial head.

OCD's can be divided into three types. Type I lesions are intact and show no evidence of displacement and no evidence of fracture of the articular cartilage. Treatment involves rest and avoidance of all vigorous activities. Protection of the elbow should be continued until there is radiographic evidence of revascularization and healing. Type II lesions show evidence of fracture or fissure of the articular cartilage or partial detachment of the lesion. If the lesion is large enough to fix the fragment adequately, the lesion should be pinned in situ. If the fragment is small and pin purchase is tenuous, single excision to prevent future loose body formation and burring of the base is undertaken. Type III lesions are completely detached and lie free in the joint. Usually the loose body is hypertrophied and rounded, and the crater is obscured by fibrous tissue and is much smaller than the loose body. Treatment usually consists of removal of the loose body by arthrotomy or arthroscopy with or without drilling and curettage. Excision of loose bodies usually relieves the pain; however, there may be no improvement in the range of motion, and late degenerative changes may still be the eventual outcome.

20. What is ulnar neuritis, and how should it be treated?
The ulnar nerve sits in a shallow groove behind the medial epicondyle. The nerve may get irritated with repeated throwing. Ulnar neuritis may occur in three different settings: (1) hypermobile nerve with anterior subluxation, (2) ulnar nerve traction due to valgus instability of the elbow, and (3) cubital tunnel irritation without instability.

Some athletes have the disadvantage of a hypermobile nerve, which may subluxate out of the cubital tunnel with rapid elbow flexion and extension. This condition may prove to be a serious deterrent to pitching. Most players with persistent ulnar neuritis have accompanying medial collateral ligament instability, accounting for the increased traction on the tethered nerve. The swollen inflamed tissues surrounding the injured medial collateral ligament also contribute to compression. When ulnar neuritis and instability are encountered, several months of rest with a complete overhaul of the throwing technique are suggested. Ulnar neuritis without instability is unusual and carries a better prognosis. After rest and nonsteroidal anti-inflammatory medication, return to pitching is allowed when light tossing produces no symptoms.

21. How often and how much should a child pitch?
Pre-adolescent throwing pains are common, but significant injuries are rare. Adolescent baseball brings several new challenges to pitchers. The field is bigger, and the hitters have more time to react to the pitches. Smaller rosters are thus common and place added expectations on available pitchers. Following is a table for adolescent pitching limits by age.

Adolescent Pitching Limits

TEAM	AGE GROUP	PITCHING LIMITS
Little League Minors	10–12	6 innings per week; local restriction—4 innings per game
Little League Majors	11–12	6 innings per week
Little League Juniors	13–14	9 innings per week
Pony League	13–14	7 to 10 innings per week; no adjacent days
Dixie Youth	13–14	10 innings per week
Little League Seniors	14–15	9 innings per week
American Legion	15–18	12 innings per week
American Amateur Baseball	17–18	Unlimited

22. What are the risks to the hand and wrist in children during sports?
In most sports, the hand and wrists are exposed, causing them to have a very high incidence of injury. Zariczny and colleagues found that 30% of all injuries in children were to the hand and wrist, with boys having twice the number of injuries. Chambers, studying a group of military children, found that 65% of all injuries were to the hand and wrist, with basketball and football causing the highest incidence. The thumb is most commonly injured in the adolescent skier, and 50% of all skateboarding fractures occur in the hand. Overall, the incidence of injuries to the hand and

wrist depend on the amount of contact and stress loading applied to the limb. Injury rates range from 3 to 65%, with swimming and soccer having the lowest incidence and football and basketball having the highest.

23. How should nailbed injuries be treated?

The treatment of the nailbed injury must allow for optimum nailbed function. If the nail is not avulsed and the subungual hematoma is less than one third of the nail, simply draining the hematoma and treating the fracture, if present, is adequate. If hematoma is greater than one third or if the nail is partially avulsed, a significant tear in the nailbed is assumed. Under metacarpal block, the nail is removed, and the nailbed is repaired with fine chromic suture. The nail is then cleaned, and several holes are made in it for drainage. It is then placed back into the nail fold. The nail is the best protection for the bed and an excellent splint for the fracture. Antibiotic coverage should be used in all open fractures for at least 3 days. The nail injuries and the associated fractures remain tender 3–6 weeks. The patient should be told to expect some residual nail deformity.

24. What is a mallet finger and how is it treated?

The most common injury to the distal interphalangeal (DIP) joint is a bony or tendinous mallet finger. It is most commonly seen in athletes who are forced to catch objects. Mallet finger results from forced hyperflexion of the DIP joint. The patient is unable to extend the DIP joint actively but has full passive extension. Unless there is subluxation of the DIP joint, all these injuries can be treated with splinting of the DIP joint in full extension, not hyperextension, for 6 weeks. If the patient has active extension at 6 weeks, flexion exercises can be started, and a splint is worn for another month during athletic activities. If an extension lag is present at 10 weeks, terminal tendon repair can be considered. This is usually not necessary in children or adolescents. Large displaced epiphyseal fractures should be treated with open versus closed reduction and internal fixation.

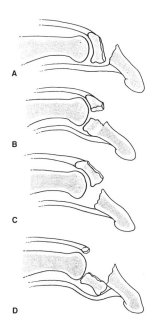

"The "mallet-equivalent" fractures types A–D.

25. What is rugger jersey finger and how is it treated?

Avulsion of the flexor digitorum profundus is the most common closed flexor tendon injury in the adolescent athlete. This injury most commonly occurs to the ring finger. The injury results when a hyperextension force is applied to the DIP joint with concomitant attempted flexion of the flexor digitorum profundus. This happens almost exclusively in football or rugby as the finger catches on the opposing player's jersey while attempting to tackle. On physical examination, the patient

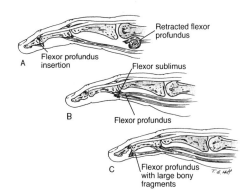

The classification system proposed by Leddy and Packer for flexor digitorum profundus (FDP) avulsion injuries. A, Type I: FDP rupture and retraction into the palm. B, Type II: The FDP ruptures and retracts to the level of the proximal interphalangeal joint. A flake of bone may be present. C, Type III: A large bony fragment is avulsed along with the FDP.

will not be able to flex the DIP joint with the proximal interphalangeal (PIP) joint in full extension. The avulsed tendon classically retracts into one of three levels: (1) just distal to the A4 pulley, often with a chip of bone, which is the level of the DIP flexion crease; (2) at the level of the PIP joint; or (3) within the palm. The treatment for this injury in the acute situation is to repair the tendon. The difficulty with flexor digitorum profundus avulsion occurs when the initial diagnosis is delayed. If the diagnosis is made within 3 weeks, the tendon can usually be reattached. If the diagnosis is not made until 6 weeks, it is virtually impossible to repair the tendon because the tendon has retracted into the palm and has become fibrotic.

26. What is a "coach's finger," and how is it treated?
The "jammed finger" is the most common joint injury in the child and the adolescent. This hyperextension injury to the PIP joint can happen in any ball or contact sport. This injury results from an axial compressive force being applied to the end of the digit and can result in PIP joint hyperextension with or without dislocation. This injury is called "coach's finger," since the injury is usually treated by the coach on the sideline by in-line traction and "popping" the finger back into place. Treatment of dorsal dislocation of the PIP joint is closed reduction and proper evaluation. First, radiographs are obtained to look for displaced fractures. Then the joint is placed through an active range of motion to see if redislocation occurs. Lateral stress testing is also performed in both directions. In stable cases, the initial treatment is 2–3 days of PIP splinting in 30° of flexion to allow for pain and edema control. A dorsal splint is better tolerated than a volar splint because it allows metacarpophalangeal joint flexion and use of the fingertips. This is followed by buddy taping during athletic activities for 6 more weeks to permit protected range of motion. These injuries can produce persistent pain and swelling for up to 6 months.

27. What is gamekeeper's thumb and how is it treated?
Gamekeeper's thumb describes acute and chronic injury to the ulnar collateral ligament at the thumb metacarpophalangeal (MP) joint. The thumb MP joint is the most commonly injured joint in downhill skiers from ages 11 to 16. These injuries result from an excessive radial deviation force on the thumb after falling on the outstretched hand with the thumb in abducted position. This results in either a Salter-Harris fracture or ligamentous injury (less common in children). Salter-Harris II fractures are common in children, whereas adolescents typically present with a Salter-Harris III fracture. With the typical history, radiographs must be obtained first, since stressing the joint could theoretically displace a nondisplaced fracture.

Nondisplaced Salter-Harris I and II fractures should be treated with a short-arm thumb spica cast. Displaced fractures should be treated with closed reduction and casting. Nondisplaced or minimally displaced Salter-Harris III or IV fractures can be treated with a short-arm thumb spica cast. If the fracture fragment is displaced, open reduction and internal fixation are required.

If radiographic findings are negative, the integrity of the ulnar collateral ligament must be assessed. This is accomplished by radially deviating the MP joint in full extension and 30° of flexion. The opposite side must be used as comparison. If there is no firm end point, there is a complete tear of the ulnar collateral ligament, and surgical repair is indicated. If there is a firm end point, the thumb can be treated in a short-arm thumb spica cast for 6 weeks for ligamentous healing to occur.

28. What is Kienböck's disease?

Kienböck's disease is avascular necrosis of the lunate. It is rare in the immature carpus but does occur in the adolescent. The goals of treatment for Kienböck's disease are to reduce pain, maintain wrist motion, promote revascularization of the lunate to prevent carpal collapse, and prevent secondary arthritis.

In patients with this disease, a return to preinjury status is unpredictable.

Classification of Kienböck's Disease

STAGE	PAIN	PLAIN RADIOGRAPHS	LUNATE COLLAPSE	CARPAL COLLAPSE	ARTHRITIS
1	+	−	−	−	−
2	+	+	−	−	−
3	+	+	+	±	−
4	+	+	+	+	+

Kienböck's disease can be classified according to radiographic finding. Stages 1, 2 and 3 are most likely in the adolescent age group.

Treatment of Kienböck's Disease

STAGE	PROCEDURE	LUNATE COLLAPSE	CARPAL COLLAPSE	ULNAR VARIANCE	RADIOLUNATE ARTHRITIS	RADIOSCAPHOID ARTHRITIS
1 and 2	Radial shortening ⎱	N	N	− or neutral	N	N
	Ulnar lengthening ⎰	N	N	+	N	N
3	Radial shortening	Y	None or moderate	− or neutral	N	N
	Ulnar lengthening	Y	Y-Severe	Ms> or +	N	N
4	STT arthrodesis; excision of lunate, no silicone	Y	Y	− or +	Y	N
	Fibrous arthroplasty or Radiocarpal fusion	Y	Y	− or +	Y	Y

STT, Scaphoid-trapezial-trapezoid; N, no; Y, yes; −, negative, +, positive.

29. How do stress injuries to the distal wrist manifest?

Roy and colleagues in 1985 reported on 21 gymnasts who sustained stress injuries to the distal radial epiphysis. These gymnasts practiced more than 36 hours per week. Stiffness and pain with dorsiflexion were presenting symptoms. Radiographs demonstrated widened epiphysis, cystic changes, and beaking of the distal metaphysis. There is evidence that repeated dorsiflexion stress loading of the wrist leads to partial distal radial growth arrest, creating a positive ulnar variance. Although no cases of severe distal radial or ulnar epiphyseal growth arrest have been reported, if a child develops changes of the distal radius or the ulna, the family should be informed that growth arrest may be significant enough to require future surgical intervention.

BIBLIOGRAPHY

1. Andrews JR: Bony injuries about the elbow in the young throwing athlete. Instr Course Lect 34:323–331, 1985.
2. Backx FJ, Erich BM, Kemper AB, et al.: Sports injuries in school-aged children: an epidemiologic study. Am J Sports Med. 17:234–240, 1989.
3. Burkhead WZ, Rockwood CA: Treatment of instability of the shoulder with an exercise program. J Bone Joint Surg 74A(6):890–896, 1992.

4. Green DP: Operative Hand Surgery. New York, Churchill-Livingstone, 1993.
5. Hawkins RJ, Kennedy JC: Impingement syndrome in athletes. Am J Sports Med 8(3):151–157, 1980.
6. Leddy JP, Packer JW: Avulsion of the profundus tendon insertion in athletes. J Hand Surg 2:66–69, 1977.
7. McCue FC, Baugher WH, Kulund DN, et al.: Hand and wrist injuries in the athlete. Am J Sports Med 7:275–286, 1979.
8. Pappas AM: Elbow problems associated with baseball during childhood and adolescence. Clin Orthop 164:30–41, 1982.
9. Rockwood CA, Jr.: Fractures and dislocations of the ends of the clavicle, scapulae and glenohumeral joint. In Rockwood CA, Wilkins KE, Beatty JH (eds), Fractures in Children, Vol. 3. Philadelphia, J.B. Lippincott Co., 1996.
10. Sharrard WJW: Pediatric Orthopaedics and Fractures. London, Blackwell Scientific Publications, 1993.
11. Tibone JE: Shoulder problems of adolescents: how they differ from those of adults. Clin Sports Med 2:423–427, 1983.
12. Stanitski CL, DeLee JC, Drez D: Pediatric and Adolescent Sports Medicine. Philadelphia, W. B. Saunders Co., 1994.
13. Wilkins KE: Fractures and dislocations of the elbow region. In Rockwood CA, Wilkins KE, Beatty JE (eds): Fractures in Children. Philadelphia, J. B. Lippincott Co., 1996.

43. LOWER EXTREMITY SPORTS INJURIES

Michael T. Busch, M.D.

1. What is an apophysis?

Apophyses are specialized growth centers of the immature skeleton that occur around joints. Major muscles or muscle groups take origin or insert into these areas, where they are prone to a variety of injuries in youths participating in sports.

2. What apophyses are located about the hips and pelvis, and what inserts or originates in these locations? (see Figure)

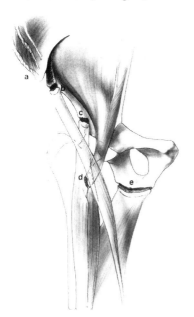

There are several apophyses in the area of the hip and pelvis. Avulsion fractures and overuse syndrome of these apophyses are fairly common in youth sports injuries. The muscle origin and insertion are illustrated. (a) The abdominal wall muscles insert into the iliac crest apophysis. (b) The sartorius originates from the anterior superior iliac spine apophysis. (c) The direct head of the rectus femoris originates from the anterior inferior iliac spine apophysis. (d) The iliopsoas tendon inserts into the lesser trochanteric apophysis of the proximal femur. (e) The hamstrings originate from the ischial apophysis. (From Busch MT: Sports medicine. In Morrissy RT (ed): Lovell and Winter's Pediatric Orthopaedics, 4th ed. Philadelphia, Lippincott-Raven, 1996, with permission)

Apophysis	Origin/Insertion
Iliac crest	External oblique muscle of the abdomen
Anterior superior iliac spine	Sartorius
Anterior inferior spine	Direct head of the rectus femoris
Lesser trochanter	Iliopsoas
Greater trochanter	Gluteus medius
Ischium	Hamstrings

3. How are most apophyseal avulsion fractures treated?

Most apophyseal avulsion fractures around the pelvis do not displace significantly. The periosteum is usually in continuity with the fragment, so with time the fracture will heal satisfactorily. Even with moderate displacement, surgical fixation is rarely indicated. [Complications are rare.] Crutches help to rest the area and the muscles around the hip. Sports activities should be terminated or significantly modified until healing has completed, which can take from 4–12 weeks. Premature return to sports is associated with a high incidence of recurrent symptoms.

4. Which two fractures of the hip and pelvis are most often associated with sports injuries?

Traumatic posterior dislocations of the hip, usually produced by an axial load applied to the adducted hip, frequently occur in football players. The dislocation is often accompanied by a fracture of the posterior wall of the iliac portion of the acetabulum. If the fragment is small, it may heal without compromising the stability of the acetabulum. If larger open reduction and internal fixation may be necessary.

Occasionally, pathological fractures of the femoral neck occur. These are typically secondary to benign lesions such as simple bone cysts, aneurysmal bone cysts, fibrous dysplasia, and sometimes stress fractures.

5. What are the two most common serious complications arising from traumatic hip dislocation?

Small fracture fragments are sometimes difficult to visualize with plain radiography. The source of these includes the posterior margin at the acetabulum, the femoral head, and the origin of the ligamentum teres from the acetabular fossa. If trapped in the joint and left unrecognized, these can lead to severe arthrosis.

Avascular necrosis (AVN) of the femoral head can occur after any traumatic hip dislocation. In youth sports, the hip will often spontaneously reduce on the field. This makes diagnosis more difficult, and must therefore, be kept in mind. The longer the hip is dislocated, the higher the rate of AVN. However, it can even occur in cases of spontaneous (immediate) reduction. Radiographic evidence of AVN is usually evident after one year, but can take up to two years to present. Early bone scan and magnetic resonance imaging (MRI) have a high rate of false positives and negatives.

6. How soon can a player return to sports following a quadriceps contusion?

While technically a bruise, this injury has a wide spectrum of severity. Players with mild bruises can return to sports almost immediately, while these with severe contusions may be out for more than 6 weeks.

7. How is a quadriceps contusion initially treated? How is its progress monitored?

Acutely: rest, ice, compressive wrap, and elevation are used to reduce bleeding. The three most important parameters to follow are pain, swelling, and restriction of passive knee flexion. The ability to fully flex the knee is the last function to return to normal, and is, therefore, the best indicator for return to sport.

8. What is the consequence of premature return to participation following a quadriceps contusion?
Repeat interstitial hemorrhaging. This can lead to significant exacerbation of the injury with marked delay in subsequent resolution. It is very important to be sure that this injury has completely resolved before returning an athlete to sports, particularly contact sports.

9. If a teenage athlete presents with pain and swelling in his/her anterior thigh without a clear history of significant trauma, what should be considered in the differential diagnosis?
Quadriceps contusions sometimes result from fairly minor injuries. Interstitial muscle tears, particularly of the rectus femoris, can present as a spontaneous bleed in the thigh as well. More serious problems, however, need to be investigated, especially in teenagers: rhabdomyosarcoma of the quadriceps, Ewing sarcoma, and osteosarcoma should be considered. At a minimum, plain radiographs should be obtained. If soft tissue sarcoma is suspected, the patient should undergo MRI.

10. How do meniscal tears present in young patients?
Meniscal tears in youths are usually associated with significant injuries that result from a *memorable event*. They produce pain, swelling, and limping. They rarely result from *trivial episodes* as can happen in adults. There is often associated injury to the ligaments in youths, particularly the anterior cruciate ligament and the medial collateral ligament. The youth with spontaneous or gradual onset of joint line pain in the knee rarely has a torn cartilage.

11. At what age do meniscal tears begin to occur?
Tearing of a normal meniscus rarely occurs under 12 years of age. A discoid meniscus is a congenitally abnormal cartilage and can present at almost any age.

12. How does a discoid meniscus become symptomatic?
Discoid menisci can be thick and bulbous (Wrisberg's ligament) which causes them to snap when the knee performs a range of motions. Discoid menisci can also tear spontaneously in children as young as 7 or 8 years of age.

13. What portion of the meniscus has a blood supply that aids in the healing process, either spontaneously or with surgical repair?
Microangiographic studies have shown that the menisci are not completely avascular structures, as was once thought. Approximately 30% of the meniscus closest to the capsule has a blood supply that facilitates healing. Children and adolescents have a high percentage of detachments and longitudinal tears near the capsular margin, both of which are good candidates for repair. Repair yields an 80–90% success rate with minor deterioration over time.

14. What is the expected outcome of meniscectomy in youths?
Initially, meniscectomy is supposed to relieve the symptoms of a torn cartilage. A small percentage of patients then begin to develop symptoms between 3–5 years of age. Seventy-five percent of these patients will show degenerative articular changes radiographically, although only 30% will be clinically symptomatic. Presumably, most of these patients will develop debilitating arthritis in their 40s and 50s. The long-term affects of arthroscopic partial meniscectomy are still not known, but may not be completely favorable. All reasonable efforts should be made to preserve a torn meniscus in a young person.

15. Name the naturally occurring plicae of the knee.
- Suprapatellar plica
- Medial patellar plica
- Infrapatellar plica (see Figure)

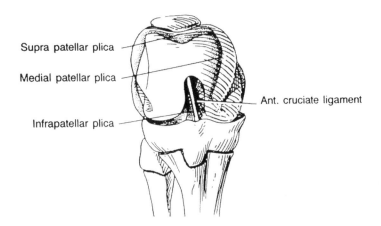

Supra patellar plica

Medial patellar plica

Ant. cruciate ligament

Infrapatellar plica

Plicae are synovial folds, and three major ones are commonly present in the knee. A suprapatellar plica can partially or completely divide the suprapatellar pouch from the rest of the knee joint. The medial patellar plica is the one that most commonly becomes symptomatic. The infrapatellar plica (ligamentum mucosum) lies directly in front of the anterior cruciate ligament. (From Busch MT: Sports medicine. In Morrissy RT (ed): Lovell and Winter's Pediatric Orthopaedics, 4th ed. Philadelphia, Lippincott-Raven, 1996, with permission)

16. Which plica is most often symptomatic?
Plicae are normally occurring structures that are remnants from the embryologic development of the knee joint. Initially, three cavities form, and as these coalesce, their fusion is incomplete; the remaining small septae form the plicae. Plicae are rarely symptomatic, with the exception of the medial plica.

17. Name the two most common ways for a symptomatic medial plica to present.
    Acute: Often plicae become symptomatic after sustaining a direct blow to the area (e.g., a fall). It is believed that the plica and overlying synovium become thickened and then begin to catch or impinge where they previously had not. The youngster may experience persistent pain with attempts to resume activities, and occasionally, presents with an acutely "locked" knee. The knee is typically held in flexion with the youngster refusing to fully extend it—blocking because of pain.
    Chronic: Characterized by a gradual onset of pain this is particularly associated with sports that involve running. Patients who pronate as they walk and run may develop pain symptoms over the anteromedial portion of the knee joint. This usually follows the onset of a new sports season or with a sudden increase training levels. Participants in track, cross-country, soccer, football, and cycling are especially vulnerable.

18. True or false: The anterior cruciate ligament (ACL) is rarely ruptured in children because the physeal plates are weaker and break first, thereby acting as a "safety valve."
False. Although the physeal plates of the distal femur and proximal tibia can act as the "weak link in the chain" and may fracture prior to disruption of the ACL, concurrent injuries **do** occur, although rarely in children under the age of 8. Rupture of the ACL should always be considered in the differential diagnosis of a young person with an acute knee injury and swelling. ACL's are sometimes associated with femur fractures, but this usually requires significant trauma to produce.

19. Should an ACL sprain be treated by casting of the knee?
As in adults, the ACL has very limited capacity to heal. The blood supply comes from each end and is often disrupted with the sprain because it is located in the center of the knee joint. Rigid immobilization has not been shown to improve outcome. Following acute injury, the knee is

rested with a brace or knee immobilizer until the swelling and pain begin to subside. Aspiration may be indicated for a very tense and painful hemarthrosis. As the knee recovers from this acute phase a definitive treatment plan may be formulated and the injury better evaluated.

20. Can the ACL be safely reconstructed in a skeletally immature person?

In order to best restore the biomechanical properties of the ACL, a graft must be placed in as nearly an anatomical location as possible. Nonanatomic reconstructions (such as iliotibial band tenodesis) almost always stretch out and fail due to their anisometric nature. The ACL is a structure which spans from epiphysis to epiphysis. Most anatomical reconstruction techniques require the placing of drill holes through the proximal tibia and distal femur. In the skeletally immature individual, these cross the physeal plates and therefore are at risk for a growth plate injury which could result in either the shortening or angular deformity of the limb. Most studies of ACL reconstruction in young adolescents suggest that in spite of this, physeal disruption is uncommon. Be sure, however, that the graft does not position a bone block across the physeal plate which would promote the development of a physeal bar. Hamstring tendons are the preferred graft in skeletally immature individuals. The safety of these transphyseal reconstructions in boys under 12 and girls under 10 is not well documented.

21. Is surgical intervention necessary for posterior cruciate ligament (PCL) injuries in youths?

Fortunately, PCL injuries are much less common than ACL injuries in children and adults. They can be associated with bony avulsions from either the femoral or tibial ends. Bony avulsion is an indication for primary repair of a posterior cruciate ligament injury in a skeletally immature individual. Midsubstance ruptures are treated expectantly—reconstruction in boys <12 and girls <10 is rarely necessary.

22. Compared to the other ligaments about the knee, what is unique about the tibial insertion of the medial collateral ligament (MCL)?

Distally, the MCL inserts into the metaphysis of the proximal tibia. Its femoral origin is from the epiphysis of the femur. The lateral collateral ligament originates from the epiphysis of the femur and inserts into that of the fibula. Only the tibial end of the MCL inserts into a metaphysis spanning the physeal plate.

23. What inexpensive test can be performed if a severe grade MCL sprain is suspected in a skeletally immature individual?

Plain radiographs should always be performed when looking for physeal and epiphyseal fractures in skeletally immature individuals with instability at the knee. Since physeal fractures are much more common than complete MCL sprains in youths, a valgus stress radiograph should be obtained if the knee is clinically unstable and the plain radiographs appear normal. This should not be done so forcefully as to potentially further injure the physeal plate.

24. What is the most likely diagnosis for a 14-year old male basketball player who sustains an inversion injury of the ankle and presents with lateral swelling and tenderness?

Most males are still skeletally immature at 14 years of age, and if the physeal plate of the distal fibula is still open, fracture is a strong possibility. The other likely diagnosis is sprain of the anterior talofibular ligament. In more severe ankle sprains, the calcaneal fibular ligament can be involved as well.

25. Can there be a fracture present in the distal fibular physis in spite of a normal radiograph?

The most common physeal fracture pattern from an inversion injury of the ankle is a Salter-Harris type I injury. These are often nondisplaced and result in a normal-looking bone. The diagnosis of fracture in these cases is made primarily based upon the physical examination findings.

26. What physical exam finding best differentiates a physeal fracture of the distal fibula from an ankle sprain?

While there may be generalized swelling that is diffusely tender, one should specifically examine for tenderness to percussion over the physeal plate typically about 15 mm proximal to the tip of the fibula). Comparing the tenderness in the area of the anterior talofibular ligament to the pain produced with gentle digital percussion is often helpful.

27. What congenital foot anomaly is associated with an increased incidence of ankle sprains?

Talar coalitions, anomalies resulting from failure of segmentation of the hindfoot bones. The two most common are the calcaneocuboid and talocalcaneal (subtalar) coalitions. Motion of the subtalar joint is particularly important for compensating inversion and eversion moments produced in walking on uneven surfaces and the action mechanisms of many sports. By restricting intrinsic hindfoot motion, talocalcaneal coalitions increase inversion and eversion stresses at the ankle joint, and are thereby associated with an increased rate of ankle sprains and recurrent injury.

28. What other fractures are typically associated with inversion injuries of the foot and ankle?

Fractures at the base of the fifth metatarsal often result from inversion mechanisms. Originally, these were thought to result from an avulsion mechanism based upon pull of the peroneus brevis. Current studies suggest that the culprit is actually the band of the lateral plantar fascia which inserts on the plantar base of the fifth metatarsal. In runners, the proximal portion of the fifth metatarsal can be an area of stress concentration (and stress fracture) resulting from excessive training. This can subsequently fracture, either from repetitive use or an inversion injury.

29. How are fractures at the base of the fifth metatarsal treated?

Identifying the fracture is important. Transverse fractures through the metaphysis that extend from lateral to medial above the articulation with the cuboid are referred to as Jones fractures. When associated with a chronic stress reaction, these fractures are very prone to delayed union and nonunion. The most common treatments are nonweightbearing immobilization in a cast for 6–12 weeks and acute internal fixation with a screw if indicated.

More proximal fractures often heal with minimum treatment, including compressive wraps and hard-soled shoes; however, delayed unions and refractures can occur, particularly in highly active young athletes such as gymnasts. For these individuals, cast immobilization is warranted until radiographic healing is evident.

30. What normal structure can be mistaken for a fracture of the base of the fifth metatarsal?

The apophysis at the base of the fifth metatarsal typically appears in girls 9–11 years of age and in boys 11–14 years of age. The small ossified portion can be mistaken for a fracture fragment; however, the apophysis runs parallel to the shaft of the fifth metatarsal, while most fractures are perpendicular to the longitudinal axis of the metatarsal.

BIBLIOGRAPHY

1. Busch M: Sports Medicine. In Morrissy, RT (ed): Lovell and Winter's Pediatric Orthopaedics, 4th ed. Philadelphia, Lippincott-Raven, 1996.
2. Jackson D, Feagin J: Quadriceps contusions in young athletes. J Bone Joint Surg 55A(1):95, 1973.
3. Metzmaker J, Pappas A: Avulsion fractures of the pelvis. Am J Sports Med 13(5):349, 1985.
4. Smith R, Reischl S: Treatment of ankle sprains in young athletes. Am J Sports Med 14(6):465, 1986.
5. Quill G: Fractures of the proximal fifth metatarsal. Orthop Clin North Am 26(2):353, 1995.

44. ANISOMELIA

Robert M. Bernstein, M.D., and Colin F. Moseley, M.D., C.M., FRCS(C)

1. What is a leg-length discrepancy (LLD)?
We define this as a measurable difference in the overall lengths of the two legs. This can be subdivided into true, apparent, and functional leg-length discrepancies.

2. What is true leg-length discrepancy?
This is the measurable difference in the overall lengths of the two legs from the anterior superior iliac spine (ASIS) to the medial malleolus.

3. What is apparent leg-length discrepancy?
This is the measurable difference in the two legs from the umbilicus or xiphisternum to the medial malleolus.

4. Why might the true and apparent LLDs be different?
There are times when these measurements are not equal. This occurs when the overall lengths of the two legs may be the same, but, because of a contracture around the hip, knee, or ankle, one leg "seems" short. For example, a child with two limbs of equal length but an abduction contracture of the right hip will have an apparent leg-length discrepancy, with the left leg "seeming" to be short.

5. What is the functional leg-length discrepancy?
This is best determined clinically by placing blocks under the short leg of the patient to level the pelvis while standing. This discrepancy is what the patient notices in the upright position.

6. Which is more important?
All are important, but functional discrepancy is what is most important to the patient.

7. How do you assess for an LLD?
- Clinically
  Level the pelvis with blocks under the short leg.
  Measure the distance from ASIS to medial malleolus (true LLD).
  Measure the distance from umbilicus or xiphisternum to medial malleolus (apparent LLD).
  Observe for Galeazzi sign.
- Radiographically
  Scanogram.
  Teleoroentgenogram.
  Orthoroentgenogram.
  CAT scan.

8. What is a teleoroentgenogram?
This is a single 3-foot radiograph taken of the lower extremities. The advantages of this are that malalignments or lesions in the bone will appear on the film and measurements are not affected by patient movement. The disadvantage is that it distorts the results by magnification at the upper and lower ends of the film; as the child gets bigger, the distortion gets bigger. In addition, the large film size makes storage difficult.

9. What is an orthoroentgenogram?
This is also a 3-foot radiograph, but it is taken in three separate exposures, with the beam directly over the three joints to avoid the magnification problems seen with teleoroentgenograms. Again, the large film size makes storage difficult.

10. What is a scanogram?

This is currently the most popular way of measuring the lengths of the femur and tibia. It is a series of radiographs of the hips, knees, and ankles exposed separately in order to avoid magnification errors, taken with the child lying supine next to a radiographic tape measure. The machine and film are moved to take each set of x-rays. A small, easily stored and handled film is produced. Problems with this method are that the child can move in between radiographs and that a knee or hip flexion contracture can distort the results by magnification. Malalignments and intraosseous lesions may also be missed, since the entire extremity is not included on the film.

11. How are limbs measured on a CT scan?

A scout film of the leg is taken. The technician places points on the ends of the bones, and the computer measures the distance between points. There is less potential for error because of angular deformities.

12. What are the causes of an LLD?

Acquired	Congenital
Traumatic	Hemihypertrophy
Femoral or tibial length malunion or overgrowth	Congenital short femur
Growth due to growth plate fracture	Proximal femoral focal deficiency
Paralytic (reduces the growth rate of a limb)	Fibular hemimelia
Polio, cerebral palsy	Hip dislocation
Vascular	Posteromedial bow of the tibia
Hemangioma	
Klippel-Trenaunay-Weber syndrome	**Positional**
Neoplastic	Pelvic obliquity
Wilms' tumor	Hip contracture
Radiation treatment	
Infectious	

13. At what age is overgrowth of a fractured femur a problem that can result in an LLD?

The problem of growth acceleration is most consistent between 2–10 years of age. There seems to be a potential for overgrowth of the fracture limb; thus, the recommendation is to accept fractures that are healing approximately 1–1.5 cm short in order to avoid an LLD at skeletal maturity.

14. Why does overgrowth occur after a fracture?

This may be related to local hyperemia induced by the fracture and remodeling.

15. What is the Galeazzi sign?

Have the child lie supine with the knees flexed and the feet on the table. If the knees are at different heights, this implies that one leg is shorter than the other.

16. What are the consequences of an LLD in a child?

Small amounts are of little consequence (0–2 cm). Larger amounts are more difficult to hide and result in a larger energy expenditure during gait because of the up-and-down motion of the body mass.

      < cm: Probably of no consequence. Many people don't even know that they have one.

  1–3 cm: Easily hidden by the child slightly bending one knee, hiking the pelvis, or walking on tiptoe.

  > 3 cm: The child must walk with significantly more knee flexion and hip flexion or up on tiptoe.

17. What are the consequences of an LLD in an adult?

As the ratio of body mass to muscle strength increases, the ability of the person to compensate for the discrepancy decreases. Thus, a child might be able to hide a 5-cm discrepancy by bending the knee, but a full-grown adult cannot and pistons up and down, utilizing significantly more energy to walk.

18. Is an LLD ever beneficial?
When the short leg is stiff or weak and a brace is required to stiffen the knee, hip, or ankle, it can be an advantage to be a little short (1–2 cm) so that the limb does not scuff the ground.

19. What kinds of problems can an LLD cause?
Very small LLDs (< 1 cm) do not cause any problem.
- Inefficient gait: As the discrepancy gets larger, the gait gets less efficient.
- Cosmetic problems: As children get older, they may not like how they look.
- Arthritis: There is "soft" evidence that the hip of the longer leg is less covered and may be predisposed to arthritis.

20. Does an LLD cause scoliosis?
When a patient with an LLD is standing with both feet on the ground, there is pelvic obliquity and subsequent "functional" scoliosis to keep the trunk upright. Little time is spent in this position, however; thus, the effects on the spine are probably minimal. Keep in mind that some diseases that cause an LLD can also cause scoliosis (e.g., polio).

21. Does an LLD cause back pain?
This is controversial. An LLD up to 2.5 cm is unlikely to cause back pain.

22. Who should manage this?
A pediatric orthopaedic surgeon versed in the treatment of LLDs and limb lengthening procedures.

23. What are the guidelines for selecting the appropriate treatment?

LLD at maturity	Treatment options
< 2 cm	No treatment required
2–6 cm	Shoe lift, epiphyseodesis, or femoral shortening to equalize the leg lengths.
6–20 cm	Either a leg lengthening procedure or a combination of leg lengthening and shortening of the opposite side.
> 20 cm	Amputation and prosthetic fitting.

24. What are the limitations of a shoe lift?
Shoe lifts < 2 cm can fit inside a shoe and thus may be moved into a different pair of shoes. Shoe lifts > 2 cm must be attached to the sole of the shoe and thus are permanent and may be unsightly. If the lift is > 5 cm, it can potentiate ankle instability.

25. What means are available to perform an epiphyseodesis?
1. Phemister technique: A rectangular block of bone, 2/3 on the metaphyseal side and 1/3 on the epiphyseal side, is removed and replaced in the reverse position.
2. Staples: Blount introduced the use of three medial and three lateral staples to arrest growth with the assumed advantage that the procedure is potentially reversible by removal of the staples. Permanent epiphyseodesis occasionally occurred, however, and the staples sometimes backed out and required reoperation.
3. Percutaneous: This method involves the destruction of the growth plate medially and laterally under fluoroscopic guidance by means of a drill.

26. What are the limitations of femoral shortening?
A femur can be acutely shortened up to approximately 5 cm. Any more than this and the quadriceps may not recover its preoperative strength. The wound also becomes more difficult to close.

27. What are the contributions of the major physes in the total growth of the lower extremity?

    Proximal femur (capital physis): 10%
    Distal femur: 40%
    Proximal tibia: 30%
    Distal tibia: 20%

28. How much does the femur grow from its proximal and distal physes?

    Proximal: 30%
    Distal: 70%

29. How much does the tibia grow from its proximal and distal physes?

    Proximal: 55%
    Distal: 45%

30. What work-up should a patient with hemihypertrophy undergo?

Because of the association between Wilms' tumor and hemihypertrophy, a patient with the diagnosis of hemihypertrophy should undergo an abdominal ultrasound yearly until the age of 5 years.

31. How can you predict the ultimate leg-length discrepancy at maturity?

    There are currently three methods in widespread use: the Green-Anderson method, the Moseley straight-line graph, and the Menelaus method. Both the Green-Anderson method and the Moseley straight-line graph method utilize the information published by Anderson and Green in 1948 and 1964. They compiled information relating the leg lengths of children to chronologic and skeletal age. From these graphs, one can determine the growth percentile of the child and the growth remaining in the long leg. Both the Green-Anderson and the Moseley methods utilize exactly the same information, just in different ways.

    The Menelaus method is based on the assumption that the distal femur grows approximately 3/8″ per year and the proximal tibia grows 2/8″ per year; that boys stop growing at age 16 and girls at age 14; and that the discrepancy increases by 1/8″ per year. Using this method, one can make fairly good predictions for those patients whose skeletal maturity corresponds to their chronologic age and who are in their later years of growth.

32. What are the advantages of a leg lengthening procedure?

There are two distinct advantages to leg lengthening. One is that the procedure is performed on the abnormal (short) limb. Parents are much more likely to understand and accept this. The other advantage is that the patient retains his preprogrammed height at the end of the procedure.

33. What are the disadvantages of a leg lengthening procedure?

These are numerous and very significant. First and foremost is that on average, at least one major complication occurs during a lengthening procedure. These include mechanical failure, hypertension, deep infection, nerve injury (from the application of the fixator or from the distraction), knee subluxation, ankle equinus, and delayed union. Also, the patient will be in an external fixator for many months and thus will be unable to participate in sports or many other normal activities. A lengthening is painful and thus should be reserved for older children (we use 12 years as a rough threshold) who can understand the long-term benefits in the face of short-term discomfort. In addition, any family turmoil (obvious or hidden) will often be potentiated by this difficult treatment, further complicating the treatment.

34. How is a bone lengthened?

The bone is cut at the area to be lengthened, and a lengthening device is attached to the bone above and below this cut (osteotomy) by either wires or pins. After waiting a few days for healing to begin, the device is slowly distracted, lengthening the bone with it.

35. What types of lengthening devices are available?

There are a number of lengthening devices on the market. All are similar in that 1) they must be fixed to the bone above and below the site to be lengthened and 2) they utilize one or more threaded rods that are turned gradually to achieve the desired length. The devices differ in complexity and the method of fixation.

Simple lengthening devices

These allow only distraction at the lengthening site. In general, they are "half-pin" external fixators that are attached to the bone by large threaded pins. The pins stick out through the skin on one side of the leg and are attached to the device. Once attached, they do not allow angular or rotational changes of the bone. Examples include the Wagner and Orthofix devices.

Complex lengthening devices

These allow gradual angular and rotational changes as well as distraction to lengthen the bone. In general, they are attached to the bone by thin, tensioned wires that are inserted completely through the limb. The wires are attached to "rings" that surround the limb. The rings are attached to each other by threaded rods and hinges. Using these devices, complex deformities can be corrected at the same time as the bone is lengthened. Examples include the Ilizarov and Monticelli-Spinelli devices.

36. How fast should a limb be lengthened?

In general, the soft tissues are the rate-limiting factor. Since the nerves are the most sensitive to stretch and seem to regenerate at approximately 1 mm/day, most lengthenings are now performed at this rate.

37. How long will an external fixator need to be used?

The fixator needs to remain on the limb long enough for the bone to mature enough to tolerate full weightbearing without external support. This works out to be approximately 1 month/cm lengthened, including the time during the lengthening. Thus, for a 60-mm lengthening, the fixator would be on 60 days for the lengthening plus an additional 120 days for the bone to mature. Keep in mind that this is a rule of thumb and thus an approximation. Radiographic appearance of the lengthening site is also important in making the decision to remove the fixator.

38. When a patient is undergoing a lengthening procedure, why should you always check the blood pressure?

Acute hypertension can occur. The mechanism is not clear, but shortening the lengthening gap resolves this problem reliably. After the blood pressure has returned to normal, the lengthening can be resumed, and the hypertension may not recur.

39. What are some of the most common pitfalls in the treatment of an LLD?

- Making mistakes in arithmetic. Always be sure to write the measurements on the x-ray film with a soft lead pencil and to check and recheck the measurements and the math on all scanograms prior to making a clinical decision.
- Correcting the current discrepancy in a growing child instead of the predicted discrepancy at maturity.
- Assuming that the measurement difference on the scanogram equals the LLD. Remember that in some patients the pelvis may be small (polio) or the hindfoot could be short (post-talectomy).
- Assuming that the child grows at the mean (Green-Anderson method). When using this method to determine the projected LLD at maturity, it is imperative to plot the current femoral and tibial lengths on the distribution of lengths chart to determine the rate of growth of the normal leg. Then, using this information, determine the amount of growth remaining.

BIBLIOGRAPHY

1. Anderson M, Green W, Messner M: Growth and predictions of growth in the lower extremities. J Bone Joint Surg [Am] 45:1, 1963.
2. Anderson M, Messner M, Green W: Distributions of the lengths of normal femur and tibia in children from one to eighteen years of age. J Bone Joint Surg [Am] 46(6):1197, 1964.
3. Gross RH: Leg length discrepancy: how much is too much? Orthopedics 1:307, 1978.
4. Menelaus M: Correction of leg length discrepancy by epiphyseal arrest. J Bone Joint Surg [Br] 48:336, 1966.
5. Moseley C: A straight-line graph for leg-length discrepancies. J Bone Joint Surg [Am] 59(2):174, 1977.
6. Moseley C: Leg length discrepancy and angular deformity of the lower extremities. In Morrissy RT, Weinstein SL (eds): Lovell & Winter's Pediatric Orthopaedics, 4th ed. Philadelphia, J.B. Lippincott Co., 1996, pp 849–901.
7. Rang M: Leg length discrepancy. In Wenger DR, Rang M: The Art and Practice of Children's Orthopaedics. New York, Raven Press, 1993, pp 508–533.

45. LEG ACHES

Richard E. McCarthy, M.D.

1. What are leg aches?

"Leg aches" is a term that has been proposed by some to replace the often misunderstood disease entity referred to as "growing pains." Leg aches refer to generalized pains or discomfort generally felt in children's legs bilaterally late in the day or at night. They occur in 13% of boys and 18% of girls and have a benign nature and an idiopathic origin. No functional disability or objective signs are associated with leg aches, and they generally resolve spontaneously with the completion of growth. Leg aches may be due to an as-yet-unknown specific syndrome, and most authors feel that discounting leg aches as "growing pains" does an injustice to children. It is important that this diagnosis be made by excluding all other possible causes.

2. What age is most affected by leg aches?

Leg aches generally start about the age of 4 years, when the discomfort is most pronounced, but they can affect children up to 12 years of age. Pain in the limbs accounts for 7% of pediatrician visits every year.

3. What are the most common causes of leg aches?

The cause is unknown, but the pattern of pain supports the commonly held theory that this is due to fatigue of the muscles in the thighs and calf.

4. What are the usual patterns of pain?

The most common sites of pain are at the front of the thighs, in the calves, and behind the knees. Occasionally, pains are felt in the groin. The pain is generally outside the region of the joints. The pain is typically bilateral; this is important because serious causes of pain in the limbs are usually unilateral. Leg aches usually occur late in the day and in the evening, occasionally awakening a child from sleep. The pain typically is gone in the morning and does not limit the child's activities during the day.

5. What should be asked of the parents when taking a history of a patient with leg aches?

Certainly the time of day of occurrence and area of localization of the pain are important. The words used to characterize the pain may reflect a cramping pain of muscle fatigue or the deep, aching pain of bone tumors. Certainly the location is important, whether it be bilateral or unilateral or localized to one region of the limb. Whether this is associated with swelling or affects gait or overall health is also noted. The date of onset of the pain may correspond with initiation of a new sports activity. How long the pain has been present and whether it is a daily pain felt for a few minutes or for hours may shed some light on how serious this problem is. Whether medication helps to relieve the pain may pinpoint the diagnosis; for example, pain secondary to a benign osteoid osteoma typically abates with salicylates. The child's overall constitution needs to be questioned; poor general health and an attitude of malaise may indicate that a hematologic disorder such as leukemia causes the leg aches.

6. How does one examine a child for leg aches?

Examination of the child begins with initial observation. The child who sits in the corner of the examination room playing quietly with toys, then stands to stroll casually or even run toward the parent may indicate a more benign pattern to the disorder. The movements of the legs or back may be restricted in situations of infection or neurologic disorders. Distracting the child and getting him or her to play with toys or walk along with the parent will give the examiner an indication of how fluid and natural the gait may be. Range of motion through the hips, knees, and ankles should be checked as well as examination of the joints to look for swelling, especially along the medial aspect of the parapatellar border. Starting the examination of the limbs away from the areas of complaint will yield more information, saving a potentially tender area for the last part of the examination. Asking the child to stand on tiptoes and heels and making a game of the examination is especially helpful for determination of muscle function. Reflexes, including abdominal reflexes, must be checked in order to rule out any spinal cord abnormalities. The circumference of the thighs and calves may indicate atrophy or hypertrophy of musculature when comparing one side with the other. Measurement of leg lengths may indicate a leg length inequality such as one might expect with a hemangioma near a growth plate or with atrophy due to a tethered spinal cord. Any restriction in the range of motion, whether it be due to contracture or guarding from pain, may indicate joint disease rather than simple leg aches.

7. What is the differential diagnosis for leg aches?

Most unknown causes will fall into the categories of congenital, infectious (inflammatory), metabolic, tumor, or traumatic (CIMTT). Utilizing the CIMTT mechanism for approach to unknown causes allows one to consider the differential diagnosis in an orderly fashion. Congenital causes would include disorders such as clubfeet or dislocated hips, which may have produced subtle deformities as yet not diagnosed. Infections, including Brodie's abscesses, may also cause leg aches. Inflammatory disease, including monoarticular juvenile rheumatoid arthritis and other forms of arthritis, should be considered as well as tumors, local or remote. Osteoid osteoma in the upper femur may be hard to diagnose without ancillary studies. Tumors of the spinal cord may produce leg symptoms as well. Other spinal disorders including tethering must be considered. Traumatic causes, including stress fractures, may be subtle; a bone scan may be helpful in making this diagnosis. Specific diseases about the hip must also be considered, such as toxic synovitis, Perthes' disease, and slipped capital femoral epiphyses, which often present with a limp or pain in the thigh.

8. What ancillary studies will help in the initial evaluation of leg aches?

If there is any question about the motion, function, or tenderness of a specific area, then x-rays must be considered. Knee pain in a child is often referred from the hip. Therefore, when ordering x-rays for knee pain in children, an anteroposterior (AP) pelvis film should be considered as well. When considering a hip disorder, a frog lateral film is also helpful, especially when diagnosing a subtle slipped capital femoral epiphysis. A full-length AP view of the pelvis and both legs can easily be acquired in the smaller child to assess both legs fully. If there is any doubt regarding the diagnosis or if the parents are expecting an x-ray, one should proceed with the study. Blood studies including a complete blood count with differential and sedimentation rate may be helpful in certain cases to eliminate the possibility of hematologic disorders such as leukemia or to eliminate suspicion of infectious causes. The use of a bone scan may be necessary when persistence of the symptoms necessitates further examination. Certainly, one would utilize follow-up repeat examinations and attempts at simple treatment before proceeding to the second line of tests, which would include bone scans, MRIs and CT scans. If one is considering the possibility of a spinal cord origin for the leg aches, then inclusion of the entire spine will put the matter to rest, since it is possible that a syringomyelia can cause distal symptoms from its location in the spinal cord.

9. Do medications help in the treatment of leg aches?
Some physicians have recommended the use of salicylates or other anti-inflammatories at bedtime to help with treatment of leg aches with an evening or a nocturnal pattern. Others have utilized stretching exercises in conjunction with the anti-inflammatories.

10. What are the danger signs to watch for?
A persistent pattern of night pain waking the child from sleep, especially with a unilateral location, is worrisome. One might fear the presence of a tumor such as a benign osteoid osteoma. In that case, bone scan results would generally be positive.

11. What is the expected outcome for the child with simple leg aches?
Children outgrow leg aches and grow into normal adults without any restrictions in activities.

12. What is the most important fact to remember about leg aches?
It is critical not to write these off as simply "growing pains." A careful history and physical examination may be all that is necessary. Reassurance of the parents and an invitation to return should the pattern of the pain change or persist may be sufficient treatment. For the worrisome child, follow-up visits off the opportunity for repeat examination and further history-taking. For the child with a limp or functional limitation, additional tests will certainly be necessary to rule out other possible causes. The greatest diagnostic error is to make the diagnosis of "growing pains" while overlooking a serious underlying condition.

BIBLIOGRAPHY

1. Bowyer SL, Hollister JR: Limb pain in childhood. Pediatr Clin North Am 31(5):1053, 1984.
2. Peterson H: Growing pains. Pediatr Clin North Am 33(6):1365, 1986.
3. Staheli LT: Fundamentals of Pediatric Orthopaedics. New York, Raven Press, 1992.
4. Wenger DR, Rang M: The Art and Practice of Children's Orthopaedics. New York, Raven Press, 1993.

46. LIMPING

Jon R. Davids, M.D.

1. What is a limp?
"Limp" refers to an abnormal gait pattern due to pain, weakness, or deformity of the musculoskeletal system. Dysambulation is a more concise descriptor of the clinical circumstance commonly described as a limp.

2. How can limping be classified?
Limping may be classified by (1) description of the abnormal gait pattern, (2) the absence or presence of pain, (3) the age of the child at the time of presentation, and (4) the anatomic region involved.

3. What are the most common abnormal gait patterns associated with limping?
A *painful or antalgic* gait pattern is characterized by a decreased duration of stance phase on the

affected side. This deviation is present because loading and weightbearing on the affected limb are painful. Weakness (or poor control) of muscles about the hip, knee, and ankle cause distinct gait patterns. Inadequate strength of the hip abductor muscles is the most common cause of a *trunk shift* gait pattern (also known as an abductor lurch, compensated gluteus medius lurch, or Trendelenberg gait). In this deviation, the trunk shifts over the stance-phase limb to decrease the load on the ipsilateral hip abductor muscles. Weakness of the knee extensors (quadriceps muscle) is compensated for by keeping the knee extended (or stiff) during stance phase. Toe walking, or *equinus* gait, is associated with poor motor control and muscle imbalance about the ankle. Structural deformity of the musculoskeletal system may result in a functional leg-length inequality. A *short leg* gait is characterized by an apparent trunk shift (or increased downward pelvic obliquity in the coronal plane) over the short leg during stance phase and deviations such as circumduction (increased hip abduction, upward pelvic obliquity, and increased pelvic rotation on the sound side during swing phase) and vaulting (early heel rise on the short side during stance phase) to facilitate clearance of the sound (i.e., long) side in swing phase.

4. What are the most important points in taking a clinical history?

It is essential to establish whether the limp is associated with pain. When pain is present, its location, duration, and aggravating and ameliorating factors should be established. It is also helpful to perform an appropriate review of systems to determine if any signs of systemic illness are present.

When the limp is not associated with pain, the clinical history should establish when the limp was first appreciated, who noticed it, whether it is associated with certain activities or shoe wear, and whether it is consistently or inconsistently present.

5. What are the most important points in the physical examination?

The physical examination should be systematic, anatomically based, and comprehensive. The examination should begin at the spine and work its way down through the pelvis, hips, knees, ankles, and feet. Each bone should be palpated, and each joint should be placed through a passive and active range of motion. Stress testing should be performed on all ligamentous and tendinous structures. Common pitfalls include failure to examine the sacroiliac joints following complaints of back pain and failure to examine the hip in the child who presents with complaints of thigh or knee pain.

6. How do I use observational gait analysis?

Observational gait analysis should be performed with the child wearing the least amount of clothing possible. It should be done in a long hallway, and the child should be observed in both the coronal (i.e., walking toward and away from the observer) and sagittal (i.e., walking past the observer in both directions) planes. Global assessment should focus on speed, stability, balance, and symmetry. Observations of the ankle in the sagittal plane should include (1) heel strike at initial contact, (2) flat foot in midstance, (3) the timing of heel rise (just prior to the opposite swing limb contacting the floor), and (4) the alignment in swing phase. The foot-progression angle and hindfoot alignment in stance and swing are the most important observations made of the foot and ankle in the coronal plane. The knee is observed primarily in the sagittal plane. Attention should be directed to its position (1) at initial contact (extended), (2) during loading response (a small flexion wave), and (3) during swing phase (a large flexion wave). The hip should be fully flexed at the beginning of stance phase and fully extended at the end of stance phase. The pelvis should exhibit minimal dynamic deviations in all planes. The trunk should be stable throughout the gait cycle. The upper extremity should exhibit a reciprocal swinging pattern that is out of phase with the ipsilateral lower extremity.

7. What is the clinical algorithm for the evaluation of a painful limp?

Once the clinical history has established that the limp is associated with pain, the differential diagnosis should focus on trauma, infection, inflammation, and tumor. The physical examination should emphasize careful observation for swelling or discoloration, palpation for tenderness, and limitation of joint range of motion. Appropriate diagnostic laboratory studies include the complete blood count (for infection and hematologic malignancies), the erythrocyte sedimentation rate (ESR, a nonspecific indicator of infection, inflammation, and certain skeletal tumors), and the C-reactive protein (similar to the ESR, but more acutely responsive). In general, an ESR > 30 should be considered a sign of a musculoskeletal infection until proven otherwise. While the presence of other serologic indicators of rheumatologic disease (such as antinuclear antibody, rheumatoid factor, and HLA-B27) may be helpful clinically, the absence of these markers does not rule out the presence of this group of diseases. When the principally affected anatomic area is known, appropriate imaging studies include plain radiographs, CT scan (the best study for analysis of bony skeletal structures), and MRI (the imaging modality of choice for examining soft tissue structures). When the location of the cause of a painful limp cannot be determined, which may be the case in infants and younger children, a nuclear medicine scan (usually a 3-phase technetium scan) is the most effective imaging study.

8. What is the clinical algorithm for the evaluation of a nonpainful limp?

Once the clinical history has established that the limp is not associated with pain, the differential diagnosis should focus on structural musculoskeletal (congenital and developmental), neurologic, and metabolic diseases. The physical examination should emphasize the assessment of limb length and limb girth and the neurologic evaluation. Limb length is best assessed with the patient standing and the examiner palpating the iliac wings. Wooden blocks are placed beneath the short side until the limb lengths are equalized. This method relies upon both proprioception and visual assessment and is more accurate than methods that involve measuring from either the umbilicus or the anterior superior iliac spine to the medial malleolus when the patient is supine. The neurologic examination should include assessment of muscle strength and selective control (manual muscle testing), sensation, spasticity, and deep tendon reflexes. Diagnostic laboratory studies are appropriate only when considering muscle and metabolic diseases. Plain radiographs are appropriate when considering structural problems such as hip dysplasia or femoral hypoplasia. Limb lengths may be determined by plain radiography (orthoroentgenography) or by CT scan. Electrodiagnostic studies (nerve conduction studies, electromyography), muscle biopsy, and chromosomal analysis are appropriate only after the more common problems have been ruled out.

9. What are the most common causes of a limp in a child 0–5 years of age?

This may be the most difficult age at which to evaluate a child for a limp, since many are not yet able to walk. These children may instead present with refusal to stand or irritability. The history is often vague, and the child may not cooperate with the physical examination. The physician's goal should be to identify the more mundane causes of a limp in this age group, such as new shoes or skin blisters, and to rule out serious conditions such as infection, hip dysplasia, fracture, tumor, and nonaccidental trauma. Remember that mild cerebral palsy, particularly spastic hemiplegic type, is often not appreciated until the child begins to walk and run. Occasionally, follow-up clinical examination over a period of 1–2 weeks is necessary to make the correct diagnosis.

ANKLE/FOOT	KNEE/TIBIA	HIP/FEMUR	PELVIS/SPINE	OTHER
Clubfoot	Septic arthritis	Hip dysplasia	Discitis	Nonaccidental
Osteomyelitis	Osteomyelitis	Synovitis	Osteomyelitis	trauma
Juvenile rheumatoid	Toddler's fracture	Septic arthritis		Cerebral palsy
arthritis	(tibia)	Osteomyelitis		Acute lymphocytic
	Discoid lateral			leukemia
	meniscus			Congenital limb
	Congenital patellar			length inequality
	dislocation			(femoral, tibial,
	Juvenile rheumatoid			fibular)
	arthritis			Acquired limb
	Infantile tibia vara			length inequality
	(blount disease)			(Ollier's disease,
				neurofibromato-
				sis)

10. What are the most common causes of a limp in a child 5–10 years of age?

ANKLE/FOOT	KNEE/TIBIA	HIP/FEMUR	PELVIS/SPINE	OTHER
Calcaneal apophysitis (Sever's disease)	Tibial tubercle apophysitis (Osgood-Schlatter disease)	Perthes' disease	Discitis	Muscular dystrophy
Navicular osteochondritis (Köhler's disease)	Osteochondritis dissecans	Synovitis	Osteomyelitis	Hereditary motor sensory neuropathy (Charcot-Marie-Tooth disease)
Tarsal coalition	Growing pains	Septic arthritis	Septic arthritis	Friedreich's ataxia
Trauma (fractures sprains)	Trauma (fractures, sprains)	Osteomyelitis	Spondylolysis	
Juvenile rheumatoid arthritis	Tumor (osteochondroma, unicameral bone cyst, nonossifying fibroma, Ewing's sarcoma, osteogenic sarcoma)	Tumor (unicameral bone cyst, nonossifying fibroma, Ewing's sarcoma, osteogenic sarcoma)		
Osteomyelitis				
Cavus				

Children in this age group are generally able to give a good clinical history and to cooperate with the physical examination. Although infection is still a common cause of limping in these children, other conditions related to growth (e.g., apophysitis) and increased physical activity (e.g., fractures and sprains) are frequently seen. This is the most common age group for presentation of Perthes' disease, transient synovitis of the hip, and Duchenne's muscular dystrophy.

11. What are the most common causes of a limp in a child 10–15 years of age?

Limping in this age group is more commonly due to acquired causes related to increased levels of physical activity; also known as overuse injuries, particularly about the hip and knee. The adolescent growth spurt is often accompanied by apophysitis and the peripatellar pain syndrome. Once the physes have closed, athletic injuries in teenagers become similar to those seen in adults. This is the most common age group for the presentation of slipped capital femoral epiphysis and spondylolysis or spondylolisthesis. Children who develop Perthes' disease at this age have a distinctly worse outcome than those who present in the younger age group.

ANKLE/FOOT	KNEE/TIBIA	HIP/FEMUR	PELVIS/SPINE	OTHER
Tarsal Coalition	Tibial tubercle apophysitis (Osgood-Schlatter's)	Slipped capital femoral epiphysis	Pelvic apophyseal avulsions/apophysitis	Hereditary motor sensory neuropathy (Charcot-Marie-Tooth)
Accessory navicular	Patellar apophysitis (Sindig-Larson)	Perthes'	Osteitis pubis	
Calcaneal apophysitis (Sever's)	Peripatellar pain syndrome	Hip dysplasia (subluxation)	Spondylolysis	
5th metatarsal apophysitis	Patellar dislocation (acute, recurrent)	Tumor (Ewing's, Osteosarcoma)	Spondylolisthesis	
Stress fracture (calcaneus, metatarsals)	Ligament/injuries		Lumbar scheurmann's	
Trauma (fractures, sprains)	Osteochondritis dissecans		Diastematomyelia	
	Meniscal/injuries		Tethered cord	
	Tumor (osteochondroma, Ewing's, Osteosarcoma)			

BIBLIOGRAPHY

1. Bucholz RW, Lippert FG, Wenger DR, Ezaki M: Orthopaedic Decision Making. St. Louis, C.V. Mosby Co., 1984.

2. Lloyd-Roberts GC, Fixsen JA: Orthopaedics in Infancy and Childhood, 2nd ed. London, Butterworth-Heinemann, 1990.
3. Phillips WA: The child with a limp. Orthop Clin North Am 18:489–501, 1987.
4. Scoles PV: Pediatric Orthopedics in Clinical Practice, 2nd ed. Chicago, Year Book Medical Publishers, Inc., 1988.
5. Staheli LT: Fundamentals of Pediatric Orthopedics. New York, Raven Press, 1992.
6. Sutherland DH: Gait Disorders in Childhood and Adolescence. Baltimore, Williams & Wilkins, 1984.
7. Tolo VT, Wood B: Pediatric Orthopaedics in Primary Care. Baltimore, Williams & Wilkins, 1993.
8. Wenger DR, Rang M: The Art and Practice of Children's Orthopaedics. New York, Raven Press, 1993.

47. INTOEING AND OUT-TOEING

Lynn T. Staheli, M.D.

1. What is intoeing?

Intoeing is a medial rotation of the foot in the transverse plane relative to the direction in which the child is walking. Sometimes when families describe their child's problem as a *turning in of the feet,* this may describe either intoeing or flatfeet. Ask for more information to make this distinction.

2. How common is intoeing?

Intoeing is very common; torsional problems account for the greatest number of referrals of children to orthopaedists.

3. Is intoeing abnormal?

Usually not. We define abnormal conditions as those that fall beyond 2 standard deviations (SD) from the mean. Many normal children who intoe fall within the normal range and may be considered to have a *developmental variation,* i.e., a variation of normal that resolves spontaneously. If the rotational deformity is severe and falls outside this 2-SD range, we describe the condition as a *torsional* deformity.

4. What is the natural history of intoeing?

The lower limb shows a triphasic sequence of rotational development.

Embryonic phase. Initially, the limb bud is formed with the great toe in a preaxial position, i.e., with the great toe pointing laterally. Over the next few weeks of embryonic development, the limb rotates medially to bring the great toe to the midline.

Fetal phase. The second phase includes the remainder of intrauterine life and early infancy. During this intrauterine period, the lower limbs are positioned in lateral rotation in the uterus. This results in a lateral rotation contracture of the hips. This lateral rotational contracture resolves during early infancy.

Childhood phase. The third phase occurs during infancy and childhood. Both the tibia and the femur gradually rotate laterally with growth.

5. What is the background of the conditions that cause intoeing?

There are several known causes of rotational deformities.

Developmental variations. The reason for the wide range of normal is unclear. We are not aware of any functional reasons to account for this development sequence. Normal variability accounts for the majority of rotational problems.

Genetic causes. In other children, the pattern of limb development appears to be genetic. Medial femoral torsion is often seen in both a girl and her mother. Medial tibial torsion has been described to run in certain families. It is likely that we inherit the shape of the lower limbs just as we do any other physical characteristic. Examining the parents of children with rotational problems often uncovers a more subtle rotational deformity similar to that of the child.

Intrauterine position. Intrauterine position is the likely cause of lateral rotational contracture of the hip, metatarsus adductus, and possibly medial tibial torsion.

6. What conditions cause intoeing?

The clinical conditions include medial femoral torsion, medial tibial torsion, and forefoot adductus. Often deformities are multiple. For example, in the infant, forefoot adduction (metatarsus adductus) and medial tibial torsion often exist together, each contributing to the degree of intoeing.

7. What is the rotational profile?

The different conditions that cause intoeing can be differentiated by measuring the child's *rotational profile* and comparing these values with published normal values. This profile is determined by physical examination. The values may be measured but for practical reasons are usually estimated and are expressed in degrees. These values document the level and severity of the problem. The rotational profile includes several measurements.

- Foot progression angle (FPA). This is the number of degrees the foot turns in or out relative to the direction of walking. Intoeing values have a minus sign ($-$) preceding the number of degrees. Usually, mild intoeing is $-0°$ to $-10°$, moderate is $-10°$ to $-20°$, and severe is more than $-30°$ of intoeing. Most children and adults will walk in an out-toeing with a FPA between $0°$ and $30°$. When estimating the FPA, focus on one foot at a time. Because the FPA will often change with each step in the infant or young child, make your estimates based on an average number of steps.
- Arc of hip rotation. This measures the arc of motion with the child prone. Flex the knees to a right angle and rotate both thighs concurrently. Let the limbs fall to the level of maximum

ROTATIONAL PROFILE

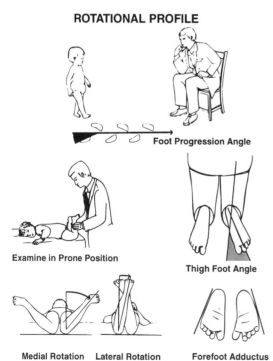

Foot Progression Angle

Examine in Prone Position

Thigh Foot Angle

Medial Rotation   Lateral Rotation   Forefoot Adductus

Rotational profile. Each element of the rotation profile should be determined and recorded.

rotation without force. If necessary, rotate both limbs concurrently to level of the pelvis. Measure both medial rotation (MR) and lateral rotation (LR). When measuring lateral rotation, it is necessary for the legs to be crossed. Measure the maximum rotation as the vertical-tibial angle. The normal values change with age. The arc of hip rotation during early infancy is primarily lateral due to contracture secondary to the intrauterine position. In late infancy and early childhood, the arc shows similar values for MR and LR. Later in childhood and the teen years, LR exceeds MR as the femur rotates laterally, which is associated with declining degrees of femoral anteversion. During childhood, the upper range of medial rotation is about 70° for girls and 60° for boys. Girls tend to intoe slightly more than boys. Normally the total arc of motion is about 90°, but this will be greater in individuals with ligamentous laxity and less in tight-jointed individuals. Beware of asymmetric hip rotation. This is often a sign of hip disease and is the basis of the hip rotation test (HRT) used for screening hip disease. Asymmetric hip rotation is an indication for radiography of the pelvis.

- Thigh-foot angle (TFA). This is a measure of tibial rotation. With the foot in a quiet resting position, estimate this angle by comparing the axis of the foot with that of the thigh. Precede the number of degrees with a minus sign (−) if the axis of the foot is turned in (medial) compared with the axis of the thigh. The TFA rotates laterally with increasing age. A minus value for TFA is often seen in infants. A minus value during childhood or the teen years that falls outside the normal range is referred to as *medial tibial torsion* (MTT). The upper range of normal is about +30°. Values beyond that level are abnormal and are described as *lateral tibial torsion* (LTT).
- Foot. The shape of the sole of the foot is easily assessed with the patient prone. Normally, the lateral border is straight. A convex lateral border is indicative of forefoot adductus (right foot in illustration).

8. What are the pitfalls of diagnosis?
To avoid overlooking underlying disease when assessing a child with a rotational problem, first order a screening examination to make certain that the rest of the musculoskeletal system is normal. Assess hip abduction and symmetry to rule out hip dysplasia. Be aware that children with mild diplegia or hemiplegia (cerebral palsy) may present with a rotational problem. Outtoeing in the older child or teenager may be a sign of slipped capital femoral epiphysis.

9. Is age at presentation useful in diagnosis?
Yes. In early infancy, inward rotation of the feet is usually due to metatarsus adductus. In the toddler, intoeing is most likely due to medial tibial torsion. Intoeing in early childhood (especially in girls) is most likely due to medial femoral torsion.

10. Does intoeing require treatment?
Not usually. The vast majority of cases will resolve spontaneously over time. The conditions that are most likely to require treatment are rigid forefoot adductus (metatarsus varus) and severe intoeing that persists into late childhood or the teen years.

11. Are shoe modifications, braces, or night splints useful?
No, with one exception: in metatarsus varus. In the past, intoeing children were prescribed all sorts of devices: twister cables, night splints, shoe wedges and inserts, and so forth. Every study has shown these devices to be ineffective. These conditions improve spontaneously; the improvement is due to natural history, not to *treatment*. Not only are the devices ineffective and usually unnecessary, but they probably also harm the child and are expensive for the family.

12. Does intoeing ever persist and cause disability?
Yes. Like everything else in medicine, exceptions do occur. Rarely, metatarsus varus, medial tibial torsion, and femoral torsion may persist. The frequency of persistent disease severe enough to produce symptoms is less than 1%. I believe that these severe persistent deformities are often genetically based and are different from the usual developmental variations. The disability is usually functional and cosmetic.

13. Does a rotational deformity at one level cause problems in other joints or the spine?

No. This *cascading* of problems is frequently described to justify various treatments but is unfounded.

14. Is surgical correction of intoeing ever necessary?

Rarely. Operative rotational osteotomy of the femur or tibia is indicated only for severe disabling deformity that persists beyond the age of 10 years.

15. How can I convince the family that observation is best?

1. *Take the family's concerns seriously.* This is a real concern to them. See what is bothering the family. For example, if the family members are concerned about how much the child intoes while running, watch the child run.

2. *Make an accurate diagnosis* by performing a screening examination and the rotational profile. Thoroughness will instill confidence. Knowing the cause of the rotational problem makes possible more accurate prediction of the natural history.

3. *Provide reassurance.* Explain the natural history and the reason why letting the condition resolve without interference is best for the child.

4. *Offer to follow* the progress if the family wishes.

16. How long do rotational problems take to resolve?

Resolution is often slow and usually occurs over months or sometimes several years. When told that the condition will resolve on its own, many parents expect this to take only a few weeks or a few months. Orthopaedic time is slow!

17. When should I refer the child to the orthopaedist?

1. *For additional reassurance.* The most common indication will be a family who requires additional reassurance. Make certain that you inform the orthopaedist of the reason for the referral—to reassure the family and not necessarily for treatment.

2. *Uncertain diagnosis.* If the findings are not clear or an abnormality is found on the screening examination that poses a problem, referral is indicated.

3. *Older infant or child with stiff forefoot adductus.* The child may be a candidate for cast or brace treatment.

4. *Older child or adolescent with disability due to a rotational problem.* If the problem appears to be permanent and disabling, operative correction may be necessary.

18. If the family insists that something be done, what should I do?

Prescribe a healthy lifestyle for the child: exercise through play activities, limited television watching, and healthy diet. Avoid mechanical devices, since these can be harmful in addition to being ineffective.

19. Do sprinters intoe?

In our study of high school sprinters, we found that sprinters have a smaller thigh-foot angle than controls and tend to intoe more often than nonsprinters while running. This suggests that mild medial rotation of the tibia enhances running. We concluded that slight medial rotation allows the toe flexors to be more effective in enhancing pushoff.

FOREFOOT ADDUCTUS

20. What is forefoot adduction?

Forefoot adductus is a transverse plane deformity in which the forefoot is medially angulated relative to the hindfoot. Forefoot adductus may be due to metatarsus adductus or metatarsus varus or may be part of the skewfoot deformity.

21. What is metatarsus adductus?

Metatarsus adductus is a common flexible form of forefoot adduction secondary to intrauterine positioning. Like other positional deformities, it improves spontaneously and resolves in the first months or year of life. Treatment is usually unnecessary.

22. What is metatarsus varus?

Metatarsus varus is an uncommon form of forefoot adduction that is stiff and is more persistent than the common form. In some cases, the first cuneiform is triangular in shape. Persisting deformity produces little disability. It is not a cause of bunions. Since the disability is only cosmetic, correction with serial corrective casts or bracing may be appropriate. Operative correction should be avoided because the risk of complications exceeds the benefits.

23. What are skewfeet?

Skewfeet (Z feet, serpentine feet) are a rare complex deformity including forefoot adduction, mid-foot abduction, and heel valgus. This deformity is often present in loose-jointed children, is sometimes familial, is often bilateral, but is often asymmetric in severity. The natural history is poorly understood, and the potential for disability in adult life is uncertain. Nonoperative treatment is not effective. Delay operation correction until midchildhood, and correct the deformity by lengthening the calcaneus and first cuneiform.

24. How should flexible forefoot adductus in the infant be managed?

First examine the hips to rule out hip dysplasia. Note the degree of flexibility of the foot. The more flexible the foot, the more rapid the resolution. Some physicians ask the parents to massage or stretch the foot. I don't recommend this because it is unlikely to make any difference, and, if the condition persists, the parent will feel responsible for the *failure of treatment*. The severity can be documented by clinical description, tracing the shape of the foot on paper, recording the shape of the foot with a copy machine, or photography. Radiographs are not appropriate. See the infant again in 3–4 months. Most will improve. Stiff adductus or a failure of improvement are indications for treatment. Most primary care physicians will elect to refer infants requiring treatment to an orthopaedist.

Braces or casts that extend above the knee are most effective. The knee is flexed to 90°, and the foot is laterally rotated to the position of maximum comfort. This stabilizes the hindfoot. The forefoot is then abducted and held in either the cast or a long-leg brace. Short-leg braces or casts are much less effective because the rotation of the hindfoot is poorly controlled.

TIBIAL TORSION

25. What is tibial torsion?

Tibial torsion is a deformity in which the horizontal plane of the tibia is rotated medially or laterally beyond the normal range (+2 or −2 SD). The deformity may be medial (internal) or lateral (external). Medial tibial torsion is common in the toddler. Lateral tibial torsion is most common in late childhood or adolescence. In contrast to femoral torsion, tibial torsion is often asymmetric and may be unilateral. Since the human tibia tends to rotate to the right, unilateral medial tibial torsion is more common on the left and lateral tibial torsion is more common on the right.

26. Should tibial torsion be treated with a night splint?

This is controversial. The evidence indicates that resolution occurs with or without treatment. Splints are a hassle for the family and the child. If you use splints, restrict their use to nighttime only. Daytime devices are clearly much more harmful because they may limit play and alter the child's self-image. I do not recommend treatment of tibial torsion during infancy or early childhood.

27. When is surgical correction necessary?

Operative correction of tibial torsion is rarely necessary. Medial tibial torsion continues to improve until growth is complete. Lateral tibial torsion increases with growth, is more serious, and is more likely to require operative correction than medial tibial torsion. The severity of deformity that requires correction is influenced by the rotational status of the femur, since femoral rotation can aggravate or compensate for tibial torsion. Generally, if the TFA is more medial than −10° or more lateral than +40°, operative correction may be considered.

28. How is tibial torsion corrected surgically?

The tibia is divided transversely and is rotated to correct the deformity. The osteotomy is best performed in the tibia about 2 cm above the distal growth plate. The osteotomy is fixed with crossed smooth pins, which are left protruding through the skin for ease in removal. If rotation of more than 25° is required, the fibula may also require division. A long-leg cast is necessary to supplement the cross-pin fixation. The leg is immobilized 7–8 weeks. Both tibias can be corrected at the same time, but the child will require a wheelchair for mobility while the osteotomies heal. Although correction can also be achieved with proximal tibial osteotomy, upper tibial osteotomy is more likely to be complicated by compartment syndrome or peroneal nerve palsy.

FEMORAL TORSION

29. What is femoral torsion?

Femoral torsion is an abnormal twisting (rotation in the transverse plane) of the femur. This femoral twisting is defined as the angular difference between the axis of the upper femur and that of the knee. Since the hip is a ball-and-socket joint that allows about 90° of rotation, the axis of the upper femur rather than the joint serves as the proximal point of reference. Normally, the upper femur is anteverted, i.e., the head and neck are angled forward relative to the rest of the femur. Increased anteversion allows increased medial hip rotation equivalent to a medial rotational deformity. The upper femur may be retroverted or angled posteriorly. Retroversion is uncommon and results in increased lateral rotation of the hip. An abnormal increase in anteversion or retroversion is sometimes called *antetorsion* and *retrotorsion*. For consistency, we prefer the terms *medial femoral torsion* and *lateral femoral torsion*.

30. What is the natural history of anteversion?

At birth, femoral anteversion averages 40°. Anteversion spontaneously decreases with growth and averages 10° for adult men and 15° for adult women.

31. What are the clinical features of medial femoral torsion?

Medial femoral torsion (MFT) usually first becomes clinically noticeable in early childhood. We believe that MFT is not seen in infancy because it is masked by the lateral rotation contracture of the hip. As this contracture resolves, abnormalities in the shape of the femur become apparent, and the clinical features of MFT may develop.

MFT is more common in girls and may be familial. It is not uncommon for the mother to describe having the same problem as a child. Examination of the parents often shows a milder degree of MFT. The child with MFT intoes and stands with the patella pointing medially, which is sometimes described as the *cross-eyed* or *squinting* patella. Running is awkward and is described as an *eggbeater* running style. The child sits with the legs medially rotated, described as the *reverse tailor* or *M* position. Medial rotation of the hip is increased, and lateral rotation is decreased. Usually, we consider MFT as mild if medial hip rotation is 70°–80°, moderate if between 80° and 90°, and severe if more than 90°

32. Are radiographs or other imaging studies necessary?

Usually not. Although the degree of femoral anteversion can be measured with special imaging studies, imaging is not necessary unless hip rotation is asymmetric or operative correction is planned.

33. What happens without treatment?

Medial femoral torsion usually peaks in severity between the ages of 4 and 6 years, then improves. After that, the condition becomes muted. In less than 1% of cases, the condition is severe, and disability persists into late childhood or adolescence. The child continues to intoe, running is awkward, and the altered function and appearance pose a problem. For these rare cases, operative correction may be appropriate.

34. Does the use of twister cables or night splints change the natural history of MFT?

No. Such treatment simply adds another disability for the child and should be avoided.

35. Does MFT cause osteoarthritis of the hip or functional problems in adult life?

No. In the past, MFT was thought to cause arthritis and severe functional problems in adult life. We studied the relationship between measured anteversion in adults with osteoarthritis and controls and found no relationship. We also found no relationship between anteversion and physical performance in adults. Operative correction of MFT should not be considered *prophylactic*.

36. How should I manage femoral torsion?

Manage the family's concerns, as described previously. Emphasize the natural history of spontaneous resolution. Encourage the family and child not to focus on the problem. Discourage the family from telling the child, *"Turn your feet out,"* or *"Don't sit that way."* Do not allow them to insist that the child take ballet lessons. Encourage the family to explain the reasons for this method of management to other family members or the preschool staff. Offer to discuss the problems with other concerned adults. If the family insists on doing something, encourage a healthy lifestyle for the child, as discussed previously. If additional reassurance is necessary, it may be time to get a second opinion from an orthopaedist who deals with such problems frequently.

37. Are orthotics useful in the management of MTF?

No. Changing the position of the foot will not affect the bony configuration of the femur. In addition, MFT does not lead to foot deformities, and foot problems do not cause MFT.

38. How is MFT corrected surgically?

Medial femoral torsion may be corrected operatively if the deformity is severe (i.e., MR of 90°, LR of 0°) and if the child has a significant cosmetic and functional disability and is older than 10 years. The correction is achieved with a rotational femoral osteotomy. This may be performed at any level, but we have found that correction at the proximal femoral level is best. The femur is divided transversely and the distal fragment rotated 45° laterally. Whether a cast is necessary depends on the rigidity of the internal fixation. Operative correction is effective and permanent, usually corrects the problem, and improves function but is not without risks; it should be undertaken only for a severe deformity.

OUT-TOEING

39. What is out-toeing?

The feet are normally turned out in relation to the direction of walking. We naturally out-toe. The normal range throughout most of life is from neutral position to about 30° of out-toeing.

40. What are the causes of out-toeing?

Physiologic lateral rotation contracture of infancy. Most infants' feet turn out when first supported in the upright position. This pattern resolves during the first year. We often see infants because one foot turns out. This is usually due to the combination of bilateral physiologic lateral rotation contracture of infancy and unilateral medial tibial torsion on the *opposite* side. It is usually the right foot that is turned out, since unilateral medial tibial torsion is more common on the left side. No treatment is required.

Lateral tibial torsion (LTT). This can be a major problem. Since the tibia normally rotates laterally with growth, LTT tends to become worse. Sometimes it becomes severe enough to require correction with a tibial osteotomy.

Lateral femoral torsion (LFT) or retrotorsion. This condition is very rarely severe enough to require operative correction. It may be a risk factor in developing a slipped capital femoral epiphysis. Some evidence suggests that it may increase the risk of osteoarthritis of the hip in later adult life.

TORSIONAL MALALIGNMENT

41. What is the torsional malalignment syndrome (TMS)?

The combination of medial femoral torsion and lateral tibial torsion is the most common form.

The foot progression angle is normal, but the knee is rotated medially during walking or running. A less common form is the reverse: lateral femoral torsion and medial tibial torsion.

42. What are the clinical features of TMS?

Torsional malalignment syndrome is usually seen in teenaged patients who complain of knee pain. The pain is patellofemoral in origin with symptoms of chondromalacia patellae, sometimes patellar subluxation, or, rarely, dislocation. Because the knee is rotated medially, the quadriceps tends to displace the patella laterally, causing or aggravating patellofemoral instability.

43. How should TMS be managed?

First, apply the routine treatment for chondromalacia, i.e., activity modification or restriction, nonsteroidal analgesics, and so forth. Avoid lateral releases. In rare situations, correction with a double osteotomy may be required to correct the underlying bony deformity.

44. Can TMS be prevented?

Not at present. We are unable to predict which children are likely to develop TMS. Nonoperative management does not change the torsion of the femur or tibia, and prophylactic single-level osteotomy would likely cause a great number of complications. Possibly in the future, prospective natural history studies will make it possible to predict which children are at risk, and we will be able to selectively correct single-level torsional deformities before compensatory deformity develops.

BIBLIOGRAPHY

1. Cooke TD, Price N, Fisher F, Hedden D: The inwardly pointing knee. An unrecognized problem of external rotational malalignment. Clin Orthop 260:56, 1990.
2. Dietz FR: Intoeing—fact, fiction and opinion. Am Fam Physician 50:1249, 1994.
3. Driano AN, Staheli LR, Staheli LT: Psychosocial Development and "Corrective" Shoewear Use in Childhood. Rosemont, IL, American Academy of Orthopedic Surgeons, 1997.
4. Fabry G, MacEwen GD, Shand AR: Torsion of the femur; a follow-up study in normal and abnormal conditions. J Bone Joint Surg 55A:1726, 1973.
5. Heinrich SD, Sharps CH: Lower extremity torsional deformity in children: a prospective comparison of two treatment modalities. Orthopedics 14:655, 1991.
6. Hubbard DD, Staheli LT, Chew DE, Mosca VS: Medial femoral torsion and osteoarthritis. J Pediatr Orthop 8:540, 1988.
7. Knittle WF, Staheli LT: The effectiveness of shoe modifications for intoeing. Orthop Clin North Am 7:1019, 1976.
8. Krengel WF, Staheli LT: Tibial rotational osteotomy for idiopathic torsion: a comparison of the proximal and distal osteotomy levels. Clin Orthop 283:285, 1992.
9. Meister K, James SL: Proximal tibial derotational osteotomy for anterior knee pain in the miserably malaligned extremity. Am J Orthop 24:149, 1995.
10. Shim LS, Staheli LT, Holm BN: Surgical correction of idiopathic medial femoral torsion. Int Orthop 19:220, 1995.
11. Somerville EW: Persistent foetal alignment of the hip. J Bone Joint Surg 39B:106, 1957.
12. Staheli LT, Lippert F, Denotter P: Femoral anteversion and physical performance in adolescent and adult life. Clin Orthop 129:213, 1977.
13. Staheli LT, Clawson DK, Hubbard DD: Medial femoral torsion; experience with operative treatment. Clin Orthop 146:222, 1980.
14. Staheli LT, Corbett M, Wyss C, King H: Lower-extremity rotational problems in children. J Bone Joint Surg 67A:39, 1985.
15. Staheli LT: Rotational problems in children. J Bone Joint Surg 75A:939, 1993.
16. Svenningsen S, Terjesen T, Apalset K, Anda S: Osteotomy for femoral anteversion—a prospective 9-year study of 52 children. Acta Orthop Scand 61:360, 1990.
17. Wedge JH, Munkacsi I, Loback D: Anteversion of the femur and idiopathic osteoarthrosis of the hip. J Bone Joint Surg 71A:1040, 1989.

48. BOWLEGS AND KNOCK-KNEES

Peter M. Stevens, M.D.

1. What should be asked in the history?

The **family history** is relevant and may highlight the parents' concerns. Persistent familial angular deformities, especially those affiliated with short stature, should raise concerns about metabolic disorders or inheritable skeletal dysplasias. On the other hand, spontaneous resolution of deformities in siblings or parents may prove to be reassuring. The pre- and perinatal history, along with information about **growth and developmental milestones,** is also relevant. Early walking may be associated with bowlegs; late walking may imply neuromuscular disease. The **age at presentation** and the observed trend (worsening versus improving) are critically important. Up until the age of 2, there is a prevalence of physiologic bowlegs. Between the ages of 3 and 6, knock-knees are exceedingly common. The onset or persistence of angular deformities after these respective ages should be viewed with suspicion. Likewise, **asymmetric deformities** and those associated with **functional impairment** or **pain** should be investigated and documented radiographically. A history of trauma, infection, or tumor may account for local or regional growth disturbance, causing clinical deformity.

2. What are the physical findings?

Bowlegs: When a person stands erect with his or her feet together and ankles touching, the knees should touch as well. Any separation between the knees is indicative of bowlegs; the greater the distance, the more serious the implications. While one can make a qualitative assessment of infants, this deformity is not typically noted before the child can stand. In these young children, physiologic ligamentous laxity will accentuate the bow. Documented by tape measure (or fingerbreadths) as the **intercondylar distance,** this is a very reproducible measurement that even the parents can monitor. Concomitant torsional deformities often include outward torsion of the femora and inward torsion of the tibiae, each of which contributes to the bowed appearance. The child usually has an intoeing gait pattern and may be prone to tripping. The findings are typically symmetric and the limb lengths are equal. Progressive, asymmetric, or unilateral bowing or associated limb-length discrepancy should raise suspicion regarding underlying disease and should prompt further investigation.

Knock-knees: The distance measured between the ankles when the child is standing erect with knees touching reflects the presence and severity of knock-knees. Once again, ligamentous laxity, particularly in younger children, will accentuate the deformity. The **intermalleolar distance** may be readily measured and recorded by the parents, serving as an indicator of severity and progression. There is often coexisting outward torsion of the femur or tibia. In adolescence, the combination of inward femoral torsion and outward tibial torsion known as "miserable malalignment" may produce the appearance of knock-knees. In more severe cases, one may note lateral tilt and even instability of the patella. The gait pattern is marked by circumduction, which is more pronounced with running. When knock-knee is unilateral or associated with limb-length inequality, there may be underlying disease and progressive deformity. Idiopathic genu valgum developing or persisting in a teenager is unlikely to resolve spontaneously.

3. What imaging studies are appropriate?

A **standing full-length AP radiograph** of the lower extremities, with both knees extended and the patellae pointing straight forward, will provide useful information pertaining to the major joints and their respective epiphyses. The tilt of the pelvis and the comparative length of the long bones are readily ascertained, noting the contour of the shaft as well as the quality of the trabecular bone and the growth plates. By drawing a "plumb line" from the center of each femoral head to the center of the ankle, one may readily see where the center of gravity passes relative to the knee. By adolescence, this line, which is called the **mechanical axis,** should bisect the knee (see Figures). The angle subtended by the articular surfaces of the tibia and femur and their respective shafts are also measured.

In a symptomatic patient with knock-knees, a patellar sunrise view, taken with the knees flexed 30°, may reflect the degree of lateral patellar tilt of subluxation.

For persistent or increasing clinical deformities, follow-up radiographs are indicated annually to document progression and to plan intervention. In adolescents, the status of the growth plates should be noted, particularly if hemiepiphysiodesis is being contemplated. It is helpful to obtain an AP radiograph of the hand to assess skeletal maturity. Other imaging studies such as scanography CT, or MRI are seldom beneficial.

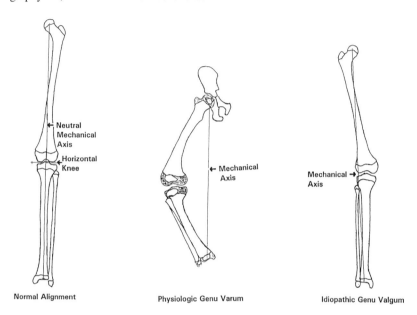

Normal Alignment   Physiologic Genu Varum   Idiopathic Genu Valgum

4. Are laboratory studies useful?

In rare cases, when metabolic disturbances are suspected to be the cause of the deformity, it is helpful to assess serum and urinary calcium and phosphate, along with alkaline phosphatase. Genetic anomalies may also be documented via chromosomal analysis in selected patients.

5. Do these conditions require treatment? By whom?

Primary care providers or trained health care professionals may safely triage and manage most patients, referring only those with suspicious or recalcitrant deformity. The overwhelming majority of bowlegs presenting before the age of 2 and knock-knees presenting before 6 will resolve spontaneously. The natural history of each condition is typically benign because the deformities are self correcting. Therefore, the current philosophy is that "corrective shoes" and bracing are superfluous and represent an unnecessary expense. Despite parental education and reassurance, it is still wise to see the children annually until your prediction is fulfilled and their legs are straight.

The minority of children who do not follow the expected course or those with unilateral deformity, limb-length inequality, or pain should be referred for evaluation by an orthopaedist. His or her role is to determine the cause and to intervene judiciously. The goal of intervention is to achieve and maintain straight legs of equal length, alleviating (or averting) pain and instability. The historic approach of applying braces has yielded to an all-or-nothing philosophy; physiologic deformities are best observed while pathologic problems are treated surgically.

6. What are the controversies with bracing?

Parental anxiety, often compounded by pressure from grandparents, may produce an atmosphere of "don't just stand there, *do something!*" Often a parent or relative wore braces or corrective shoes and obtained a good result. It may prove difficult to convince them that the outcome was despite, rather than due to, the treatment. Having excluded pathologic bowing or knock-knee, the managing physician must educate the concerned parents regarding the benign natural history of these deformities. I find it helpful to date and label a diagram of the legs, comparing sequential measurements on a semiannual or annual basis. For the extreme skeptics, I am apt to show them before and after radiographs of another child who outgrew the problem without treatment. I further explain that bracing requires three-point fixation with the knee locked in extension—a very unphysiologic situation. Pointing out the ligamentous laxity at the knee, I explain that bracing may exacerbate ligamentous stretch without documented beneficial effect upon the growth plates. The cost of unnecessary bracing is an important consideration.

A lingering controversy is the potential benefit of bracing children with bowleg(s) due to type one (mild) Blount disease. This is a pathologic condition involving the posteromedial growth plate of the proximal tibia. Given the difficulties of radiographic analysis, many of these children may actually have physiologic bowing and be destined for spontaneous resolution.

Adolescent idiopathic knock-knees behave differently; these patients frequently have anterior knee pain and functional limitations. One controversy pertains to the type and severity of symptoms deemed worthy of intervention. Recognizing that **"conservative" management such as exercises, physical therapy, and bracing are of no lasting benefit,** one is left with the options of limiting sports and activities versus surgical intervention.

Most patients are unwilling to accept the deformity and adopt a sedentary lifestyle, hoping to reduce symptoms and avoid arthritis. Furthermore, activities of daily living such as kneeling, squatting, sitting, and descending stairs may produce pain. These patients are apt to seek out more aggressive treatment.

7. What about epiphysiodesis?

Another controversy pertains to the preferred timing and technique of epiphysiodesis to change the angle of growth, thereby straightening the limb. The traditional method of surgical ablation of the physis, be it by open or percutaneous technique, produces permanent closure. Therefore, timing must be perfect to avoid overcorrection. Unfortunately, estimation of skeletal maturity is imprecise (+/− one year), so one must follow these patients closely and be prepared to arrest the opposite side of the growth plate(s) to preserve a neutral mechanical axis. If this opportunity is missed, the patient may have to undergo corrective osteotomy.

8. What about stapling?

Stapling offers an attractive alternative. By placing one or more staples *around* a physis, one may induce an angular change with continued growth. Provided that the periosteum is carefully spared, this method is the only reversible means of manipulating growth. Therefore, timing is not so critical. Slight overcorrection may resolve with rebound growth following staple removal. While this technique may be successfully applied to younger children, the literature states that it is best reserved for adolescence. Detractors of stapling have expressed concerns about permanent closure and the need to remove the staples. I find that it is a more forgiving and versatile procedure with respect to timing, however, and may safely be repeated if deformities recur.

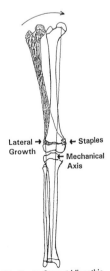

Lateral → Growth

← Staples

← Mechanical Axis

Stapling to Correct Idiopathic Genu Valgum

9. What about osteotomy?

Osteotomy of the tibia and fibula or the femur should be reserved for more severe deformities and, when possible, may be delayed until skeletal maturity. Preoperative planning should be employed to preserve equal limb lengths and a horizontal knee while neutralizing the mechanical axis. Osteotomies of the proximal tibia have earned a reputation for frequent complications, most notably compartment syndrome and peroneal nerve injury.

10. What is the prognosis?

The prognosis is determined by the stability of the knee (including the patella), the orientation of the joint surface (parallel to the ground), and the location of the mechanical axis at maturity (females, age 14; males, age 16). With these attributes and good musculature, the knees should function well for decades.

Bowlegs: If the mechanical axis falls in the medial compartment or medial to the knee, regardless of the cause, eccentric and pathologic compression of the medial meniscus and articular cartilage will accelerate the degenerative process, leading to secondary arthritis. In advanced cases, the lateral ligaments yield to excessive tensile forces, exacerbating this process. Once the medial articular cartilage has worn away, bone erosion ensures.

Knock-knees: With significant knock-knee deformities, the mechanical axis may produce pathologic compression of the lateral compartment, combined with tensile stresses on the medial ligaments and shear forces on the patella. The net result is patellar tilt and, in some instances, instability along with accelerated water and degenerative arthritis involving the patellofemoral joint and the lateral compartment of the knee.

BIBLIOGRAPHY

1. Brooks W, Gross R: Genu varum in children: diagnosis and treatment. J Am Acad Orthop Surg 3(6):326–335, 1985.
2. Heath DH, Stahell L: Normal limits of knee angle in children; genu varum and genu valgum." J Pediatr Orthop 13:259–262, 1993.
3. Kling T, Hensinger R: Angular and torsional deformities of the lower extremities in children. Clin Orthop 176:136–147, 1983.
4. Mielke C, Stevens P: Hemiepiphyseal stabling for knee deformities in children younger than ten. J Pediatr Orthop 16:423–429, 1996.
5. Salenius P, Vankka E: The development of the tibiofemoral angle in children. J Bone Joint Surg 57:259–261. 1975.
6. Shopfner CE, Colin CG: Genu varus and valgus in children. Radiology 92:723–732, 1969.
7. Zuege R, Kempken TG, Blount WP: Epiphyseal stapling for angular deformity at the knee. J Bone Joint Surg 61:320–329, 1979.

49. FOOT PAIN

James C. Drennan, M.D.

1. How do children present with foot pain?

Infants will withdraw the limb when the foot is touched or manipulated. Toddlers may limp or refuse to bear weight. Older children demonstrate an antalgic limp and may be able to isolate the pain to a specific site.

2. What are the physical findings?

Most causes of foot pain are unilateral. This permits comparison between the two feet. The involved foot may be swollen, warm, red, or locally tender. Both acute and chronic problems may demonstrate limited motion, particularly in the subtalar joint. The normal callus distribution between the hindfoot and forefoot may be changed if there is a chronic problem leading to an abnormal weightbearing position for the foot.

3. What are the most common causes of pain?
- Flatfeet may reflect generalized ligamentous laxity or may be an acquired problem that causes pain or restriction in joint motion. "Growing pains" are associated with flatfeet with ligamentous laxity.
- Trauma, including stress fractures and foreign bodies.
- Juvenile rheumatoid arthritis.
- Congenital, e.g. tarsal coalition.
- Infection, including pyogenic arthritis and osteomyelitis.
- Pediatric foot tumors, e.g., osteoid osteoma or synovial sarcoma.

4. What is the most common cause of pain in toddlers and young children?
"Growing pains" (ages 2 to 7 years) describe lower extremity discomfort in young children that develops during or following vigorous physical activity and can be equated to adult 'shin splints.' The healthy child goes to sleep in the evening only to awaken 1–2 hours later crying in pain and complaining of anterior calf discomfort. In another scenario, the child may prematurely stop participating in a strenuous activity and localize the pain to the anterior leg. The calf muscles, particularly the tibialis anterior, are subject to increased compartmental pressure. Alternatively, the child's behavioral response may be similar but the complaint may focus on foot, knee, or thigh symptoms. Children with "growing pains" generally have flexible flatfeet and demonstrate normal shoe or sneaker wear. In most children, the problem spontaneously resolves by the age of 8 years, as the foot loses its excessive ligamentous laxity. Parents generally report that they have been using local massage, a hot tub, or analgesics to relieve the complaint. The prophylactic use of custom shoe inserts or orthotics placed inside inexpensive sneakers leads to symptomatic relief in nearly all cases. The inserts can be discontinued at any age, and a clinical trial can be performed to determine the need for their continued use.

5. What happens if there is no treatment?
The symptoms in the young child will persist. A flexible flatfoot is characterized by sufficient length of the tendo Achillis to permit at least 10°–15° of dorsiflexion of the ankle beyond neutral when the knee is extended and the subtalar joint is held in a neutral position.

There is a small group of patients with a flexible flatfoot who gradually develop a shortened tendo Achillis, which limits hindfoot dorsiflexion. The heel becomes locked in valgus and equinus by the shortened heelcord. Pedal dorsiflexion during the stance phase of gait is transferred forward to the midfoot, leading to a flattened medial longitudinal arch and a painful callus beneath the talar head. Associated forefoot pronation creates a painful rigid flatfoot. Weightbearing x-rays of this type of flatfoot show plantar sag in the midfoot. When a heelcord stretching program is unsuccessful, there is the occasional need for a calcaneal lengthening osteotomy and tendo Achillis lengthening both to relieve the hindfoot equinus and to lengthen the lateral column of the foot.

6. What are the most common sports-related heel injuries?
These include Achilles tendinitis, retrocalcaneal and Achilles bursitis, plantar fasciitis, calcaneal bursitis, calcaneal apophysitis, and calcaneal stress fracture. The specific diagnosis is made according to the anatomic location of pain, which may be accompanied by local swelling.

7. What other conditions can cause heel pain?
Soft tissue and osseous infections (e.g., a nail puncture wound) can occur. Bony tumors are uncommon, and malignant tumors are especially rare. Benign osteoblastoma, osteoid osteoma, and calcaneal cysts can occur. Ewing's sarcoma involving either the calcaneus or the talus is the most common hindfoot osseous malignancy. A tarsal tunnel syndrome can develop from a bony prominence (talocalcaneal coalition) or from mechanical stress to the posterior tibial nerve in the tarsal tunnel.

8. What types of problems limit subtalar motion?

These include congenital conditions (e.g., tarsal coalition); trauma, especially occult calcaneal fractures; and acquired inflammatory conditions, including pauciarticular juvenile rheumatoid arthritis, inflammatory bowel disease, spondyloarthropathies, and juvenile onset ankylosing spondylitis. These conditions can present with insidious onset of pain, swelling, and restricted inversion and eversion in the subtalar joint.

9. What is tarsal coalition?

A tarsal coalition represents a failure of complete segmentation between two or more tarsal bones. Calcaneonavicular and talocalcaneal forms are the most common. They occur in approximately 1% of the population with a 2:1 male-to-female distribution. The tarsal bars become symptomatic at the time of ossification, with the calcaneonavicular coalition presenting between 8 and 12 years and the talocalcaneal coalition presenting between 12 and 16 years. Pain is the initial complaint and is usually insidious in onset. The pain in the talocalcaneal coalition can be poorly localized in the hindfoot, whereas calcaneonavicular coalition usually causes pain laterally in the area of the coalition. Subtalar motion is restricted to absent. The hindfoot is usually in valgus, and the peronei may be contracted. Calcaneonavicular coalitions can be visualized on an internal oblique radiograph of the foot, while coronal plane CT scans are necessary to document the talocalcaneal coalition, which is most commonly located in the area of the sustentaculum tali (see Figure). Symptomatic coalitions are best managed by excision of the bar. Triple arthrodesis is reserved for major coalitions involving more than one joint or for symptomatic degenerative arthritis.

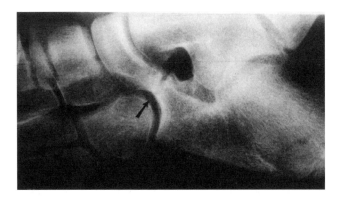

Tarsal coalition. The 45° oblique radiograph illustrates the calcaneonavicular bar.

10. What conditions can cause pain in the midfoot?

Köhler's disease (avascular necrosis of the navicular bone) presents with pain localized to the medial border of the midfoot and can be confused with juvenile rheumatoid arthritis. Clinical onset usually occurs between the ages of 3 and 10 years and is particularly common in athletic males. Physical findings may include soft tissue swelling, erythema, and tenderness at the talonavicular or naviculocuneiform joint, with pain elicited on manual forefoot pronation and supination. Radiographic findings include flattening and patchy ossification of the navicular bone with preservation of its joint surfaces. The condition is managed with cast immobilization and rest. The use of custom shoe inserts after resolution of the acute symptoms will protect the navicular bone while revascularization is occurring. Radiographic improvement is noted over the following year, and most youngsters have an excellent clinical outcome (see Figure). Physical activity can gradually be reintroduced after symptoms have subsided and there is radiographic evidence of revascularization.

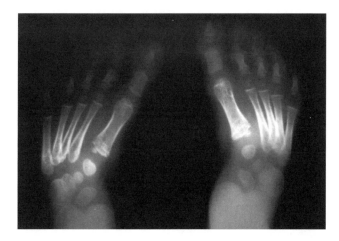

Köhler's disease. The avascular navicular bone demonstrates bony resorption and sclerosis but retains its articular relationships.

11. What is an accessory navicular?
An accessory navicular bone is another unique midfoot problem and occurs in 10% of patients older than the age of 5 years, with symptoms more commonly developing in girls. Pain and tenderness are localized to the prominent medial accessory navicular. An external oblique x-ray may be needed to visualize this accessory ossification center. Technetium bone scanning may show local increased uptake. Conservative management includes short-term use of a walking cast or foot orthotic. Occasionally, this condition requires surgical resection because of the bursitis that develops between the navicular and its accessory bone.

12. What are causes of pain in the forefoot?
Freiberg's disease (metatarsalgia) usually presents with unilateral foot pain that develops during athletic activities, with the pain later being noted during all ambulatory activities. This is most commonly encountered in the 13–18 year age group and has a predilection for female athletes. Local tenderness can be demonstrated, usually at the second metatarsophalangeal joint or occasionally at the third metatarsophalangeal joint. Many of these patients have a relatively long first metatarsus. This clinical finding should lead to radiographic evaluation and the diagnosis. The x-rays may demonstrate sclerosis of the metatarsal epiphysis, particularly on its dorsal surface, and eventually the metatarsal head becomes flattened, enlarged, and irregular. A painful plantar callus develops under the adjacent metatarsal heads owing to excessive weightbearing. This condition is managed by discontinuing sporting activities and immobilization. Use of a metatarsal pad immediately proximal to the joint is effective once the process is no longer painful. Surgery is reserved for chronic problems.

13. What are stress fractures?
Stress fractures in the young athlete generally involve the diaphysis of the metatarsi. Initially, the pain is present with activity, but later it becomes constant with all weightbearing. Physical examination will demonstrate well-localized pain. Swelling may not be a prominent finding. Repetitive running activities are more likely to lead to a metatarsal fracture, while basketball is associated with fractures of the hindfoot. This is particularly true in the older child with a less flexible foot and greater bone rigidity. Nondisplaced fractures can be treated with rest and decreased activity for 6 weeks. More symptomatic stress fractures may require cast immobilization.

14. What are unique problems causing ankle pain?

Osteochondritis dissecans of the talus occurs in adolescent athletes and is more frequently found in males. A deep aching sensation that is poorly localized may be the presenting complaint. This can be clinically distinguished from a chronic ankle sprain by the absence of tenderness over the anterior talofibular ligament. Swelling, bruising, and limited range of motion of the ankle may be noted. A bone scan may be diagnostic if routine x-rays fail to demonstrate the lesion. Arthroscopic management may be required.

Dysplasia epiphysealis hemimelica is an uncommon skeletal lesion that describes isolated overgrowth of either the medial distal tibia or the talus. Children present within the first few years of life with an asymmetric swelling of the joint with associated limited range of motion or pain. Radiographs demonstrate an irregular enlargement of the involved growth center. Treatment depends on the symptoms and degree of deformity, and the process completes its course at skeletal maturity. Attempts at surgical excision of the immature mass may lead to regrowth of the lesion and may also remove normal articular cartilage from the joint surface.

15. What are other unusual causes of foot pain?

Reflex sympathetic dystrophy can result from minor trauma and is associated with localized skin blanching or venous discoloration, increased or decreased skin temperature, and exquisite local tenderness and pain out of proportion to the original injury. Alternating contrast baths and the use of medication may be required in addition to immobilization in a weightbearing cast.

A crushing type of pedal injury may result in a compartment syndrome. Pain on passive dorsiflexion of the foot and evidence of decreased circulation are important clues. Increasing pain in the foot with complaints of numbness or tingling in the toes is worrisome. The presence of pulses should not preclude this diagnosis, which can be confirmed by increased compartment pressure measurements. Prompt fasciotomy will be required to avoid amputation.

16. How should pediatric infections be assessed?

Infectious processes include septic arthritis, acute hematogenous osteomyelitis, puncture wounds, and infections of the skin and nail. A personal history should include questions about recent or current infections as well as recent pedal trauma. Physical examination of a septic arthritis wound demonstrates an elevated temperature, tenderness, and restriction of motion of the joint along with pain, warmth, and erythema. Osteomyelitis would present with localized bone pain, warmth, swelling, and erythema.

Basic laboratory studies for both conditions would reveal an elevated white blood cell count and erythrocyte sedimentation rate. Blood cultures reveal the responsible organism in 40–50% of soft tissue and bony infections. Radiographic lytic changes of bone destruction do not become apparent for 7–10 days after the onset of osteomyelitis. Bone scans are reasonably accurate in isolating (and corroborating the suspicion of) pediatric osteomyelitis but are less reliable in neonates. Technetium bone scanning is reserved for cases in which the diagnosis is not clear.

17. What types of tumors can occur in children?

There are a variety of benign bone tumors in the pediatric population. Osteoid osteoma is most common in the first decade, and the foot and tarsal bones are a common site. The radiographs demonstrate a radiolucent nidus generally surrounded by dense reactive bone. An osteoid osteoma generally presents with pain, classically greater at night, and is relieved by salicylates. The tumor can be managed by surgical resection, or the pain can be controlled with nonsteroidal anti-inflammatory medication. Osteoblastoma of the hindfoot and enchondroma of the metatarsi or proximal phalanges are also found. The calcaneus is the most common pedal site of a unicameral bone cyst. An aneurysmal bone cyst is an expansile cystic lesion that presents in the first two decades of life with swelling and pain and is generally localized in the metaphysis of the phalanges or the calcaneus.

Leukemia and Ewing's sarcoma are the two most frequent causes of malignant bony lesions. Synovial sarcoma is the most common of malignant and neoplasm of soft tissue. Its average age of presentation is 13 years, and it generally occurs in the soft tissues of the midfoot and hindfoot.

This is a slow-growing lesion that presents as a painless enlarging mass in close proximity to a joint. Radiographic analysis reveals a soft tissue mass arising in proximity to a joint or tendon sheath, which may have some calcification. An MRI will show an oval tumor with the same density as muscle.

BIBLIOGRAPHY

1. Angermann P, Jensen P: Osteochondritis dissecans of the talus: long term results of surgical treatment. Foot Ankle 10:161–163, 1989.
2. Gould N, Moreland M, Alvarez R, Trevino S, Fenwick J: Development of the child's arch. Foot Ankle 9:241–245, 1989.
3. Harris RI, Beath T: Hypermobile flat-foot with short tendo-Achillis. J Bone Joint Surg 30A:116–138, 1948.
4. Ippolito PT, Pollini R, Falez R: Köhler's disease of the tarsal navicular: long-term follow-up of 12 cases. J Pediatr Orthop 4:416–417, 1984.
5. Jacob RF, McCarthy RE, Elser JM: Pseudomonas osteochondritis complicating puncture wounds of the foot in children: a 10 year evaluation. J Infect Dis 106:657–661, 1989.
6. Kirby EJ, Sheref MJ, Lewis MM: Soft tissue tumors and tumor-like lesions of the foot. An analysis of eighty-three cases. J Bone Joint Surg 71A:621–626, 1989.
7. Mosca VS: Flexible flatfoot and skewfoot. J Bone Joint Surg 77A:1937–1945, 1995.
8. Murari TM, Callaghan JJ, Berrey BH Jr, Sweet DE: Primary benign and malignant osseous neoplasms of the foot. Foot Ankle 10:68–80, 1989.
9. Olney BW, Asher MA: Excision of symptomatic coalition of the middle facet of the talocalcaneal joint. J Bone Joint Surg 69A:539–544, 1987.
10. Scott RJ: Acute osteomyelitis in children: a review of 116 cases. J Pediatr Orthop 10:649–652, 1990.
11. Staheli LT, Chew DE, Corbett M: The longitudinal arch. A survey of eight hundred and eighty-two feet in normal children and adults. J Bone Joint Surg 69A:426–428, 1987.
12. Wenger DR, Mauldin D, Speck G, Morgan D, Lieber RL: Corrective shoes and inserts as treatment for flexible flatfoot in infants and children. J Bone Joint Surg 71A:800–810, 1989.

50. BUNIONS

Hamlet A. Peterson, M.D.

1. What is a bunion?

Technically, a bunion is an abnormal prominence on the medial side of the first metatarsal head, with its accompanying bursa. From the perspective of an orthopaedist, a bunion is associated with an increased first cuneiform-first metatarsal angle, metatarsus primus varus, hallux valgus, and malrotation of the great toe.

2. How is the deformity documented?

A standard anteroposterior radiograph of the foot taken while standing allows measurement of multiple parameters and best depicts the deformities. The most notable and commonly recorded measurements (see Figure) are (*a*) the first-second metatarsal angle, (*b*) the first metatarsal-proximal phalanx angle, and (*c*) the first-second intrametatarsal distance. The length of the first metatarsal (*d*) as it relates to the length of the second metatarsal is also important.

3. What is the distal metatarsal articular angle (DMAA)?

The DMAA is the same as the metatarsophalangeal angle measured in a different way.

4. Are there other means of documenting the deformity?

Yes. Tracing around the foot with the patient standing, standing footprints recorded in ink, and

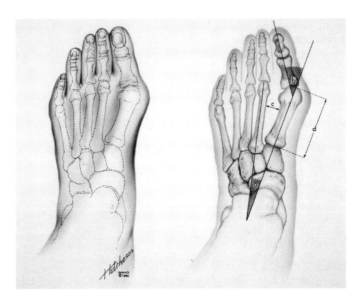

Left: Bunion deformity with underlying bone. *Right*: Radiographic bunion deformity measurements. *a,* First-second metatarsal angle. *b,* First metatarsal-proximal phalanx angle. *c,* First-second intermetatarsal distance. *d,* Length of first metatarsal.

photographs are all used, particularly to display pre- and postoperative changes. Tomograms, bone scans, CT scans, and MRI add no additional information.

5. What is the cause of bunions?
Although the cause is unknown, there is an increased familial incidence. In the typical patient, there is no congenital abnormality or underlying neurologic deficit. Bunions are commonly found in patients with neuromuscular disease (e.g., cerebral palsy), connective tissue disorders (e.g., Ehlers-Danlos syndrome), or relative shortening of the second metatarsal (e.g., multiple hereditary osteochondromata).

6. What is the incidence of adolescent bunions?
Bunions have been reported to affect 22–36% of adolescents. The population chosen for study, the methods of gathering the information, and the definition of deformity determined by the specific radiographic measurements used all have a significant impact on determining the prevalence. These figures seem high, although one report from Great Britain recorded more than 2000 adolescent feet operated on for hallux valgus per year.

7. What complaints accompany bunions?
The two most common complaints, pain and shoe-fitting difficulties, are interrelated. Pain in the prominent bursa over the medial side of the head of the first metatarsal is the first symptom noted and is usually due to external pressure from shoes. In long-standing cases, pain can be due to first metatarsophalangeal joint irritation, which can eventually develop into degenerative arthrosis. Cosmetic concerns are frequently important to adolescents. A teenager's desire to wear footwear similar to that of peers is great. As females get older, the increasing desire to wear higher heels and stylish shoes increases shoe-fitting difficulties. Parental concern about cosmesis and future functional impairment is common and is difficult to separate from more objective concerns. Functional impairment associated with bunions is extremely rare in adolescents.

8. What are the choices for management?

The patient may move to a climate conducive to the use of sandals or no shoes, may adapt the footwear to avoid pressure over the bunion, or may consider corrective surgery. Most patients (85% in our study) are successfully managed nonoperatively.

9. What are the choices for nonoperative treatment?

The only nonoperative treatment of benefit is to remove the pressure applied to the medial site of the great toe. This can best be accomplished by going barefoot (which in most parts of the United States is not culturally feasible). Finding shoes that are wide enough in the forefoot yet narrow enough to hold the heel comfortably is difficult. Mechanically stretching the forefoot width of the shoe or cutting a hole in the medial side of the shoe effectively reduces external pressure. Use of a variety of splints to hold the great toe in a more neutral position has not been found to have a lasting corrective effect.

10. What types of operations are available for treatment of bunion deformity?

More than 130 operations have been described for the treatment of bunions. These can be divided into several major groups: simple bunionectomy (surgical excision of the prominent exostosis); soft tissue procedures such as tenotomies; lateral capsular release or medial capsular tightening to align the metatarsal-phalangeal (MP) joint; osteotomies to change bone alignment; arthroplasty (both bone resection and replacement with artificial substances); and arthrodesis.

11. Why are there so many operations?

This suggests that a universally satisfactory operation is not available and that different manifestations of the problem require different operations. It is well known that the risks of a poor outcome and complications are higher in adolescent patients.

12. Why are surgical results less good in adolescents than adults?

The possibilities include a tendency among surgeons to use a more plastic, less invasive, and less corrective procedure in adolescents; recurrence of deformity with additional growth; and an increased use of poor shoes with pointed toes as the patient proceeds into adulthood.

13. Which of the surgical procedures seems to work best for adolescents?

Metatarsal osteotomy. There are many types of osteotomy. Most (e.g., Chevron, Mitchell) procedures reposition the metatarsal head to straighten the toe. The most natural anatomic goal is to maintain the articular congruence and the capsular structures about the MP joint. This is best accomplished with a closing wedge osteotomy of the distal first metatarsal. If this were the only procedure accomplished, the big toe would be in relative varus to the other four toes with a gap between the first and second toe. Thus, an accompanying open-wedge osteotomy at the base of the first metatarsal is necessary to make it parallel to the second metatarsal. The same wedge of bone that is excised in the distal closing wedge osteotomy can be used to hold the proximal osteotomy open.

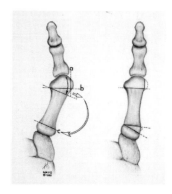

Left: First metatarsal double osteotomy. *a*, Excision of metatarsal head prominence. *b*, Closing wedge osteotomy (excision of medially based wedge). *c*, Transverse osteotomy in proximal metatarsal.

Right: Distal osteotomy closed. The wedge of bone removed from the distal closing metatarsal osteotomy is inserted into the proximal metatarsal and becomes an opening wedge osteotomy, which makes the first ray parallel to the second ray. The MP joint relationships (DMAA) are unchanged. Mathematically there is no shortening of the first metatarsal, since the wedge removed distally is placed proximally. The first-second intermetatarsal angle, the first metatarsal-phalangeal angle, and the first-second intermetatarsal distance are all decreased.

14. What are the disadvantages of corrective osteotomies?

They are major procedures, require 2–3 days of hospitalization, and, if done bilaterally, require nonweight-bearing for 2–4 weeks. Patients who have an osteotomy of any type usually note loss of plantar flexion in the MP joint. There is usually no loss of dorsal flexion or of plantar flexion strength, and running and jumping abilities are not altered. The loss of plantar flexion has little if any accompanying functional impairment (the only one being the inability to flex the toe down, e.g., over a starting platform for competitive swim races).

15. Which procedures do not work well in adolescents and why?

Simple bunionectomy (removal of the medial side of the head of the first metatarsal) is associated with poor results primarily because of increasing deformity, since the patient has many years to live. Resection arthroplasty and fusion of the joint reduce function, which is usually unacceptable in young patients who desire to be active.

16. What are the disadvantages of resection arthroplasty?

Procedures that remove the proximal end of the first phalanx to straighten the toe make it floppy and weak. Walking on tiptoes without shoes is difficult, and the remaining proximal end of the phalanx may eventually rub against the head of the first metatarsal, causing degenerative changes.

17. What is the difficulty with fusion of the MP joint?

Fusion of the joint determines permanently the angle of alignment between the proximal phalanx and the first metatarsal. The height of the heel of the shoe must always be the same thereafter to accommodate this angle. For a male, an angle of a few degrees of dorsiflexion can be determined for normal shoewear. The female would be limited in the choice of shoe heel height.

18. What happens if the condition is not treated?

The condition will not spontaneously improve. With properly modified shoewear, the patient may live a reasonably normal life, although progression of the deformity in middle age is common, especially if other middle-aged members of the family have noted progression of deformity.

BIBLIOGRAPHY

1. Beadling L: Juvenile hallux valgus: adapt surgery to address DMAA. Orthop Today, October 1995, p 26.
2. Bordelon RL: Evaluation and operative procedures for hallux valgus deformity. Orthopedics 10(1):38–44, 1987.
3. Geissele AE, Stanton RP: Surgical treatment of adolescent hallux valgus. J Pediatr Orthop 10:641–648, 1990.
4. Helal B: Surgery for adolescent hallux valgus. Clin Orthop 157:50–63, 1981.
5. Luba R, Rosman M: Bunions in children: treatment with a modified Mitchell osteotomy. J Pediatr Orthop 4:44–47, 1984.
6. Mann RA: Etiology and treatment of hallux valgus; bunion surgery: decision making. Orthopedics 13(9):951–957, 1990.
7. Peterson HA, Newman SR: Adolescent bunion deformity treated with double osteotomy and longitudinal pin fixation of the first ray. J Pediatr Orthop 13:80–84, 1993.
8. Zimmer TJ, Johnson KA, Klassen RA: Treatment of hallux valgus in adolescents by the Chevron osteotomy. Foot Ankle 9(4):190–193, 1989.

51. TOE DEFORMITIES

Peter L. Meehan, M.D.

CURLY TOES

1. What is a curly toe?
A toe whose distal portion is flexed, medially deviated, and externally rotated. As a result, the toenail is directed laterally and plantarward (see Figure). Such toes may underlie or less commonly overlie the adjacent toe(s). Curly toes are usually familial, bilateral, symmetric, and asymptomatic. They are the most common variant of normal seen in a child's foot.

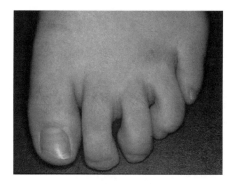

Curly toes involving second, third, and fourth toes.

2. Do curly toes require treatment?
The goals of management of foot problems are threefold: The foot should be painless, plantargrade, and able to accommodate normal shoes. Curly toes rarely interfere with normal foot function.

3. Are x-rays necessary for the evaluation of a child with curly toes?
No. The diagnosis is based on physical exam. Usually, the fourth and fifth toes and less often the third toe is involved. The toes are flexible when the child is examined in a supine position. The deformity is accentuated with weightbearing.

4. Does strapping of the toes work?
Strapping or taping of the toes has not proved effective.

5. What happens to these toes with time?
One study found spontaneous improvement in 25% of children. For the rare child who has persistent pain due to the deviation of their toes in shoes, release of the long toe flexor either alone or in combination with release of the short flexors of the toes is a proven procedure.

OVERRIDING FIFTH TOE

6. What is an overriding fifth toe?
A fixed deformity of the fifth toe in which it overrides the fourth toe (see Figure). It is a familial problem that may affect one foot or both feet. The fifth toe is externally rotated. As a result, the toenail is directed laterally.

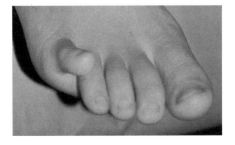

Overriding fifth toe.

7. How is this different from a curly toe?

Curly toes usually deviate medially but underlie the adjacent toe. The primary difference is that the curly toe is flexible whereas this type of deformity is rigid.

8. Does this require treatment?

As with all foot deformities and variants of normal, the patient's symptoms determine whether treatment is indicated.

9. Are patients likely to have pain?

About half of patients will have difficulty with footwear. Most patients can be managed by being fit with shoes of appropriate width.

10. What are the treatment alternatives for the patient who has persistent pain with proper-fitting shoes?

There is no effective nonoperative method of management. This is a rigid deformity that has fixed contracture of the long extensor tendon and the joint capsule. Such rigid deformities require surgical release.

11. Is removal of the proximal phalanx of the fifth toe advised?

A group of patients managed with this method was studied 3.5 years after surgery. One fourth of the study group had developed pain over the fifth metatarsal head and a bunionette deformity. In addition, a hammer toe deformity developed in one third of the patients. There are other procedures available that do not have these accompanying problems. The Butler procedure can effectively correct the deformity and avoid these problems.

SUBUNGUAL EXOSTOSIS

12. What is subungual exostosis?

A benign tumor of bone found on the distal and dorsal aspect of the toe, usually beneath or immediately adjacent to the nail. It can occur in the upper extremity but usually is found on the great toes. Patients present with deformity of the nail, pain, or ulceration and secondary infection. Exostoses may be mistaken for ingrown toenails.

13. How is the diagnosis made and what is the treatment?

A plain x-ray of the toe or finger in the lateral projection will demonstrate the lesion (see Figure). These exostoses originate from the dorsal aspect of the distal phalanx distal to the physeal plate. Surgical excision is necessary.

Subungual exostosis on the dorsum of the terminal phalanx of the great toe.

FREIBERG'S INFRACTION

14. What is Freiberg's infraction?
A rare abnormality of unknown cause that involves the metatarsal heads of adolescents and results in deformity of the metatarsal head and pain. The second metatarsal head is usually involved. This process less commonly affects the third and fourth metatarsal heads. Patients present with pain and stiffness of the foot. The involved metatarsophalangeal (MP) joint has restricted motion. There will be palpable stiffness of the joint.

15. How is the diagnosis made?
A plain x-ray will demonstrate an irregular metatarsal head that is enlarged and flattened. The cartilage space of the MP joint will be narrowed, an indication of joint destruction. Abnormality of the adjacent proximal phalanx will be seen as well.

16. What is the preferred treatment?
For the patient who presents with acute pain and disability, a short-leg cast will provide relief of symptoms and will allow the patient to ambulate. Following cast removal, a molded foot orthotic can be constructed to relieve pressure on the affected metatarsal head. The orthotic alone may be sufficient for the patient whose symptoms are mild.

17. What can be done if these methods do not provide adequate relief of pain?
Surgical exploration will usually demonstrate loose bodies in the MP joint. These are removed, the deformed metatarsal head is shaved, and the adjacent portion of the proximal phalanx is removed. This method is preferred by some because it does not disturb the weightbearing forces on the plantar aspect of the foot. An alternative procedure is simple excision of the affected metatarsal head. There is no long-term study that clearly defines which approach is superior.

HAMMER TOES

18. What is a hammer toe?
A hammer toe is one in which the metatarsophalangeal joint is extended, the proximal interphalangeal (PIP) is flexed, and the distal interphalangeal (DIP) joint is either normal or extended. This is a congenital problem usually involving one or two toes and not associated with other disease processes. It is important to be able to distinguish the hammer toe from a claw toe, which is often associated with underlying neurologic disease. The claw toe deformity will be accentuated with weightbearing, placing the nail in a weightbearing position.

19. Do hammer toes require treatment?
Unless symptomatic, no treatment is indicated.

20. Where do patients have problems with hammer toes?

The PIP joint is usually irritated by shoes. The toenail may become deformed and irritated because it is in a weightbearing position.

21. What can be done for the symptomatic patient?

In a young child, the deformity will often be passively correctable. If the MP joint is flexed, the PIP joint can often be extended. In this case, the long and short toe flexors can be released through a transverse incision at the proximal phalanx.

For the older child or the child with a fixed deformity of the PIP joint, fusion of the PIP joint together with release of the MP contracture is an effective alternative.

CLAW TOES

22. What are claw toes?

A deformity in which there is extension of the metatarsophalangeal joint with flexion of the proximal interphalangeal and distal interphalangeal joints (see Figure). Usually, all toes of the foot are involved. One or both feet may be involved. These deformities may be flexible or rigid.

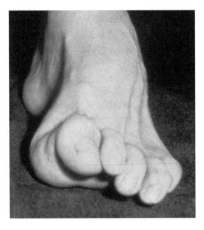

Cavus foot and claw toes.

23. What is the importance of claw toes?

Claw toes are usually associated with cavus feet and are secondary to the deformity of the forefoot. Since 80% of cavus feet in some series have an identifiable underlying neurologic cause, it is important to recognize the association between claw toes, cavus feet, and the possibility of underlying neurologic disease.

24. Are other tests necessary when claw toes have been identified?

A high percentage of such patients will be found to have an underlying neurologic problem. A plain radiograph of the spine should be obtained to look for radiographic signs of spinal dysraphism. These signs include congenital vertebral body anomaly, spina bifida occulta at a level other than S1, and interpedicular widening.

25. Do all claw toes require treatment?

Unless symptomatic, claw toes do not require treatment. Milder deformities usually do not cause symptoms. When pain is present, it typically occurs over the PIP joints owing to problems with footwear.

26. If a patient has persistently painful claw toes, what can be done?

For the patient whose claw toes are flexible, these deformities usually improve when the forefoot deformity of the cavus foot is corrected surgically.

If the claw toes are rigid, fusion of the PIP joints, release of the contracted dorsal capsule of the MP joint, transfer of the long toe extensor to the metatarsal neck, and suture of the distal portion of the long extensor to the short extensor provide reliable correction of the deformity. This procedure is usually done after the cavus foot has been treated surgically.

27. Are claw toes ever treated surgically before surgery for a cavus foot?

If a patient is symptomatic at the PIP joints and if there is no indication for surgical management of the associated cavus foot, surgery could certainly be done on the toes only.

POLYDACTYLY

28. What is polydactyly?

Polydactyly is a relatively common congenital problem. It usually is a familial problem with duplication of the ulnar digit of the hand and the fifth digit of the foot. It is not associated with other conditions. When the duplication involves the first ray of the foot, hallux varus is usually seen.

29. Does polydactyly require treatment?

With duplication of the toes, there may be associated duplication of the metatarsals. The result is a widened forefoot. It may be difficult to find shoes that will accommodate the widened forefoot.

30. What can be done surgically?

Surgical excision of the duplicated digits and associated metatarsals can narrow the forefoot sufficiently to allow the child to wear normal shoes.

31. Is this an easy procedure?

Some of the duplicated digits are relatively easy to remove surgically, while others involve duplication of joint surfaces, which are more difficult to reconstruct. In addition, the lateralmost digit is not necessarily the digit that requires removal. At times, osteotomy of a normal metatarsal is necessary in order to narrow the forefoot adequately to accommodate normal shoes.

HALLUX VARUS

32. What is hallux varus?

Hallux varus is a congenital deformity of the foot characterized by medial deviation of the great toe. It is usually associated with either complete or partial duplication of the great toe (see Figure). There may be a palpable band of soft tissue over the medial aspect of the foot. Usually, the deformity is fixed. Plain x-rays may demonstrate a widening of the first metatarsal or other radiographic evidence of partial duplication.

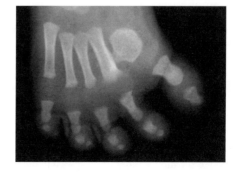

Congenital hallux varus.

33. What are the problems in management?

The components of hallux varus are contracture of the soft tissues medially; contracture of the MP joint medially; presence of a fibrous, cartilaginous, or bony anlage of a partially formed duplicate of the first ray; and a variety of potential bony and joint deformities.

34. Is surgery necessary for these patients?
If the deformity is rigid, it will interfere with shoe fitting. If there is an anlage of a duplicated digit in the medial soft tissues, the deformity is not likely to improve. For these reasons, surgery is often necessary to correct the deformity.

35. Are there situations in which a child may have hallux varus and not have long-term difficulties?
Yes. The foot of the normal child will usually be adducted with some element of hallux varus. These feet and great toes are flexible, however. Spontaneous correction is expected.

SYNDACTYLY

36. What is syndactyly?
Syndactyly is a situation wherein the skin of the toes did not separate, and two toes became "webbed." Simple syndactyly of the toes is an isolated deformity that does not limit function or interfere with shoe fitting. Only the skin is joined together in simple syndactyly. Complex snydactyly is present when the failure of separation involves the bony structure. Simple syndactyly does not require treatment, since it does not cause problems.

37. Since fingers that have simple syndactyly are routinely surgically separated, why are toes not routinely surgically separated?
The technique of surgical separation of phalanges joined by simple syndactyly often requires skin grafting and can be complex. Scar tissue is the result of any surgical procedure. Since the foot is weightbearing, it would not be desirable to have painful scar tissue develop in an area that would have been pain free otherwise.

38. When the bones are joined together in complex syndactyly, is surgical separation necessary?
If the failure of separation of the phalanges results in abnormal growth of the toes and in deformity that interferes with shoe fitting and causes pain, surgical separation is indicated.

INGROWN TOENAILS

39. What causes an ingrown toenail?
The encroachment of the soft tissues either medially or laterally onto the toenail. As the nail grows, it creates a mechanical irritation of the soft tissue. These areas become secondarily infected. The great toe is usually involved.

40. What are the contributing preventable causes?
Improper nail trimming allows the corner of the nail to grow into the soft tissues. The toenail may be traumatized by wearing shoes that are too short or too narrow. Stockings may also be too tight, compressing the soft tissues against the nail.

41. What is the proper way to trim the toenail?
The great toenail should be trimmed straight across. It should not be rounded; this can cause the distal end of the nail to become embedded into the medial or lateral soft tissues.

42. Are there other contributing causes?
Some patients have malformation of the nail, which results in its being U-shaped. Patients with this anatomic situation are often predisposed to problems with ingrown toenails.
Subungual exostosis is a rare cause of nail inflammation.

43. What is the normal anatomy of the toenail pertinent to this problem?
The space between the nail margin and the nail groove is about 1 mm. This groove is lined with a thin layer of epithelium and lies immediately under and to the sides of the nail margin.

44. What is the initial treatment?

Initial treatment depends on the severity of involvement, specifically the presence of active infection. For the patient whose problem is primarily mechanical irritation, placement of gauze under the leading edge of the nail together with daily warm-water soaks followed by application of an antibiotic ointment is sufficient. Since the toenail grows at a rate of 2 mm per month, this requires continued treatment until the toenail is able to grow out beyond the end of the soft tissue on either the medial or the lateral edge of the nail. Activities should be restricted, since mechanical trauma aggravates the problem.

45. What is recommended when there is evidence of active cellulitis?

If there is evidence of active cellulitis, an oral antibiotic with *Staphylococcus aureus* coverage is advised as well.

46. What should be avoided?

It is tempting to remove the lateral margin of the nail that is embedded in the soft tissues. Since the nail originates from the germinal matrix located at the base of the distal phalanx, the nail will continue to grow at its original width. By trimming the medial or lateral margin of the nail, the problem has been prolonged, since the nail will regrow at its normal width because the germinal matrix has not been altered.

47. Should the nail be removed?

Nail avulsion is not advised unless it is deemed necessary to control infection. Avulsed great toenails often grow back deformed.

48. What should be done if the problem is the result of bony deformity of the distal phalanx?

If the nail is U-shaped and if there have been persistent problems with infection, it may be appropriate to narrow the nail by surgically excising a portion of either the medial or lateral germinal matrix and associated nail. By removing a portion of the germinal matrix, the corresponding portion of the nail will not regrow. The nail will therefore be made narrower.

BIBLIOGRAPHY

1. Cockin J: Butler's operation: an over-riding fifth toe. J Bone Joint Surg 50B:78–81, 1968.
2. Dixon GL Jr: Treatment of ingrown toenails. Foot Ankle 3(5):254–260, 1983.
3. Janecki CJ, Wilde AH: Results of phalangectomy of the fifth toe for hammer toe. The Ruiz-Mora procedure. J Bone Joint Surg 58A:1005–1007, 1976.
4. London GC, Johnson KA, Dahlin DC: Subungual exostosis. J Bone Joint Surg 61A:256–259, 1979.
5. Margo MK: Surgical treatment of conditions of the forepart of the foot. J Bone Joint Surg 49A:1665–1674, 1967.
6. Meehan PL: The cavus foot. In Morrissy RT (ed): Pediatric Orthopaedics, 3rd ed. Philadelphia, J.B. Lippincott Co., 1990, p 971–981.
7. Meehan PL: Other conditions of the foot. In Morrissy RT (ed): Pediatric Orthopaedics, 3rd ed. Philadelphia, J.B. Lippincott Co., 1990, pp 1009, 1011–1012, 1017.
8. Pollard JP, Morrison PJM: Flexor tenotomy in the treatment of curly toes. Proc R Soc Med 68:480–481, 1975.
9. Ross ERS, Menelaus MB: Open flexor tenotomy for hammer toes and curly toes in childhood. J Bone Joint Surg 66B:770–771, 1984.
10. Sweetnam R: Congenital curly toes. An investigation into the value of treatment. Lancet 2:398–400, 1958.
11. Venn-Watson EA: Problems in polydactyly of the foot. Orthop Clin North Am 7:909, 1976.

52. NAIL PUNCTURE

Peter L. Meehan, M.D.

1. What is the most likely cause of a puncture wound of the foot?
Nails are the most likely source. In a large series by Fitzgerald and Cowan, 869 of 887 puncture wounds to the foot were caused by nails.

2. What is the preferred initial management of the wound?
Local wound care with cleaning of the adjacent tissues is advised. In addition, plain radiographs of the foot should be obtained if there is suspicion of a possible retained foreign body. Plain radiographs can provide limited information. Wood, unleaded glass, and pieces of sock and shoe are radiolucent.

3. What is the role of prophylactic antibiotics?
There is no proven efficacy for prophylactic antibiotics. The use of antibiotics may suppress a potentially destructive infection of a bone or joint.

4. What instructions should be given to the family?
Pain and tenderness in an uncomplicated puncture wound should resolve quickly. If there is persistent or increasing pain, erythema, swelling, or drainage, the patient should return to the orthopaedist for evaluation. Systemic signs such as fever are unlikely even when there is an infection.

5. What is the usual outcome?
In the series previously mentioned, 132 of 887 developed cellulitis, and 16 developed osteomyelitis. Most of those with cellulitis developed signs and symptoms within 24–48 hours of the injury. Those with osteomyelitis did not return with problems for 7–10 days.

6. What should be done if a retained foreign body is suspected at the time of initial presentation?
The patient should be taken to the operating room for wound exploration, débridement, and culture. It is only in this controlled environment with use of a tourniquet that an adequate, thorough, and safe exploration of the foot can be done. Foreign material, parts of the patient's socks, shoe, gravel, rust, dirt, and other material may be found. In addition, cultures should be taken to look for aerobic, anaerobic, fungal, and acid-fast organisms. The latter is most important if the injury occurred outside with possible soil contamination. If it is suspected that bone has been penetrated, it is important to curet that bone. If the injury is adjacent to a joint, the joint should be explored to be certain that penetration has not occurred. Over the forefoot, dorsal and plantar incisions may be appropriate in order to explore that portion of the foot adequately, safely, and thoroughly.

7. What should be done if a patient returns with evidence of cellulitis?
Surgical exploration of the wound with culturing should be done. It osteomyelitis is suspected, the bone should be curetted and cultures taken. A large needle can be used to aspirate the bone, and the aspirate should be placed in blood culture bottles. This method may have a greater yield in culture results.

8. Are there areas of the foot that are more difficult to manage?
Puncture wounds of the forefoot may be more difficult to manage because of the proximity of multiple vital structures. These wounds have the potential to affect two joints as well as bone. Since the foot is thinner in this area, the nail may almost penetrate through the dorsal skin. Therefore, in order to explore this area thoroughly, both a plantar and a dorsal incision may be neces-

sary. Injuries of the heel may penetrate the calcaneus, and those of the midfoot may penetrate the midtarsal joints.

9. Why can a patient not be placed on antibiotics alone if there is evidence of cellulitis?
The potential organisms that need to be considered include both gram-positive and gram-negative bacteria. In addition, there may be a rare child with an atypical acid-fast organism as an associated pathogen. It is only with good surgical culturing that the proper choices of antibiotics can be made. The antibiotics used for the gram-negative organisms have potential adverse reactions. In addition, many patients of Fitzgerald and Cowan were found to have a foreign body at the time of surgical exploration. Therefore, although broad-spectrum antibiotics may treat some patients, they may only suppress an infection in others or may potentially mask a bone or joint infection.

10. Is a bone scan indicated for the patient who returns with evidence of cellulitis?
Some authors do recommend a bone scan, but the suggested management is surgical exploration in order to debride the wound and obtain cultures.

11. What are the most likely organisms to be involved in infections of this type?
For those patients who have cellulitis, only gram-positive organisms are likely, but when osteomyelitis or septic arthritis is the problem, *Pseudomonas aeruginosa* has been a commonly isolated pathogen. Therefore, until culture reports are available, patients should receive antibiotics that will cover both possibilities.

12. What is the source of the *Pseudomonas*?
The source is not known. It does not seem to be part of the normal flora of the foot, metal nails, or the sole of tennis shoes. It has been cultured from the inner foam layer of tennis shoes, however.

13. What should be done if the initial culture shows *Pseudomonas aeruginosa* and I have placed the patient on an appropriate antibiotic based on sensitivities, but the patient is not getting well?
Consider another pathogen that may not have grown initially owing to an overwhelming infection of one pathogen or insufficient culture time. Atypical mycobacteria are soil pathogens and may be the source of the problem in addition to a retained foreign body. Re-exploration of the foot would be appropriate. If the lesion is over the forefoot and the injury has been explored through only a plantar incision, consider making a dorsal incision as well, and vice versa.

14. What are the complications of puncture wounds of the foot?
Cellulitis, osteomyelitis, and septic arthritis are possible complications of puncture wounds of the foot. Septic arthritis with destruction of a joint has the potential to cause the greatest long-term morbidity.

BIBLIOGRAPHY

1. Fitzgerald RH, Cowan JDE: Puncture wounds of the foot. Orthop Clin North Am 6:965–972, 1975.
2. Jarvis JG, Skipper J: Pseudomonas osteochondritis complicating puncture wounds in children. J Pediatr Orthop 14:755–759, 1994.

53. METATARSUS ADDUCTUS

James C. Drennan, M.D.

1. What is metatarsus adductus?

Metatarsus adductus is a common foot deformity that presents in the newborn period. The condition is generally benign and describes adduction of the metatarsi at the tarsometatarsal joints associated with normal alignment of the hindfoot and midfoot. In utero positioning is the most likely cause. The problem is more frequent in firstborn children because primigravida mothers have stronger muscle tone in the uterine and abdominal walls, and this results in more compact positioning of the fetus. The incidence is reported to be 1:1000 live births, with 50% having bilateral involvement. There is an equal frequency of occurrence in males and females.

2. What are the clinical characteristics?

The hindfoot and midfoot have no deformity. The forefoot is adducted and slightly supinated (see Figure). The lateral border of the foot has a convex contour with prominence of the base of the fifth metatarsus. Tickling the bottom of the foot may lead to a dynamic separation of the first and second toes caused by the active contracture of the abductor hallucis muscle. This dynamic medial movement of the great toe spontaneously stops when the stimulation is discontinued. Patients who require treatment generally have a noticeable medial skin crease at the level of the tarsometatarsal joints. Passive forefoot abduction may accentuate a palpably contracted abductor hallucis muscle. Internal tibial torsion is frequently associated with metatarsus adductus.

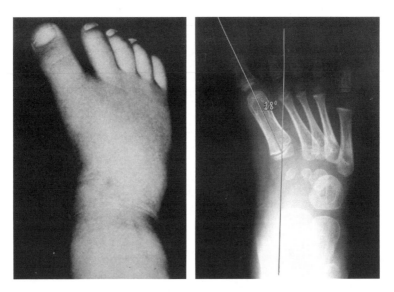

Metatarsus adductus. The clinical and radiographic findings document that the adduction occurs at the metatarsocuneiform joints.

3. How does the condition differ from talipes equinovarus and the skewfoot?

A rigid clubfoot has a hindfoot that is fixed in equinus and inversion and generally has conspicuous deep posterior heel and medial midfoot skin creases. The fat pad below the heel crease is devoid of bone, since the calcaneus is actually located at the level of the skin crease. The entire foot is supinated, has a rigid convex outline to its lateral border, and may have a shortened first ray.

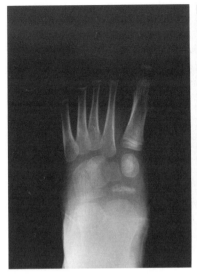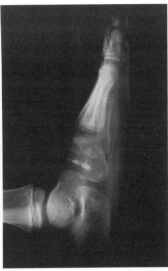

Serpentine foot. The AP radiograph demonstrates hindfoot valgus, lateral subluxation of the navicular bone, and adduction of the forefoot localized to the cuneonavicular joint.

Metatarsus varus (skewfoot) is more difficult to distinguish on infant examination. Its medial skin crease is located at the more distal naviculocuneiform joint. The heel in the skewfoot is in valgus, and this condition rarely has an associated contracture of the abductor hallucis muscle. This complex foot deformity combines heel valgus with a lateral subluxation of the talonavicular joint (midfoot) and adduction of the forefoot, which explains its common nickname of the Z foot (see Figure). The differentiation of metatarsus adductus from metatarsus varus is important because serial casting of the skewfoot is inappropriate and could lead to the development of a significant iatrogenic flatfoot as the congenital midfoot lateral subluxation becomes exaggerated.

4. What is the outcome without treatment?

The vast majority of cases of metatarsus adductus spontaneously resolve, and clinical observation is sufficient. The presence of a skin crease on the medial aspect of the midfoot coupled with a contracture of the abductor hallucis muscle should warrant consideration of serial corrective casting. Extension of the abnormal medial skin crease onto the plantar surface should signal the physician that there is an associated contracture of the plantar fascia (cavus), which can significantly lengthen the period of serial casting.

5. Who should care for this condition?

The primary care physician should be responsible during the first 3 months unless there is a passive stretching program, which is usually performed at diaper changes. The parents are taught to hold the heel in neutral position and manually abduct the forefoot using their thumb placed over the lateral cuboid as the fulcrum for correction. The exaggerated forefoot abduction position should be maintained for a few seconds and the stretching repeated 10 times at each session.

6. Are any additional studies needed?

X-rays offer limited information in the skeletally immature foot. The radiographic medial soft tissue outline may help distinguish metatarsus adductus from the more complex skewfoot in the newborn. Use of x-rays should be limited to situations in which there is a clinical suspicion of a more complex foot deformity.

BIBLIOGRAPHY

1. Berg EE: A reappraisal of metatarsus adductus and skewfoot. J Bone Joint Surg 68A:1185–1196, 1986.
2. Ghali NN, Abberton MJ, Silk FF: The management of metatarsus adductus et supinatus. J Bone Joint Surg 66B:376, 1984.
3. Mosca VS: Flexible flatfoot and skewfoot. J Bone Joint Surg 77A:1937–1945, 1995.
4. Peterson HA: Skewfoot (forefoot adduction and heel valgus). J Pediatr Orthop 6:24–30, 1986.

54. CLUBFOOT

Norris C. Carroll, M.D., FRCSC

1. What is clubfoot?

A congenitally deformed foot that points downward and inward.

2. How common is clubfoot?

The overall incidence of clubfoot in the general population is 1.24 per thousand live births.

3. Is clubfoot more common in boys or girls, and are both feet deformed?

Boys are affected twice as often as girls, and 50% of cases are bilateral.

4. When a boy is born with a clubfoot, what are the chances that a baby brother or baby sister will have a clubfoot?

The chances are 1 in 40 that a baby brother will be affected and very low that a sister will be affected.

5. If a girl is born with a clubfoot, what are the chances that a new brother or a new sister will have a clubfoot?

About 1 in 16 that the new brother will have a clubfoot, and about 1 in 40 that the new sister will have a clubfoot.

6. If both the parent and a child have clubfeet, what are the chances that another baby will be affected?

The chances are 1 in 4.

7. What are the causes of clubfoot?

No one knows for sure.

8. What are the etiology theories?

Fetal developmental arrest, germ plasm defect, retracting fibrosis, and neurogenic and myogenic theories.

9. What is the pathoanatomy?

The talus has an abnormal shape, and all the relationships of the talus are abnormal. The plantar flexors and invertors are shortened, there is thickening of the tendon sheaths, and the joint capsules ligaments and fascia are contracted.

10. When should treatment begin?

As soon as possible after the baby is delivered.

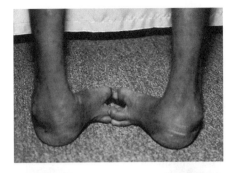

Anterior view of the feet shows untreated clubfeet in an adolescent boy. Note the severe equinovarus deformity with load bearing on the dorsum of the foot. (Courtesy of John Roberts, M.D.)

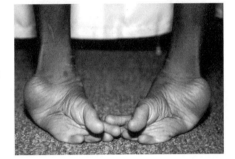

Posterior view showing the lack of load bearing on the sole of the foot. (Courtesy of John Roberts, M.D.)

11. Are all clubfeet the same?
No, there are various degrees of severity.

12. How do you classify the severity of a clubfoot?
There is no universal standard. The simplest classification is mild, moderate, or severe. I have tried to classify clubfeet according to the presence or absence of the following assessment criteria.

- Calf atrophy
- Posterior displacement of the fibula
- Creases (medial, plantar, and posterior)
- Curved lateral border
- Cavus

- Fixed equinus
- Navicular fixed to medial malleolus
- Os calcis fixed to fibula
- No midtarsal mobility
- Fixed forefoot supination

13. How does one treat a clubfoot?
Initial treatment is manipulation to stretch the soft tissues in an attempt to realign the bony architecture. A cast is then applied to maintain the position obtained with the manipulation.

14. How often is the cast changed?
I change the cast biweekly at first, weekly at 1 month, and every 2 weeks when maintaining the correction obtained.

15. How successful is manipulation and casting?
Figures in the literature are all over the place from 50% to 5% but as a rule, the stiffer the foot, the less likely it is to be corrected by manipulation.

16. What do you do if you can't correct the foot with manipulation and casting?
If after 3 months of manipulation and casting, the foot is still not corrected, I advise the parents to schedule surgical correction of the deformity.

17. What is the goal of surgery?
To restore the bony architecture to normal and to balance the muscle forces.

18. How do you restore the bony architecture to normal?
The plantar fascia and tight intrinsic muscles are divided, a Z-plasty is performed of the tendo Achillis and tibialis posterior, and the tight capsules are divided so that the navicular can be reduced onto the head of the talus, the cuboid can be reduced onto the end of the calcaneus, and the whole foot can be brought out of equinus. The lengthened tendons are then sutured with the foot held in a plantigrade position.

19. Are there imaging studies that can help you determine whether there is good correction of the deformity?
Yes, I like to have an AP and lateral x-ray of the foot with the posterior cortex of the fibula in line with the posterior cortex of the tibia. On the lateral view, the talus should align with the first ray and the calcaneus should be out of equinus. On the AP view, there should be divergence between the talus and the calcaneus, the first ray should align with the talus, and the lateral border of the foot should be straight with the cuboid sitting on the end of the calcaneus.

20. What is the after treatment? Do you apply the cast immediately?
No, at the time of surgery the alignment of the bony architecture is maintained with K-wires across the talonavicular and calcaneocuboid joints. The limb is immobilized in a soft dressing from the groin to the tip of the toes. This is done to maintain good blood flow to the foot and to promote wound healing. One week postoperatively, the child is taken back to the operating room for a short anesthetic and application of the definitive cast.

21. How long do you maintain the plaster immobilization postoperatively?
I change the initial cast in 4 weeks, and another plaster cast is applied for another 4 weeks. Then the foot position is maintained in an ankle-foot orthosis until the child is walking and the foot is plantigrade with a good progression angle.

22. How successful is the overall treatment for a clubfoot?
The initial casting and surgical treatment should be successful in about 85% of cases.

23. What are some of the pitfalls?
An incomplete correction, for instance, not recognizing the cavus component and lengthening the plantar fascia, or not recognizing medial displacement of the cuboid at the time of the initial surgery. Another problem is overcorrection of the deformity.

24. How do you avoid overcorrection of the deformity?
By preserving the anterior deep portion of the deltoid ligament and the interosseous ligament between the talus and calcaneus, by being careful not to overdisplace the navicular laterally, and by not overlengthening the tibialis posterior and tendo Achillis. Finally, when I apply the postoperative cast, I make sure that the foot is not placed in an overcorrected position.

25. How do you classify residual deformity?
Dynamic or fixed.

26. What do you mean by dynamic deformity?
I can grasp the foot and place it in a fully corrected position.

27. What is the most common dynamic deformity?
Adduction and supination of the forefoot due to an imbalance between the peroneus longus and the tibialis anterior.

28. How do you correct this deformity?
If the deformity is not corrected with appropriate orthotic care, then it can be corrected by a split tibialis anterior tendon transfer.

29. How do you analyze a clubfoot with a residual fixed deformity?
I do a careful examination of the hindfoot, the midfoot, and the forefoot and decide which components of the deformity are acceptable and which must be fixed. Standing, AP, and lateral x-rays of the foot and an axial view of the os calcis help me in my decision-making.

30. What do you look for in the hindfoot?
First, I assess the range of motion in the ankle. I look to see if the talus and calcaneus are still parallel and if the talus is misshaped (e.g., is the top of the talus flat?). Then I look to see if the heel is in varus, valgus, equinus, or calcaneus position.

31. What about the midfoot?
I look to see where the navicular bone is lying in relation to the head of the talus. Is it medial, dorsal, or dorsal lateral? Where does the cuboid sit in relation to the calcaneus?

32. What deformities do you look for in the forefoot?
I look to see if there is adduction, supination, pronation, or abduction of the forefoot.

33. When treating a recurrent clubfoot with a fixed deformity, what are your goals?
I want to balance the medial and lateral columns of the foot so that the foot is plantigrade and balance the muscle forces so that the foot stays plantigrade.

34. What do you mean by the medial and lateral columns?
The medial column consists of the talus, the navicular, the three cuneiforms, and the first three metatarsals. The lateral column consists of the calcaneus, the cuboid, and the fourth and fifth metatarsals. In most recurrent deformities, the medial column is shortened and the lateral column is elongated.

35. What are some of the common procedures done to correct a residual fixed deformity?
Correct heel varus with a sliding calcaneal osteotomy. Correct forefoot adductus by either reducing the navicular on the head of the talus or shortening the lateral column by removing a wedge of bone from the cuboid and lengthening the medial column by an open wedge osteotomy of the medial cuneiform.

36. Is it sometimes necessary to do even more surgery?
Yes, some feet will require a wedge tarsectomy to correct the forefoot deformity, and some severely deformed feet can only be corrected with a triple arthrodesis or the application of an Ilizarov frame.

37. Is there information that it is important to communicate to the family up front?
It is especially important to tell the family that there will be calf atrophy, that the calf atrophy was already present at birth, and that the clubfoot will be smaller than the normal foot.

38. What are the controversies?
   1. The timing of surgery. Should it be in the first 6 months of life or at 1 year of age? I prefer to do the surgery early, when the bony architecture of the foot has its greatest remodeling potential.
   2. The surgical approach. The two common surgical exposures are the Cincinnati exposure and the two-incision exposure. I prefer the two-incision exposure because the tendon sheaths behind the medial malleolus are preserved.

3. What should be released at the time of surgery? I believe in a à la carte approach and release only those structures that are preventing the bony architecture from assuming a normal position.

4. Should pins be used at the time of surgery? It is my position that pins are important to maintain the exact interosseous relationship.

39. Who is the author of the oldest written description of clubfoot and its treatment?
Hippocrates (460–377 B.C.) stated, "Manipulate the foot as if molding a wax model, not by force, but gently."

BIBLIOGRAPHY

1. Carroll NC: Controversies in the surgical management of clubfoot. In Pritchard DJ (ed): Instructional Course Lectures, Vol. 45. Rosemont, IL, Amer Acad Orthop Surg. 1996, pp 331–337.
2. Carroll NC: Surgical treatment for talipes equino-varus. Op Tech Orthop 3(2):115, 1993.
3. Crawford AH, Marxen JL, Osterfeld DL: The Cincinnati incision: a comprehensive approach for surgical procedures of the foot and ankle in childhood. J Bone Joint Surg [Am] 64:1355, 1982.
4. Evans D: Relapsed clubfoot. J Bone Joint Surg [Br] 43:722, 1961.
5. Goldner JL: Congenital talipes-equino varus—15 years of surgical treatment. Curr Prac Orthop 4:61, 1969.
6. Herzenberg JE, Carroll NC, Christofersen MR, et al.: Clubfoot analysis with three-dimensional computer modeling. J Pediatr Orthop 8(3):257–263, 1988.
7. McKay DW: New concepts of an approach to clubfoot treatment, section 1—principles and morbid anatomy. J Pediatr Orthop 2:347, 1982.
8. McKay DW: New concept of an approach to treatment, section 2—correction of clubfoot. J Pediatr Orthop 3:10, 1983.
9. Ponseti IV: Congenital Clubfoot, Fundamentals of Treatment, New York, Oxford University Press, 1996.
10. Simons GW: Complete sub-talar release in clubfeet, part I—a preliminary report. J Bone Joint Surg [Am] 67:1044, 1985.
11. Simons GW: Complete sub-talar release in clubfeet, part II—comparison of less extensive procedures. J Bone Joint Surg [Am] 67:1056, 1985.
12. Tarraf YN, Carroll NC: Analysis of the components of residual deformity in clubfeet presenting for re-operation. M Pediatr Orthop 12(2):207, 1992.
13. Turco VJ: Resistant congenital clubfoot—one stage posterior medial release with internal fixation, a follow-up report of 15 years experience. J Bone Joint Surg [Am] 61:805, 1979.

55. FLATFOOT

Vincent S. Mosca, M.D.

1. What is a flatfoot?
"Flatfoot" is used to describe a foot shape in which the medial longitudinal arch is depressed toward the ground. There is a sagging of the midfoot, valgus alignment of the hindfoot, abduction of the forefoot on the hindfoot, and supination of the forefoot in relation to the hindfoot. There are no universally accepted clinical or radiographic criteria for differentiating a foot with a low normal arch from a flatfoot.

2. How common are flatfeet?
It's hard to say with certainty because a strict definition does not exist. Nevertheless, flatfeet are seen in more than 20% of adults, according to Harris and Beath. Based on footprint and radiographic studies, flatfeet are much more common in children than in adults.

3. Are there different types of flatfeet?
The flatfoot shape can be seen in otherwise normal individuals as well as in those with underlying neuromuscular disorders. There are three types of flatfoot in normal individuals: hypermobile or flexible flatfoot, flexible flatfoot with a short Achilles tendon, and rigid flatfoot.

4. Why is it important to classify flatfoot into different types?

To help with prognosis. The flexible flatfoot accounts for approximately two thirds of flatfeet in adults and a greater of percentage of flatfeet in children and is of little or no clinical concern as a potential cause of disability. The flexible flatfoot with a short Achilles tendon accounts for about 25% of flatfeet in adults and a smaller percentage of flatfeet in children and has the potential for causing disability. The third and least frequent type of flatfoot is the rigid type, which is seen with tarsal coalition. Pain and disability are evident in about one quarter of affected individuals.

5. How do you differentiate the types of flatfoot on clinical examination?

A flexible flatfoot has good mobility of the subtalar joint. The foot has the characteristic flat appearance when the individual stands still. The hindfoot inverts to neutral (or even varus) and the medial longitudinal arch elevates when the heel is elevated during toe standing. The arch is also evident when the foot is dangling in the air, as when the individual is seated with the foot off the ground. The common benign flexible flatfoot has normal excursion of the ankle joint and Achilles tendon (triceps surae musculotendinous complex). In order to assess this accurately, the subtalar joint is inverted to neutral position and the ankle is dorsiflexed with the knee held in flexion. The knee is then extended while maintaining inversion of the subtalar joint and attempting to maintain dorsiflexion of the ankle. The ankle should maintain at least $10°$ of dorsiflexion with the knee extended. A flexible flatfoot with less than $10°$ of dorsiflexion due to contracture of the Achilles tendon is more likely to cause pain and disability than one with more excursion. A rigid flatfoot has a stiff subtalar joint that does not change shape during toe standing. The heel will of course elevate, but the sagging of the midfoot and the valgus alignment of the hindfoot will still be evident.

6. What causes a flexible flatfoot?

The height of the longitudinal arch is determined by the shapes of the bones and the laxity of the ligaments of the foot. Muscles are important for balance and function, but not for structure. Flexible flatfeet often run in families and are more common in certain ethnic and racial groups.

7. What is the natural history of arch development in the child?

There is spontaneous elevation of the longitudinal arch of the foot in most children during the first decade of life. Clinical footprint and radiographic studies confirm this finding.

8. Can shoes, braces, and orthoses affect the natural history of arch development?

No. Only two prospective controlled studies have been performed to answer this question, and both found no beneficial effect of shoes or orthoses in the development of the longitudinal arch.

9. What causes a rigid flatfoot?

The most common cause of a rigid flatfoot is a tarsal coalition, an autosomal dominant failure of differentiation and segmentation of the primary mesenchyme forming the tarsal bones. The most common sites for a coalition are between the calcaneus and navicular and between the talus and calcaneus. The coalitions undergo metaplasia from fibrous (syndesmosis) to cartilaginous (synchondrosis) to osseous unions (synostosis) during childhood and adolescence.

Other causes of a rigid flatfoot include congenital vertical talus, juvenile rheumatoid arthritis, septic arthritis, and traumatic arthritis following intra-articular fracture of the subtalar joint.

10. What is the most likely cause of progressive flattening of the longitudinal arch in a child?

A tarsal coalition produces a progressive flattening of the longitudinal arch in childhood. A flexible flatfoot, with or without a short Achilles tendon, is almost always present from birth and shows a progressive elevation of the arch or no change in height during growth of the child.

11. Should radiographs be obtained when evaluating the flatfoot?

Radiographs are not indicated when evaluating the asymptomatic flatfoot in a child who presents because of parental concern about the shape of the foot. Physical examination is all that is required. Radiographs may be indicated for the child with a flexible flatfoot or flexible flatfoot with a short Achilles tendon who has foot pain, particularly if the symptoms are excessive and unrelated to activities and if other signs or symptoms are present.

Weightbearing anteroposterior, lateral, oblique, and axial Harris view radiographs are appropriate for the adolescent with a painful rigid flatfoot. A calcaneonavicular coalition is best seen on the 45° oblique radiograph. The axial Harris view may show a talocalcaneal coalition, but the definitive imaging study for demonstration of a coalition at this site is the CT scan.

12. Is it true that flexible flatfeet never hurt?
No. Many individuals with flexible flatfeet have generalized laxity of their ligaments. Activity-related pain and fatigue as well as aching pain at night in the feet, ankles, and legs will sometimes be reported. It is thought that these symptoms represent an overuse syndrome caused by muscles overworking to compensate for the excessively lax ligaments. In these situations, use of over-the-counter or, less commonly, molded foot orthoses can diminish or eliminate symptoms.

13. Are there other benefits from the use of orthoses?
Yes. Orthoses may change the pattern of wear and increase the useful life of shoes.

14. How does pain manifest in the flexible flatfoot with a short Achilles tendon?
There is pain, redness, and callus formation in the arch area under the plantar-flexed head of the talus. This is a specific site of pain and tenderness, which differentiates it from the activity-related, generalized aching occasionally seen in the flexible flatfoot in which there is good excursion of the Achilles tendon.

15. What can be done for pain and disability in the flexible flatfoot with a short Achilles tendon?
Foot orthoses may exacerbate symptoms in this condition and are not recommended. Pressure is already being concentrated under the head of the talus because the tight Achilles tendon is forcing it to the ground. An arch support will increase the pressure in this area and cause more pain. Stretching the Achilles tendon may be beneficial. A block is placed under the first and second metatarsal heads in order to invert the subtalar joint. The knee is extended. The child leans into a wall, keeping the heel on the ground. Aching is experienced in the popliteal fossa and proximal calf during effective stretching.

16. What are the operative management principles for the two types of flexible flatfoot?
Surgery is rarely, if ever, indicated for the flexible flatfoot.

Surgery is indicated for a flexible flatfoot with a short Achilles tendon when prolonged attempts at nonoperative treatment have failed to relieve the pain and callosities under the head of the plantar-flexed talus. Surgery may be as simple as an Achilles tendon lengthening if the flatfoot deformity is very mild. With more severe deformity, Achilles tendon lengthening should be accompanied by one or more osteotomies that preserve joint motion while correcting deformity. Arthrodesis, even of the small joints of the foot, should be avoided in the child. The technique of placing Silastic plugs in the subtalar joint has been popular among podiatrists but has not been embraced by most pediatric orthopaedic surgeons because of the risks of infection and foreign body reaction.

17. What are the treatment principles for the rigid flatfoot?
A tarsal coalition may become painful as it changes from a cartilaginous to a bony union. This generally occurs between 8–12 years of age for calcaneonavicular coalitions and between 12–16 years of age for talocalcaneal coalitions. Only symptomatic coalitions should be treated, because approximately 75% of coalitions do not cause pain or disability. A radiographically confirmed, painful tarsal coalition is treated with a below-the-knee walking cast for 4–6 weeks. The pain should be relieved immediately, thereby confirming that the coalition is the cause of the pain and not just an incidental finding. An over-the-counter or molded arch support is recommended following removal of the cast. There is a 30–68% chance that the child will remain free of pain after

removal of the cast and return to regular activities. Surgery is indicated if symptoms recur. Resection of the coalition with interposition of fat, muscle, or tendon is the procedure of choice in most cases. The long-term results of this procedure for calcaneonavicular coalition are very good. The long-term results for talocalcaneal coalitions have not been reported but are probably less favorable.

Osteotomy may be used for the correction of severe deformity. Triple arthrodesis should be considered for the foot with established and documented severe painful degenerative osteoarthrosis of the subtalar joint complex. It should, therefore, rarely be used in children.

BIBLIOGRAPHY

1. Gould N, Moreland M, Alvarez R, Trevino S, Fenwick J: Development of the child's arch. Foot Ankle 9:241–245, 1989.
2. Harris RI, Beath T: Army Foot Survey, An investigation of foot ailments in Canadian soldiers, Vol. 1. Ottawa, National Research Council of Canada, 1947.
3. Harris RI, Beath T: Etiology of peroneal spastic flatfoot. J Bone Joint Surg 30B:624–634, 1948.
4. Harris RI, Beath T: Hypermobile flat-foot with short tendo Achilles. J Bone Joint Surg 30A:116–138, 1948.
5. Leonard MA: The inheritance of tarsal coalition and its relationship to spastic flat foot. J Bone Joint Surg 56B:520–526, 1974.
6. Mosca VS: Flexible flatfoot and skewfoot. An instructional course lecture of the American Academy of Orthopaedic Surgeons. J Bone Joint Surg 77A:1937–1945, 1995.
7. Mosca VS: Flexible flatfoot and tarsal coalition. In Richards BS (ed): Orthopaedic Knowledge Update: Pediatrics. Rosemont, IL, American Academy of Orthopaedic Surgeons, pp 211–218, 1996.
8. Staheli LT, Chew DE, Corbett M: The longitudinal arch. A survey of eight-hundred and eighty-two feet in normal children and adults. J Bone Joint Surg 69A:426–428, 1987.
9. Vanderwilde R, Staheli LT, Chew DE, Malagon V: Measurements on radiographs of the foot in normal infants and children. J Bone Joint Surg 70A:407–415, 1988.
10. Wenger DR, Mauldin D, Speck G, Morgan D, Lieber RL: Corrective shoes and inserts as treatment for flexible flatfoot in infants and children. J Bone Joint Surg 71A:800–810, 1989.
11. Wray JB, Herndon CN: Hereditary transmission of congenital coalition of the calcaneus to the navicular. J Bone Joint Surg 45A:365–372, 1963.

56. CAVUS FOOT

Vincent S. Mosca, M.D.

1. What is a cavus foot?

Cavus refers to a fixed equinus (plantar flexion) deformity of the forefoot in relation to the hindfoot, resulting in an abnormally high arch. The high arch may be along the medial border of the foot or across the entire midfoot. The heel may be in neutral, varus, valgus, calcaneus (dorsiflexed), or equinus position. There may be an accompanying clawing of the toes.

2. What causes cavus deformity?

Cavus is a manifestation of a neuromuscular disease with muscle imbalance, unless proven otherwise. Various patterns of muscle imbalance due to weakness or spasticity cause the various types or patterns of cavus deformity.

3. What are some specific diagnostic causes of bilateral cavus foot deformity?

Charcot-Marie-Tooth (CMT) disease
Dejerine-Sottas interstitial hypertrophic neuritis
Polyneuritis

Friedreich's ataxia
Roussy-Lévy syndrome
Spinal muscular atrophy
Myelomeningocele
Syringomyelia
Spinal cord tumor
Diastematomyelia
Spinal dysraphism—tethered cord
Muscular dystrophy
Cerebral palsy—diplegia or tetraplegia (although usually planus deformities)
Familial (consider CMT)
Idiopathic (diagnosis of exclusion; very rare)

4. What are some specific diagnostic causes of unilateral cavus foot deformity?
Traumatic injury of a peripheral nerve or spinal nerve root, poliomyelitis, syringomyelia, lipomeningocele, spinal cord tumor, diastematomyelia, spinal dysraphism—tethered cord, tendon laceration, overlengthened Achilles tendon, cerebral palsy—hemiplegia, old treated or untreated clubfoot, compartment syndrome of the leg, severe burn of the leg, crush injury of the leg.

5. What are typical presenting complaints?
Patients typically complain of difficulty with shoe fitting, with pressure and pain over the dorsum of the midfoot; pain and callosities under the metatarsal heads and lateral to the base of the fifth metatarsal; clawing of the toes with pain and callosities over the interphalangeal joints; inversion instability with frequent falling; and a feeling that ankles are "giving out." There is often a history of repeated ankle sprains.

6. Why should you take a family history?
Charcot-Marie-Tooth disease is an autosomal dominant disorder and is a common cause of cavus foot deformity. You should also examine the feet of parents and other family members if possible.

7. What are you looking for on examination?
First, examine the foot with the child standing. Note the varus, neutral, or valgus alignment of the heel. Severe cavus may give the impression of ankle equinus when in fact the equinus is entirely in the forefoot. Therefore, with the child seated, obscure the forefoot from view with your hand and assess dorsiflexion and plantar flexion of the ankle. Then attempt to dorsiflex the forefoot onto the hindfoot and note, by palpation, the tightness of the plantar fascia. Flexibility of the subtalar joint can be assessed by manually inverting and everting the hindfoot with the ankle in neutral alignment. The Coleman block test can also be used to assess flexibility of the subtalar joint; it has the advantage of permitting the assessment with the foot in a weightbearing position. Rigid plantar flexion of the first metatarsal and pronation of the forefoot precede rigid inversion deformity of the subtalar joint of the hindfoot. The block test is performed by placing a block under the lateral border of the foot. By thus allowing the forefoot to pronate, a flexible subtalar joint will correct to neutral position and a rigid one will not. This information gives an indication of chronicity and is important for operative planning. Carefully note the areas of excessive callusing on the plantar aspect of the foot. Also note calluses on the dorsum of the interphalangeal joints of the toes. Perform a careful motor, sensory, and reflex examination of the foot and leg. Include tests for position and vibratory sensation.

Examine the spine. Look for scoliosis, kyphoscoliosis, lateral translation of the shoulders with an oblique take-off of the spine from the pelvis, diminished flexibility, and paraspinal muscle rigidity. Note any midline defects, abnormal hairy patches, or dimpling. Check the abdominal reflex. Inquire about urinary incontinence and anal sphincter control.

Examine the upper extremities for neurologic abnormalities (specifically wasting and weakness of the interosseous muscles of the hand, as seen in CMT).

8. What radiographs should be obtained?

Standing AP and lateral radiographs of the spine are more important in the initial evaluation of the child with a cavus foot than are radiographs of the foot. Look for widening of the inter-pedicular distance, congenital malformations, atypical-pattern scoliosis (left thoracic), pelvic obliquity with lateral translation of the shoulders over the pelvis, and an opaque central bone spike (as may be seen with diastematomyelia).

Foot radiographs should include *standing* AP and lateral views. As a simple rule of thumb, a straight line normally passes through the axes of the talus and the first metatarsal on the AP and lateral images. Varus angulation of the axis of the first metatarsal in relation to the axis of the talus on the AP view and plantar angulation of the axis of the first metatarsal in relation to the axis of the talus on the lateral view are characteristic of a cavus deformity. More detailed and specialized radiographs may be obtained by the treating orthopaedic surgeon.

9. What other studies should be performed?

Unless there is a known cause of the cavus foot, such as poliomyelitis or myelomeningocele, an electromyogram and nerve condition velocity study are indicated. Creatinine phosphokinase and aldolase blood levels may be calculated. One may choose to obtain a consultation with a pediatric neurologist at this point. Magnetic resonance imaging of the spine and brain may also be appropriate in certain circumstances.

10. How is the cavus foot deformity treated?

Once the deformity has been identified, the underlying cause needs to be ascertained. If the underlying cause is untreatable, such as Charcot-Marie-Tooth disease, the child should be referred to an orthopaedic surgeon for foot surgery. If the underlying condition is treatable, such as a spinal cord tumor, treatment of that condition should precede treatment of the foot deformity.

11. What is the role of nonoperative management of the cavus foot?

There is little role for nonoperative management of the cavus foot deformity because most are progressive and of advanced severity at the time of diagnosis. The worse the deformity, the more complex is the operative reconstruction. Arch supports and shoe modifications may be used in the earliest stages of a developing cavus foot deformity, but this decision should be made by the orthopaedic surgeon, who will know when to proceed with surgery.

12. What are some relative indications for operative intervention?

Painful calluses under the metatarsal heads and over the claw toes, difficulty with fitting shoes, abnormal and excessive shoe wear, and painful ankle instability are some indications that surgery should be performed.

13. What are the principles of operative management?

There are two principles: The first is to correct the deformity, and the second is to balance muscle forces so as to maintain deformity correction and prevent recurrences. These two components of the operative management are carried out concurrently, in either one or two closely timed operative sessions.

Correction of the deformity involves release of soft tissue contractures and realignment osteotomies. The contracted plantar fascia is always released. The abductor hallucis is released from the calcaneus in a foot with mild adductus deformity. Capsulotomy of the talonavicular joint with release of the spring ligament and the long and short plantar ligaments is carried out if the subtalar joint does not evert to neutral position. The joints should be aligned following these soft tissue releases. The foot is then evaluated for residual bony deformity, which is corrected using one or more osteotomies. These may be placed in the medial cuneiform, the base of the first metatarsal, the cuboid, or the calcaneus. The techniques for correction of deformity are based on the shape and the rigidity or flexibility of the foot, not on the muscle imbalance.

The choices for tendon transfers relate directly to the specific pattern of muscle imbalance in the child's foot. Consideration must be given to the present and expected future pattern of muscle weakness.

14. What about arthrodesis?

The final principle is that arthrodesis should be reserved as a salvage procedure for severe degenerative osteoarthrosis and should not be used as a primary reconstructive technique. Arthrodesis causes stress shifting and premature degenerative osteoarthrosis in adjacent unfused joints.

BIBLIOGRAPHY

1. Tachdjian MO: Pes cavus. In Clinical Pediatric Orthopedics: The Art of Diagnosis and Principles of Management. Stamford, CT, Appleton and Lange, 1997, pp 48–55.
2. Thometz JG, Gould JS: Cavus deformity. In Drennan JC (ed): The Child's Foot and Ankle. New York, Raven Press, 1992, pp 343–354.

57. TOE WALKING

Jose Fernando De la Garza, M.D.

1. Is there another name for idiopathic toe walking?

This entity was first described by Hall, Salter, and Bhalla in 1967 by the name congenital short tendon calcaneus, also known as habitual toe walking or tiptoe walking.

2. Before what age in normal gait development is toe walking considered a normal condition?

Toddlers may walk with the foot in equinus when beginning independent walking. At the age of 2, children develop walking patterns similar to adults, and by the age of 3 a mature gait pattern is established. This means that the heel-strike gait should occur by age 3.

3. What is the main reason for consultation?

Persistent bilateral toe walking after age 3 in a developmentally normal child who can usually stand flat-footed when not walking.

4. How often does this condition have a positive family history?

Kallen's series found that 71% of the patients had a positive family history.

5. What are common causes of an equinus gait?

CATEGORY	DIAGNOSIS
Congenital	Clubfoot
Idiopathic	Gastrocnemius contracture
	Accessory soleus muscle
	Generalized triceps contracture
Neurologic	Cerebral palsy
	Poliomyelitis
Myogenic	Muscular dystrophy
Functional	Hysterical toe walking

6. What are the main conditions in the differential diagnosis?

Cerebral palsy, particularly in a mildly diplegic child

Spinal cord tumor

Spinal dysraphism

Muscular dystrophy	Diastematomyelia
Tethered cord syndrome	Acute myopathies
	Idiopathic toe walking (diagnosis of exclusion)

7. What are the differences between cerebral palsy and toe walking?

	CEREBRAL PALSY	IDIOPATHIC TOE WALKING
Spasticity	Usually present at ankle, knee, or hips	Negative
Gait	Permanent equinus	Occasional equinus
Standing	Equinus	Foot flat standing
Neonatal history	Can be positive or preterm delivery or neonatal asphyxia	Negative

8. What are the most important aspects of the history?
Prenatal history
Perinatal data, including gestational age at birth and Apgar scores
Presence of delayed neuromotor skills
Family history

9. If by definition idiopathic toe walkers do not have a central problem, where is the problem?
In the Achilles tendon, which is short due to shortening of the soleus or gastrocnemius muscles.

10. Are there any other diagnostic modalities that help in the differential diagnosis between idiopathic toe walking and mild cerebral palsy?
Dynamic electromyography (EMG)
Computerized gait analysis

11. What are the main findings in the dynamic EMG and the computerized gait analysis?
The data demonstrate lack of heel strike in association with knee flexion at the end of the swing phase in patients with cerebral palsy.

12. How many degrees of ankle dorsiflexion are needed for a normal gait (heel-toe walking)?
10° or more.

13. What are the treatment strategies for toe walking?
1. Strengthening exercises
2. Serial stretching casts every 2 weeks for 6–10 weeks
3. Night braces after the stretching cast to maintain the dorsiflexion
4. Ankle-foot orthotics
5. Heelcord lengthening

14. What is the best way to maintain the dorsiflexion after the stretching exercises or the stretching cast?
Place the foot in an ankle-foot orthosis (AFO) in an attempt to break the toe-walking pattern.

15. When is surgery indicated for idiopathic toe walking?
Surgery is reserved for patients in whom physical therapy (stretching exercises), casts, and orthotics have not been successful. Achilles tendon lengthening is the usual procedure performed to obtain the necessary dorsiflexion for the heel-toe gait pattern.

16. What is the main complication of surgical treatment?
Overlengthening of the Achilles tendon producing a calcaneus gait, which is worse than the equinus gait.

CONTROVERSY

17. Is idiopathic toe walking a diagnosis of exclusion or is it really an unknown central nervous system deficit?

EMG studies were conducted in which children with idiopathic toe walking behaved similarly to patients with cerebral palsy and equinus deformities and differently from the toe-walking control group. Other reports exist in which muscle biopsy specimens in operated patients showed features suggesting a neuropathic process, including predominance of type I muscle fibers and atrophic angulated fibers, thus suggesting a possible neurogenic basis for the condition.

BIBLIOGRAPHY

1. Eastwood DM, Broughton NS, Dickens DRV, Menelaus MB. Idiopathic toe-walking: does treatment alter the natural history? J Bone Joint Surg 78B(suppl I):77, 1996.
2. Griffin PP, Wheelhouse WW, Shiavi R, Bass W: Habitual toe walkers: a clinical and electromyographic gait analysis. J Bone Joint Surg 59A:97–101, 1977.
3. Hall JE, Salter RB, Bhalla SK: Congenital short tendo calcaneus. J Bone Joint Surg 49B:695–697, 1967.
4. Kalen V, Adler N, Bleck E: Electromyography of idiopathic toe walking. J Pediatr Orthop 6:31–33, 1986.
5. Morrissy R, Weinstein S: Lovell and Winter's Pediatric Orthopaedics, Vol. 2, Philadelphia, J. B. Lippincott, 1996.
6. Staheli L: Fundamentals of Pediatric Orthopedics. New York, Raven Press, 1992.
7. Wanger D, Rang M: The Art and Practice of Children's Orthopaedics. 1993.

58. KNEE PAIN

Carl L. Stanitski, M.D.

1. What is the most common type of knee pain?

Adolescent, nonspecific, anterior knee pain is most common. It is often erroneously referred to as "chondromalacia."

2. Why is the term "chondromalacia" a misnomer for this condition?

The articular surfaces of the patella, femur, and tibia are pristine, and the source of pain is not the chondral zone. The condition should be considered idiopathic, and diagnostic efforts should be made to establish a specific diagnosis.

"Chondromalacia" should be eliminated as a diagnostic term for this nonspecific complaint.

3. What is the most common mistake made in the diagnosis of chronic knee pain?

Failure to evaluate the hip as a source of pain. Referred pain from the hip can masquerade as knee pain in such conditions as Perthes' disease and chronic slipped capital femoral epiphysis.

4. What is the most helpful technique to evaluate knee pain?

Clinical evaluation by history and physical exam including assessment of the hip and contralateral knee.

5. What should routine radiographic views of the knee include?

When possible, weightbearing AP, lateral, skyline (patellar profile) and tunnel (notch) views. Comparison views of the opposite knee are not routinely done.

6. When should comparison views of the opposite normal knee be taken?

To assess physeal status following an acute injury or for follow-up of a previous physeal injury. They are also used to compare congenital anomaly status (e.g., bipartite patella, discoid meniscus).

7. When should a bone scan be ordered to help assess knee pain?
Bone scintigraphy is helpful when a stress fracture is suspected. The study is also used in cases of reflex sympathetic dystrophy but in this condition, bone scan results are highly dependent on the stage of the disorder. Quantitative bone scans may be helpful to predict healing potential in cases of osteochondritis dissecans.

8. When should an MRI be ordered?
MRI is a powerful tool in knee disorder diagnosis. Unfortunately, it is commonly misused. The test should be done only after a thorough clinical examination and standard radiograph review are unable to provide a specific diagnosis. The MRI examination should be ordered by the individual with the expertise to correlate the pertinent clinical findings with the imaging study and who can provide the appropriate specific treatment for the specific diagnosis. Knee MRI should not be looked upon as a screening examination. Continued progress is being made with MRI technology, but false-positive and false-negative readings do occur, and clinical correlation, as with results of all studies, is mandatory.

9. What are pertinent points to be evaluated during history-taking?
Pain characteristics: onset, duration, change with activity or rest, night pain; effect of previous treatments; swelling; giving way; locking; trauma; and growth velocity.

10. Physical examination should include what assessments?
The patient must be appropriately garbed (preferably in shorts) for an accurate exam to be done. Exam should include analysis of gait, lower extremity weight-bearing alignment, muscle definition, leg lengths (by block test), generalized laxity, range of motion (active/passive), swelling (extra-intra-articular), focal tenderness (physes, patella, joint lines, tibial tubercle, collateral ligaments), patella tracking, and stability (anteroposterior, rotatory, and mediolateral).

11. What repetitive stress (overuse) problems can manifest as knee pain?

Osgood-Schlatter disease	Sindig-Larsen-Johansson's disease
Stress fractures	Jumper's knee (patellar Tendinitis)
Minor patellar maltracking	Pathologic plica

12. What intra-articular conditions should be considered in the differential diagnosis?

Osteochondritis dissecans	Discoid meniscu
Pathologic plica	Meniscal tears
Meniscal cyst	Cruciate ligament injury

13. What inflammatory causes should be considered in the assessment?

Juvenile rheumatoid arthritis	Hemophilia
Pigmented villonodular synovitis	Septic arthritis
Osteomyelitis	

14. Are tumors a likely source of knee pain?
Benign and malignant tumors are uncommon causes of knee pain. Benign lesions include osteochondroma, nonossifying fibroma with stress fracture, osteoid osteoma, and chondroblastoma. Malignant tumors, though rare, can cause knee symptoms, especially in adolescence. These include osteosarcoma and Ewing's sarcoma. In very young children, metastases from a neuroblastoma can also cause pain.

15. What are common presenting complaints in patients with Osgood-Schlatter disease?
The condition usually is seen in active young adolescent males undergoing a period of rapid growth. Activity-related pain is present at the tibial tubercle with complaints of "good days and bad days." Pain is particularly aggravated with kneeling, squatting, or jumping. Parents are often concerned about a tumor because of the tubercle's prominence.

16. Are radiographs needed in patients with suspected Osgood-Schlatter disease?

Even though the diagnosis usually appears straightforward, radiographs confirm the diagnosis (tubercle enlargement, fragmentation) and may show uncommon, unsuspected additional sources of pain, such as tumors or infections.

17. What treatment is recommended for Osgood-Schlatter disease?

Patient and parental reassurance about the benign nature of the condition is paramount. They also should be counseled about the cyclic nature of the symptoms and the 12–18 months required for resolution (i.e., the approach of skeletal maturity). Symptomatic treatment with ice massage, knee pad, anti-inflammatory medication, hamstring and quadriceps flexibility exercises, and activity modification (not elimination) leads to satisfactory resolution in most cases. Steroid injections into the tubercle are to be condemned. If a separate ossicle persists, surgical excision may be required.

18. What is the difference between Sindig-Larsen-Johansson's disease and "jumper's knee"?

The former is a sequela of traction on the immature distal patellar pole by the patellar tendon. It is analogous to Osgood-Schlatter disease and is seen in the pre-teen age group. The treatment is similar. The latter, seen in adolescents, is an inflammation of the proximal patellar tendon brought about by repetitive stress from jumping. The condition may progress to produce intratendinous degeneration and necrosis.

19. What other evaluations should be considered in a patient with suspected juvenile rheumatoid arthritis?

In addition to evaluation of laboratory parameters (sedimentation rate, rheumatoid factor, etc.) and synovial fluid analysis, slit lamp examination should be included in the assessment of these patients, because children with pauciarticular or monoarticular arthritis are at increased risk of developing iridocyclitis.

20. What is the cause of a "snapping knee" in a 6 to 10 year-old?

A discoid meniscus commonly presents with complaints of snapping at the knee. The condition may be asymptomatic (other than the auditory nuisance). Pain and mechanical symptoms result if a tear is present in the abnormally shaped meniscus or if the meniscus is unstable because of congenital absence of the menisco tibial ligament.

21. What is the treatment of a symptomatic discoid meniscus?

Treatment is dependent on the meniscal morphology and stability. If the meniscus is stable and without a tear, reconfiguration of the meniscus by means of surgical debulking, usually by arthroscopic techniques, results in a more normal meniscus shape and size. If a tear is present, either repair or excision (arthroscopically) is done. If the meniscus is unstable, surgical stabilization is done. All efforts are directed at preserving as normal a meniscus as possible so that its weightbearing function may continue and prevent premature onset of degenerative joint disease.

22. How does one know that one is dealing with a bipartite patella and not a fracture?

Bipartite patellae are common incidental radiographic findings and should not be confused with an acute injury. Radiographic characteristics of a bipartite patella (as opposed to an acute fracture) include regular, smooth fragment margins; no evidence of soft tissue swelling; and enlarged total size of the patella (main plus accessory fragment). Clinically, there is no pain or tenderness at the site. One caveat: An acute separation following trauma can occur at the junction of the fragment and the main patellar body. In this case, clinical signs of acute injury are present, and immobilization is undertaken. If there is no clinical evidence of injury, the condition is considered a radiologic curiosity with no intervention required other than informing the patient and family of the condition's presence to avoid future confusion.

23. What is the prognosis for osteochondritis dissecans?

The primary prognostic factors are patient age and skeletal maturity. The less mature, the better the prognosis, with best results seen in the juvenile form (i.e., before adolescence), where full recovery is the usual outcome. In the adolescent type (i.e., partial skeletal maturity), outcome is unpredictable. With the adult type (i.e., skeletally mature), a guarded prognosis is the rule.

24. What are common presenting symptoms in a patient with osteochondritis dissecans?

Mechanical-type pain (increased with activity, diminished with rest) and intermittent effusion are the most frequent complaints. Locking or catching due to fragment instability are uncommon findings.

25. What is a knee plica, and how does it cause symptoms?

The knee has normal synovial folds, which are residual embryonic remnants from when the knee cavity was a septated structure. As such, these folds (plicae) are common findings and are considered variants of normal anatomy. Occasionally, pathologic conditions occur within the plica when the synovium is inflamed owing to acute, direct, or repetitive microtrauma. The inflamed plica becomes enlarged and is trapped between the patella and the femoral condyle. This impingement sets up further inflammatory changes. The thickened plica may cause secondary abrasive injury to the underlying articular surfaces.

26. How can one diagnose a pathologic plica?

The diagnosis is made on clinical grounds. The patient complains of snapping and catching when the knee is in a specific position of flexion. The pain and snapping are reproduced by direct palpation over the plica when the knee is taken through a flexion arc, usually from 30° to 70°. Standard radiographs show normal findings.

27. What is the treatment for adolescent anterior knee pain?

If possible, a specific diagnosis is made, e.g., Osgood-Schlatter disease. If objective review does not provide a specific diagnosis, the patient and family should be reassured of the nonfatal nature of the condition. A multitude of nonspecific treatments (taping, braces, exercises, physical therapy modalities) have made claims of efficacy, but objective evidence is lacking.

28. How common is reflex sympathetic dystrophy in this age group?

This diagnosis is being made with increasing frequency as awareness of the condition in this age group is becoming more widespread. Unfortunately, it is still commonly missed with resultant delay in diagnosis and treatment. The diagnosis must be suspected in any patient whose complaints of pain and disability are out of proportion to the precipitating event or injury. Hypersensitivity to the slightest touch is a common finding. The skin vasomotor changes are of late onset, and their absence should not invalidate the diagnosis. Familial and school problems are common associated findings in this poorly understood condition.

29. What is the prognosis for reflex sympathetic dystrophy in children?

The prognosis is usually quite good in children as opposed to adults. Most childhood disease is seen in the lower extremity. Hallmarks of treatment include physical therapy focused on progressive function, anti-inflammatory medication, and counseling.

30. What is the role of surgery in treating adolescent anterior knee pain?

Surgery has a very limited role. Indications for surgery are based on specific objective findings. Pain alone is not an indication for surgery.

BIBLIOGRAPHY

1. Bourne MH, Bianco AJ Jr: Bipartite patella in the adolescent: results of surgical excision. J Pediatr Orthop 10:69–73, 1990.

2. Crawford EJ, Emery RJ, Aichroth PM: Stable osteochondritis dissecans: does the lesion unite? J Bone Joint Surg 72B:320, 1990.
3. Dietz FR, Mathews KD, Montgomery WJ: Reflex sympathetic dystrophy in children. Clin Orthop 258:225–231, 1990.
4. Johnson BL, Eastwood DM, Witherow PJ: Symptomatic synovial plicae of the knee. J Bone Joint Surg 75A:1485–1496, 1993.
5. Kelly MA, Flock TJ, Kimmel JA, et al.: MR imaging of the knee: clarification of its role. Arthroscopy 7:78–85, 1991.
6. Krause BL, Williams JP, Catterall A: Natural history of Osgood-Schlatter disease. J Pediatr Orthop 10:65–68, 1990.
7. Stanitski CL: Anterior knee pain syndromes in the adolescent. J Bone Joint Surg 75A:1407–1416, 1995.

59. PATELLOFEMORAL DISORDERS

Robert E. Eilert, M.D., and Mark A. Erickson, M.D.

1. In acute dislocation of the patella in a child, what is the appropriate treatment?

The outcome of nonoperative treatment in children and adolescents is similar to that obtained with acute surgery, and nonoperative treatment carries far less risk of possible complications such as hemarthrosis, nerve damage, and scarring.

Nonoperative treatment consists of a short period of joint rest followed by a vigorous rehabilitative effort. Using a knee immobilizer or splint during the period of joint rest for 1–2 weeks allows early movement of the joint and isometric exercises while the initial swelling and pain resolve. As soon as the patient begins to tolerate isometric exercise, this can be supplemented by weight resistance in a short arc mode as well as electrical stimulation to the vastus medialis obliquus, which was inhibited by the joint swelling and by the stretching associated with lateral dislocation of the patella.

A reasonable argument can be made for removal of osteochondral fragments, which may be detached either at the time of dislocation or during relocation of the patella. This can be done arthroscopically and does not require initial open surgery.

2. What is the most common physical finding associated with anterior knee pain in adolescents?

Hamstring contracture is frequently associated with an episode of rapid growth. Resolution of this contracture reliably resolves the symptoms of anterior knee pain. The course of stretching exercises necessary to lengthen the hamstring and increase the range of straight leg-raising takes about 6 weeks to complete. The exact mechanism by which stretching of the hamstring contracture relieves anterior knee pain is not proven but seems biomechanically related to decrease in the patellofemoral reaction force by means of reducing the relative knee flexion at heel strike. Hamstring contracture produces chopped strides clinically, especially noted when the patient runs.

3. By what mechanism does lateral release relieve knee pain?

Theoretically, lateral release improves anterior knee pain by altering the alignment of the patella. Another theory is that the release divides nerve fibers in the lateral retinaculum and capsule that are the source of the pain. The other theory is that it changes the pressure relationships under the patella, therefore altering the pain symptoms.

These theories must be correlated with the clinically apparent relief of symptoms following the operative procedure in selected patients. Operative candidates are patients showing decreased medial mobility (as evidenced by the inability to separate the lateral border of the patella from the lateral condyle of the femur) and in whom a vigorous program to strengthen the vastus medialis obliquus and stretch contractures around the knee does not resolve knee pain.

4. When do you perform a distal versus proximal reconstruction for a dislocating patella?

The most common reconstruction performed for recurrent dislocation of the patella is a proximal one, which involves lateral retinacular release and some type of medial tightening operation—whether it be plication of the medial capsule or a more sturdy medial vector reconstruction, such as use of the semimembranosus tendon routed through the patella (using the method of Putti and Dewar).

Distal reconstruction is reserved for those patients in whom the tibial apophysis has closed and there is an increased Q angle. The tibial apophysis is shifted medially while its anterior position is preserved in order to reduce the Q angle and valgus shift at the patella. The Goldthwait procedure, performed with partial medial routing of the patellar ligament, has been condemned as producing many complications in the skeletally immature.

5. Can you clinically diagnose a plica syndrome as a cause of anterior knee pain?

A plica is a normal structure that represents a fold in the synovium of the knee. If the plica is thickened because of fibrosis due to injury or inflammation, it may become more rigid and cause abrasion of the underlying medial femoral condyle or the patella. The plica is recognizable clinically as a tender band across the medial condyle that moves with flexion and extension of the knee, coming in contact with the medial femoral condyle during the flexion arc between 30° and 60°. This tender band can be rolled beneath the finger and is well localized as the site of pain in the affected patient. Improvement may occur with decrease in the inflammation as a result of rest and anti-inflammatory drugs. The diagnosis may be confirmed by arthroscopy, at which time the plica should be seen as a thick band. The area of rubbing and abrasion should be apparent either on the medial femoral condyle (which is the most common location) or on the undersurface of the medial facet of the patella.

6. What common conditions produce referred pain to the knee in children?

One should always be suspicious of more proximal lesions that can refer pain to the knee. The obturator nerve, which innervates both the hip and the knee joint, can cause confusing pain patterns, which are commonly perceived on the medial side of the knee. Perthes' disease in the younger child or slipped capital femoral epiphysis in the adolescent may present as knee pain. Other diseases such as osteoid osteoma, which often occurs in the region of the lesser trochanter, likewise can be referred distally, so any child with knee pain should have a careful hip examination. Because of suspicion of a proximal lesion, x-rays should include the entire femur in any case in which symptoms are not resolving with knee treatment. The cardinal sign of an abnormal hip exam may be decreased internal rotation as detected by the log roll test, which is performed by rolling the lower extremity medially and laterally with the hip in extension.

7. Can a meniscal tear masquerade as patellofemoral pain in adolescents?

A tear of the anterior horn of the meniscus can imitate patellofemoral pain, since the pain symptoms are located anteriorly and may have mechanical symptoms similar to those generated during ascending or descending stairs. Therefore, if arthroscopy is performed for delineation of patellofemoral pain, the anterior compartment of the joint should be carefully examined to rule out tear of the anterior horn of the meniscus as well as possible pinching of a hypertrophic fat pad or Hoffa's disease. Fibrotic nodules in the anterior portion of the joint are another mime that may mimic patellofemoral pain and that can be detected by viewing the anterior compartment from a superior portal.

8. When should you place a patient with Osgood-Schlatter disease in a cast?

Rarely should you use a cast for a child with Osgood-Schlatter disease, which is a developmental variation based on a stress reaction in the area of the tibial tubercle due to a relative overuse syndrome. In these individuals, the strength of the tibial tubercle can be exceeded by the activity of the individual's quadriceps, such as in vigorous sports activities, running, or jumping. The primary form of treatment is alteration of activities. In the most extreme cases, a splint may be necessary, but it can be removed for active use of the joint and muscles to prevent atrophy and stiffness. The splint may be worn at night with good relief of symptoms in the daytime. Use of a cast results in disuse and stiffness and tends to compound the situation more than it helps.

9. Is arthroscopy ever indicated to evaluate chondromalacia patellae?

The term "chondromalacia patellae" should probably be replaced in the literature by "patellofemoral pain" or even by the more general term "anterior knee pain," since the findings of softening of the patellar cartilage and pain do not correlate well. There are patients in whom arthroscopy demonstrates a softening of the articular cartilage under the patella, which may be an incidental finding when arthroscopy is performed for another reason. In contradistinction, patients with patellofemoral pain may have normal-appearing articular cartilage without softening. The mechanism of pain production is debatable but does not appear to be related to the anatomic abnormality of softened articular cartilage. In the past, the pathologic term had been applied to all anterior knee pain, but this led one away from a specific diagnosis. In each case, a specific diagnosis should be sought even if the therapy (such as stretching and strengthening) is nonspecific.

10. What is the difference between Osgood-Schlatter disease and the Sinding-Larsen-Johansson lesion?

The lesion described by Osgood and Schlatter is pain in the area of the tibial tubercle caused by microfractures in the area of the apophysis that are associated with activity-related stress on this region. A similar condition occurs at the other end of the patellar ligament, which is the lower pole of the patella. Traction in this area may also be associated with pain and fragmentation of small bones. Both conditions are time limited and associated with rapid growth and immature bone maturation in the middle teenage years. What separates Osgood-Schlatter disease from Sinding-Larsen-Johansson lesion is the patellar ligament, the two conditions occur at opposite ends of the ligament.

11. Can vastus medialis obliquus deficiency be corrected with exercise?

Vastus medialis obliquus (VMO) deficiency can be congenital or associated with injury or inflammation about the knee. In the case of injury or inflammation, the VMO deficiency may be corrected with rest, anti-inflammatories, and an exercise program to include electrical stimulation. Even for congenital cases, a conscientiously followed exercise program may strengthen whatever muscle is present and may help to rebalance the patella. There is some evidence that patellar subluxation occurs when there is an asymmetric firing of the VMOP and the vastus lateralis. This tendency for firing out of sequence, that is, the vastus lateralis firing before the VMO in terminal extension, can be corrected by exercise training with or without biofeedback.

12. Are x-rays necessary in the evaluation of patellofemoral pain syndromes?

Plain x-rays can be valuable to rule out less common causes such as tumor, osteochondritis dissecans, or unsuspected fracture. X-rays have been promoted for evaluation of patellar tilt and stability. The difficulty is in the use of static x-rays to attempt to measure dynamic function. Many of the causes of anterior knee pain operate in the last few degrees of extension between $0°$ and $30°$ which is impossible to visualize on plain x-ray films. Serial CT scans or MRI may be necessary to evaluate the patellofemoral relationship in small degrees of flexion between $0°$ and $30°$.

13. What characterizes congenital dislocation of the patella?

In the first type of congenital dislocation, the patella is fixed and permanently dislocated laterally. These children present with a flexion contracture and delay in walking. The definitive diagnosis may require an MRI because the patella is unossified and difficult to palpate.

In the second type, there is an obligatory dislocation of the patella as it shifts laterally from an underdeveloped trochlea with each flexion and extension cycle of the knee. More commonly, the patella is tethered laterally as the knee flexes and reduces in full extension, but the reverse may also be true. These children usually present at a later age because this condition does not usually delay walking. They have the striking physical finding of a "popping" patella that shifts laterally each time they flex and extend their knee.

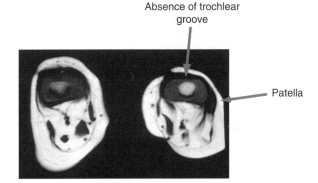

Absence of trochlear groove

Patella

MRI demonstrating persistent (fixed) congenital lateral dislocation of the patella in a 1-year-old child.

14. What is an apprehension test?
To perform the apprehension test, the examiner attempts manually to subluxate the patella laterally. The test is performed with the knee relaxed in an extended position. In a positive test, the patient suddenly becomes "apprehensive" and resists any further lateral motion of the patella. The apprehension test is commonly positive in patients with recurrent patellar instability.

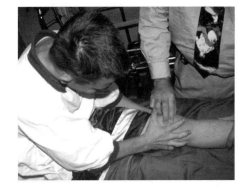

Positive apprehension test.

15. What is a Q angle?
The Q angle is a clinical measurement. A line from the anterior superior iliac spine to the center of the patella is created. A second line is drawn from the center of the patella to the center of the tibial tubercle. The angle formed at the intersection of these two lines is the Q angle. Normal Q angles range from 10° to 20°. An increased Q angle creates a lateral force on the patella as the knee is extended and is a predisposing factor for patellar instability.

16. What anatomic variations can predispose a patient to patellofemoral instability?
Increased Q angle	Genu valgum
Deficient vastus medialis obliquus	Increased femoral anteversion
Tight lateral retinaculum	External tibial torsion
Hypoplastic lateral femoral condyle	Patella alta

17. What is the significance of a bipartite patella?
A bipartite patella is usually an asymptomatic, incidental radiographic finding that may be misdiagnosed as an acute fracture. The reported incidence ranges from 1–5%. The most common location is the superolateral patella.

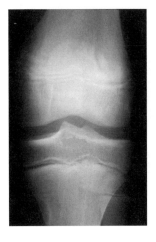

Note the smooth edges and contour of this bipartite patella, which distinguish it from an acute fracture.

BIBLIOGRAPHY

1. Fulkerson JP: Diseases of the Patellofemoral Joint, 2nd ed. Baltimore, Williams & Wilkins, 1980.
2. Fulkerson JP, Shea KP: Mechanical basis for patellofemoral pain and cartilage break down. In Ewing JW (ed): Articular Cartilage and Knee Joint Function: Basic Science and Arthroscopy. New York, Raven Press, 1990, pp 93–101.
3. Hoffa A: The influence of the adipose tissue with regard to the pathology of the knee joint. JAMA 43:795, 1904.
4. Jacobson KE, Flandry FC: Diagnosis of anterior knee pain. Clin Sports Med 8:179, 1989.
5. Kolowich PA, Paulos LE, Rosenberg TD, et al.: Lateral release of the patella: indications and contraindications. Am J Sports Med 18:359, 1990.
6. Leveau BF, Rogers C: Selective training of the vastus medialis muscle using EMG biofeedback. Phys Ther 60:1410, 1980.
7. Lindberg U, Lysholm J, Gillquist J: The correlation between arthroscopic findings and the patellofemoral pain syndrome. Arthroscopy 2:103, 1986.
8. McManus F, Rang M, Hesling DJ: Acute dislocation of the patella in children: the natural history. Clin Orthop 139:88, 1979.
9. Merchant AC: Classification of patellofemoral disorders. Arthroscopy 4:235, 1988.
10. Morshuis WJ, Pavlov PW, DeRooy KP: Anteromedialization of the tibial tuberosity in the treatment of patellofemoral pain and malalignment. Clin Orthop 255:242, 1990.

60. CONGENITAL HYPEREXTENSION OF THE KNEE

N.M.P. Clarke, Ch.M., FRCS, and Klaus Parsch, M.D.

1. Are there other terms that describe this problem?
Synonyms include *congenital genu recurvatum, congenital dislocation of the knee (CDK), and hyperextended knee.*

2. What is a hyperextension deformity?

In normal babies up to the age of 3 months, there is a knee flexion contracture of about 20°–30° (i.e, the knees do not straighten fully). In breech babies, the knees may hyperextend 20° beyond the straight position (genu recurvatum). In such circumstances, the anterior articular surfaces of the tibia have continuous contact with the articular surface of the distal femur, distinguishing the physiologic deformity from congenital subluxation and dislocation of the knee.

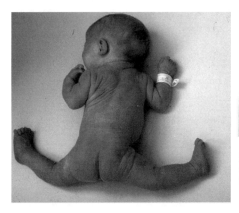
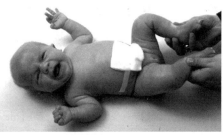

(Left) Bilateral hyperextension of the knees at 10 days of age. (Right) Same infant at 5 weeks of age following conservative treatment.

3. How often does one see hypextended knees at birth?

About 2 in 100,000 children are born with a hyperextended knee. Only half true subluxation or frank dislocation, while the majority show simple hyperextension without anterior tibial displacement. We see not more than one child with congenital genu recurvatum for every hundred with developmental dysplasia of the hip.

4. What are the clinical types?

Physiologic genu recurvatum is common in molded babies. Pathologic hyperextension deformities embrace a spectrum of anatomic displacements from subluxation to dislocation. In congenital subluxation, there is some contact maintained between distal femoral and proximal tibial articular surfaces. Conventionally, the severity of deformity is graded from I to III.

Grade I is most common (50%). The joint can be passively flexed to 45°–90°.

Grade II is less common (30%). The tibia is displaced anteriorly on the femur, although there is still some retained anticular contact. Clinically, there is perhaps 45° of hyperextension, and the knee will flex only to the neutral position.

Grade III is least common (20%), with total displacement of the proximal tibia and no contact between the articular surfaces. The knee is in severe hyperextension with the toes often in contact with the face. There is often wrinkling of the skin over the patella, and there may be associated angular deformity of the knee.

5. What are the causes?

Intrauterine breech malposition is a common cause of genu recurvatum. It has been proposed that absence of the cruciate ligaments permits knee dislocation. Fibrosis of the quadriceps mechanism has also been incriminated. It is, however, difficult to differentiate primary causative factors from secondary adaptive changes.

6. What is the pathology?

In pathologic as opposed to physiologic displacement, the upper end of the tibia is anterior to the distal end of the femur. There may be associated lateral subluxation or angular deformity of the knee, and contraction of the lateral soft tissue structures may be encountered. As a consequence of the bony displacement, the hamstrings may be displaced anteriorly and may effectively function as extensors of the knee joint. The patellar tendon and quadriceps are usually contracted. Often, the patella is hypoplastic. The cruciate ligaments are elongated but always present. No associated neurovascular abnormalities have been reported.

7. What imaging methods are used?
Plain radiographs do not reveal very well the amount of subluxation present at birth because the femoral and tibial physes are not yet ossified. Arthrography has some value and was used in the past to identify the underlying disorder. Ultrasound is very useful in identifying the position of the tibia against the femur and is also an efficient method of monitoring the reduction achieved during conservative treatment. MRI has similar value but is more expensive and less available.

8. What is the natural history?
It is usual for simple genu recurvatum deformities to resolve spontaneously (in 50%). Active treatment is necessary for subluxation and dislocation. In the most severe cases, surgical correction of the contracture of the quadriceps mechanism and relocation of the joint should allow the patient to walk normally and retain reasonable knee function.

9. What are the associated problems?
Other congenital malformations. Hyperextension may be a component, for instance, of Larsen's syndrome, which is characterized by multiple joint dislocations. The most frequent association (45%) is with developmental dysplasia of the hip, perhaps as a consequence of the generalized molding deformity. Congenital foot deformities and congenital dislocation of the elbow are also recognized as associations, as are cleft palate and imperforate anus. Hyperextended knees are frequently seen in arthrogryposis. Finally, joint dislocations in general can be related to syndromes incorporating generalized joint laxity, such as Down or Ehlers-Danlos syndromes.

10. What is the management in the newborn?
It is not necessary to begin active treatment for simple congenital hyperextension deformities, since they will resolve spontaneously. Gentle active physiotherapy may hasten resolution of the deformity. In congenital subluxation and dislocation, treatment is commenced as soon as possible. Reduction may be achieved by manipulation of the joint into flexion, held by plaster casts. Serial changing of the cast allows a gradual increase in the range of flexion. Joint stability is achieved by 6–8 weeks, after which the position is held by means of a Pavlik harness. The splint is primarily used for treatment of developmental dysplasia of the hip but does allow dynamic movement at the knee while maintaining flexion. It may be necessary to maintain harness treatment for 2–3 months. If reduction cannot be achieved by conservative means or satisfactory flexion obtained, operative treatment is necessary. Open surgical reduction of the knee displacement is required.

11. Are there alternative conservative methods of treatment?
Traction in the prone position used on an inpatient has proven to be successful.

12. What should be done with knees that cannot be reduced by conservative treatment?
Knees that are irreducible after a course of conservative treatment require surgical reduction. Lengthening of the quadriceps tendon is performed in combination with a medial and lateral release of the patellar retinaculum. In cases with additional lateral dislocation of the patellar insertion, the patellar tendon is lengthened as well. The elongated cruciate ligaments are placed in their anatomic position. After reduction, the leg is held in a plaster cast for a period of 6 weeks. It may not be possible to hold the leg in 90° of flexion owing to pressure on the skin anteriorly. If this is the case, the best possible position is obtained and the patient is brought back at 1 to 2 weeks for further manipulation, until 90° of flexion is obtained.

13. What happens to the cruciate ligaments in congenital dislocation of the knee? Do these knees become stable?
We have never seen a child with CDK without cruciate ligaments. The anterior and posterior cruciates can be elongated and thinned out. This is especially true for complete irreducible disloca-

tions and children with Larsen's syndrome. It is obvious that after considerable cruciate ligament elongation, the knee will not have normal stability after reduction. Additional instability may be caused by the medial and lateral release necessary for otherwise irreducible knees. We have seen meniscal tears arising in adolescence as a late sequela of the initial instability.

14. What is the final functional outcome in CDK?
The functional outcome after conservative or surgical treatment is variable. Some children achieve full flexion with normal extension and show no further disadvantage. The majority will live with a restricted flexion of around 90°. In addition, lack of stability may be seen in children who needed surgical reduction owing to the necessary medial and lateral releases. Quadriceps muscle power can be reduced in children who have had late reduction of the displaced knee. The majority, however, show normal motor power in their knee extensors.

15. How is the knee treated in Larsen's syndrome?
In Larsen's syndrome, there is a combination of knee dislocation and other malformations like developmental dislocation of the hips and facial anomalies. Conservative treatment cannot reduce the knee joint. It seems wise to support the child's motor activity by stimulating exercises in the first 1–2 years of life. Open reduction with quadriceps lengthening is needed, most likely in combination with a realignment of the patellar tendon.

BIBLIOGRAPHY

 1. Austwick DH, Dandy DJ: Early operation for congenital subluxation of the knee. J Pediatr Orthop 3:85–87, 1983.
 2. Bell MJ, Atkins RM, Sharrard WJW: Irreducible congenital dislocation of the knee. J Bone Joint Surg Br 69:403–406, 1987.
 3. Bensahel H, Dal Monte A, Hjelmstedt A, Bjerkheim I, Wientraub S, Matasovic T, Porat S, Bialik V: Congenital dislocation of the knee. J Pediatr Orthop 9:174–177, 1989.
 4. Curtis B II, Fisher RL: Congenital hyperextension with anterior subluxation of the knee: surgical treatment and long term observations. J Bone Joint Surg [AM] 51A:255–269, 1969.
 5. Katz MP, Grogono BJS, Soper KC: The etiology and treatment of congenital dislocation of the knee. J Bone Joint Surg [Br] 49:112–120, 1967.
 6. Larsen LJ, Schottstaedt ER, Bost FC: Multiple congenital dislocations associated with characteristic facial abnormality. J Pediatr 37:1–8, 1950.
 7. Laurence M: Genu recurvatum congenitum. J Bone Joint Surg [Br] 49B:121–134, 1967.
 8. Leveuf J, Pais C: Les dislocations congénitales du genou (genu recurvatum, subluxation, luxation). Rev Chir Orthop 32:313–350, 1946.
 9. Niebauer JJ, King DE: Congenital dislocation of the knee. J Bone Joint Surg [Am] 42:207–225, 1960.
10. Nogi J, MacEwen GD: Congenital dislocation of the knee. J Pediatr Orthop 2:509–513, 1982.
11. Parsch K, Schulz R: Ultrasonography in congenital dislocation of the knee. J Pediatr Orthop [Br] 3:76–81, 1994.

61. TIBIAL BOWING

Edilson Forlin, M.D., M.Sc.

1. What is bowleg?
Bowleg (genu varum) is a varus angulation of the knee or the leg. It is associated with some degree of internal rotation of the leg.

2. Is bowleg always an abnormal finding?
No, some degree of genus varum is normal up to the age of 2 years.

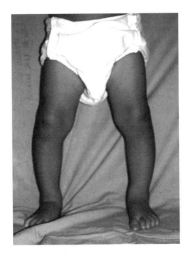

An 18-month old girl with symmetric varus knees.

3. What is the normal development of the leg in children?

We know that children are born with a varus tibial-femoral angle. Its value decreases with age. By 18–24 months of age, the knee is straight. At the age of 3–5 years, valgus angulation became more pronounced. From that point to the end of growth, there is a normal valgus angulation of the knee around 5°–10°. Of course, development can vary in normal children; for example, the Japanese population has a higher percentage of varus knee in adulthood.

4. How do I differentiate clinically physiologic tibia vara from other diseases with bowing legs?

In physiologic tibia vara, the child has no other findings, and stature and development are within normal range. Also, bowing has to be symmetric, not intense. It improves up to the age of 18–24 months.

5. When is radiography of a bowleg required?

Most children referred to an orthopaedic surgeon will not require radiography. There are some situations in which I find it necessary, if there is unilateral bowing, if there is any feature not associated with physiologic bowing (like short stature), or if it progresses faster than expected. In tibia vara (Blount disease), radiographic features are present only after the age of 18 months.

6. What diseases are associated with marked tibia vara?

Blount disease, skeletal dysplasias, rickets, or fibrocartilaginous dysplasia of the tibia.

7. What is Blount disease? What is its pathogenesis?

It is growth disorder of the medial part of the proximal tibial physis, epiphysis, and metaphysis that causes a medial angulation and rotation of the tibia.

The pathogenesis may be repetitive trauma to the medial and posterior physeal area due to walking with a varus knee. Most histologic changes are localized at the zone of resting cartilage.

8. How do I differentiate physiologic bowing from Blount disease?

Usually patients with Blount disease are obese and walked early, before the age of 1 year. Also, blacks are affected more often than white children. In Blount disease, deformity is progressive, while physiologic varus may improve until 18 months of age. We should be aware that differentiation is difficult before the age of 18 months, and observation is required.

9. How does imaging help to differentiate physiologic bowing from Blount disease?

After the age of 18 months, imaging studies can be useful. Blount disease can show an irregularity of the medial aspect of the proximal tibia. Also useful is the metaphyseal-diaphyseal angle, which is the angle formed by a line parallel to the top of the proximal tibial metaphysis and a line perpendicular to the lateral cortex of the tibial shaft (see Figure). If the angle is greater than 11°, Blount disease is the probable diagnosis. Because errors of measurement may occur, I believe we should find an angle greater than 15° to establish a diagnosis of Blount disease.

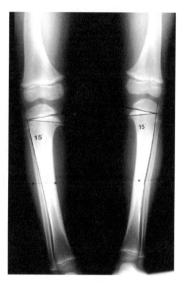

Metaphyseal-diaphyseal angle of 15°. There is a deformity on the medial side of the epiphysis. These findings suggest Blount disease.

10. What is the natural history of Blount disease?

In the infantile form (before age 3 years), spontaneous resolution is very uncommon, and most cases progress to deformity with marked varus angulation and internal torsion. The medial part of the tibial epiphysis becomes depressed and fuses with the metaphysis by the age of 10–13 years. In the juvenile and adolescent types, these deformities are less pronounced.

11. What is the treatment for Blount disease?

Conservative treatment is recommended in children younger than 3 years. I have found the knee-ankle-foot orthosis to be most efficient. Although it seems reasonable that best results would be obtained by using it during the daytime, this may be difficult for some children, and nighttime use may be an option. The orthosis may have a system that forces valgus angulation of the knee.

If the disease progresses and the child is older than 3 years, or if there are moderate changes of the medial aspect of the proximal tibia, surgery is indicated.

12. What type of surgery should be performed for Blount disease?

In most instances, a single proximal osteotomy of the tibia is appropriate. The osteotomy is done distal to the tibial tubercle to avoid damage to the tibial apophysis. Osteotomy of the fibula is also performed to allow correction of the varus and internal rotation.

As the children get older and the deformity progresses, more complex procedures may be necessary. Bar resection and elevation of the medial plateau can be associated with the valgus osteotomy. Epiphysiodesis of the lateral tibial physis and proximal fibula may be necessary in older children with a large medial physeal bridge that cannot be resected.

13. What is the worst complication of the proximal tibial osteotomy?

Compartment syndrome. To prevent it, I recommend fasciotomy of the anterior compartment at the time of the osteotomy.

14. What should I tell parents of children with probable physiologic tibial bowing?
It must be made very clear to parents that physiologic tibial bowing carries an excellent prognosis and should not be considered a disease. Close follow-up will rule out pathologic changes.

BIBLIOGRAPHY

1. Greene WB: Infantile tibia vara. J Bone Joint Surg 75A:130–143, 1993.
2. Johnston CE II: Infantile tibia vara. Clin Orthop 255:13–23, 1990.
3. Langenskiöld A: Tibia vara (editorial). J Pediatric Orthop 14:141–142, 1994.
4. Levine AM, Drennan JC: Physiological bowing and tibia vara. The metaphyseal-diaphyseal angle in the measurement of bowleg deformities. J Bone Joint Surg 64A:1158–1163, 1982.
5. Morrissy RT, Weinstein SL (eds): Lovell and Winter's Pediatric Orthopaedics, 4th ed. Vol. 1. Philadelphia, Lippincott-Raven, 1996, pp 322–329.
6. Salenius P, Vanka E: The development of the tibiofemoral angle in children. J Bone Joint Surg 57A:259–261, 1975.

62. CONGENITAL PSEUDOARTHROSIS OF THE TIBIA

Edilson Forlin, M.D., M.Sc.

1. What is congenital pseudoarthrosis of the tibia?
Dysplasia of the bone and soft tissue of the leg with failure of normal bone formation, anterolateral angulation, and pathologic fractures.

2. Can we assume that the pseudoarthrosis is present at birth?
No, the term "congenital pseudoarthrosis of the tibia" is widely used among orthopaedic surgeons, but it is not correct. In most patients, pseudoarthrosis is not present at birth. Some authors have proposed the term "infantile pseudoarthrosis."

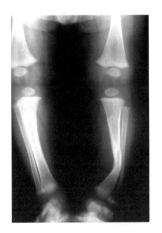

A young child with anterolateral angulation. The disorder can be classified as sclerotic type (sclerosis without narrowing).

3. What is the clinical picture?
Unilateral anterolateral bowing is noticed in the first year of life. The apex is in the distal part of the leg. In most patients, a nontraumatic fracture occurs by 2–3 years of age. Leg-length inequality is an important feature.

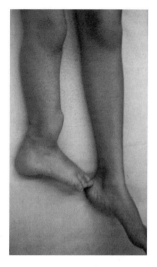

A 10-year-old boy with congenital pseudoarthrosis of the tibia. There is severe deformity and shortening.

4. What is the other form of leg angulation in a newborn?
Posteromedial angulation. It is very different from congenital pseudoarthrosis of the tibia. The correction is spontaneous, and there is no tendency to fracture. The only problem that may result is a mild leg-length discrepancy (3–6 cm).

5. What diseases are frequently associated with congenital pseudoarthrosis of the tibia?
The most common is neurofibromatosis. In published series, around 50% of children with congenital pseudoarthrosis of the tibia had a diagnosis of neurofibromatosis. The second most common associated disease is fibrous dysplasia.

6. What are the histologic findings?
Hamartomatous tissue.

7. How is congenital pseudoarthrosis of the tibia classified?
Boyd and Anderson classifications are based on the radiographic features.
Dysplasic type. There is narrowing with sclerosis of the tibia (associated with neurofibromatosis).
Cystic type. This resembles fibrous dysplasia and has a better prognosis.
Sclerotic type. There is sclerosis without narrowing.
Early type. Pseudoarthrosis is present at birth.

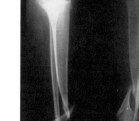

A dysplastic type of congenital pseudoarthrosis. This patient had neurofibromatosis as well.

8. What is the natural history?

After a fracture, there is no tendency to heal. As the child grows, the index of consolidation improves.

9. Can we prevent a fracture? How?

Yes, we can prevent it by using a brace. The most often recommended is a long-leg brace. Prophylactic grafting is controversial, and most authors do not recommend its use. Corrective osteotomy before fracturing should not be performed.

10. What are the goals of treatment when pseudoarthrosis is established?

   Obtain union.
   Maintain the union.
   Correct the deformity.
   Obtain leg-length equality.

11. What are the principles and techniques of surgery?

   The principles of most techniques are resection of the dysplastic segment and use of autologous bone grafting.

   Currently there are three methods that are considered the most successful:
   - Intramedullary rod: corrects the deformity, prevents refracture, and is easily performed. It does not provide correction of the leg-length inequality.
   - Vascularized fibular graft: very specialized technique with high success rate but adds only a small amount of length.
   - Ilizarov technique: allows compression of pseudoarthrosis and lengthening but carries a high rate of refracture.

12. When is amputation indicated? What type should be performed?

Amputation is indicated in a patient with repeated surgical failures who has ankle stiffness or severe deformity. An ankle disarticulation (Boyd and Syme procedure) is preferred rather than amputation through the lesion, because it avoids problems such as spike formation, provides good end-bearing skin, and gives some length.

13. What is your personal view of surgical treatment?

Treatment of congenital pseudoarthrosis of the tibia is challenging. In most patients, several operations may be necessary. The results can be so disappointing that some surgeons have recommended the use of a brace without trying to achieve union surgically. In some instances, amputation may be the final (and best) option. I have preferred using a combination of intramedullary rod placement with Ilizarov technique. In young children, I prescribe a brace and wait as long as I can before surgery.

BIBLIOGRAPHY

1. Anderson DJ, Schoenecker PL, Sheridan JJ, et al.: The use of intramedullary rod for the treatment of congenital pseudoarthrosis of the leg. J Bone Joint Surg 74A:161–178, 1992.
2. Anderson KS: Congenital pseudoarthrosis of the leg. J Bone Joint Surg 58A:657–662, 1976.
3. Boyd HB: Pathology and natural history of congenital pseudoarthrosis of the tibia. Clin Orthop 166:5–13, 1982.
4. Morrissy RT, Weinstein SL (eds): Lovell and Winter's Pediatric Orthopaedics, 4th ed. Vol. 1. Philadelphia, Lippincott-Raven, 1996, pp 322–329.
5. Tachdjian MO: Pediatric Orthopaedics, 2nd ed. Vol. 1. Philadelphia, W.B. Saunders Co., 1990, pp 651–685.
6. Weiland AJ, Weiss APC, Moore JR, et al.: Vascularized fibular grafts in the treatment of congenital pseudoarthrosis of the tibia. J Bone Joint Surg 72A:654–662, 1990.

63. HIP PAIN

John Charles Hyndman, M.D., FRCS (C)

1. Where is hip pain usually felt?

Most commonly, hip pain is felt in the knee or in the distal thigh, usually medially. Hip pain can also be experienced in the groin or in the anterior and anterolateral portion of the hip area. It is unusual for hip pain to be experienced in the patient posteriorly, since this usually reflects either back or pelvic problems. Pain in the knee always demands evaluation of the hip.

2. When is hip pain significant?

Hip pain is particularly significant when it is associated with other physical findings, such as limp. Hip limps are usually seen as one of the earliest representations of hip disease and are character-ized by lateral translation or trunk shift of the upper body toward the affected side during walk-ing. This type of limp is a strategy that is automatically adopted by the patient because it decreases the force on the hip and thereby decreases the pain. Associated night pain, particularly night pain that awakens the patient from sleep, is a very significant historical feature and is frequently asso-ciated with significant underlying disease.

3. When is hip pain an emergency?

Hip pain associated with the inability to walk is always a pediatric orthopaedic emergency. There are many disorders that must be defined urgently if the child is significantly affected, such as be-ing unable to bear weight. In those children who cannot walk, hip disease will usually be associ-ated with a significant decrease in the range of motion. Commonly, in children particularly, range of motion (ROM) can appear to be more than it is as a result of the flexibility of the adjacent lum-bar spine. It is important in quantifying the decreased range of motion, particularly in serial ex-amination to ensure that the lumbar spine is fixed, such as in the Thomas test. The ability to as-sess accurately whether the ROM is increasing or decreasing allows definition of the longitudinal evaluation of the hip disease and its rate of progression.

4. What is the most useful investigation in the evaluation of hip pain?

A single AP pelvis x-ray is essential in evaluation of hip pain. It is cheap, and will define any sig-nificant disorders such as tumors, Perthes' disease, slipped epiphysis, or chronic inflammatory conditions such as osteoid osteoma. All patients who have limp and hip pain should have an AP pelvis x-ray as part of the initial evaluation. Some early cases of slipped epiphysis will require a lateral exam to confirm this diagnosis, but the AP film is generally abnormal too.

5. What other investigations are helpful in the evaluation of hip pain?

Analysis of the complete blood count, sedimentation rate, and C-reactive protein is useful in defin-ing infections, nonspecific inflammatory conditions and, rarely, unusual and significant haema-tologic conditions such as granulocytic leukemia, which sometimes presents as hip pain and arthritis. The absence of abnormality in the test results, however, does not preclude the presence of disease. Another investigation that is very helpful in the evaluation of hip pain is a bone scan. Bone scanning is nonspecific in terms of its ability to define disease but is very sensitive in lo-calizing abnormal foci of bone physiology. Less commonly, CT is helpful in defining areas lo-calized by the bone scan or plain x-ray, and it is particularly useful in preoperative planning. It is not particularly helpful in defining disease in patients who have normal plain x-rays. MRI scan-ning is particularly helpful when soft tissue problems are the predominant problem. In addition, MRI scanning is very useful in the definition of blood supply to the femoral head and may be the earliest indicator of abnormalities in such conditions as Perthes' disease. Abnormalities involv-ing the marrow cavity, such as other infection and tumor, are readily seen on MRI films well be-fore x-ray changes appear.

6. Is ultrasound useful in hip pain evaluation?

Small quantities of fluid can be detected with ultrasonography. Whether the nature of the fluid (e.g., pus versus blood) can be defined remains debatable. Prospective studies have not shown ultrasonography to be more sensitive than clinical evaluation. Careful clinical evaluation therefore remains the standard for detecting and following hip pain associated with fluid in the hip.

7. Can hip pain by psychologic?

In children, particular young children, hip pain is rarely psychologic. It is true that in older children, if there has been careful evaluation with no evidence of disease, hip pain can be of a psychogenic nature. It is important to remember, however, that this is a diagnosis of exclusion. One must remember that hip pain, particularly hip pain associated with limp and objective physical findings, usually has a definable pathologic cause. A careful history and physical examination coupled with well-selected investigations will usually easily define the nature of this disorder.

8. When should the patient with hip pain be referred?

It should be emphasized that those children who are unable to walk require careful and urgent determination of the cause of this inability. Additionally, if there is a suspicion that the patient may have an early slipped epiphysis—as manifested by the typical clinical findings, the presence of a limp, or a questionable x-ray—he or she should be urgently referred for further evaluation because of the serious consequences of progressive slip. These patients should be protected from weightbearing as soon as the question arises and referred promptly for further evaluation.

9. Do age and sex influence the disorders that present with hip pain?

Many childhood hip disorders definitely have predilections for certain ages and sexes. For example, Perthes' disease is more common in boys between the ages of 3–7 years. Slipped epiphysis typically affects a preadolescent, often obese child, who is more commonly a male. Transient synovitis on the other hand, follows a similar age and sex distribution to Perthes' disease. Conditions such as osteoid osteoma are more commonly seen in the older child or young adolescent. Infectious diseases cover the whole age range of childhood, as do developmental abnormalities of the hip.

10. What is the most sensitive indicator of disease in patients with hip pain?

In my experience, there is essentially no hip disorder that it *not* associated with limp. Frequently the limp is not noticed, often because the patient's gait is not examined carefully in a hallway but rather is assessed in a small examining room. The presence of limp virtually always precedes pain and is always associated with thigh atrophy secondary to the limp. Careful evaluation for these clinical findings will strengthen the clinical suspicion that true disease exists and will encourage a more aggressive investigation of the problem. On the other hand, if on careful evaluation there is no limp and no atrophy, questionable results on imaging studies are more usually benign.

BIBLIOGRAPHY

1. Mukamel M, Litmanovitch M, Yosipovich Z, Grunebaum M, Varsano I: Legg-Calvé-Perthes disease. Clin Pediatr (Phila) 24(11):629–631, 1985.

64. TRANSIENT SYNOVITIS

John Charles Hyndman, M.D., FRCS (C)

1. What is transient synovitis?

Transient synovitis is a condition that commonly affects children, particularly boys between the ages of 3–7 years. It has had many names, including observation hip and toxic synovitis, but "transient synovitis" best describes its natural history.

It presents with acute pain, limp, and sometimes the inability to talk, and presents most commonly in the morning. There may be no prodrome. Generally, the patient is not sick, and results of nonspecific investigations such as CBC and sedimentation rate are either normal or show slight deviations. X-rays and bone scans are usually normal or show nonspecific signs.

2. What causes transient synovitis?

The cause of transient synovitis is unknown. It may reflect a manifestation of a viral illness (although it is difficult to explain the strong male predilection) or it may relate to some form of trauma.

3. What is the differential diagnosis of transient synovitis?

Transient synovitis is often confused with more significant pathologic conditions such as septic arthritis. These conditions require urgent and aggressive treatment, whereas the treatment for transient synovitis is expectant. The clinician therefore must make a clear distinction between septic arthritis and transient synovitis. Other less acute conditions such as Perthes' disease can be confused, at least initially, with transient synovitis. Rarely, osteomyelitis adjacent to the hip joint in either the pelvis or the neck of the femur may have an associated synovitis that is nonspecific. Bone tumors near the hip may also present with limp, although range of motion of the hip is more likely normal.

4. How do you distinguish septic arthritis from transient synovitis?

The patient with transient synovitis is not sick, and, if there is a fever, it is usually of a low grade. Similarly, the WBC tends not to be elevated as much as it would be in the case of acute infection. Serial examinations form a very important part of the evaluation, since it is not unusual for transient synovitis to be worse in the morning and better as the day progresses. In the case of infection, the patient will always get worse. In those patients who appear to be in significant distress, who have marked restriction of range of motion, and who are unable to walk, it may be necessary to aspirate the hip in order to define whether pus is present. Transient synovitis usually has an amber-colored effusion as opposed to a purulent one. Intra-articular pressure on occasion can be quite high. In some instances, this increased intra-articular pressure may be associated with a falsely positive bone scan indicating the possibility of avascular necrosis or early Perthes' disease. Photopenia on bone scan is not diagnostic of avascular necrosis.

5. Does transient synovitis cause Perthes' disease?

The association between transient synovitis and Perthes' disease has long been discussed. Generally, it is not currently believe that there is a relationship between transient synovitis and Legg-Calvé-Perthes disease. In less than 5% of cases, however, transient synovitis can be followed by Legg-Calvé-Perthes disease months later. Whether this is a cause-and-effect relationship is unknown, but clinicians should be aware that there may be a soft relationship between the two. Parental education is prudent.

6. How do you treat transient synovitis?

Once the diagnosis of transient synovitis has been made, all that remains is to follow the patient through the expected natural history of this condition. This is a benign process, and there will generally be no residua from transient synovitis. There is no good evidence that any of the more conventional forms of treatment such as traction or anti-inflammatory drugs will affect the natural history of this condition. Therefore, the treatment is expectant, with continued vigilance to ensure that the diagnosis is indeed correct.

7. Is traction commonly used?
Traction has been traditional even though there is no good evidence to support its use. Several studies have pointed out that placing the hip in extension increases significantly the intra-articular pressure. Whether this has adverse consequences is unknown; however, theoretically, given the knowledge that increased intracapsular pressure may be associated with avascular necrosis, traction probably is unnecessary. More practically, I find that patients in traction don't get examined as often or as well as those who are not.

8. When should a patient with transient synovitis be hospitalized?
In the past, it was not infrequent that children with transient synovitis would be admitted to the hospital. Currently, however, careful management on an outpatient basis, particularly of those patients who can walk, can be safely carried out expectantly on an outpatient basis, particularly since it is not believed that traction is absolutely indicated. Parents can be instructed that if the inflammatory condition gets worse, it will be readily apparent in that the child will have an increased limp or indeed will not walk at all. It is our belief that admission for transient synovitis should be limited to those children who cannot walk and who must be urgently investigated and frequently re-examined.

9. When does a child with transient synovitis return to normal activity?
Generally, return to normal activities, including gym, is restricted until the presenting complaints, specifically the hip pain or limp, disappear. Furthermore, full range of motion should be established prior to undertaking normal activities because occasionally, increasing activities will result in aggravation of the synovitis and subsequent confusion of the evolution of the natural history. This may result in reinvestigation and admission of the patient.

10. What is the usual time frame for recovery?
Outpatient follow-up of these patients usually shows that the return to completely normal range of motion is in 2–3 weeks. Persistence, particularly of a significant restriction of motion beyond this time, should cause concern that the diagnosis is incorrect, and the possibility of a nonspecific inflammatory condition such as juvenile rheumatoid arthritis should be entertained.

11. Is transient synovitis a recurrent disease?
Recurrent bouts are unusual. Children who experience repeated bouts of inflammatory arthritis of the hip should probably be investigated further, with the question of juvenile rheumatoid arthritis (JRA) or some other collagen vascular disease being entertained. JRA is an elusive diagnosis occasionally taking months to define.

12. Is transient synovitis bilateral?
Rarely. Ultrasonography may suggest abnormality on the contralateral side, but bilateral transverse synovitis is extremely unusual—so unusual that a high index of suspicion of the diagnosis should be encouraged.

13. Is aspiration of the hip beneficial?
Some studies have suggested that the course of the illness is shortened after aspiration. Given the cost benefit of aspiration, it is our belief that aspiration should be reserved for those cases in which the diagnosis is in doubt and significant concern regarding septic arthritis is apparent.

BIBLIOGRAPHY

1. Del-Baccaro MA, Champoux AN, Bockers T, Mendelman PM: Septic arthritis versus transient synovitis of the hip; the value of screening laboratory tests. Ann Emerg Med 12:1418–1422, 1992.

2. Egund N, Wingstrand H, Forsberg L, Pettersson H, Sunden G: Computed tomography and ultrasound for diagnosis of hip joint effusion in children. Acta Orthop Scand 57(3):211–215, 1986.
3. Haueisen D, Weisner D, Weiner S: The characterization of "transient synovitis of the hip in children". J Pediatr Orthop 6(1):11–17, 1986.
4. Kesteris U, Wingstrand H, Forsberg L, Egund N: The effect of arthrocentesis in transient synovitis of the hip in the child: a longitudinal sonographic study. J Pediatr Orthop 16(1):24–29, 1996.
5. Mcgoldrick F, Bourke T, Blake N, Fogarty E, Dowling F, Regan B: Accuracy of sonography in transient synovitis. J Pediatr Orthop 10(4):501–503, 1990.
6. Miralles M, Gonzales G, Pulpeiro JR, Millan JM, Gordillo I, Serrano C, Olcoz F, Martinez A: Sonography of the painful hip in children: 500 consecutive cases. Am J Roentgenol 152(3):579–582, 1989.

65. DEVELOPMENTAL DYSPLASIA OF THE HIP

G. Dean MacEwen, M.D., and Martin J. Herman, M.D.

1. What is developmental dysplasia of the hip?

DDH comprises a wide spectrum of hip abnormalities, ranging from complete dislocation of the femoral head to mild acetabular abnormality or laxity of the hip joint. Previously referred to as congenital dysplasia of the hip (CDH), this newer terminology better describes the dynamic nature of the condition. Diagnostic clinical findings may not be evident until after walking age. Repeat examination at each well baby evaluation until after walking age is mandatory.

2. What are the typical categories of DDH?

- *The dislocated hip.* The hip is dislocated (no contact between the femoral head cartilage and the acetabulum) in a resting position.
- *The dislocatable hip.* The hip rests in a reduced or located position. With stressing of the joint in flexion and adduction, the hip can be dislocated.
- *The subluxatable hip.* The hip rests in a reduced or located position. With stressing of the hip in flexion and adduction, the hip can be subluxated (with partial contact between the femoral head cartilage and the acetabulum), but it does not dislocate.
- *The dysplastic hip.* The hip shows no signs of instability with stress maneuvers. The femoral head and acetabulum are abnormally shaped or developed, however. These hips may or may not develop instability through growth.

3. What are some of the risk factors for DDH?

First-born female infant, breech presentation, and a positive family history for developmental dysplasia of the hip.

4. What other orthopaedic conditions are associated with DDH in the infant?

Congenital muscular torticollis, skull or facial abnormalities, congenital hyperextension of the knee, metatarsus adductus, and clubfoot deformities.

5. What are the differences between developmental dislocation of the hip and teratologic dislocation of the hip?

A teratologic dislocation of the hip is usually associated with other neuromuscular abnormalities, most commonly arthrogryposis or myelomeningocele. These dislocations occur early in intrauterine life. At birth, they are typically stiff, high-riding, irreducible dislocations with severe dysplasia of the hip joint. The typical hip in DDH is supple and usually easily reducible with gentle flexion and abduction. The acetabulum and femoral head in this type of dislocation are close to normal shape and configuration compared with the teratologic dislocation.

6. What physical findings are seen in the newborn with DDH?

The newborn with DDH generally has no fixed contracture of the hip joint. The skin folds about the proximal thigh and labia are often asymmetric. On flexing the child's hips to 90° and adducting them both to the midline, the child's knees do not line up; that is, the length of the femur on the dislocated side often appears to be shorter (a positive Galleazzi sign).

7. What are the Ortolani and Barlow tests? What is their significance in the clinical evaluation of DDH?

The Ortolani test is performed sequentially on each hip (see Figure). The child is placed supine on an exam table and the flexed knee on the side to be examined is cradled, with the thumb on the medial side of the thigh and the middle and index fingers along the greater trochanter. The pelvis is supported by the opposite hand. The hip is then brought from the midline in 90° of flexion and is abducted. The greater trochanter is gently lifted superiorly. In the infant with a dislocated hip, a palpable sensation will be appreciated at the fingertips as the femoral head is seated into the acetabulum (positive Ortolani test). This indicates a dislocated hip that is reducible.

The Barlow test is a stress test of the hip joint (see Figure). This test is also done sequentially on the newborn's hips. With hands held in a fashion similar to the Ortolani maneuver, the hip is placed in 90° of flexion and is brought from abduction to adduction. Just beyond neutral adduction, a gentle posterior pressure is applied to the thigh. The sensation of the femoral head moving posteriorly out of the acetabulum indicates a positive Barlow test. The amount of displacement appreciated determines whether the hip is completely dislocatable or only subluxatable. In a normal examination, there is no sense of instability during this test.

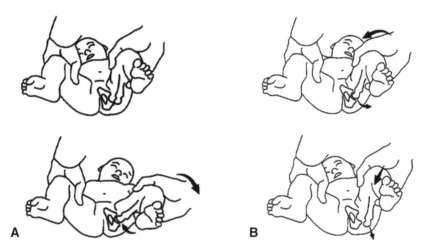

A   **B**

The Ortolani Test (A). This maneuver reduces a posteriorly dislocated hip. The affected hip is gently abducted while the femoral head is reduced with an anteriorly directed force provided by the fingers placed over the greater trochanter. **The Barlow Test (B).** This maneuver tests for dislocation or subluxation of a reduced hip. This is done by gently adducting the examined hip while directing a posterior force across the hip.

8. What is a hip click?

"Hip click" is used to describe a palpable or audible sensation about the infant's hip joint during physical examination. The term refers specifically to physical findings in a hip that has no signs of instability (negative Ortolani and Barlow tests). A hip click is most likely caused by intra-articular synovial folds, the ligamentum teres, or extra-articular structures such the iliotibial band moving over the greater trochanter or lateral condyle of the femur. A hip click requires no treatment. Follow-up is important to establish that the examination remains negative for instability. The hip click generally disappears within the first 4–6 months of age.

9. What is the Pavlik harness?

It is a flexion-abduction orthosis. The harness (see Figure) consists of a chest strap, anterior flexion straps, and a posterior abduction strap. The device is designed to maintain the affected hip in 90°–100° of flexion and to limit adduction. Because the device is not rigid, the child's own musculature aids in maintaining the hip in a reduced position. The device is not intended to hold the hip in forced flexion and abduction to insure stability but instead is designed to allow for motion of the hip within the range of reduction stability.

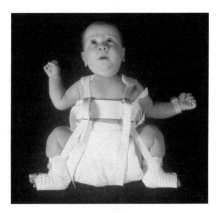

Child in Pavlik harness. Note the flexed and abducted position of the lower extremities.

10. What are the indications for use of the Pavlik harness in treating DDH?

The Pavlik harness is the treatment of choice for the child with a dislocated, dislocatable, or subluxatable hip identified in the newborn period. The harness is applied at the time of diagnosis and is used for a period of 8–12 weeks to allow for stabilization of the unstable hip. The Pavlik harness is not indicated in the infant with teratologic dislocation of the hip. Children older than 6 months of age are rarely successfully managed with the Pavlik harness.

11. How successful is the Pavlik harness in managing DDH? What are the complications?

The Pavlik harness is successful in treating DDH in the newborn in 90–95% of cases. Infants with bilateral hip dislocations, those in whom a diagnosis of DDH was made beyond 6–7 weeks of age, and those with an irreducible dislocation (a negative Ortolani sign) at the time of presentation are at highest risk for failure of the Pavlik harness. Complications include femoral nerve palsy secondary to hyperflexion and brachial plexopathy due to a high-riding chest strap, both of which resolve with proper readjustment of the device. Failure to recognize persistent dislocation of the hip after a 2 to 3-week period in the Pavlik harness can lead to fixed posterior dislocation of the hip and potential damage to the posterior acetabulum ("Pavlik harness disease"). An infrequent complication of treatment with a Pavlik harness is growth disturbance of the proximal femur, which occurs in less than 5% of patients.

12. What is the role of ultrasound in the evaluation and treatment of DDH in the newborn?

In the infant less than 6 months of age, imaging of the acetabulum and proximal femur is best achieved with ultrasound. Within this age range, the femoral head and acetabulum are primarily cartilaginous. Thus, ultrasound can provide details of femoral head and acetabular configuration, including the relationship between these structures, that cannot be obtained with plain radiography. Valuable information about the stability of the hip reduction can be obtained with real-time dynamic imaging of the infant hip while stress maneuvers such as the Barlow test are being performed.

Ultrasound evaluation of the child's hip can be done while the child is in a Pavlik harness. Success of the harness in maintaining hip reduction can be easily determined by serial evaluation during the first few weeks of treatment. Near the conclusion of treatment, final stability of the reduction can be determined with a dynamic ultrasound evaluation of the hip joint.

13. What is the role of plain radiography?

The AP view of the child's pelvis taken with the hip extended and the lower extremities held in neutral rotation is valuable in the assessment of the child with DDH after the newborn stage (see Figure). This imaging method is most valuable in the child older than 4–6 months of age whose femoral head has begun to ossify. An ossifying femoral head beneath the ilium pointed toward the triradiate cartilage and an intact Shenton's line are indicative of a reduced hip joint. The acetabular index provides a quantitative measurement of acetabular development. In the majority of cases, DDH can be reliably diagnosed. Especially in the infant with a cartilaginous femoral head, however, plain radiography may be difficult to interpret definitively.

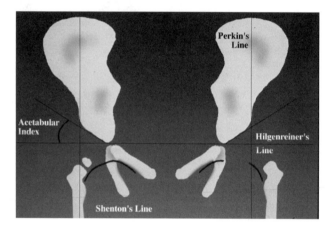

Radiographic findings in DDH. Left hip with DDH shows delayed femoral head ossification, discontinuity of Shenton's line, and an increased acetabular index (the angle between Hilgenreiner's line and a line drawn parallel to the acetabulum) compared with normal right hip.

14. What physical findings are seen in the 6-month-old child with DDH?

The dislocation of the hip in the older infant can be difficult to diagnose. The child with DDH most commonly will have no symptoms related to the disease. In the case of unilateral DDH, a limp may be detected only rarely, secondary to a leg-length discrepancy. The child with bilateral DDH often has no limp but demonstrates a waddling gait and a hyperlordotic (extended) lumbar spine. On physical exam, a child with a unilateral process may have asymmetry of skin folds in the groin. A positive Galleazzi sign may or may not be present. The only physical finding that is consistent is asymmetry of abduction of the hips. As little as 10° loss of abduction compared with the opposite side warrants radiographic evaluation. The child with bilateral DDH will commonly have symmetric abduction, but it will usually be less than 60° on each side.

15. What are the treatment options for the 6- to 18-month-old child newly diagnosed with DDH?

Closed reduction of the affected hip with application of a spica cast is the treatment of choice. First there is a short period of skin traction. The child is then examined under general anesthesia, and arthrography of the affected hip, with possible adductor tenotomy, is performed in the operating room. If a concentric stable reduction has been achieved, the child is then placed in a spica cast in the "human" position of Salter with hips flexed 90°–100° and abducted to a maximum of approximately 45°–60°. Postreduction CT scan or tomograms are helpful to confirm maintenance of reduction in the cast. The cast is worn 8–12 weeks. The cast generally needs to be changed at the 4- to 6-week interval to accommodate growth of the child.

16. What are the indications for open reduction of DDH?

Open reduction of DDH is indicated when an attempt at closed reduction under general anesthesia has failed. Open reduction of the hip, sometimes combined with a femoral shortening procedure, is the primary treatment of DDH diagnosed in the child older than 18–24 months of age.

17. What are the risks and benefits of the two common surgical approaches to open reduction of DDH?

Two common methods of open reduction are the medial approach and the anterolateral approach to the hip joint. The medial approach is performed through a medial groin incision. The capsule is approached medially between the adductors. The iliopsoas tendon and adductor longus are incised. A medial capsulotomy is then performed to achieve reduction. This approach is indicated in children younger than 4–6 months of age. The medial femoral circumflex artery is at risk during this surgical approach.

The anterolateral approach to the hip is done through a "bikini" incision, developing the tensor fascia-sartorious interval. The ilium is subperiosteally exposed medially and laterally, and the hip capsule is cleared anteriorly and posteriorly. The acetabulum is opened through a capsular incision, the head is reduced under direct vision, and a capsular repair is then performed. This approach provides wide access to the hip joint and facilitates the performance of pelvic osteotomies, if indicated. This method, however, requires an extensive exposure through a larger incision. The iliac crest apophysis is split or is displaced in its entirety. The femoral neurovascular bundle is at risk in the most medial part of the exposure.

18. What is the Salter innominate osteotomy? What are the indications for its use in the treatment of DDH?

The Salter innominate osteotomy is indicated in the child with a dislocated hip and associated mild-to-moderate acetabular dysplasia to increase stability of the hip at the time of open reduction. The Salter innominate osteotomy is also indicated in the 2- to 3-year-old child treated previously with a Pavlik harness or with closed reduction who has residual mild-to-moderate acetabular dysplasia and a congruent reduction of the hip joint.

The Salter osteotomy is performed through an anterolateral approach. A single pelvic cut is made from the sciatic notch to just below the anterior superior iliac spine. The acetabulum is then hinged anteriorly and laterally, pivoting on the pubic symphysis. The displacement is maintained by a wedge of iliac crest bone graft and is fixed with pins.

19. Name and briefly describe indications and techniques for other pelvic procedures used in the treatment of DDH.

- **The Pemberton osteotomy.** The Pemberton osteotomy has indications similar to those for the Salter innominate osteotomy. This osteotomy, however, is indicated in the child with more severe acetabular dysplasia that may not be completely corrected by the Salter osteotomy. This osteotomy is performed through the anterolateral approach. The ilium is cut to the triradiate cartilage. The acetabulum is then hinged anteriorly and laterally on the flexible triradiate cartilage. This displacement is maintained by a wedge of iliac crest bone graft.
- **Steel osteotomy.** The Steel triple innominate osteotomy is indicated in the older child with severe acetabular dysplasia who has minimal mobility in the pubic symphysis or triradiate cartilage. The ilium is cut in a fashion similar to the Salter osteotomy. Two additional cuts, one through the ischium and one through the superior pubic ramus, are then made. The en-

tire acetabulum is then rotated in the position that provides maximum acetabular coverage of the femoral head, as determined by arthrographically preoperative evaluation of the hip joint.
- *Chiari osteotomy.* The Chiari osteotomy is indicated for severe acetabular dysplasia in which adequate coverage of the femoral head cannot be achieved with other repositional pelvic osteotomies, or in which a nonconcentric reduction of the femoral head exists. The Chiari osteotomy also serves as a salvage procedure in the hip with subluxation and early osteoarthritis. The procedure is done through an anterolateral approach. An osteotomy is made obliquely through the ilium at the level of the anterior inferior iliac spine. The acetabulum is then medially displaced. The ilium abuts the superior and lateral capsule and acts as act as a shelf to cover the lateral aspect of the uncovered, subluxated femoral head.
- *The Shelf procedure.* The Shelf procedure is performed through an anterolateral approach. This procedure augments the existing acetabulum by slotting iliac crest bone grafts into the lateral aspect of the ilium at the level of the acetabular margin. The Shelf procedure is indicated in a hip with residual dysplasia and lateral subluxation with uncovering of the femoral head in which a congruous reduction of the hip joint cannot be achieved with other redirectional osteotomies.

20. What is the natural history of untreated DDH?

The child with unilateral DDH may have a leg-length discrepancy and Trendelenburg type of limp. A painless functional range of motion is generally maintained through early adulthood, however. Osteoarthritis of the hip joint can be expected in the fifth decade of life. Those patients who have not developed a false acetabulum in the wing of the ilium are less likely to develop degenerative arthritis in early adulthood than those with a false (pseudo) acetabulum. Hip fusion and total hip arthroplasty are treatment options for the symptomatic hip in adulthood.

Patients with bilateral DDH often have no leg-length discrepancy and functional symmetric range of motion. These patients tend to walk with extension of the lumbosacral spine (i.e., hyperlordosis) and have a waddling gait. As in the case of unilateral DDH, the patient with bilateral DDH is at risk for osteoarthritis. Total hip arthroplasty in adulthood is the treatment of choice for symptomatic bilateral DDH.

21. What is the most serious complication associated with DDH?

Proximal femoral growth disturbance is the most serious complication. It is seen only with treatment of the disease and is not part of the natural history of DDH.

22. What are treatment options for the painful hip in the adolescent or young adult with residual acetabular dysplasia and subluxation?

Redirectional pelvic osteotomy can be used to improve the coverage of the femoral head and thus reduce the abnormal stresses across the acetabulum. This procedure can be done in conjunction with femoral osteotomy. In a patient with severe incongruity and deficient lateral coverage, the Shelf or Chiari osteotomy may improve the symptoms and delay the onset of debilitating osteoarthritis. In the patient with advanced osteoarthritis and acetabular dysplasia or subluxation, a hip fusion or total arthroplasty is the best treatment option.

BIBLIOGRAPHY

1. Fish DN, Herzenberg JE, Hensinger RN: Current practice in the use of prereduction traction for congenital dislocation of the hip. J Pediatr Orthop 11:149–153, 1991.
2. Galpin RD, Roach JW, Wenger DR, et al.: One-stage treatment of congenital dislocation of the hip in older children, including femoral shortening. J Bone Joint Surg 7A:734–741, 1989.
3. Harcke HT, Kumar SJ: The role of ultrasound in the diagnosis and management of congenital dislocation and dysplasia of the hip. J Bone Joint Surg 73A:622–628, 1991.
4. Ilfeld W, Westin GW, Makin M: Missed or developmental dislocation of the hip. Clin Orthop 203:276–281, 1986.

5. Kalamchi A, MacEwen GD: Avascular necrosis following treatment of congenital dislocation of the hip. J Bone Joint Surg 62A:876–888, 1980.
6. Malvitz TA,, Weinstein SL: Closed reduction for congenital dysplasia of the hip: functional and radiographic results after an average of thirty years. J Bone Joint Surg 76A:1777–1792, 1994.
7. Salter RB: Innominate osteotomy in the treatment of congenital dislocation and subluxation of the hip. J Bone Joint Surg 43B:518–539, 1961.
8. Viere RG, Birch JG, Herring JA, et al.: Use of the Pavlik harness in congenital dislocation of the hip: an analysis of failures of treatment. J Bone Joint Surg 72A:238–244, 1990.
9. Weinstein SL, Ponseti IV: Congenital dislocation of the hip: open reduction thorough a medial approach. J Bone Joint Surg 61A:119–124, 1979.

66. LEGG-CALVÉ-PERTHES DISEASE

J.A.Herring, M.D.

1. What is Legg-Calvé-Perthes disease?
Legg-Calvé-Perthes disease is idiopathic avascular necrosis of the femoral head (also called the capital femoral epiphysis) that occurs in children.

2. What ages of children are affected?
The most common ages are 5–9 years, but children as young as 18 months and as old as 18 years can develop the problem.

3. Why does it have such a weird name?
It was discovered by Arthur Legg of Boston, Jacques Calvé of France, and Georg Perthes of Germany in 1909. Each worked at a hospital for children with tuberculosis, and each had a newfangled x-ray machine. With this magic machine, the authors found a subset of children who had mild symptoms and no tuberculosis. Actually, Dr. Waldenstrom of Sweden wrote about it in the preceding year, but he called it mild tuberculosis.

4. Does it have a nickname?
It is commonly referred to as Perthes' disease, especially by the Germans, or as LCP.

5. What causes it?
We are still not sure. The most recent work suggests that it occurs in children with abnormalities of thrombolysis. These children are deficient in either protein S or C or in thrombolysin. The femoral head changes may be due to arterial or venous infarction, the latter being most likely.

6. Is it a bad problem?
It is not the worst thing that can happen to a child. Most have a year or two of stiffness, limp, and some pain in the hip, and then return to normalcy. A few have minimal symptoms, and a few have continued disability.

7. Which children are prone to develop it?
There is a typical patient profile. He (boys outnumber girls 4:1) is a wiry, thin, very active boy who is noticeably smaller than his age mates. Of course, some children who develop the symptoms do not fit this profile.

8. How do I make the diagnosis?
The parent reports that the child limps and complains of occasional pain, either in the hip or in the knee. The patient often denies hurting but will point to the hip or knee when pinned down.

This may have been going on for weeks or even months, and the parents often relate it to an injury. The examination shows a mild limp and decreased range of motion of the hip. Internal rotation is especially limited.

9. What studies should be performed?

The best initial study is an AP and lateral pelvis x-ray. The early film will show an increase in the density of the femoral head compared with the asymptomatic side (see Figure). If that is negative and the symptoms are very recent, the x-ray should be repeated in a month. A technetium bone scan or even an MRI will yield an earlier diagnosis than an x-ray, but since there is no advantage to earlier treatment, these studies are not really necessary.

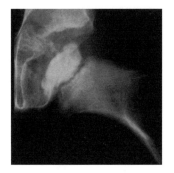

A radiograph of a child with early Legg-Perthes, with symptoms present for 1 month. There is uniform increased density in the femoral head.

10. How does the disease progress?

There are four stages. 1. *Initial* stage, in which the femoral head is dense. 2. *Fragmentation* stage, in which the femoral head is soft and deforms (see Figure at left). 3. *Healing* stage, in which new bone grows into the femoral head (see Figure at right). 4. *Residual* stage, in which the femoral head is healed with some deformity.

Clinically, in the early stages there is intermittent synovitis with pain, limp, and irritability of the hip. These symptoms increase with activity and diminish with rest. As the head fragments and deforms, there is more definite loss of motion, especially internal rotation and abduction. After about a year of symptoms, the patient gradually improves. After 2 years he is usually back to normal activities with little in the way of complaints.

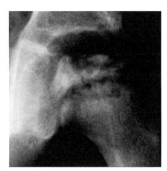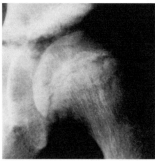

A radiograph of a child who has had Legg-Perthes for 8 months. There is fragmentation of the femoral head with lucency in the center of the head. A radiograph of the hip in Figure 2, now 3 years after onset. The hip has healed, and the roundness has gradually improved.

11. What is the natural history?

In the short run, the natural history is very favorable. Most patients go through adolescence and most of adulthood with either no symptoms or mild transient aches and pains. By the fifth decade, half the patients will have developed degenerative arthritis and will be in need of hip replacement. The other half will remain asymptomatic through adulthood (as far as we know).

12. How is the natural history influenced by age at onset?
The age at onset is a very significant prognostic factor. The older the child, the worse the outcome. This is probably due to the ability of a mostly cartilaginous femoral head of a 3-year-old to remodel compared with the limited remodeling capacity of a 16-year-old's bony femoral head. Those with onset earlier than 6 years usually require little treatment and do well, with a few exceptions. Those with onset between 6 and 8 years do well with treatment. Those with onset at 9 years or older have more severe symptoms and loss of femoral head roundness and may or may not respond to treatment.

13. How is the severity classified?
The current favorite classification method is the lateral pillar classification. Group A femoral heads have no change in the lateral pillar (the lateral one third or so of the femoral head) and do well without treatment. Group B heads have partial (up to 50%) collapse of the lateral buttress of the femoral head and have an intermediate prognosis. Group C heads have more than 50% collapse of the lateral pillar and do not do well in general.

14. What is the appropriate early treatment?
The proper early approach is to observe the child and restrict him or her from vigorous sports. If the symptoms continue or worsen, short periods of rest may help along with anti-inflammatory medications. Crutches may be used if the symptoms are really severe.

15. How soon should a patient be referred?
A reasonably early referral is appropriate, but this is not an emergency. The child can be seen by a pediatric orthopaedist in a week or two with no harm done.

16. Can the other hip become involved?
Sequential involvement of the other hip happens in about 10% of children. When both hips are simultaneously involved, one should consider the diagnosis of epiphyseal dysplasia.

17. Are there other diseases that could be confused with Legg-Perthes?
Multiple epiphyseal dysplasia, spondyloepiphyseal dysplasia, and the mucopolysaccharidoses have abnormalities in femoral head ossification that can resemble avascular necrosis. Hypothyroidism may mimic Legg-Perthes, and other causes of avascular necrosis such as steroid therapy and hemoglobinopathies should be considered.

CONTROVERSIES

18. Is surgical treatment more effective than medical treatment?
At this point, the exact efficacy of treatment is still in question. I have coordinated a multicenter study that so far suggests that surgical treatment is better for about two thirds of the children. Children with group A hips (see question 13) need no treatment. Children with group B hips with a bone age of more than 6 or group C hips do better with early surgery, either femoral or pelvic osteotomy.

19. Is nonsurgical treatment better than surgical treatment?
Nonsurgical treatment is better for the children who are young (i.e., less than 6 years) or who do not meet the surgical criteria outlined in question 18. This usually amounts to activity reduction and use of nonsteroidal anti-inflammatory drugs.

BIBLIOGRAPHY

1. Calve J: On a particular form of pseudo-coxalgia associated with a characteristic deformity of the upper end of the femur. Clin Orthop 150:4–7, 1980.
2. Catterall A: The natural history of Perthes' disease. J Bone Joint Surg 53B:37–53, 1971.

3. Glueck CJ, Crawford A, Roy D, et al.: Association of antithrombotic factor deficiencies and hypofibrinolysis with Legg-Perthes disease. J Bone Joint Surg 78A:3–13, 1996.
4. Hall DF: Genetic aspects of Perthes' disease: a critical review. Clin Orthop 209:100–114, 1986.
5. Herring JA: Legg-Calve-Perthes disease: a review of current knowledge. In Barr JS Jr (ed): Instructional Course Lectures XXXVIII. Park Ridge, IL, American Academy of Orthopaedic Surgeons, 1989, pp. 309–315.
6. Herring JA: Legg-Calve-Perthes disease. Monograph Series. Rosemount, IL, American Academy of Orthopaedic Surgeons, 1996.
7. Herring JA, Neustadt JB, Williams JJ, et al.: The lateral pillar classification of Legg-Calve-Perthes disease. J Pediatr Orthop 12:143–150, 1992.
8. Landin LA, Danielson LG, Wattsgard G: Transient synovitis of the hip: its incidence, epidemiology, and relation to Perthes' disease. J Bone Joint Surg 69B:238–242, 1987.
9. Loder RT, Schwartz EM, Hensinger RN: Behavioral characteristics of children with Legg-Calve-Perthes disease. J Pediatr Orthop 12:598–601, 1993.
10. McAndrews MP, Weinstein SL: A long-term follow-up of Perthes disease treated with spica casts. J Pediatr Orthop 3:160–165, 1983.
11. Roy DR: Perthes-like changes caused by acquired hypothyroidism. Orthopedics 14:901–904, 1991.
12. Stulberg SD, Cooperman DR, Wallensten R: The natural history of Legg-Calve-Perthes disease. J Bone Joint Surg 63A:1095–1108, 1981.

67. SLIPPED CAPITAL FEMORAL EPIPHYSIS

S. *Terry Canale*, M.D.

1. What is slipped capital femoral epiphysis?

Slipped capital femoral epiphysis (SCFE) is a displacement or "slipping" of the proximal femoral epiphysis on the femoral neck. The displacement usually is posterior.

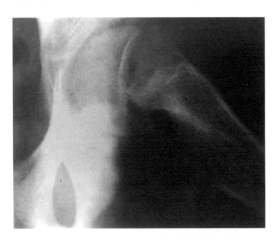

Acute SCFE with moderate displacement.

2. How frequently does SCFE occur, and who is most at risk?

SCFE is the most common hip disorder in adolescents, with a prevalence that varies greatly by geographic locale. In the United States, rates vary from approximately 2 in 100,000 to 10 in 100,000. Boys aged 9–16 years and girls aged 8–15 years are most at risk; it occurs approximately two to three times as often in boys as in girls. Most children with SCFE are obese, with at least half weighing more than 95% of children in their age group. "Red flags" that should alert the physician to the possibility of SCFE are (1) older children or adolescent, especially male; (2) obesity; (3) limp; and (4) pain in the hip, groin, thigh, or knee.

3. Is slipping of the epiphysis caused by a traumatic event?

Rarely, extreme trauma may cause an acute physeal fracture that results in displacement of the epiphysis, but most children do not recall a specific traumatic event. The exact cause of SCFE is still unclear. In addition to trauma, suggested causes have included mechanical factors, inflammation, endocrine and renal disorders, nutritional deficiencies, and irradiation therapy. Because many children with SCFE are large for their age and excessive proximal femoral retroversion is common in children with SCFE, mechanical factors appear to play a significant role. High shear forces applied to a normal physis may make it unstable and prone to slipping.

4. What are the clinical features of SCFE?

The onset of symptoms may be sudden or may occur insidiously over many months. Symptoms are variable but usually include pain in the groin, medial thigh, or knee and limitation of hip motion, especially internal rotation. Patients with chronic slips may have mild or moderate shortening of the affected extremity.

5. What is the role of imaging studies SCFE?

Anteroposterior (AP) and lateral radiographs are the most important imaging studies for diagnosis and treatment. The earliest radiographic finding on the AP view usually is slight widening and fuzzy irregularity of the physis. The central height of the epiphysis may be slightly less than in the contralateral hip. The lateral view will show the posterior position of the capital epiphysis. In chronic slips, callus formation at the inferomedial head-neck junction and "rounding off" of the superior proximal edge of the head-neck junction can be seen on the lateral view. When acute slipping of a chronic slip occurs, the acute physeal separation can be superimposed on the osseous remodeling in the metaphysis. Subtle slipping is best appreciated on "frog-leg" lateral comparison views. Ultrasonography, bone scanning, and CT scanning have been reported to aid in early diagnosis and to provide more quantitative accuracy, but these imaging studies are not necessary for diagnosis and treatment.

6. How is SCFE classified?

SCFE can be classified by duration of symptoms: acute (sudden onset of symptoms for 2 weeks or less), chronic (symptoms for more than 2 weeks and radiographs showing callus formation and attempted remodeling), acute-on-chronic (symptoms for longer than 1 month with sudden exacerbation of pain), or preslip (essentially a radiographic finding of irregularity, widening, and fuzziness of the physis).

The amount of displacement also may be classified as mild (1/3 or less of the femoral head diameter), moderate (1/3 to 1/2 of femoral head diameter) or severe (more than 1/2 of femoral head diameter).

A more recent classification system uses only two designations: stable (child can bear weight with or without crutches) and unstable (severe pain makes weightbearing impossible even with crutches). Approximately 85% of patients have stable slips.

7. If SCFE is present in one hip, is it likely to be present or develop in the contralateral hip? Is prophylactic pinning warranted?

The prevalence of bilateral SCFE has reportedly ranged from 21–80% and was recently reported to be 37% in children with symptomatic slips; if asymptomatic slips are included, the prevalence rate probably is higher. Nearly all patients who develop SCFE in the contralateral hip do so within 18 months of diagnosis of the first slip. Therefore, patients with unilateral SCFE should be followed closely to detect the development of SCFE in the opposite hip. Prophylactic pinning generally is not recommended. Bilateral SCFE is present in approximately 60% of patients with endocrine disorders, however, and prophylactic treatment of the opposite hip should be considered.

8. What is the most effective treatment?

The primary goals of treatment are stabilization of the slipping process and premature closure of the physis. Currently, the most often used treatment method for stable slips is percutaneous in situ single-screw fixation under fluoroscopic control. A 6- or 7-mm cannulated screw, either partially or fully threaded, is inserted into the center of the epiphysis. Because the epiphysis is posterior; screw insertion begins on the anterior aspect of the femoral neck (see Figure);

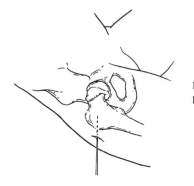

Kirschner wire inserted percutaneously to estimated starting point on femur for insertion of cannulated screw.

the more severe the slip; the more anterior the screw insertion. For unstable slips, a period of preoperative traction can be used for reduction of the slip before fixation. Often, an unstable slip will spontaneously reduce with the induction of anesthesia and patient positioning on the operating table. Open reduction rarely is required if closed reduction cannot be obtained.

9. What can go wrong during in situ pinning, and how can errors be avoided?

Incorrect pin placement probably is the most common error. Either the pin may be passed obliquely toward the anterior surface rather than the center of the femoral head, or it may pass out the posterior neck and into the head. This can be avoided by selecting a starting point on the anterior femoral neck so that the device enters the center of the femoral head perpendicular to the physeal surface. The more posterior the slip, the more anterior the starting point should be. Pin penetration can be avoided by advancing the pin tip to 8 mm or to one third of the femoral head radius from subchondral bone, whichever projection is closest. This places the pin tip 7 to 8 mm from the subchondral bone, a safe margin.

10. When is realignment osteotomy indicated?

Some form of reconstructive procedure often is necessary in moderately or severely displaced chronic slips that have produced permanent irregularities in the femoral head and acetabulum. Os-

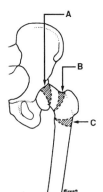

Osteotomies of SCFE. *A,* Through neck near epiphysis. *B,* Through base of neck. *C,* Through trochanteric region. (Redrawn from Crawford AH: The role of osteotomy in the treatment of slipped capital femoral epiphysis. AAOS Instr Course Lect 38:273, 1989.)

teotomy (see Figure) may be indicated to restore the normal relationship of the femoral head and neck to delay the onset of degenerative joint disease. Problems with gait, sitting, or cosmetic appearance 1 year after stabilization as well as malunion of a chronic slip in poor position are indications for osteotomy.

11. What type of osteotomy is best to correct the deformity?

This question is still somewhat controversial. The advantage of femoral neck osteotomy is correction of the deformity itself; however, postoperative avascular necrosis has been reported in 2–100% of patients. This procedure is contraindicated when the proximal femoral physis is closed.

Proponents of compensatory osteotomy at the base of the femoral neck believe it is safer because it is distal to the major blood supply in the posterior retinaculum; avascular necrosis and chondrolysis are infrequent after this type of osteotomy. The production of a compensatory deformity shortens the femoral neck to some degree, however.

Intertrochanteric or subtrochanteric osteotomies can provide good reorientation of the capital physis with little risk of avascular necrosis, but the compensatory deformity at the osteotomy makes subsequent total hip replacement more difficult.

12. What complications should be expected after treatment?

The most serious is osteonecrosis, which rarely occurs in untreated slips and is relatively infrequent after in situ fixation of stable slips. Recent reports indicate that osteonecrosis occurs in nearly 47% of unstable slips that are not reduced before fixation. Reduction of stable slips via aggressive manipulation should not be done because of the likelihood of disrupting the tenuous blood supply to the capital epiphysis. Chondrolysis is a less frequent complication (3–7% in most series).

13. Does the development of osteonecrosis require early reconstructive surgery?

The natural history of osteonecrosis after SCFE appears to be that of gradual degenerative changes, for which reconstructive surgery most often can be delayed until adulthood. In a group of 22 patients (24 hips) evaluated at an average of 31 years after treatment of SCFE, we found that only nine had undergone reconstructive surgery: four during adolescence and five during adulthood. The remaining 13 patients (15 hips) had no further surgery, but all showed degenerative changes on radiographs. Early operative treatment of osteonecrosis recently has been advocated by some authors, but no long-term results of such treatment have been reported.

BIBLIOGRAPHY

1. Aronson DD, Carlson WE: Slipped capital femoral epiphysis: a prospective study of fixation with a single screw. J Bone Joint Surg 74A:810–819, 1992.
2. Blanco JS, Taylor B, Johnston CE II: Comparison of single pin versus multiple pin fixation in treatment of slipped capital femoral epiphysis. J Pediatr Orthop 12:384–389, 1992.
3. Carney BT, Weinstein SL, Noble J: Long-term follow-up of slipped capital femoral epiphysis. J Bone Joint Surg 73A:667–674, 1991.
4. Dietz FR: Traction reduction of acute and acute on chronic slipped capital femoral epiphysis. Clin Orthop 302:101–110, 1994.
5. Jerre R, Billing L, Hansson G, et al.: The contralateral hip in patients primarily treated for unilateral slipped upper femoral epiphysis: long-term follow-up of sixty-one hips. J Bone Joint Surg 76B:563–567, 1994.
6. Kallio PE, Mah ET, Foster BK, Paterson DC, LeQuesne GW: Slipped capital femoral epiphysis: incidence and clinical assessment of physeal instability. J Bone Joint Surg 77B:752–755, 1995.
7. Krahn TH, Canale ST, Beaty JH, Warner WC, Lourenço P: Long-term follow-up of patients with avascular necrosis after treatment of slipped capital femoral epiphysis. J Pediatr Orthop 13:154–158, 1993.
8. Loder RT, Richards BS, Shapiro PS, et al.: Acute slipped capital femoral epiphysis: the importance of physeal stability. J Bone Joint Surg 75A:1134–1140, 1993.
9. Loder RT, Wittenberg B, DeSilva G: Slipped capital femoral epiphysis associated with endocrine disorders. J Pediatr Orthop 15:349–356, 1995.

10. Ward WT, Stefko J, Wood KB, et al.: Fixation with a single screw for slipped capital femoral epiphysis. J Bone Joint Surg 74A:799–809, 1992.

68. BACK PAIN

B. *Stephens Richards*, M.D.

1. How common is back pain in children and adolescents?

In a review of several large community studies, it appeared that 10–30% of children (including adolescents) experience back pain. Back pain in childhood and adolescence is less common than it is during adulthood. In children, underlying disease is frequently detectable by obtaining a careful history, by performing a complete examination, and, as needed, by using various imaging studies.

2. How often can the cause of back pain be identified in children?

Several studies reported finding a definite diagnosis in 63–84% of children with back pain. A recent study, however, reported finding a definite diagnosis in only 22% of those who presented with pain. In general, if young children and toddlers, who are unlikely to exaggerate symptoms or physical findings, are thoroughly evaluated, an abnormality is likely to be found.

3. What should be asked when taking a history?

By emphasizing the initial onset and duration of symptoms, the presence of trauma or infection, the location of the pain, and the frequency and intensity of the pain, enough information is often gained to form an initial impression.

4. What is looked for during the physical examination?

Initially, a general examination with the child gowned or in shorts should be done to rule out any associated abnormalities (systemic or neurologic). Once done, specific attention can be focused on the child's back to assess posture, alignment, and skin condition. The forward bending test assesses for thoracic and lumbar asymmetry and flexibility. Underlying disease should be suspected with the presence of localized tenderness, exaggerated stiffness of the lumbar spine, pronounced thoracic kyphosis, midline skin defects (sinuses, hemangiomas, or hair patches), excessive hamstring tightness, or neurologic abnormalities (asymmetric abdominal reflexes, clonus, gait disturbances, and motor or sensory deficiencies).

5. What types of imaging studies are helpful in the assessment of back pain?

Plain radiographs, technetium bone scans, single photon emission computed tomography (SPECT), computed tomography (CT) scans, and magnetic resonance imaging (MRI) scans are all valuable tools. Rarely would all be needed together.

6. When should plain radiographs be ordered?

These are consistently found to be the most helpful imaging study in children with back pain. Anteroposterior and lateral radiographs of the thoracolumbar spine should be obtained during the initial evaluation in children who are age 4 or younger, who have had pain longer than 2 months, who have pain that awakens them from sleep, or who have associated constitutional symptoms. Disk space narrowing, vertebral end plate irregularities, vertebral scalloping, bone defects, and scoliosis are several detectable abnormalities. Additional oblique radiographs will provide further detail in areas of concern (e.g., spondylolysis). Adequate visualization of the pelvis is required because some conditions involving the pelvis, such as osteoid osteoma, may lead to complaints of back pain.

7. When should bone scans be ordered?

If suspicion of an abnormality is high, but the neurologic examination and the plain radiographs are normal, a technetium bone scan should be the next imaging study obtained. This should include the entire spine and pelvis, but a total body scan is not necessary. Although this test is not specific, it is quite sensitive for infection, benign and malignant neoplasms, and occult fractures. SPECT scans may be useful when the plain bone scan is equivocal, since it is superior in precisely locating lesions within the spine (e.g., spondylolysis).

8. When should an MRI scan be ordered?

If the neurologic exam is abnormal, then the spinal cord and canal should be evaluated with MRI. This has replaced CT myelography as the optimal study for assessing the neural axis, particularly in the evaluation of spinal cord tumors, syringomyelia, and disk herniations. MRIs must be carefully interpreted to avoid "overreading" positive disk disease and thereby making the assumption that this is responsible for the back pain.

9. When are CT scans helpful?

When a bone lesion has been identified on plain radiographs or a bone scan, a CT scan remains the best imaging study to clarify the extent of the disease. CT myelography may still provide additional useful information in adolescent patients with difficult-to-evaluate disk herniations.

10. What are useful laboratory studies?

A complete blood count with differential and an erythrocyte sedimentation rate are the most useful screening tests. These should be obtained early in young children, those complaining of night pain, and those with constitutional symptoms in whom infection, lymphoma, or leukemia may be suspected. If a rheumatologic disorder is suspected, further helpful tests include analysis of rheumatoid factor, antinuclear antibody, and HLA-B27.

11. What is included in the differential diagnosis?

Developmental:	Scheuermann's kyphosis	**Neoplastic:**	Benign
	Painful scoliosis		Osteoid osteoma, osteoblastoma,
Infectious:	Diskitis and vertebral		aneurysmal bone cyst
	osteomyelitis		Histiocytosis
	Tuberculous spondylitis		Malignant
Traumatic:	Muscle strain		Leukemia, lymphoma, sarcoma
	Spondylolysis and	**Visceral:**	Renal abnormalities
	spondylolisthesis		Gynecologic abnormalities
	Herniated disk		
	Slipped vertebral		
	apophysis		
	Fractures		

12. After muscle strain, what are the more common causes of back pain in the young?

Diskitis, spondylolisthesis, and Scheuermann's kyphosis.

13. What can be done for back pain secondary to muscle strain?

Rest from activities that led to the back pain and the use of nonsteroidal anti-inflammatory medication are usually sufficient. Recovery should be expected within several weeks. If pain persists and further work-up has ruled out causes other than muscle strain, physical therapy instruction in back stretching and strengthening exercises may be helpful.

14. What is diskitis?

This is thought to represent infection within the disk space, usually with *Staphylococcus aureus*. It is the most common cause of back pain in the very young child and occasionally can lead to osteomyelitis of the adjacent vertebrae.

15. When should diskitis be suspected?
Diskitis typically affects children 1–5 years of age. The child may complain of pain in the back or abdomen, may refuse to walk, or may present with a limp. Some may appear ill, but fewer than half will be febrile. Often, movement of the spine is limited and is accompanied by tenderness to palpation of the lower back. The child may refuse to bend over to retrieve a toy from the floor.

16. What kind of work-up is needed if diskitis is suspected?
A plain lateral radiograph of the thoracolumbar spine may demonstrate disk space narrowing, and the erythrocyte sedimentation rate will be elevated. Radiographic findings frequently lag behind the clinical picture, however. If it is early in the disease process, disk space narrowing and subsequent adjacent vertebral end plate erosions will not yet be evident. A bone scan, demonstrating increased uptake in the disk, will confirm the diagnosis. MRI imaging will also pick up the abnormalities in the disk and adjacent vertebrae but is not necessary if a positive bone scan has been obtained. A needle biopsy of the disk space should be considered *only* if the child does not respond to treatment.

17. What treatment is needed for diskitis?
Intravenous antibiotics, usually first-generation cephalosporins, and bed rest are recommended by most authors. The antibiotics can be changed to the oral route after 7–10 days and should be continued 3–4 weeks. Immobilization in a brace or cast may provide some comfort. Biopsy or débridement is reserved for those whose conditions do not improve with treatment or who are shown on imaging studies to have abscess formation.

18. What is spondylolisthesis?
Spondylolisthesis represents a forward slippage of part of one vertebra upon another. This occurs in the low back region, most commonly when the fifth lumbar vertebra slips forward on the sacrum. For this to happen, a stress fracture of the pars interarticularis (spondylolysis) is necessary, which weakens the structural support of the spine. Spondylolysis and spondylolisthesis are the most common causes of identifiable lumbar back pain in adolescents. Generally, the symptoms begin during the adolescent growth spurt.

19. What causes the stress fracture of the pars to occur?
Repetitive activities that involve an increased amount of lumbar lordosis lead to stress on the pars (a part of the posterior element of each vertebra). Several examples include gymnastics, dancing, diving, and weightlifting.

20. What are the symptoms and signs of spondylolisthesis?
Lower back or buttock pain is most common. Occasionally, this will be accompanied by pain radiating into the legs. The discomfort is associated with activity, particularly those activities that involve hyperextension or twisting of the lumbar spine. Flattening of the normal lumbar lordosis, localized tenderness to palpation, hamstring tightness, and a shuffling gait are the more common clinical signs.

21. How is spondylolisthesis diagnosed?
Spondylolisthesis is readily recognized on a lateral radiograph of the lumbar spine (see Figure). If spondylolysis is suspected but there is no spondylolisthesis, however, then oblique radiographs of the lumbar spine will often provide a clear picture of the abnormality. If these radiographs are equivocal but suspicion remains high, then a bone scan is often helpful in identifying an occult pars fracture. SPECT imaging offers superior visualization. CT and MRI imaging are not needed.

22. What treatment is needed for spondylolisthesis?
If the abnormality has been noticed incidentally, the patient is asymptomatic, and the amount of slip is mild (less than 50%), then no active treatment is needed. If the adolescent is symptomatic, activity modification and nonsteroidal anti-inflammatory medication are used. Additionally, a lumbosacral corset may be used to provide minimal immobilization. In most adolescents, this will

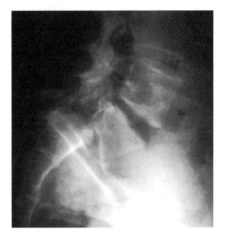

Lateral radiograph of a 15-year-old female with spondylolisthesis of L5 onto the sacrum. The displacement measures approximately 50%. She underwent posterolateral fusion between L5 and the sacrum because of persistent symptoms.

be sufficient. Some will continue to experience significant low back pain, however. These adolescents, along with those whose slips have been noted to worsen progressively on serial radiographs and those who upon initial diagnosis have severe slips (> 50%), will require surgical fusion in the lower back. Excellent long-term results can be expected.

23. Does scoliosis cause back pain in children?

Generally, children and adolescents with scoliosis (idiopathic type being the most frequently encountered) present for evaluation because of cosmetic concerns rather than back discomfort. If discomfort is present in this group of children, it usually is mild, nonspecific, intermittent, and nonradiating. It resolves with rest and does not limit activities. Further investigation of the discomfort is usually not necessary. When persistent severe back pain is the prominent complaint and a scoliotic deformity is noted secondarily, however, a thorough investigation into the source of pain is needed. Painful scoliosis is not a specific diagnosis, but it is a physical finding that may be associated with many underlying abnormalities and can affect any age group.

BIBLIOGRAPHY

1. Karol L: Evaluation of back pain. In Richards BS (ed): Orthopaedic Knowledge Update—Pediatrics. Rosemont, IL, American Academy of Orthopaedic Surgeons, 1996, pp 11–18.
2. King H: Back pain in children. In Weinstein SL (ed): The Pediatric Spine: Principles and Practice. Vol. 1. New York, Raven Press, 1994, pp 173–183.
3. Koop SE: Scheuermann's disorder. In Richards BS (ed): Orthopaedic Knowledge Update—Pediatrics. Rosemont, IL, American Academy of Orthopaedic Surgeons, 1996, pp 125–128.
4. Mayfield JK: Spondylolysis and spondylolisthesis. In Richards BS (ed): Orthopaedic Knowledge Update—Pediatrics. Rosemont, IL, American Academy of Orthopaedic Surgeons, 1996, pp 129–138.
5. Ring D, Johnston CE, Wenger DR: Pyogenic infectious spondylitis in children: the convergence of discitis and vertebral osteomyelitis. J Pediatr Orthop 15:652–660, 1995.
6. Thompson GH: Back pain in children. In Schafer M (ed): Instructional Course Lectures 43. Rosemont, IL, American Academy of Orthopaedic Surgeons, 1994, pp 221–230.

69. IDIOPATHIC SCOLIOSIS

Denis S. Drummond, M.D.

1. What is idiopathic scoliosis?
Scoliosis is a deformity of the spine marked by a lateral curvature that occurs in the frontal plane and is thus seen best on an anteroposterior radiograph. In reality, the deformity is expressed in three planes. Idiopathic means without cause; however, we now know that idiopathic scoliosis has a genetic basis.

2. What happens to the spine?
It becomes deformed in three planes. For example, with scoliosis involvement in the thoracic spine, one can observe on the anteroposterior radiograph that the vertebra are deviated from the midline as a bend or curve. Examination of the lateral radiograph shows a flattening of the normal thoracic kyphosis. Further rotation of the vertebrae at the apex of the curve can be seen in the AP view, particularly with the more extreme curves. The rotation is partially responsible for the chest wall rib hump or prominence, usually noted on the convex side of the curve.

3. What is the pattern of inheritance?
Although incompletely worked out, inheritance appears to be autosomal dominant, which means that the risk for child with one involved parent is 50%.

4. How common is idiopathic scoliosis?
If one considers all curves of 11° or more, the prevalence of idiopathic scolisis in children in early adolescence is 2%, and the likelihood of having a curve that will progress or worsen enough to require treatment is 0.2%. Therefore, idiopathic scoliosis is relatively common, but most curves do well without treatment. Although the gene is inherited equally by both girls and boys, the most important and progressive deformities occur in girls.

5. When does it occur?
Idiopathic scoliosis occurs in childhood but is detected at different ages. Generally, the earlier it is diagnosed, the more aggressive the deformity and the more likely that treatment will be necessary. Thus, the condition is classified according to the age at diagnosis.

Infantile	0–3 years
Juvenile	3–10 years
Adolescent	>10 years

6. How does one diagnose scoliosis?
First, examine the patient from behind with the back exposed. Observe the two shoulders for asymmetric height. Then observe the top of the pelvis for similar asymmetry. Examine the scapu-

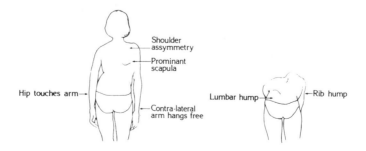

Scoliosis screening test showing the most important diagnostic features.

lar region to detect posterior protrusion, which is suggestive of rib cage deformity accompanying the spinal curvature. Finally, examine the patient bending forward from the waist, which highlights rib cage deformity, asymmetry, and elevation. This is the Adams forward bending test, and it is the definitive clinical test.

7. What is the best way to document scoliosis?

A radiograph of the spine. The exam is done on a long cassette with the x-ray beam directed in an anterioposterior or posteroanterior direction with the patient standing. The curve can then be identified and measured. The standard for measurement is the Cobb method, in which an angle is drawn from lines extending from the upper and lower surfaces of the vertebrae at the ends of the curve (see Figure). The Cobb angle is described in degrees, thus providing an objective measurement of curve size and a baseline with which follow-up studies can be compared.

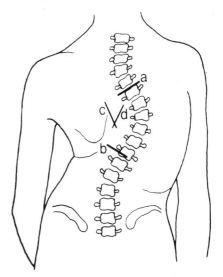

How to draw and measure the Cobb angle.

8. What problems can arise for patients with scoliosis?

Patients who develop large curves approaching 50° can develop back pain, though seldom prior to the fourth decade of life.

Patients with thoracic scoliosis and a large and rigid curve frequently have a measurable decrease in pulmonary function, although by itself this is seldom a clinical problem. For example, a curve that has progressed to 50° will be associated with pulmonary volumes that are about 77% of established norms.

Also, the larger curves (50° or more) will most likely continue to progress or worsen during the adult years and may cause the greatest cosmetic concern for patients, at times negatively affecting their perception of their own body image.

9. What is the likelihood that a curve will progress?

Risk factors include young age, female gender, and an already well-established curve that is at least 11°. When seen at maturity, curves less than 30° seldom progress, curves 50° or more invariably do worsen, and those in between may or may not change.

10. Which patients are at greatest risk for progression?

The risk is greatest for growing girls with an established curve of 11° or more. Progressive curves are seven times more likely to occur in girls than boys. Also, risk is associated with immaturity, being greatest in prepubertal children and in those with signs of skeletal immaturity. The easiest method to determine skeletal maturity from the radiograph is to examine the top of the iliac crests of the pelvis. As maturity approaches, the growth center for the ilium (apophysis) begins to os-sify progressive from the lateral end.

11. What is the goal of treatment?
My philosophy is that **no child should enter adult life with a curve of 50° or more.**

12. How is idiopathic scoliosis treated?
In a growing child, progression of idiopathic scoliosis can be arrested but not improved with a body brace. Bracing is most effective for moderate-sized and flexible curves in growing ado-lescents. The goal of a brace program therefore is controlling the progression. The success rate for properly managed brace programs in compliant adolescent is approximately 80%. The risk of failure is greater in children with juvenile idiopathic scoliosis.

Small and moderately sized progressive curves (25° to 40°) that occur in a growing child can be treated with a brace. Brace management cannot eradicate a curve, but bracing can prevent the progression. Holding the curve is the goal of orthotic management. Bracing programs usually be-gin with full-time wear. This is variously defined as 16–23 hours, depending on the treatment cen-ter. Usually as skeletal maturity approaches, the regimen can be reduced to nighttime wear only.

Larger curves may require surgical treatment. This means correction with spinal instrumen-tation and spinal arthrodesis or fusion.

13. What are the indications for a brace?
In general, brace treatment is reserved for patients who are still growing when it can be anticipated that the risk for a significant deformity exists. My own indications for initiating brace management are a growing child with a curve of 30° at the first visit or with a progressing curve between 20° and 30°.

14. Who needs surgery?
Those patients with an established curve of 50° or more and those with a somewhat smaller curve (40°–50°) that is progressive enough to become 50°.

15. What is involved with a spinal fusion with corrective instrumentation?
A spinal fusion or arthrodesis is a surgical procedure in which the vertebral segmental levels involved in the deformity are fused together to form one long rigid area. With addition of cor-rective instrumentation, this usually achieves a permanent correction.

Most recent techniques of instrumentation use multiple implants such as hooks, which are in-serted into the back of the spine and attached to long rods. Through these implants, corrective forces can be applied to the spine. The instrumentation also provides stability to the corrected spine while the spinal fusion matures to create a permanent correction.

BIBLIOGRAPHY

1. Fowles JV, Drummond DS, Roy L, L'Ecuyer S: Scoliosis in adults. Clin Orthop 134:212, 1978.
2. Lonstein JE, Carlson JM: The prediction of curve progression in untreated scoliosis during growth. J Bone Joint Surg 66A:1061, 1984.
3. Lonstein JE, Winter RB: Milwaukee brace treatment of adolescent idiopathic scoliosis—review of 1020 patients. J Bone Joint Surg 76A:1027, 1994.
4. MacEwen GD, Cowell H: Familial incidence of idiopathic scoliosis. J Bone Joint Surg 54A:1451, 1972.
5. Rogala E, Drummond DS, Gurr J: Scoliosis incidence and natural history: a prospective epidemilogical history. J Bone Joint Surg 60A:173, 1978.
6. Tolo VT, Gillepie R: The characteristics of juvenile idiopathic scoliosis and results of treatment. J Bone Joint Surg 60B:181, 1978.
7. Winter RB, Lovell WW, Moe JA: Excessive thoracic lordosis and loss of pulmonary function in patients with idiopathic scoliosis. J Bone Joint Surg 57A:972, 1975.
8. Weinstein SL, Ponsetti IV: Curve Progressive in idiopathic scoliosis. J Bone Joint Surg 65A:447, 1983.

70. KYPHOSIS AND LORDOSIS

Jeroen G. V. Neyt, M.D., and Stuart L. Weinstein, M.D.

1. What is kyphosis?

A curvature of the spinal column viewed from the side (the sagittal plane). It originates from the Greek word *kyphos*, meaning *humpbacked*. It refers to a curve pointing backwards (the apex of the curve is posterior), as in a diver ready to dive into a swimming pool.

2. What is lordosis?

Lordosis refers to a curve pointing forward (the apex of the curve is anterior). The Greek word *lordos* means *curved forward*.

3. What is a normal spinal curvature?

In the frontal plane, the normal pediatric and adult spines are relatively straight. In the sagittal plane, the neonate has a single kyphotic spinal curve. As the infant starts to gain head control, cervical lordosis develops. With progressive biped ambulation, the toddler starts to assume an upright position. At the age of 6 years, the single curve has become a quadruple one: thoracic and sacral kyphotic curves and cervical and lumbar lordotic curves. Structural wedging of the vertebral bodies contributes to most of the primary kyphotic curves. The lordoses of the cervical and lumbar curves, however, are created by the adjacent vertebrae being angulated with respect to each other. The disks rather than vertebral bodies are wedged. In a normal school-aged child, kyphotic and lordotic curves seem to balance each other in that the head is well aligned over the pelvis in the lateral projection.

4. How do you measure kyphosis and lordosis?

It is virtually impossible to measure these "sagittal" curves on a purely clinical basis. One can appreciate the sagittal alignment of a patient in a standing or sitting position, but only a standardized radiograph of the spine in the lateral projection allows one to quantify these parameters objectively. The radiograph is taken in the standing (looking straight forward) position with the arms elevated to 90° (resting on a stand). The knees and hips should be fully extended. The universally used Cobb method of measurement requires a goniometer and a pencil. The vertebral end plates are used as reference points. One should include the most inclined end vertebrae in the measured curve (see Figure). There is some variability in measuring these angles; the interobserver range of measurement is 5°–10°. Sacral inclination is measured by drawing a line parallel to the

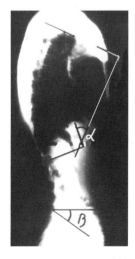

Lateral radiograph of the spine showing normal spinal curvature. Method of measurement: Cobb angle. Draw lines parallel to the selected end plates. Measure the angles in the frame of the radiograph. α angle measures thoracic kyphosis. β angle measures sacral inclination.

end plate of the first sacral vertebra and measuring the angle formed between this line and a horizontal one. It is important to be aware of the three-dimensional aspect of some spinal deformities. A lateral radiograph supplies two-dimensional information. Therefore, a posteroanterior radiograph of the spine is also usually taken.

5. What is normal kyphosis and lordosis?

Normal sagittal spinal alignment is not easily defined. The four curves (cervical/lumbar lordosis and thoracic/sacral kyphosis) vary significantly among individuals. Normal cervical sagittal alignment has been reported as $-14.4°$ measured from C2 to C7. The angular value for the thoracic kyphotic curve should be $20°–40°$ measured from T5 to T12. Kyphosis between $40°$ and $50°$ is borderline normal. Values below $20°$ are referred to as hypokyphosis and above $50°$ as hyperkyphosis. Normal levels for lumbar lordosis fall between $20°$ and $55°$ measured between L1 and L5. A line parallel to the end plates of L3 should point to 3 o'clock, and one drawn parallel to L4 should point to 4 o'clock. No data are available on the normal pelvic tilt or sacral inclination. The curves tend to balance each other, in that an increased pelvic tilt is accompanied by lumbar hyperlordosis. In a normal standing individual, a plumb line dropped from the middle of the C7 body falls within 2.5 cm of the posterosuperior corner of the first sacral body.

6. What are the causes of kyphosis?

Kyphosis is a normal component of the human spinal curvature, but some pathologic conditions may lead to hyperkyphosis or hypokyphosis.

KYPHOSIS	HYPERKYPHOSIS	HYPOKYPHOSIS
Physiologic (thoracic/sacral)	Congenital	
	Failure of formation	
	Failure of segmentation	
	Neuromuscular	
	Static encephalopathy	
	Neurofibromatosis/arthrogryposis	
	Poliomyelitis	
	Postural	Scoliosis
	Scheuermann's disease	Iatrogenic (spinal
	Juvenile rheumatoid arthritis/ankylosing	fusion)
	spondylitis	
	Posttraumatic	
	Metabolic	
	Osteopenia/osteoporosis	
	Osteogenesis imperfecta	
	Collagen diseases	
	Sponydylolisthesis at the lumbosacral junction	
	Postinfectious (tuberculosis)	
	Tumor/irradiation	
	Iatrogenic (laminectomy)	

7. What are the causes of lordosis?

Lordosis is also a normal component of the human spinal curvature, but increased or decreased lordosis may be seen in some diseases.

LORDOSIS	HYPERLORDOSIS (SWAYBACK)	HYPOLORDOSIS
Physiologic	Flexible lumbar curve in late childhood (normal)	
	Skeletal dysplasia (e.g., achondroplasia)	
	Spina bifida (e.g., myelomeningocele)	
	Hip joint contractures	Posttraumatic (e.g., whiplash injury)
	Juvenile rheumatoid arthritis	Iatrogenic (flat back)

8. What is the three-column spine concept?

A better understanding of sagittal deformities of the pediatric spine is possible by applying the biomechanical concept of three columns. Originally, the concept was described in 1983 by Dr. Francis Denis to study and classify acute thoracolumbar spinal injuries.

The *anterior column* is formed by the anterior longitudinal ligament, the anterior annulus fibrosus, and the anterior half of the vertebral body.

The *middle column* is formed by the posterior half of the vertebral body, the posterior annulus fibrosus, and the posterior longitudinal ligament.

The *posterior column* consists of the posterior bony complex (posterior arch) alternating with the posterior ligamentous complex. The ligamentous complex is formed by the supraspinous and interspinous ligaments, the facet joint capsule, and the ligamentum flavum.

Normal spinal growth requires many features. The balanced growth of each column of each vertebra adds to the overall increase in length and shape of the spine. Inadequate formation of and injury or damage to one or more segment(s) of the columns can alter the development of normal spinal alignment.

9. What causes congenital kyphosis?

Failure of formation of whole vertebrae or parts of them can result in deficient anterior and middle column support and congenital hyperkyphosis. If some vertebrae fail to separate and the cell masses remain fused, as in block vertebrae or in bar conditions, normal anterior column spinal growth may be impaired as well. Failure of formation of various portions of the posterior elements results in spina bifida, as in meningocele or meningomyelocele. If this happens at the cervical or thoracic level, the lack of stabilizing posterior column structures may result in congenital hyperkyphosis.

10. Why can children with neuromuscular disease develop abnormal kyphosis?

In children with neuromuscular involvement, paraspinal muscle weakness and poor head, neck, and trunk control together with gravity effects may cause segmental instability, especially at the cervicothoracic and the thoracolumbar spinal junctions.

11. How can the balanced growth of the spine be altered so that hyperkyphosis develops?

Compression of the vertebral body may result in a segmental collapse of the *anterior and middle* columns of the spine and may thus result in a kyphotic deformity. This can occur with high-impact injuries (fractures) or with conditions in which the bony strength has decreased, as in osteolytic tumors, osteoporosis, infections, or osteogenesis imperfecta. Growth disturbances of the vertebral end plate can occur as sequelae of infections (pyogenic and tuberculous) or after irradiation of the spine for tumors such as neuroblastoma, Wilms' tumor, astrocytoma, or ependymoma. Any condition destabilizing the structures of the *posterior column* of the spine, however, can result in kyphotic deformities, such as decompressive laminectomy, high-impact flexion-type spinal injuries, and collagen diseases. Severe spondylolisthesis at the lumbosacral junction may result in a clinical pseudohyperlordosis, but radiographically this is a kyphotic deformity that extends over the distal lumbar vertebrae and the sacrum.

12. What is Scheuermann's disease?

Scheuermann's disease is named after Dr. Holger Scheuermann, who in 1921 described a typically juvenile (> 10 yr) kyphotic vertebral disorder. This condition is radiographically characterized by anteriorly wedged vertebrae and irregularities of the vertebral end plates. To make the diagnosis, at least three wedged (> 5°) vertebrae should be seen on the lateral radiograph of the axial skeleton. Scheuermann's kyphosis affects boys more often than girls.

13. What are Schmorl's nodes?

In adolescents with Scheuermann's disease, small rounded radiolucent erosions can sometimes be seen in the vertebral end plate. These erosions are called Schmorl's nodes, and they represent herniations of the discal nucleus pulposus into the vertebra. Related pressure phenomena may cause pain.

14. What is the clinical difference between postural kyphosis and Scheuermann's disease?

The main clinical difference is the rigidity of the curve. Both conditions occur in prepubertal and adolescent children. The otherwise healthy teenager presents with a cosmetically apparent roundback deformity or with vague back pain. Often, the parents may be affected as well.

Voluntary or forced correction of the curve is not possible in Scheuermann's kyphosis. Furthermore, the forward bending test reveals a more-or-less acute angulation of the back if observed from the side (see Figure). In postural kyphosis, the test shows normalization of the lateral spine profile (see Figure). Finally, patients with Scheuermann's disease often present with tight hamstrings or contracted pectoral muscles.

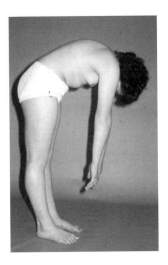 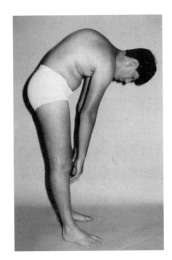

Adam's test: normal spine profile (left). Adam's test: angulated spine profile, as in Scheuermann's disease (right).

15. How do I manage a teenager with Scheuermann's disease?

The parents are most often concerned about the cosmetic deformity and potential for future problems. It is important to determine the skeletal maturity of the teenager and the flexibility of the kyphosis.

1. If pain is the major complaint and if the kyphosis of the immature spine measures less than 45° but is correctable to the normal range (with hyperextension in the supine position), a short course of nonsteroidal anti-inflammatory medication taken on a regular basis may be sufficient (10–14 days).

2. If there is no pain and if the kyphosis is mild, clinical follow-up at 6-month intervals until skeletal maturity is recommended.

3. If the deformity progresses to more than 50°, brace treatment is indicated. The most effective is the Milwaukee brace worn 23 hours a day. If unacceptable to the patient and family, try the underarm orthosis.

4. Surgery is indicated for progression despite bracing. Many authors recommend surgery for curves of more than 75°. In the absence of documented progression, continued careful follow-up should be recommended.

16. What can be done to maintain a good posture?

Many factors play a role in determining the posture of each individual child: puberty, height relative to peers, beginning breast development, self-consciousness, or genetic factors. The patient should be approached directly and engaged in an "adult-to-adult" dialogue about any postural problems. A full-length mirror can be used to provide feedback. Home exercise programs are often doomed to failure. Engaging in such activities as regular swimming is a good option (20 minutes 3–4 times/week). The value of exercises that strengthen the shoulder girdle or the back muscles in preventing adult back pain is not scientifically proven. Exercises supervised by a physical therapist are not cost effective unless paraspinal muscle weakness induced by pain is present.

17. When does hypokyphosis develop?
Hypokyphosis of the thoracic spine is usually present in idiopathic scoliosis, the most common type. It is unclear whether the more vertical alignment of the shingle-type facet joints precedes or accompanies the characteristic vertebral rotation or deformity in the frontal plane. Thoracic hypokyphosis, however, may also be an unintentional feature of posterior column fusion owing to the continued growth of the anterior and middle spinal columns. It is important for the spine surgeon to acknowledge the sagittal spinal alignment of the patient before surgery. It has been shown that the use of straight rods to correct scoliotic deformities may lead to the so-called flat back syndrome in the lumbar spine (hypolordosis).

18. Can juvenile rheumatoid arthritis change the sagittal alignment of the spine?
Juvenile rheumatoid arthritis has one of the most devastating effects on normal spinal growth. The inflammatory synovitis may decrease the height and diameters of the vertebral bodies and of the intervertebral disks. Muscle spasm, fibrous tissue contractures or ruptures, gradual facet joint destruction, and enhanced blood flow alter the growth patterns of the spine significantly. High-dosage steroid use depletes bone stock with the potential for compression fractures. Clinically, this may result in a child of short stature with a short hyperlordotic neck, thoracic hyperkyphosis, and compensatory overgrowth of lumbar vertebrae.

19. How does lumbar hyperlordosis relate to contractures about the hip joint?
Excessive lumbar lordotic posture can be due to tight hip flexor muscles. The psoas muscle originates from the proximal lumbar vertebrae. Tight rectus femoris and sartorius muscles may increase the pelvic tilt and can influence the sacral inclination. These muscular and tendinous contractures can be seen in children with skeletal dysplasia or with lumbar meningomyelocele (muscular imbalance).

20. What is the clinical relevance of rigid lumbar lordosis?
The lordosis will not reverse on the forward bending test or with the hips hyperflexed. This may suggest an intrathecal mass. A full work-up is warranted.

21. What type of imaging is useful in abnormal kyphosis or lordosis?
Radiography remains the mainstay of diagnostic imaging, but radiographs should not be routinely taken for every child with minor deviations of the normal sagittal balance found on physical exam. In a 35-kg child, a posteroanterior or lateral radiograph of the spine requires a radiation exposure of 200 mR. A chest radiograph exposes the child to 15 mR. One receives a yearly radiation exposure of 100–300 mR from the earth itself, depending on the geographic location. It is preferable to allow the consulting orthopaedic surgeon to order any imaging studies. Spine radiographs should be taken in the upright position on 36" film utilizing shielding and techniques that avoid excessive radiation exposure. The film must include the entire spine from C1 to the coccyx.

22. What does the sagittal spinal alignment on radiography reveal?
The complete or partial loss of the four physiologic curvatures may be pathologic, even in neonates, suggesting a spectrum of conditions ranging from tumors to ordinary muscle spasms. Flexion or extension views may help in determining the flexibility of an abnormal curve.

23. In a conscious patient with neck pain, what is a radiographic feature of a whiplash injury?
An abrupt deceleration of the human body as in a frontal collision may result in a forceful thrust of the head and neck. Painful contractures of muscles can produce flattening of the normal cervical lordosis.

24. Should I order laboratory tests?

In the setting of a general practice, a laboratory work-up is only occasionally necessary to rule out infections or inflammatory diseases in children with significantly abnormal sagittal alignment.

25. How do I screen children with abnormal sagittal alignment of the spine?

1. Have the child participate actively in the *inquiry* about the onset and duration of complaints, the presence of cosmetic concerns and disability, and the progression of the deformity. The *family history* can be helpful in cases of Scheuermann's disease.

2. A proper clinical examination should be done with the child wearing underwear, a swim suit, or a hospital gown that opens in the back.

3. The *chest* must be examined. Be aware that obesity can mask abnormal kyphosis or lordosis.

4. Observe the *body habitus* in the standing position from the front, the back, and the side. Ask the child to look straight forward (preferably away from the parents) and to stand with the knees fully extended.

5. Note any *shoulder asymmetry, scapular prominence, rib hump, trunk shift, pelvic tilt,* or *asymmetry.*

6. Note any *skin lesions* such as dimples, hairy patches, and hemangiomata, which are often associated with intraspinal lesions or dysraphism.

7. In the case of a *leg-length discrepancy*, use a small wooden block of appropriate size to correct the imbalance.

8. Look for *abnormalities of the feet*, knowing that cavovarus deformities suggest spinal dysraphism or neuromuscular disorders.

9. *Palpate* the prominences of the spinous processes and the paraspinal muscles.

10. Drop a *plumb line* from the C7 prominence. It should fall between the gluteal creases.

11. Assess spinal flexibility in the sagittal plane by asking the child to *hyperextend*.

12. Perform *Adam's forward-bending test*. Ask the child to assume the diving position with the feet placed together, the knees fully extended, and the palms opposed. Limited forward bending (above the midshin level) because of pain in the back or hamstrings, hesitation, or trunk shift to one side is abnormal. It may be associated with general body stiffness, diskitis or disk herniation, spinal column or cord tumors, or spondylolisthesis.

The back should curve smoothly and evenly. Sharp segmental angulation as seen in congenital kyphosis or Scheuermann's disease should be noted. Evaluate the spine in the Adam's position from the bottom, from the head, and from the side.

13. *Palpate the spine* in the prone position. If local tenderness over the midline can be elicited, ask the child to hyperextend (instability test). Note any decrease or increase in pain.

14. Do a careful *neurologic exam*. Do not forget to assess the abdominal reflexes.

26. What do I look for in children with neuromuscular disease?

1. Evaluate head-neck and trunk control and motor strength in the sitting position.

2. Look for pressure sores and skin breakdown.

3. Assess the flexibility of the curvature.

4. Examine the child in the prone position with the pelvis balancing on the edge of the table. Extend the hip. An increase in the lumbar lordosis suggests a hip flexion contracture.

5. Note any documented change in or asymmetry of neurologic integrity. Increased intracranial pressure, tethered cord syndrome, or spinal dysraphism may be present.

27. What are the pitfalls in common practice when assessing the sagittal balance of a child?

Underestimating back pain in a child with abnormal sagittal balance can lead to the major diagnostic error of missing a spinal tumor or an infection. Most back pain is related to muscle strain, and a wait-and-see period of 7–10 days would resolve most complaints. Over-the-counter nonsteroidal anti-inflammatory drugs can be taken on a regular basis with food. If pain persists or the sagittal deformity is fixed or progressive, we would recommend referral to an orthopaedic surgeon, preferably one interested in pediatric conditions.

BIBLIOGRAPHY

1. Bernhardt M: Normal spinal anatomy: normal sagittal plane alignment. In Bridwell KH, DeWald RL (eds): The Textbook of Spinal Surgery, 2nd ed. Philadelphia, Lippincott-Raven, 1997, pp 185–191.
2. Jackson RP, McManus AC: Radiographic analysis of sagittal plane alignments and balance in standing volunteers and patients with low back pain matched for age, sex and size: a prospective controlled clinical study. Spine 19:1611–1614, 1994.
3. Propst-Doctor L, Bleck EE: Radiographic determination of lordosis and kyphosis in normal and scoliotic children. J Pediatr Orthop 3:344–346, 1983.
4. Stagnara P, de Mauroy JC, Dran G, et al.: Reciprocal angulation of vertebral bodies in a sagittal plane: approach to references for the evaluation of kyphosis and lordosis. Spine 7:335–342, 1982.
5. Voutsinas SA, MacEwen GD: Sagittal profiles of the spine. Clin Orthop 210:235–242, 1986.
6. Weinstein SL (ed): The Pediatric Spine: Principles and Practice. New York, Raven Press, 1994.

71. TORTICOLLIS

Peter Pizzutillo, M.D.

1. What is torticollis?
Tilt of the head with rotation to one side.

2. What is the most common type of torticollis?
Congenital muscular torticollis.

3. What are causes of torticollis?
Temporary tilt of the head in response to fracture of the clavicle; congenital anomalies of the base of the skull; congenital anomalies of the upper cervical spine; imbalance of extraocular muscles; rotary subluxation of the atlantoaxial joints; and neoplasm of the posterior fossa, brain stem, or cervical spinal cord.

4. What is the pathophysiology of congenital muscular torticollis?
Intrauterine positioning may result in compartment syndrome of the sternocleidomastoid muscle with resultant fibrosis, which restricts normal motion of the cervical spine.

5. What are the presenting clinical signs of congenital muscular torticollis?
Persistent tilt and rotation of the head and neck.

6. What are the physical findings associated with congenital muscular torticollis?
Limited lateral rotation and lateral side-bending of the neck, flattening of the occiput on the same side of the tilt, and facial asymmetry. Occasionally, a firm nontender mass is palpable in the substance of the sternocleidomastoid on the side of the tilt. The mass spontaneously resolves in a matter of months.

7. What conditions are associated with congenital muscular torticollis?
Hip dysplasia occurs in 20% of children with congenital muscular torticollis. Although infrequent, congenital muscular torticollis may occur in association with congenital anomalies of the cervical spine.

8. What other types of physical examination are required in the patient with torticollis?
Neurologic evaluation is required to rule out an underlying neurologic cause. If indicated, obtain an ophthalmologic or neurologic consultation.

9. What imaging studies are indicated?

Routine radiographs of the cervical spine will frequently rule out congenital anomalies of the cervical spine and rotary subluxation of the atlantoaxial junction. Anteroposterior radiography of the hips and pelvis will detect subluxation or dysplasia of the hip joint.

More precise evaluation of the upper cervical spine and the base of the skull is accomplished with CT scanning. MRI is most effective in detecting neoplasms of the neurologic system.

10. What is the treatment for congenital muscular torticollis?

When other forms of torticollis have been eliminated, range-of-motion exercises of the neck to increase lateral rotation and lateral sidebending have been successful in infants younger than 1 year of age. Exercises are typically performed by the child's parents, and only rarely is formal physical therapy needed. If exercises are not successful after the age of 18 months, surgical release of the sternocleidomastoid is indicated.

11. What factors suggest a neurologic cause?

The presence of ophthalmologic dysfunction, the de novo development of torticollis after the newborn period, and recurrent torticollis in the older child.

12. What factors suggest rotary subluxation of the atlantoaxial junction?

Previous normal alignment and motion of the neck, history of recent upper respiratory infection preceding the onset of torticollis, normal neurologic examination, and spasm of the sternocleidomastoid muscle on the side opposite the head tilt. Radiographs and CT scans of the upper cervical spine will confirm the diagnosis of rotary subluxation of the atlantoaxial junction.

13. What treatment is required for rotary subluxation of the atlantoaxial junction?

If the disorder is detected within the first week of symptoms, many children respond to the use of a soft cervical collar and limitation of activities. If the subluxation does not respond to early interventions or if it is not treated until after 1 week of symptoms, inpatient treatment with halter traction is usually successful in restoring normal range of motion of the neck. Following restoration of alignment and motion, immobilization in a Minerva cast or halo cast is usually required. When subluxation has been present more than 4 weeks, maintenance of alignment may require surgical fusion of the upper cervical spine.

14. What is the treatment of torticollis due to congenital dysplasia of the base of the skull?

Observation is indicated to establish whether the condition is static or progressive. When head alignment is unacceptable or when the clinical condition is progressive, use of the halo vest with posterior occipito-cervical fusion is indicated.

15. What is the treatment of torticollis due to congenital anomalies of the cervical spine?

Most congenital anomalies of the cervical spine are rigid and not progressive. Intervention is rarely indicated. When congenital fusion of cervical vertebrae is present, it is important to evaluate hearing acuity and to rule out the existence of renal anomalies.

BIBLIOGRAPHY

1. Armstrong D, Pickrell K, Fetter B, Pitts W: Torticollis: an analysis of 271 cases. Plast Reconstr Surg 35:14, 1965.
2. Ballock RT: The prevalence of neuromuscular cases of torticollis in children. J Pediatr Orthop 16:500–504, 1996.
3. Canale ST, Griffin DW, Hubbard CN: Congenital muscular torticollis. J Bone Joint Surg 64A:178, 1986.
4. Dubousset J: Torticollis in children caused by congenital anomalies of the atlas. J Bone Joint Surg 68A:178, 1986.
5. Fielding JW, Hawkins RJ: Atlanto-axial rotary fixation. J Bone Joint Surg 59A:37, 1977.
6. Gupta AK, Roy DR, Conlan ES, Crawford AH: Torticollis secondary to posterior fossa tumors. J Pediatr Orthop 16:505–507, 1996.

7. Hensinger RN: Klippel-Feil syndrome. J Bone Joint Surg 56A:1246, 1974.
8. Hensinger RN: Changes in the cervical spine in juvenile rheumatoid arthritis. J Bone Joint Surg 68A:189, 1986.
9. Kahn ML, Davidson R, Drummond DS: Acquired torticollis. Orthop Rev 20:667, 1991.
10. Ramenofsky ML, Buyse M, Goldberg ML, Leape LL: Gastroesophageal reflux and torticollis. J Bone Joint Surg 60A:1140, 1978.
11. Rubin SE, Wagner RS: Ocular torticollis. Surv Ophthalmol 30:366, 1986.
12. Tachdijian MO, Matson DD: Orthopaedic aspects of intraspinal tumors in infants and children. J Bone Joint Surg 47A:223, 1965.

72. OBSTETRIC PALSY

M. Mark Hoffer, M.D.

1. What is neonatal brachial palsy?
Paralysis of the muscles in the upper extremity noted at birth.

2. How common is neonatal palsy?
The rate of occurrence is 0.4 per 1000 live births. The rate has not changed over the years, but the prognosis may be improving with improved obstetric care. Earlier studies have shown that complete recovery was noted in 13–18% of patients, whereas recent reports show full recovery in more than 75% of patients.

3. What are the causes of brachial palsies?
These palsies are commonly thought to be caused by pelvic dystocia. In cephalic delivery, the difficulty in delivering the shoulder after the head has been delivered may cause stretch of the upper cervical roots. In breech delivery, with the arms fully abducted, the stretch may be on the lower cervical roots and may be bilateral. On the other hand, these palsies have occurred even with cesarean section delivery. These palsies are usually milder than the others, but there is not enough information about these patients to come up with statistical conclusions.

4. What are the features of these brachial palsies?
Initially, in most cases, the involved limb appears to be completely flail. There may be an associated fracture of the clavicle. It is important to separate the real paralysis caused by the brachial palsy from the pseudoparalysis of a newborn with a fractured clavicle who hesitates to use the arm because of pain. Palsy that resolves within a few days is usually due to a fracture in the upper limb.

5. What is the natural history?
Improvement in function is the rule in these children; studies have shown that more than 75% have complete resolution of symptoms by 4 years of age. Muscle function tends to return in a relatively disorganized fashion. This is because of the differential stretch that may be placed on the various nerve roots. Most of the children have return of muscle function in the hand well before the return of function in the elbow and shoulder. The few children who end up with isolated residual palsy in the hand may have an opposite course of resolution.

6. What are the residual problems?
   Those palsies that do not resolve usually develop C5–C6 residual paralysis. This so-called *Erb's palsy* was first well described by the 19th century neurologist whose name is given to the syndrome. It involves residual weakness of the abductors, the external rotators of the shoulder,

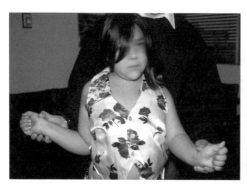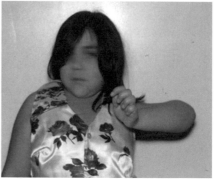

Girl with residual effects of Erb's palsy showing inadequate external rotation of the glenohumeral joint passively, measured with the arm at the side (**left**) and inadequate active shoulder abduction (**right**) as a consequence of the weakness and loss of motion.

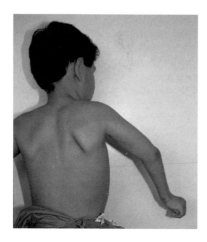

A 5-year-old-boy with Erb's palsy demonstrates the inability to abduct and externally rotate his shoulder independently of the scapula due to paralysis of deltoid and shoulder external rotator musculature.

and the elbow flexor supinator group (see Figures). Left alone, these patients can develop dislocation of the radial head posteriorly, which is of little consequence aside from positioning the forearm in pronation and flexion. A more unfortunate consequence, however, is posterior dislocation of the glenohumeral joint, which then holds the arm in adduction and internal rotation.

A rarer problem is residual weakness in the muscles of the hand related to the lower plexus, C7, C8, and T1. This results in loss of sensation in the hand and loss of finger flexor function. These children have excellent shoulder and elbow function but lose significant hand function as a consequence of the finger flexor and sensory loss.

There is a final group of mixed palsies. Although many have no organized scheme that pinpoints specific nerve damage, others have been seen involving the posterior cord (shoulder abduction, elbow extension, and wrist and finger extension).

7. Is imaging useful?

X-rays of the shoulder to determine whether the clavicle or the proximal humerus is fractured are helpful. MRI has been utilized but is inconsistent in helping to determine the level of injury.

8. What type of laboratory studies are useful?

In the past, it has been suggested that serial electromyograms are helpful in these children. This testing is done in adults with brachial plexus palsy but is very frustrating and somewhat uncomfortable for these children. The gain that one gets from analyzing these electromyograms is far outweighed by these other considerations. It is best to follow these children clinically rather than subject them to these unnecessary tests.

9. What management do these children require?

It is extremely important to keep these joints loose and to prevent dislocation, especially of the glenohumeral joint. It is also important for these children to have serial follow-up to see if they are making progress. Finally, it is important for someone to work with the family to develop appropriate programs for home therapy. Each of these children should have a pediatric orthopedic surgeon involved in his or her care. In addition, an occupational therapist should work with the family. Complex bracing in these children has been used in the past and has usually been discarded by the family and child. Ritualistic therapy in a center is inappropriate for these children. They need encouragement by the therapist, but most of the work should be done at home and should consist of range-of-motion exercises and progressive activity-of-daily-living programs.

10. What are the complications?

Complications in these children are loss of function because of muscle imbalance and loss of motion because of secondary dislocations. It is important to consider early reduction of persistent dislocations of joints that occur after loss of motion. The most important joint in this regard is the glenohumeral joint, which dislocates posteriorly, requiring surgery in some cases before full return of muscle function at 4 years of age. Another frequent joint dislocation that requires attention is anterior dislocation of the radial head in individuals who have lost elbow extension but have biceps tendon function. Finally, children with muscle imbalance need to have transfers about the shoulder, elbow, and hand to give them balanced upper extremity use. Joints left without balanced muscles eventually develop deformity and certainly function poorly.

BIBLIOGRAPHY

1. Jackson ST, Hoffer MM, Parrish N: Brachial plexus palsy in the newborn. J Bone Joint Surg [Am] 70A:1217–1220, 1988.
2. Laurent JP, Lee RT: Birth-related upper brachial plexus injuries in infants: operative and nonoperative approaches. J Clin Neurol 9:111–117, 1994.
3. Phipps GJ, Hoffer M: Latissimus dorsi and teres major transfer to rotator cuff in Erb's palsy. J Shoulder Elbow Surg 4:124–129, 1995.

73. NECK AND SHOULDER DEFORMITIES

Stephen Treadwell, M.D.

1. What is an os odontoideum?

An os odontoideum is a separate rounded ossicle positioned where the upper one third of the dens should be. It is separated from the body of the dens by a transverse radiolucent gap, which leaves the apical or upper segment unsupported and may give rise to instability that threatens the spinal cord.

2. What is the etiology of an os odontoideum?

There are three causes postulated in the literature: (1) The os odontoideum represents a previously unrecognized fracture at the base of the os odontoid that has gone on to nonunion; (2) it may represent damage to the epiphyseal plate during the first few years of life; and (3) this may be a congenital malformation of the dens itself.

3. What is the clinical significance of an os odontoideum?

Because the major portion of the dens has now been removed from the rest of C2, the cruciate ligament complex no longer provides stability for this complex. Therefore, with flexion and extension, the os odontoideum itself may stay with C1 while the hypoplastic or underdeveloped dens moves backward unconstrained by the cruciate complex, thus threatening the spinal cord.

4. What is the appropriate work-up and treatment for an os odontoideum?

The patient with an os odontoideum will often present with neck discomfort and may even present with a so-called "Lhermitte's" phenomenon or transient electric-shock–like feelings in hands or feet on sudden jerky movement. Plain x-rays plus flexion-extension lateral films will often reveal the deformity and the amount of displacement. An MRI will establish the presence or absence of chronic cord damage and may show cord impingement. For a symptomatic condition that encroaches upon the spinal cord, posterior fusion of C1 and C2 is the appropriate treatment.

5. What other clinical conditions can compromise the room available for the spinal cord at C1 and C2?

The hyperlaxity of the child with Down syndrome may produce abnormal movement at this level. Encroachment on the room available for the cord is also seen with seropositive and seronegative arthropathies. Underdevelopment of the dens and possible cord compromise can be seen with chondrodystrophy, especially involving the spine.

6. What percentage of patients with Down syndrome are at significant risk for spinal cord compromise at C1 and C2?

Although in almost 20% of children with Down syndrome, there will be 5 mm or more between the anterior arch of the atlas and the dens on forward flexion, only 5% will show enough instability to suggest cord compromise. As a result, although modification of activity may be required in some children, surgical intervention is not common.

7. What other abnormal relationships may exist in the upper cervical spine in Down syndrome?

In addition to abnormalities at the atlantodens interval, some children with Down syndrome will also show abnormal movement between the base of the skull and C1.

8. Describe the concept of the room available for the spinal cord and its relationship to the atlantodens interval. Which is more important?

In the upper cervical spine, at the C1 level, the spinal canal at age 3 is 18–23 mm in its sagittal diameter, and at age 8 it is 21–24 mm. The spinal cord is 7–10 mm at age 3 and 8–14 mm in diameter at age 8. As a "rule of thumb" about one third of the volume of the total ring of C1 is for the dens, one third is for the spinal cord, and one third is empty space to allow for movement with-

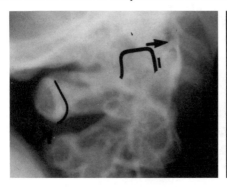 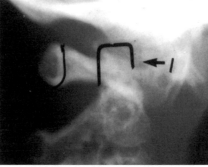

Left, Lateral view of cervical spine in extension in child with Down syndrome shows an alantodens interval of 1 mm. *Right,* In flexion the atlantodens interval increases to 10 mm.

out cord compromise. If the room available for the cord falls below 12 mm, the spinal cord is said to be at risk.

Because the atlantodens interval is visible on plain radiographs, it is often an easily acquired measurement. In the normal child, on forward flexion, there should be no more than 3 mm between the anterior arch of C1 and the dens. More than 5–6 mm difference should cause clinical concern, and more than 9 mm is usually accompanied by a significant reduction in room available for the cord. Although the atlantodens interval is a more easily acquired measurement, the room available for the cord is the more specific value and the more clinically relevant, especially when used as a surgical indicator.

9. When and how often should one order x-rays of the cervical spine in the patient with Down syndrome?
Because many children with Down syndrome are involved in an active sports program, one must assure both the parent and the sponsors that these children are not at risk. Although it is to be emphasized that a very small percentage of this population is actually at risk, it is recommended that flexion-extension lateral films for all children with this syndrome be done at or around age 4 when the child can cooperate. There is controversy whether these films should be repeated if normal. Although one cannot defend the practice with hard facts, most centers will recommend repeating the flexion-extension lateral films at around age 8 or 9 in the children who were normal at 4 years.

10. What are the common chondrodystrophies that may include compromise of C1 and C2?
The chondrodystrophies that involve the axial skeleton are spondyloepiphyseal dysplasia and the storage diseases. In these disorders, dens hypoplasia is most often seen and the cord may be at risk. The underdeveloped dens in Morquio's syndrome may also be accompanied by stenosis at C1; therefore, an MRI work-up is essential. Fusion of the C1 and C2 area in these syndromes is not necessarily indicated unless the cord is at risk, as proven by MRI studies.

11. What is the cause of the C1–C2 instability in juvenile ankylosing spondylitis or in juvenile rheumatoid arthritis?
There is a synovial joint between the cruciate ligament and the dens. This may become involved in the seropositive and seronegative arthropathies. A build-up of pannus can erode the cruciate ligament's strength and can also present as a space-occupying lesion. These children therefore may present with both instability and a build-up of tissue that compromises the room available for the cord. As in all the other syndromes, the reduction of that room to or below 12 mm is the absolute indication for surgical intervention.

12. What is the clinical triad in Klippel-Feil syndrome?
A short neck, a low posterior hairline, and marked limitation of range of motion of the neck.

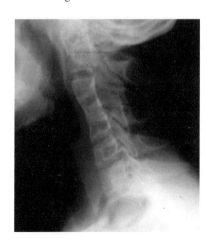

Multiple-level cervical spine fusions in Klippel-Feil syndrome.

13. What is the anatomic anomaly in Klippel-Feil syndrome?
Congenital fusion of the cervical spine. This varies from as few as two segments to the entire spine.

14. What is the medical importance of Klippel-Feil syndrome?
Because the cervical spine develops in the embryo at or about the same time as many other organ systems, patients with this anomaly often display congenital anomalies of the genitourinary system (25–35% of patients), cardiovascular anomalies (5–10%), and sensorineural hearing loss (5%). Neurologic abnormalities of movement and cord decussation within the cervical spine have been seen. The most common is termed synkinesis. This is a mirroring movement, an unconscious mimicking of the movement of the hand or foot on the other side. Miscellaneous anomalies of formation of the gastrointestinal tract are reported in a small number of cases.

15. What other skeletal anomalies can be associated with the Klippel-Feil syndrome?
Other fusions or malformations of the vertebral column are not uncommon in the Klippel-Feil syndrome. Failure of descent of the scapula or Sprengel's deformity is also seen in up to 20–30% of patients, as are cervical ribs (in up to 15%).

16. Given the wide range of anomalies in this syndrome, what is an appropriate work-up?
With the diagnosis of congenital cervical fusion comes a mandatory obligation to exclude genitourinary anomalies, usually by abdominal ultrasonography, and cardiovascular anomalies, by competent medical examination. Preschool children should have hearing testing.

Recent reports of stenosis of the cervical canal and decussation abnormalities of the spinal cord at the cervical level would also suggest that the more severely involved should have an MRI of the brainstem and cervical and upper thoracic cord.

17. Are there other syndromes than can mimic Klippel-Feil syndrome?
Children with fetal alcohol syndrome will often have congenital vertebral fusion in the neck; however, the associated anomalies are quite different. These children very often have microcephaly and very rarely have renal anomalies.

18. What is the significance of absence of the clavicle?
Symmetric clavicular absence is one of the clinical hallmarks of cleidocranial dysostosis. In addition to the absent or underdeveloped clavicles, these children have delayed ossification of the fontanelles and delayed and abnormal dentition.

19. What is the role of the orthopaedist in the management of the patient with cleidocranial dysostosis?
It behooves the orthopaedic clinician to make the family aware of the dangers of the exposed fontanelle and the advantages of protective headgear. Early pediatric dental referral is necessary to deal with the abnormal dentition. Children treated early by appropriate redirection may avoid problems in later childhood.

20. What is the significance of an asymmetric clavicular defect?
Unilateral absence of the central third of the clavicle is termed congenital pseudarthrosis. Of interest, it is almost always seen on the right side (although up to 10% of cases may be bilateral).

21. What is the clinical significance of pseudarthrosis of the clavicle?
Congenital pseudarthrosis of the clavicle is primarily a cosmetic deformity. Most children are able to function normally but present with asymmetry of the shoulder. For the small number of children with pain or whose cosmetic appearance is very objectionable, grafting of the central third of the clavicle can be attempted. One must be aware that there is a failure rate, however, and that the surgical scar may be equally objectionable from a cosmetic point of view.

22. What is Sprengel's deformity? What is the major functional difficulty encountered by patients with this problem?
Sprengel's deformity is a failure of scapular descent. From the ninth through the twelfth week of gestation, the scapula normally descends from a paramidline structure in the neck oriented in the sagittal plane to a posterior thoracic structure oriented in the coronal plane. Failure of descent will leave the scapula abnormally elevated. Because of the malposition of the shoulder girdle, decreased thoracic motion of the scapula is the common clinical finding, usually presenting as a restriction of shoulder abduction.

23. What are the classic clinical findings in Sprengel's deformity?
The scapula is usually smaller than the more normal side; it is high riding; and the interior pole is rotated medially.

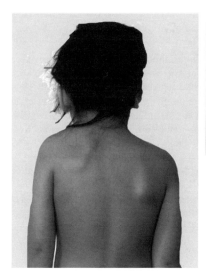
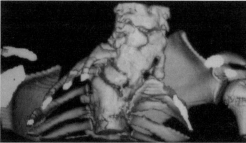

Left, Sprengel's deformity on the left side. *Above,* The three-dimensional computed tomographic reconstruction shows the elevated and hypoplastic scapula.

24. What treatment options are available for patients with Sprengel's deformity?
For those patients in whom the shoulder range of motion is functional and in whom the high elevation presents a cosmetic difficulty or causes pain, resection of the medial corner of the scapula will often produce satisfactory results.

25. What are the hazards of repositioning the scapula?
In those patients with significant shoulder girdle restriction, realignment of the scapula may be indicated; however, both the patient and the surgeon must be aware that this carries with it a risk for brachial plexus injury.

26. What is the omovertebral bone?
The omovertebral bone is an abnormal bony and cartilaginous structure extending from the upper medial border of the scapula to the spinous processes and laminae of the cervical spine. It is present in up to one third of patients with Sprengel's deformity and can contribute to the decreased motion. It also can contribute to pain. Excision is indicated when it is symptomatic.

BIBLIOGRAPHY

1. Morrissy RT (ed): Lovell and Winter's Pediatric Orthopaedics, 3rd ed. Philadelphia, JB Lippincott, 1996.
2. Weinstein, SL (ed): The Pediatric Spine, Principles and Practice. New York, Raven Press, 1994.

74. UPPER LIMB PAIN

Charles Douglas Wallace, M.D.

1. In evaluating a child with a painful extremity, what is the single most important part of the work-up?

Obtaining a thorough history. This will provide valuable insight into potential causes for the discomfort. There may clearly be a traumatic event to account for the pain or evidence of infection or overuse. Familial patterns or other involved areas of the body may aid in diagnosis.

The next step is a careful physical exam to determine the exact location of tenderness, presence of warmth or redness, inciting manipulations, and range of motion of joints. Detailed consideration must be given to the anatomic structures beneath the area of pain and tenderness.

2. I have a patient in her teens with symptoms suggestive of carpal tunnel syndrome. Does this occur in children?

Yes, carpal tunnel syndrome can occur in children and teens, although it is most frequently seen in women older than 40 years of age. Many of the potential causes of carpal tunnel syndrome seen in adults also may be found in children. These include tumors, (juvenile) rheumatoid arthritis, oral contraceptive use, pregnancy, and repetitive use and trauma. In general, treatment is conservative, utilizing activity modification, splints, nonsteroidal anti-inflammatory medications, and occasionally steroid injections into the carpal canal. Operative release of the transverse carpal ligament is reserved for cases resistant to nonoperative treatments.

3. What may cause concern in a patient who seems to have hypersensitivity to touch or manipulation after even a trivial injury?

Reflex sympathetic dystrophy is a concern. This is a poorly understood painful condition that may be progressive and debilitating following even minor trauma. The pathophysiology is not well delineated but is felt to be related to sympathetic reflex pathways. Management is difficult, with results often slow to attain. Successful outcome requires early diagnosis, a high index of suspicion, and prompt aggressive treatment.

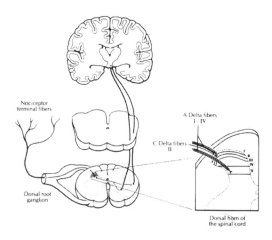

Reprinted with permission from Koman LA (ed): Infections. In Bowman Gray Orthopaedic Manual 1996. Winston-Salem, NC, Orthopedic Press, 1996.

4. What are the elements of reflex sympathetic dystrophy?

Pain, impaired function, and dystrophic changes with autonomic dysfunction. There is hyperalgesia, in which normal, generally nonpainful stimuli elicit an exaggerated sensation of pain. The dystrophic changes include stiffness of the involved joints, local edema, dermal atrophy, and osteopenia. The combination of hyperalgesia with dystrophic skin and bone changes leads to significant impairment of function. The autonomic abnormalities may be expressed as asymmetric thermal changes, sweating of the affected area, and vasomotor activity yielding skin discoloration.

5. For a patient in whom one suspects the diagnosis of reflex sympathetic dystrophy, medical intervention as well as intensive occupational therapy is often recommended. In these days of containing medical costs, is all this really necessary?

Yes! Early aggressive treatment of suspected reflex sympathetic dystrophy is the key to a successful outcome. Delay in diagnosis or in instituting treatment may allow progression of the symptom complex, making a good result less likely or much more difficult to attain. A relatively small area of involvement of the hand can easily progress to debilitate an entire extremity!

6. What are the steps in managing a patient with reflex sympathetic dystrophy?

Management of this difficult problem is multifaceted. Pharmacologic intervention may include the use of tricyclic antidepressants, such as amitriptyline; anticonvulsants; alpha antagonists; calcium channel blockers; and local anesthetics given as regional or ganglionic blocks. Early involvement of a pain specialist will aid in balancing the effects of the many medicines involved. In addition to these angles of attack, occupational therapy to maintain or gain joint motion, prevent contractures, attempt systematic desensitization, and teach strengthening exercises is critical. Therapy should involve not only the hand but also the arm and shoulder. Surgery is indicated only if a specific triggering lesion such as a neuroma can be identified. Management of reflex sympathetic dystrophy clear involves an intensive team approach.

7. How do you approach the toddler with a limp arm?

There are many conditions that may lead to a toddler's not wanting to use the arm. The first step is to rule out any history of trauma to the extremity, although a negative history does not preclude injury in this active age group. Also determine the presence or absence of any recent fevers or ear, throat, or other infections. The next step is to attempt to identify the location of the painful area (shoulder, elbow, or wrist) by first gaining the child's confidence, if possible, then manipulating only one area at a time. Plain films are taken of any areas in question. If there is no clear history of trauma, obtain a complete blood count with differential, erythrocyte sedimentation rate, and C-reactive protein level.

Diagnoses to consider include septic arthritis of the shoulder, elbow, or wrist, Fractures of the clavicle, humerus (most frequently in the supracondylar region), or along the radius or ulna may also lead to a limp arm, as well as a nursemaid's elbow from a pulling injury. Look critically at the plain films. A fat pad sign or minor wrinkle in the bone may be the only evidence of a fracture. A suspected nursemaid's elbow should resolve several minutes following a gentle flexion/supination maneuver of the elbow with pressure over the radial head. Certainly tumors are possible, although extraordinarily rare.

8. A child presents with medial elbow pain with activity, as well as radiating pain to the hand. What should be considered?

The symptoms are suggestive of ulnar nerve irritation. This may result from a previous injury to the area, such as a lateral condyle fracture malunion with a resultant fishtail deformity of the distal humerus and a tardy ulnar nerve palsy. It may also be caused by injury to the nerve from a direct blow with neuroma formation. Ongoing reinjury in the area may also lead to these symptoms. The patient may have medial epicondylitis or ulnar collateral ligament strain from repetitive throwing stress (such as in a pitcher) or a snapping ulnar nerve that subluxates out of a hypoplastic trochlear groove upon flexion of the elbow. The latter tends to be related to an anomalous portion of the triceps pushing the nerve out of the cubital tunnel, with symptoms caused by the resulting neuritis. Compression of the nerve adjacent to the cubital tunnel (such with a hypertrophied flexor carpi ulnaris), the ligament of Struthers, or the arcade of Struthers should also be considered.

9. A teen presents with a radial-side wrist pain. What should you consider?

De Quervain's stenosing tenosynovitis is one of the most common causes of radial-side wrist pain and has been known to occur in children and adolescents. The first dorsal compartment of the wrist contains the abductor pollicis longus and the extensor pollicis brevis, which may become inflamed and painful. The classic provocative test to evaluate for this condition is ulnar deviation of the thumb in a hand clenched into a fist, known as the Finkelstein test.

Management begins with application of a Velcro strap on a splint and use of nonsteroidal anti-inflammatory medications. Steroid with lidocaine injection into the first dorsal compartment of the wrist may be both therapeutic and diagnostic. Surgical release of the sheath may be indicated if conservative measures fail, with a high success rate.

Some other causes of radial-side wrist pain include radial nerve compression as well as injury to the scaphoid, trapezium, or trapezoid.

10. What is the best way to manage a painful wrist ganglion in a child?

As in adults, dorsal wrist ganglia are more common than volar ganglia. The most common site of origin is the area of the scapholunate interval. Ultrasonography provides a quick, noninvasive way to confirm the diagnosis in cases in which there may be a question as to the cause of the mass.

Conservative care with rest and splinting is the first step. This should decrease the discomfort and in a fraction of the cases may result in partial or complete resolution of the cyst. Needle aspiration should be offered to the family, with the proviso that recurrence is seen in adults in approximately 60% of cases. No good series in the pediatric population treated with aspiration alone is available for more age-specific recommendations. I do not advise steroid injection of the cyst. Surgical excision is the most reliable method to eliminate the cyst permanently, although there is still approximately a 5–15% recurrence rate despite careful removal of the cyst and its base off the capsule. I utilize a transverse incision over the mass when it is dorsal for cosmetic reasons, with care to avoid injury to the dorsal sensory branches of the radial nerve. Postoperatively, the wrist is placed in a cast flexed and extended away from the side of resection to reduce stiffness.

11. How should I approach a patient with pain along the ulnar side of the wrist?

Ulnar-side wrist pain is a distinct diagnostic challenge. One must visualize the structures beneath the skin to delineate the origins of the discomfort. Tenosynovitis of the extensor carpi ulnaris, flexor carpi ulnaris, or extensor digiti quinti may be an element of the pain. Disease in the triangular fibrocartilaginous complex due to an old injury must be considered. Lunotriquetral instability can also lead to ulnar-side wrist pain. Patients who have sustained a perhaps-forgotten forearm fracture in the past may have experienced physeal arrest of either the distal radius or the ulna, which can dramatically alter wrist biomechanics. A distal radius physeal arrest may lead to relative ulnar positivity with ulnocarpal abutment. Similarly, a distal ulnar physeal arrest can cause severe relative shortening of the distal ulna, resulting in pain and limited radial deviation of the wrist. A supinated AP film of both distal forearms should indicate either of these conditions. In addition, ganglia are rarely found in this area. Ulnar nerve compression at Guyon's canal may occur (extremely rare in children), as well as bony injuries to the carpus and distal ulna.

Evaluation should include a detailed history and careful physical exam. Diagnostic studies should start with plain radiography but may include arthrography or MRI, depending on one's specific suspicions.

12. What is thoracic outlet syndrome? How is it diagnosed and treated?

Thoracic outlet syndrome is neurovascular compression secondary to unique individual anatomy at the thoracic outlet, affecting the upper extremities. The symptoms even in adults tend to be somewhat vague and nondescript. Most frequently they include pain and paresthesias along the medial arm, although they may include the neck, chest, and lateral shoulder or arm. In children, the symptoms more frequently include aches, fatigue, and heaviness. Differential diagnosis includes any form of median or ulnar nerve compression, shoulder tendinitis, reflex sympathetic dystrophy, inflammation or tumor in the region of the brachial plexus, or cervical spine disease. This condition is rare in children, although it certainly does exist.

Anatomic sites of neurovascular compression include a cervical rib, the interscalene interval, and the area beneath the clavicle or coracoid process. Diagnosis is based on detailed physical exam and provocative clinical maneuvers as well as on plain films of the cervical spine, chest, and shoulder on the involved side. Electromyography has not proven helpful. Angiography is reserved for those with vascular alteration on provocative testing.

Management begins with a progressive shoulder strengthening program and postural reeducation. Avoiding overhead and other provocative activities has also been advocated. A 2-year trial of conservative therapy is advocated, unless symptoms are progressive. Surgical intervention is considered after failure of conservative therapy and is based on decompression of the neurovascular elements at the site of proven or suspected compression.

13. An active youth presents with shoulder pain and trouble abducting or flexing the shoulder. Does this indicate impingement syndrome or a rotator cuff tear?

The answer is most likely no. True impingement syndrome as well as rotator cuff tears are extraordinarily rare in children and adolescents. Examine the patient carefully for evidence of multidirectional instability of the shoulder as well as generalized ligamentous laxity. Shoulder pain in a ligamentously lax active young person can easily be due to a new backstroke technique, change in throwing patterns or frequency, or new exercises recently introduced into a physical training program.

The first step in attacking this problem is to identify and reduce provocative activities. Nonsteroidal anti-inflammatory drugs, rest, and ice can all be used, followed by physical therapy to address shoulder mobility and rotator cuff muscle strength and tone. The offending activity is then gradually reintroduced with modifications in technique as necessary to prevent recurrence.

14. What is of concern with lateral elbow pain in the active adolescent?

The most frequently seen condition of greatest concern in general is an overuse syndrome. Many children are in organized activities at a high level of competition. Some join multiple teams in different leagues to pursue their interest in sports. They and their parents need to be aware of the risks involved in overuse of growing and developing limbs.

While simple lateral epicondylitis is possible, treated with nonsteroidals, rest, and stretching, a more severe condition is osteochondritis dissecans of the capitellum, with possible loose body formation and collapse and fragmentation of the capitellum. MRI can be quite useful in delineating the extent of lesion found on plain radiographs as well as suggesting the integrity of the articular surface and presence of loose bodies. Drilling of the lesion as well as removal of loose bodies may be indicated. Prevention of reinjury is also important, necessitating analysis of both activity participation and environmental factors that may predispose to injury.

BIBLIOGRAPHY

1. Arner S: Intravenous phentolamine test; a diagnostic and prognostic use in reflex sympathetic dystrophy. Pain 46:17, 1991.
2. Leffert RD: Thoracic outlet syndrome. J Am Acad Orthop Surg 2:317, 1994.
3. Wilder RT, Berde CB, Wolohan M, et al.: Reflex sympathetic dystrophy children: clinical characteristics and follow-up of seventy patients. J Bone Joint Surg 74A:910, 1992.
4. Yang J, Letts M: Thoracic outlet syndrome in children. J Pediatr Orthop 16:514, 1996.

75. CONGENITAL HAND DEFORMITIES

Peter M. Waters, M.D.

1. When does the upper limb develop in utero?
The upper limb bud appears at approximately 26 days after fertilization. Progressive growth and differentiation of upper limb mesenchyme are influenced by an outer layer of ectoderm called the apical ectodermal ridge. Completion of growth and development in utero occurs by day 56 with finger separation.

2. What is the incidence of congenital upper limb anomalies?
One infant in 626 live births has been estimated to have upper extremity anomalies, but only 10% have significant functional or cosmetic deficits.

3. What other organ systems are commonly affected?
- Cardiac (ventricular and atrial septal defects, Holt-Oram syndrome)
- Musculoskeletal (VATER association: vertebral defects, anal atresia; tracheoesophageal fistula and renal and radial dysplasia)
- Craniofacial (Apert syndrome)
- Hemotalogic (thrombocytopenia with absent radii [TAR] syndrome, Fanconi's anemia)

4. What are the most common congenital anomalies?
Polydactyly (1:300 blacks, 1:3000 whites) and syndactyly (1:3000) are both inherited in an autosomal dominant fashion and occur most commonly.

5. How are congenital hand differences classified?
The presently accepted classification system of the International Society of Prosthetics and Orthotics has seven categories: failure of formation of parts, failure of differentiation of parts, duplication, overgrowth, undergrowth, constriction band syndrome, and generalized skeletal abnormalities.

6. How do you classify polydactyly?
Polydactyly is classified as preaxial (radial- or thumb-sided), central or postaxial (ulnar- or small-finger-sided).

7. What is the treatment of polydactyly?
For postaxial polydactyly, excision is preferred. For preaxial polydactyly (thumb duplication), reconstruction is necessary to combine elements from both thumbs into a single good thumb.

8. How is syndactyly classified?
Syndactyly (webbed digits) is classified in two ways. (1) Complete or incomplete. Complete syndactyly extends to the tips of the fingers, and incomplete syndactyly is partial. (2) Simple, meaning skin only, or complex, meaning conjoint bones, joints, or tendons.

9. How is radial dysplasia managed?
At birth, stretching exercises and corrective splinting or casting are begun. At approximately 1 year of age, operative correction to place the hand over the ulna (centralization or radialization) is performed. Finally, before 18 months of age, operative reconstruction of the associated thumb deficiency is performed.

10. What does syndactyly separation entail?
The skin is separated with Z-plasties to prevent late contracture. The reconstructed web is covered with vascularized flap tissue. In complete syndactyly, a full-thickness skin graft is always

necessary. The digital artery bifurcation limits the proximal separation of the digits. The digital nerve may be separated more proximally by spreading the epineurium apart.

11. What syndromes are associated with ulnar dysplasia?
Ulnar clubhand is rare, often isolated, and sporadic in presentation. It may be associated with musculoskeletal defects (ulnar-fibular syndrome) or generalized syndromes (Cornelia de Lange's syndrome).

12. How are cleft deformities inherited?
A typical cleft hand is often bilateral, associated with bilateral cleft feet, and inherited in an autosomal dominant manner. An atypical cleft hand, or symbrachydactyly, is often isolated and sporadic in presentation.

13. What is a pollicization?
An operation that converts an index finger into a thumb. By removing the index metacarpal, deepening the web space with skin flaps, and realigning tendons, the index finger is rotated into a position of opposition (see Figure). Pollicization is performed for congenital aplasia or severe hypolasia of the thumb.

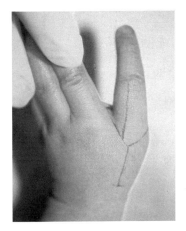 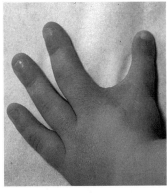

Left, Outline of incisions for pollicization of the index finger in this infant with aplasia of the thumb. *Right*, Two-year postoperative photograph of the same child.

14. What are the components of a hypoplastic thumb? How are they treated?
There are usually four components of a hypoplastic thumb: (1) weak or absent thenar muscles, (2) limited first web space, (3) unstable metacarpal phalangeal joint ligaments, and (4) stiff interphalangeal joint. Three of these four can be addressed surgically with an opponensplasty tendon transfer to improve opposition, a first web space Z-plasty to increase thumb grasp, and stabilization of the metacarpophalangeal ligaments.

15. How are thumb duplications (preaxial polydactyly) classified?
The Wassel classification defines the number of bifid or duplicated parts from proximal to distal.

16. What is the most common congenital amputation?
A forearm-level amputation occurs most commonly (1:20,000 live births). Amputations related to construction band syndrome occur in 1:15,000 live births and are now classified as deformations related to intrauterine amniotic bands.

BIBLIOGRAPHY

1. Buck-Gramcko D: Pollicization of the index finger: methods and results in aplasia and hypoplasia of the thumb. J Bone Joint Surg 53:1605–1617, 1971.
2. Buck-Gramcko D: Radialization as a new treatment for radial club hand. J Hand Surg 10A:964–968, 1985.
3. Eaton C, Lister G: Syndactyly. Hand Clin 6:555–575, 1990.
4. Foulkes G, Reinker K: Congenital construction band syndrome: a seventy-year experience. J Pediatr Orthop 14:242–248, 1994.
5. Kawabata H, Tada K, Masada K, et al.: Revision of residual deformities after operation for duplication of thumb. J Bone Joint Surg 72A:988–998, 1990.
6. Lamb D: Radial club hand: a continuing study of sixty-eight patients with one hundred and seventeen club hands. J Bone Joint Surg 59A:1–13, 1977.
7. Manske P, McCarroll H: Reconstruction of the congenitally deficient thumb. Hand Clin 8:177–196, 1992.
8. Ogino T: Cleft hand. Hand Clin 6:661–671, 1990.
9. Simmons B: Polydactyly. Hand Clin 1:545–565, 1985.

76. ACQUIRED HAND PROBLEMS

Marybeth Ezaki, M.D., and Larry H. Hollier, M.D.

1. What is camptodactly?
A nonpainful flexion deformity of the proximal interphalangeal joint unrelated to trauma.

2. How does it present?
One form of camptodactyly presents during infancy with an equal male-to-female frequency ratio. This form may be associated with syndromes with multiple contractures. A second form presents in adolescence as an isolated condition and affects primarily females.

3. What is the cause of camptodactyly?
Abnormalities in the insertion of the intrinsic and extrinsic flexor tendons as well as presumed imbalance between flexor and extensor forces in the digit have been described.

4. What is the treatment?
Treatment must balance the need for correction of the deformity with the need for continued function of the digit. Nighttime splinting with adjustable static or dynamic splints for a prolonged period of time is the standard treatment. Daytime passive stretching along with active exercises to maintain range of motion is important. A hand therapist should be involved in care whenever possible to supervise and adjust the splinting program. Nonoperative care is preferable, but surgical care may offer some improvement for those patients with severe deformities in whom splinting has failed.

5. What is Kirner's deformity?
A rare progressive deformity of the tip of the small finger. The fingernail develops a curved and clubbed appearance. It is usually bilateral and has a slight female predominance. Presentation is usually during adolescence. It is occasionally uncomfortable for the patient.

6. What causes Kirner's deformity?
Radial and palmar angulation of the distal phalanx is caused by a disruption of the radial and palmar part of the distal phalangeal growth plate.

7. What is the treatment for Kirner's deformity?

Since there is usually no pain and no functional deficit, often no treatment is needed. Splinting is ineffective. If the cosmetic deformity is significant, corrective surgical osteotomy of the phalanx may improve the appearance.

8. What is clinodactyly?

An exaggerated incurving of the little fingers toward the ring finger. This angulation may appear to increase with growth.

9. What causes clinodactyly?

These inturned little fingers are caused by a middle phalanx that is not rectangular in shape. The joints are not parallel, and the finger appears to be bent inward. The condition is most often familial. The degree of severity can vary from very mild to very bothersome.

10. Does this condition require treatment?

Most cases of clinodactyly are so mild that they are considered within the range of normal. In some cases, there may be enough overriding or underriding of the ring finger and enough functional impairment to warrant surgical correction. The deformity in this condition is primarily a bony deformity; splinting has no place in treatment.

11. What is a delta phalanx?

One that is triangular in shape. Growth of this phalanx is stunted by a "wraparound" growth plate or a longitudinally bracketed epiphysis.

12. What is macrodactyly?

Macrodactyly means "big digit." It is a condition in which there is abnormal growth of one digit or several digits.

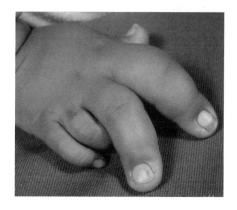

Macrodactyly with massive enlargement of fingers in an infant. The digits involved are within a "nerve territory."

13. What are the clinical features of macrodactyly?

Macrodactyly may be present at birth or may present during infancy. The rate of growth can vary from slightly disproportionate growth throughout childhood with minimal functional deficit to rapid enlargement of digits with loss of function. Growth of the affected digit stops at skeletal maturity.

14. What is the underlying disorder?

Several conditions can cause enlargement of digits. Neurofibromatosis, vascular malformations, and lymphatic abnormalities usually cause more generalized enlargement, and the deformity is not limited to the digits. The usual condition associated with macrodactyly is a nerve territory-oriented lipofibromatous hamartoma of peripheral nerve.

15. What can be done to treat macrodactyly?

There is no nonoperative treatment for this distressing condition. Surgical treatment is designed to debulk the digits and preserve function when possible. Debulking of the abnormal nerve, corrective osteotomy, and epiphysiodeses all are helpful in making these digits somewhat less unsightly.

In the case of the grossly enlarged nonfunctional digit, amputation is often a cosmetic and function-improving procedure. Remember to look for peripheral nerve compression, especially at the carpal tunnel, since there is usually enlargement of the nerve that extends more proximally.

16. What is Madelung's deformity?

A progressive deformity of the distal radius that presents during adolescence with prominence of the distal ulna, loss of forearm rotation, and discomfort at the wrist joint. Most of the patients with Madelung's deformity are female.

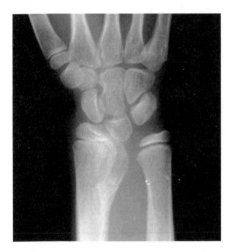

Madelung's deformity. Radiograph showing the disruption of the ulnar and palmar aspect of the distal radial growth plate. This results in progressive deformity and loss of rotation in the forearm.

17. What causes Madelung's deformity?

There is confusion about the primary lesion in Madelung's deformity. There appears to be disorganization of the growth plate at the palmar and ulnar parts of the distal radius. There is also abnormality at the proximal palmar wrist capsular structures that tethers the carpal bones into the space between the radius and the ulna. Abnormalities of the pronator quadratus muscle are also frequent.

18. What is the treatment for Madelung's deformity?

In the past, the recommended treatment was to wait until skeletal maturity and then attempt a corrective surgical procedure. It has been shown that in some cases, growth can be realigned if the diagnosis is made while the skeleton is still immature. The procedure is called an epiphysiolysis. More significant deformity requires corrective osteotomy, but it is not necessary to wait until the end of growth to do this.

19. What are the types of trigger digits?

The common trigger thumb and the less common trigger finger.

20. What is the difference?

Trigger thumbs are common and develop as early as 3–6 months of age. They are not present at birth. Trigger thumbs present either with snapping of the interphalangeal joint of the thumb or more commonly with a fixed flexion deformity of this joint.

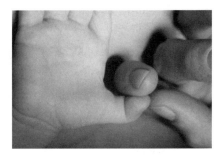

Trigger thumb. Photograph shows the limitation of extension of the thumb. This is caused by a thickening, or Notta's node, in the tendon, which prevents excursion of the tendon into the flexor sheath.

The pediatric variety of trigger digits is much less common and presents with flexion deformity of the proximal interphalangeal joint of the finger. Trigger digits are often multiple. The adult form is often related to trauma.

21. What is the cause of trigger digits?

Trigger thumb is due to a thickening of the flexor pollicis longus tendon at the entry to the flexor sheath at the metacarpophalangeal joint. This module can be quite prominent and is called Notta's node. It is unclear what causes the thickening, but it is thought that pressure or trauma plays a role.

Trigger digits are a bit more complicated and are thought to be due to an early decussation of the superficialis tendon or an abnormality in the relationship between the deep and superficial flexors, which causes a buckling of the superficialis and a snapping of the digit.

22. What is the treatment for trigger digits?

This is a mechanical problem that requires a mechanical solution. Release of the proximal annular pulley to allow the nodule unimpeded excursion is usually all that is needed to treat a trigger thumb successfully. Results of this procedure are predictably good.

Treatment of trigger digits often requires a more extensive exploration of the finger and an intraoperative decision about the need to remove one slip of the superficialis tendon. Recurrences are relatively common.

23. What is a ganglion cyst?

A fluid-filled painless cyst that arises from a synovial-lined space and presents as a hard fixed mass. The most common places for a ganglion cyst to occur are the wrist and the flexor aspect of the fingers.

24. What is the fluid in the cyst?

The content of the cyst is thick mucinous material that has the consistency of apple jelly. This material arises from periarticular or peritendinous supporting structures.

25. How is a ganglion cyst in a child different from one in an adult?

A ganglion in a child is rarely symptomatic, usually spontaneously regresses, and has a very high likelihood of recurrence with any kind of treatment. Adult ganglion cysts are often related to trauma and are frequently symptomatic. The recurrence rate in the adult form is less than that in children.

26. How is the diagnosis of a ganglion cyst made?

Transillumination of the cyst contents with an otoscope or examination by sonography. If there is doubt about the diagnosis, referral to a specialist who can rule out more serious tumors should be made expeditiously.

27. What is the treatment for a ganglion cyst in a child?

Observation is the best course, with splinting if the cyst grows with activity. Aspiration of the cyst contents is reserved for the occasional very large or symptomatic cyst. Corticosteroids play no role in the treatment of pediatric ganglion cysts.

28. What are the disorders that are associated with short metacarpals?

Trauma to the growth plate with early cessation of growth, pseudohypoparathyroidism, pseudo-pseudohypoparathyroidism, Turner's syndrome, Noonan's syndrome, and sickle cell disease.

BIBLIOGRAPHY

1. Cohn BT, Shall L: Idiopathic bilaterally symmetrical brachymetacarpia of the fourth and fifth metacarpals. J Hand Surg 11A:737, 1986.
2. Colon F, Upton J: Pediatric hand tumors: a review of 349 cases. Hand Clin 11:223, 1995.
3. Dell PC: Macrodactyly. Symposium congenital deformities of the hand. Hand Clin 1:511–524, 1985.
4. Engber WM, Flatt AE: Camptodactyly: an analysis of sixty-six patients and twenty-four operations. J Hand Surg 2:216–224, 1977.
5. Flatt AE: The Care of Congenital Hand Anomalies. St. Louis, Quality Medical Publishers, 1994.
6. Ger E, Kupcha P, Ger D: The management of trigger thumb in children. J Hand Surg 16A:944–946, 1991.
7. Miller JJ: Juvenile Rheumatoid Arthritis. Littleton, MA, PSG Publishing Company, 1994.
8. Poznanski AK, Pratt GB, Manson G, Weiss L: Clinodactyly, camptodactyly, Kirner's deformity, and other crooked fingers. Radiology 93:573–582, 1969.
9. Rodgers WB, Waters P: Incidence of trigger digits in newborns. J Hand Surg 19A:364–268, 1994.
10. Vickers D, Nielsen G: Madelung deformity: surgical prophylaxis (physiolysis) during the late growth period by resection of the dyschondrosteosis lesion. J Hand Surg 17B:401–407, 1992.

77. HAND INFECTIONS

Charles Douglas Wallace, M.D.

1. What are the hallmark signs of flexor tenosynovitis?

Kanavel's four cardinal signs of flexor tenosynovitis include (1) the digit being held in a slightly flexed posture, (2) fusiform uniform swelling along the finger (not localized), (3) intense pain on passive extension of the finger, and (4) tenderness that tracks along the course of the flexor tendon sheath, from the level of the distal interphalangeal joint down to the palm. The earliest and most sensitive sign is pain on passive extension of the finger. The most frequently found organisms include *Staphylococcus aureus, Streptococcus,* and *Pseudomonas.*

2. What are the most common organisms isolated from infections of the hand?

In one study, the most common organism cultured from hand infections was *Streptococcus,* followed by *Staphylococcus aureus, Staphylococcus epidermidis, Haemophilus parainfluenzae, Eikenella corrodens, Bacteroides melaninogenicus,* and *Peptostreptococcus.*

3. What is the best antibiotic coverage for a cat bite?

Bites from cats and dogs require coverage for an organism known as *Pasteurella multocida,* found in 50% of cat bite wounds. This gram-negative anaerobe can lead to *rapid onset* of signs and symptoms only 12–24 hours after inoculation. Penicillin is the agent of choice for these bites, coupled with a first-generation cephalosporin for improved staphylococcal coverage.

4. What is the best antibiotic coverage for a human bite?

The bite from a human can lead to infection with streptococci, staphylococci, *Eikenella, Neisseria, Bacteroides, Peptostreptococcus, Fusobacterium,* and *Veillonella. Eikenella corrodens* is resistant to cephalosporins and aminoglycosides, requiring penicillin for management. Because of frequent resistance to penicillin in some components of these polymicrobial infections, a semi-synthetic penicillin plus clavulanic acid is the drug of choice (Augmentin). Tetanus prophylaxis must be considered in every case and updated as indicated.

5. What are the deep spaces of the hand, and what is their significance in hand infections?
There are two deep bursal pockets in the hand that may become infected by direct inoculation, hematogenous seeding, or proximal extension of flexor terosynovitis. One of the thenar space, which is deep to the index flexor tendons and adjacent to the flexor pollicis longus tendon sheath. The other deep space is the midpalmar space, which is deep to the flexor tendons of the long, ring, and small fingers. A fibrous septum extending from the palmar fascia to the long-finger metacarpal separates these two spaces into distinct compartments. An infection of thenar space leads to pain and swelling over the thenar eminence and may abduct the thumb. A midpalmar space infection may cause swelling on the dorsum of the hand in addition to swelling on the palmar aspect.

6. What is the best way to drain a felon surgically?
Although fishmouth incisions have been advocated in the past, these leave a potentially painful

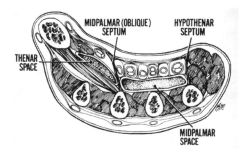

The potential midpalmar spaces. Reprinted with permission from Nevasier RJ: Infections. In Green, DP (ed): Operative Hand Surgery. New York, Churchill Livingstone, 1993.

scar on the tip of the finger. A better approach is the midlateral incision, with care to disrupt *intentionally* the fibrous septae that anchor the skin to the distal phalanx to assure adequate decompression of the abscess cavities.

7. What is the best way to decompress flexor tenosynovitis?
I prefer to use the two-incision technique. This involves feeding an irrigation catheter into the flexor tendon sheath proximal to the A-1 pulley in the palm (a #10 pediatric feeding tube is a good first try) and opening the flexor tendon sheath distally for flow-through irrigation. Saline (15–20 ml) is flushed through manually every 2–4 hours post-operatively for 36–72 hours (until the tenderness along the sheath abates).

Closed tendon sheath irrigation technique. Reprinted with permission from Nevasier RJ: Infections. In Green, DP (ed): Operative Hand Surgery. New York, Churchill Livingstone, 1993.

8. Does a septic wrist require open drainage?

The management of septic arthritis is controversial. Most surgeons feel that it is of great surgical urgency to decompress and lavage the joint. The literature also supports needle aspiration and effective antibiotic coverage. Needle aspiration may be successful in cases with low viscosity fluid, early diagnosis, and a patient willing to undergo as many serial aspirations as needed as often as needed to ensure clinical improvement. Herein lies the difficulty with needle aspiration of infected joints in children. This is the impetus to perform open irrigation of the joint, which also flushes away the neutrophil proteases and collagenases, followed by several days of suction drainage.

9. What are the sequelae of unrecognized septic arthritis of the wrist and hand?

As with septic arthritis of other joints, septic arthritis in the hand leads to proteoglycan loss, cartilage degeneration, and joint space narrowing or total loss. Pain and potential joint instability or stiffening and arthrodesis may result from unrecognized infection.

10. Does osteomyelitis occur in the hand?

Yes, generally secondary to an open fracture, rarely because of hematogenous seeding. Biopsy of the infection to determine the responsible organisms and to plan antibiotic choice and dosing is indicated. Remember the possibility of *Salmonella* in the young patient with sickle cell anemia and lytic changes in the bone.

11. What other conditions may mimic an infection in the hand?

Collagen vascular disease, foreign body reaction, inflammatory tenosynovitis, and neoplasms (very rarely). In the adult, one should also include gout and acute soft tissue calcification in the differential diagnosis.

12. What unusual infections can be seen in an infant's hand?

Herpetic whitlow can be found on the thumb or other digits frequently suckled by a child with herpes simplex infection of the mouth. The appearance of the affected digit is fairly characteristic, with multiple vesicles, some with clear fluid. Open vesicles are highly infectious. Tzanck smear should provide a diagnosis. Treatment is application of dry dressings and isolation of the digit until open vesicles close. Recurrent is anticipated, and superinfection of the whitlow with *Staphylococcus* may occur, indicating the need for oral antibiotic administration.

13. Are there any particular concerns in patients with *Varicella* infections?

Recently, patients with chickenpox have been noted to have a surprising incidence of necrotizing fasciitis and deep soft-tissue abscesses, which may extend distally to involve the forearm and hands, as well as septic arthritis and osteomyelitis. Group A beta-hemolytic streptococcus and *Staphylococcus aureus* are the primary causative organisms. Early aggressive management with débridement and lavage as well as appropriate antibiotic coverage is key to a successful outcome.

14. What is the best approach to drain a septic metacarpophalangeal joint?

An infection of the metacarpophalangeal (MCP) joint may occur owing to hematogenous seeding or direct inoculation, such as from a splinter or bite. Because of concerns regarding potential extensor tendon subluxation, the MCP joint should be approached from the dorsoulnar side, if possible.

15. Is there such a thing as extensor tenosynovitis?

This is arguable. A confined space containing the tendon and tenosynovium (i.e., the flexor sheath volarly) is required for this condition to occur. Certainly, infections of the dorsum of the hand and fingers can and do occur but would not be considered true extensor tenosynovitis. The passage beneath the extensor retinaculum is the only area in which a true tenosynovitis may occur, although this quite rare.

16. What is a horseshoe abscess?

An infection that originates in either the radial bursa (along the flexor pollicis longus) or the ulnar bursa (along the small finger flexors) may spread to the other bursae where they closely approximate each other at the wrist. The result is tenosynovitis of the thumb and small finger, which are connected near the carpal tunnel and thus form a horseshoe.

17. What is a collar-button abscess?

A collar-button abscess is in the region of the web space and often begins palmarly, spreading dorsally through the region of the transverse metacarpal ligament. The resulting dumbbell-shaped dual abscesses with connecting stalk inspired the name. These can progress to deep space infections in the palm if not adequately decompressed. Dorsal and volar incisions are necessary to address both areas.

BIBLIOGRAPHY

1. Burkhalter WE: Deep space infections. Hand Clin 5(4):553, 1989.
2. Freeland ARE, Senter BS: Septic arthritis and osteomyelitis. Hand Clin 5(4):533, 1989.
3. Neviaser RJ: Closed tendon sheath irrigation for pyogenic flexor tenosynovitis. J Hand Surg 3:462, 1978.
4. Neviaser RJ: Tenosynovitis. Hand Clin 5(4):525, 1989.
5. Schreck P, Schreck P, Bradley J, Chambers H: Musculoskeletal complications of Varicella. J Bone Joint Surg 78A:1713, 1996.

78. ARTHRITIS

David D. Sherry, M.D.

1. What is arthritis?

Arthritis is inflammation of the joint lining (synovium). The signs of inflammation include pain, warmth, swelling, redness, and limitation of function. Generally, two signs need to be present to define arthritis. Inflammatory synovial fluid is defined as that containing more than 2000 white blood cells per mm.^{3} The presence of pain alone is the definition of **arthralgia**.

2. How common is arthritis in childhood?

By various estimates, approximately 2 in 1000 children have arthritis. Arthritis is the second most common chronic condition in childhood. It is less frequent than epilepsy but more frequent than diabetes and cystic fibrosis.

3. What are some pitfalls in the initial evaluation of children with arthritis?

Frequently, physicians will think that a swollen joint is due to trauma (even without a history of injury). They will splint or cast the limb and wait for weeks for the swelling to subside. Recognizing the fact that young children get inflammatory joint disease is key. Also, physicians often will focus on the presenting joint and will not examine all the joints. Many children presenting with a single swollen joint will, on examination, have multiple-joint involvement. It is important to recognize that involved joints may have only subtle symptoms and signs of inflammation and may be painless. Many physicians also do not realize that migratory or episodic arthritis and arthralgia are features of childhood leukemia.

4. What are some tip-offs that indicate subtle joint inflammation?

Important symptoms include morning stiffness and stiffness after a nap or prolonged sitting (gelling). On examination, guarding is present, although complete range of motion may be preserved. Swelling may be minimal, so knowing the spectrum of what normal joints feel like is imperative.

5. What about painless arthritis?

The arthritis of children with juvenile rheumatoid arthritis (JRA) can be painless. Twenty-five percent of children with pauciarticular JRA may have absolutely no pain in their joints and are fully active. A few children with polyarticular or systemic-onset JRA have no pain. Sarcoidosis can also be painless and may involve multiple joints; therefore, in some patients, synovial biopsies are indicated.

6. Does painless arthritis need to be treated?

Yes. Children with painless arthritis can still develop joint contractures, muscle atrophy, and bony erosions leading to destruction of the joint.

7. What is juvenile chronic arthritis?

Chronic arthritis by definition is inflammation of the joint lasting longer than 6 weeks. Juvenile is defined as younger than 16 years old.

8. What kinds of chronic arthritis are seen most frequently in children?

Juvenile rheumatoid arthritis (pauciarticular, polyarticular, and systemic), spondyloarthopathies (Reiter's syndrome, reactive arthritis, juvenile-onset ankylosing spondylitis, and arthritis associated with inflammatory bowel disease), and psoriatic arthritis.

9. How does one classify juvenile rheumatoid arthritis?

Pauciarticular JRA involves four or fewer joints in the first 6 months of the illness. Polyarticular JRA involves five or more joints during the first 6 months of illness. Systemic JRA can involve any number of joints but is characterized by high spiking fevers, above 103°F (39.3°C).

10. What is the most common kind of JRA?

Pauciarticular (50%) is most common, followed by polyarticular (30%) and then systemic-onset (20%) arthritis.

11. What is the cause of JRA?

The cause is not known. Genetic factors seem to be closely associated with pauciarticular JRA (HLA DR 5 & 8) and with rheumatoid-factor-positive polyarticular JRA (HLA DR 4). Various infectious agents have been implicated, but proof of a causal relationship is lacking. Systemic JRA has many hallmarks of being an infection, but no one single agent has been identified.

12. What is the typical presentation of pauciarticular JRA?

Pauciarticular JRA commonly affects girls (80%); most are between the ages of 1 and 4 years. The most common joint involved is the knee, followed by the ankle and then the fingers. In 70% of these children, the antinuclear antibody (ANA) test will have positive results; almost all are rheumatoid factor negative. In 20%, there will be asymptomatic iritis, which can lead to blindness if untreated.

13. In the child with monoarticular arthritis, how can one be sure it is pauciarticular JRA?

Clues to pauciarticular JRA include a positive ANA test or the presence of chronic asymptomatic iritis. Other conditions have to be considered, especially pigmented villonodular synovitis and foreign body synovitis.

14. Can children with pauciarticular JRA present with hip or shoulder disease?

Only extremely rarely will children with pauciarticular JRA present with hip disease. Many of these children will require full antibiotic coverage so that one does not fail to treat a septic hip. Isolated shoulder disease virtually never occurs in pauciarticular JRA.

15. How should I look for iritis?

There are two kinds of iritis: chronic and acute. Chronic iritis is seen in JRA and acute iritis in those with spondyloarthropathy. Acute iritis is hard to miss—the child will have a very painful, red, photophobic eye and will seek help long before seeing an orthopaedist. Children with JRA, especially those with pauciarticular JRA, are at risk for developing chronic iritis that is totally painless and does not cause a red eye. When they present with arthritis, their eyes should be closely examined in a darkened room to make sure that the pupil is round. If there is any suggestion of irregularity, immediate ophthalmologic consultation is indicated.

16. How frequently does a patient with JRA need to see an ophthalmologist?

It depends on the child's age, type of onset, and ANA test results. Children with systemic-onset JRA need a slit lamp examination of their eyes yearly. Children who are younger than 7 years old and are ANA positive need an examination every 3–4 months for 4 years, then every 6 months for 3 years, then yearly. If the ANA is negative, they need an examination every 6 months for 7 years, then yearly. If they are older than 7 years at the onset, regardless of ANA result, an examination is needed only every 6 months for 4 years, then yearly.

17. What is the difference between iritis, iridocyclitis, and uveitis?

Many authors use these terms interchangeably. The uveal tract consists of the iris, ciliary body, and choroid. By strict definition, iritis is inflammation of the iris, iridocyclitis is inflammation of the iris and ciliary body, and uveitis is inflammation of the entire uveal tract.

18. How is iritis treated?

Steroid eyedrops and a mydriatic. Occasionally, steroid injection or immunosuppressant therapy is required.

19. What is the typical presentation of polyarticular JRA?

There are two typical groups of children who develop polyarticular JRA. The first are young girls 1–4 years of age with multiple small- and large-joint involvement. Usually, the joint involvement is symmetric. In 50%, ANA results are positive, and most are rheumatoid factor negative. Less frequently, this is complicated by asymptomatic iritis. The second are adolescent girls, again with large and small joints involved in a symmetric pattern. Up to half these girls are rheumatoid factor positive, and few are ANA positive. Rarely will these children develop asymptomatic iritis.

20. What is the typical presentation of systemic JRA?

Both boys and girls get systemic-onset JRA in equal numbers, usually between the ages of 3 and 10 years. They have high spiking fevers that start in the evenings, peak at night, and return to normal or below normal in the morning. When these children are febrile, they are very toxic appearing, have severe myalgias and arthralgias, and develop a fleeting small red macular rash, generally on the trunk. They may have sore throats and stiff necks, causing one to suspect meningitis. Other symptoms include enlarged lymph nodes (especially the axillary nodes), enlarged liver and spleen, pericarditis, myocarditis, and disseminated intravascular coagulation.

These children are rarely seen by the orthopaedist, since they tend to develop arthritis later in the course of illness (and may never get chronic arthritis).

21. What is the typical presentation of spondyloarthropathies?

These usually occur in older children (8 years of age or older) who present with predominantly lower-extremity arthritis. Both large and small joints of the legs and feet may be involved. Enthesitis is a frequent finding and most commonly occurs at the plantar fascial insertion, metatarsal heads, and sacroiliac joints. It is slightly more common in boys. Often, there is a family history of low back pain, although the parents may not readily identify back spasms or back pain that they think is due to injury as being significant. Also, ask about a family history of heel pain or spurs or of bursitis.

22. What is the cause of spondyloarthropathies?
Both genetic and infectious agents have been very closely associated with the development of spondyloarthropathies. The HLA-B27 gene (or closely linked allele) is a strong marker for the disease. In children, Reiter's and reactive arthritis frequently follow gastrointestinal infections by *Campylobacter, Salmonella, Shigella*, and *Yersinia*. In adults, there has been an association with *Klebsiella* and ankylosing spondylitis.

23. What blood tests should one order for a child with arthritis?
It is useful to obtain a complete blood count, erythrocyte sedimentation rate (or C-reactive protein), ANA, and rheumatoid factor. The vast majority of children are rheumatoid factor negative, so this test is generally more useful in older girls with polyarticular involvement who may have early-onset adult rheumatoid arthritis. Testing for HLA-B27 is helpful in children suspected of having spondyloarthopathy, since it is associated with a poorer outcome (and thus requires early aggressive treatment) and may also help confirm the diagnosis. Urinalysis can be helpful if Reiter's syndrome is suspected, since the child may have sterile pyuria without dysuria.

24. Should I get a serum uric acid level?
No. Gout or other crystal disease is almost unknown in childhood.

25. How is the arthritis portion of JRA treated?
The aim is to control the synovitis. In children with a limited number of joints involved, directly treating the joint with intra-articular corticosteroid injection (triamcinolone hexacetonide) is most useful. Generally, 1 ml (20 mg) is used in large and medium joints and lesser amounts in the smaller joints. As much as 1 mg//kg can be used in bigger children. Children with more widespread joint involvement require early treatment with methotrexate, sulfasalazine, or hydroxychloroquine to try to control the arthritis. Nonsteroidal agents are given for symptomatic relief. If a few joints continue to be inflamed, intra-articular injections can be helpful. Children with systemic JRA may require oral or parenteral corticosteroids and aggressive anti-inflammatory and immunosuppressive therapy. These children require the services of a pediatric rheumatologist.

26. How does one treat spondyloarthropathies?
If there are a limited number of involved joints, intra-articular corticosteroid injections can be used. More widespread disease may be controlled with disease-modifying agents such as sulfasalazine and methotrexate. Nonsteroidal medications are used for symptomatic relief.

27. How does one treat enthesitis?
I prefer to use indomethacin, sulindac, diclofenac, or piroxicam. Other nonsteroidal agents may be useful as well. Some patients will respond to one and not another, so several may need to be tried. Shoe inserts or heel cups to redistribute weight around tender entheses can be of great help. Injections of the entheses are fraught with difficulties and should be done only as a last resort (if at all). Occasionally, the enthesitis is severe enough to require therapy with methotrexate or sulfasalazine.

28. Are there any differences between nonsteroidal agents?
Yes. One child may respond nicely to one and not another. I prefer to use once- or twice-daily medications for most children, although liquid preparations (like ibuprofen) are useful in younger children. I rarely use naproxen, especially in fair-skinned children, owing to its association with facial scarring. I prefer indomethacin, sulindac, diclofenac, or piroxicam for the spondy-

loarthropathies and for enthesitis. An adequate therapeutic trial for each agent is 3–4 weeks at full therapeutic doses.

29. What laboratory tests are indicated for those on nonsteroidal medication?

Complete blood count (for anemia and leukopenia), aspartate aminotransferase (for hepatotoxicity), and creatinine along with urine analysis (for nephrotoxicity). These should be checked after the first month or two of therapy and then every 6–12 months (more frequently in younger children).

30. What are the side effects of intra-articular steroid injections?

The most common side effect is subcutaneous atrophy and hypopigmentation at the site of injection. This can be minimized by placing the medication well within the joint and, perhaps, limiting activity for a day or two afterward. The subcutaneous fat regrows, but this may take several years. Occasionally, the medication is irritating to the joint, and the child will have increased pain starting on the day of injection. The pain lasts 2–3 days, but the arthritis usually still subsides. Rarely (estimated to be 1:50,000 injections) septic arthritis can occur. This would manifest a few days postinjection with typical symptoms and signs of infection. Juxta-articular calcifications can occur but usually do not interfere with joint function. They are incidentally noted on subsequent radiographs. After a joint injection, the child will be steroid suppressed for about a month; if general anesthesia is required, appropriate replacement is prudent.

31. How does one inject a joint in a small child in the office?

Small children, usually those younger than 6 years old, are frequently given conscious sedation with oral midazolam, 0.25 mg/kg. After about 15 minutes, the child will become somewhat stupefied and relaxed. The joint is cleaned three times, with povidone-iodine and once with alcohol. While spraying ethyl chloride at the site, I place 1 ml of buffered lidocaine (2 ml of sodium bicarbonate in a 10-ml vial of lidocaine) under the skin as deep as a 30-gauge needle will go. Then a 1.5" 20- or 22-gauge needle is placed in the knee. Synovial fluid is aspirated and placed in an EDTA (purple top) tube. The syringe is changed to the one with medication, and the medication is injected. It should flow with ease. It is helpful, especially if repeated injections are needed, to reward the child with a small gift.

32. How frequently should one inject a joint?

We do not like to reinject the same joint more than three times within 12 months or eight or so times in total. The response to the first injection does not predict the response to the second. Rarely, the synovitis will recur quickly. If so, reinjection is indicated, since its effect may last more than a year.

33. What tests are useful on the synovial fluid that is aspirated?

Put the synovial fluid in an EDTA (purple top) or heparinized (green top) tube for cell count and differential analysis. Most children with JRA have synovial fluid cell counts of 5000–25,000. Children with systemic-onset JRA, however, can have joint fluid white blood cell counts exceeding 100,000, as can children with acute rheumatic fever. Synovial fluid protein is not helpful, nor is glucose unless infection is suspected. Culture and Gram's staining are indicated if one is concerned about possible infection. Crystal analysis is rarely indicated, since crystal disease is virtually absent in childhood.

34. What is the outcome of chronic childhood arthritis?

The arthritis can be controlled in most children. The majority (about 80%) with pauciarticular JRA generally do well but may need treatment for many years. Older children with polyarticular JRA, especially if they are rheumatoid factor positive, tend to have long-lasting disease and are at higher risk for developing erosive joint disease. Systemic JRA is both the best and the worst kind to have. In many of these children, all systemic and arthritic problems resolve after a few months to a year or so. Others have continuing destructive arthritis and frequently will require joint replacement or fusion. Although systemic JRA accounts for only 20% of all cases of JRA, 90% of those re-quiring wheelchairs and joint replacements have systemic JRA. A few children with spondy-loarthropathies will do poorly. These generally are boys with early-onset hip disease who are HLA-B27 positive.

35. In spondyloarthropathy, what (besides HLA-B27) portends a worse outcome?
Early hip disease is a poor prognostic sign. Boys tend to fare worse than girls.

36. What are the orthopaedic complications of chronic childhood arthritis?
Younger children, especially those with unilateral knee involvement, can develop overgrowth and leg-length discrepancy with an ipsilateral long leg. In older preadolescent patients who have unilateral knee involvement, the epiphysis can prematurely fuse, and they can end up with a contralateral long leg. Rarely, joint involvement can lead to subluxation. A few patients will have destructive arthritis and degenerative joint disease and will require joint replacement or fusion.

37. What is the role of synovectomy?
It is rarely indicated. It does not lead to improved joint function or long-lasting remission. How-ever, there are a few patients with a very recalcitrant joint who may benefit from synovectomy.

38. What should the family be told?
Initially, the family needs to be reassured that the child will do well and that most children with arthritis will not end up crippled. Let them know that there are numerous treatments and that most of the time the arthritis can be controlled. Prompt referral to a specialist on a multidisciplinary team who can care for both the child and the family is indicated.

39. Who should manage the problem?
Most children with chronic arthritis are best managed by a pediatric rheumatologist along with a host of pediatric health care specialists, depending on the need, including ophthalmologists, or-thopaedic surgeons, physical therapists, occupational therapists, nurse specialists, social workers, psychologists, nutritionists, and others. If a pediatric rheumatologist is not available in the area, an adult rheumatologist with experience in childhood arthritis should be consulted.

40. What are danger signs?
Red joints are extremely rare in JRA and should alert one to think of infection or another disease (such as rheumatic fever, Reiter's syndrome, lupus, leukemia, Kawasaki disease, or polyarteritis nodosa). A marked degree of disability is also rarely due to arthritis and should lead the physi-cian to consider such possibilities as subtle fractures, osteomyelitis, leukemia, disproportional pain, and tumor.

41. What are the tip-offs in distinguishing leukemia from JRA?
Most children with leukemia fall outside the typical spectrum of presentation of JRA. Specifi-cally, they are disproportionately sick or disabled, and have bone pain, episodic or migratory arthritis, hip arthritis, and nocturnal waking due to pain (especially waking after midnight). Look for discordant laboratory tests that suggest leukemia, such as a high erythrocyte sedimentation rate with normal or low white blood cell count or normal-to-low platelet count. Disproportionate anemia is also suggestive. Children with Down syndrome are especially worrisome.

BIBLIOGRAPHY

1. Cassidy JT, Petty RE: Textbook of Pediatric Rheumatology, 3rd ed. Philadelphia, W.B. Saunders, 1995.
2. Sherry DD, Mosca VS: Juvenile rheumatoid arthritis and seronegative spondyloarthropathies. In Morrissy RT, Weinstein SL (eds): Lovell & Winter's Pediatric Orthopaedics, 4th ed. Philadelphia, Lippincott-Raven, 1996, pp 393–421.

79. TUMOR EVALUATION

Ernest U. Conrad III, M.D.

1. Pediatric bone and soft tissue tumors are extremely unusual. Why is this an important topic?

While malignant tumors of bone and soft tissue are unusual, they are not rare. The typical orthopaedist will see several primary sarcomas of bone or soft tissue in his lifetime and many benign tumors. Early diagnosis and effective treatment are curative in 70–80% of children. In addition to malignant tumors or sarcomas of the musculoskeletal system, there are a large number of benign tumors that are relatively common and a source of great morbidity because of a high local recurrence rate and a high fracture rate. When these tumors occur in children, the consequences are dramatic. Early appropriate treatment is very effective. A late diagnosis or ineffective treatment will result in the loss of life, limb, or deformity; the risk of multiple procedures; or prolonged rehabilitation.

2. What are the most common musculoskeletal tumors in children?

Benign bone tumors such as the unicameral bone cyst or simple cyst, aneurysmal bone cyst,

(Left) Right proximal femoral lesion in an 18-year-old soccer player who presents with a 2-month history of hip pain. (Middle) Bone scan of the 18-year-old patient shown in previous figure. Increased uptake is seen, which is extremely suggestive of osteosarcoma (confirmed by biopsy). (Right) Distal femoral abnormalities with an eccentric metaphyseal lesion with sclerotic margins consistent with nonossifying fibroma.

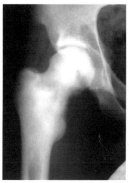
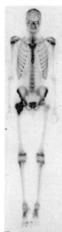
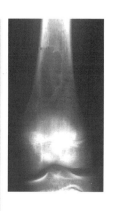

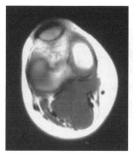
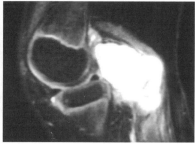

Soft tissue mass in an 8-year-old with a 10-month history of knee flexion contracture initially treated as arthritis! Popliteal mass biopsy consistent with synovial sarcoma.

and exostoses of the skeleton. Another common benign bone tumor is nonossifying fibroma, which involves the cortex of bone and is associated with a relatively high incidence of fractures.

Tumors of the soft tissues are most commonly benign lipomas, hemangiomas, or lymphangiomas. These benign soft tissue tumors are also a source of significant diagnostic challenge, morbidity, and treatment failure. Another soft tissue tumor sometimes referred to as "benign" is desmoid tumor, or fibromatosis, which behaves like a low-grade malignancy, with the highest rate of local recurrence of musculoskeletal tumors.

The most important message to convey to parents is the relatively high risk of local recurrence (10–20%) of benign soft-tissue tumors. These "benign" soft tissue tumors are also a source of significant diagnostic challenge. Approximately half of all soft tissue sarcomas are rhabdomyosarcoma, and other soft tissue sarcomas require similar treatment (chemotherapy, surgery, and radiation-therapy protocols).

Malignant soft tissue sarcomas may be recognized by the following clinical characteristics: most soft tissue sarcomas are larger than 5 cm in diameter, firmer or denser than normal muscle, nontender, and deep to the superficial fascia. Tumors with those characteristics should be evaluated with an MRI.

3. Are there certain pediatric age groups at risk for certain tumors?

Clearly, adolescents are most at risk for osteosarcoma, with a peak age of 14 years, and Ewing's sarcoma, with a peak age of 12 years. Young children (less than 10 years of age) are at less risk for sarcoma although at greater risk for a benign bone tumor, a benign soft tissue tumor, or an infection. When these tumors are located adjacent to an active physeal growth plate, the risk of growth plate injury becomes a potential significant problem. Because they are at greater risk, adolescents should be evaluated with greater caution when presenting with knee pain.

4. What is the typical history in a child presenting with osteosarcoma? How should it be evaluated?

A child with osteosarcoma will typically have deep-seated pain that is worse at night and is not typically related to physical activity. Other benign tumors may also be associated with night pain, such as osteoid osteoma. The typical history of pain in a child with osteosarcoma involves a 3-month interval of time. Children or adolescents with bony pain lasting 6 weeks or longer should be evaluated with a bone scan if a diagnosis is not clinically obvious.

Teenagers with persistent knee pain are the highest risk group development of osteosarcoma. Patients presenting with knee pain should be evaluated with a careful clinical exam and plain radiographs. Determining where the pain is located is an important and challenging part of the initial evaluation. The typical patient with osteosarcoma presents with pain of several months' duration. The distal femur is the most common location. If the plain x-ray is nondiagnostic and bony pain persists, then a technetium bone scan should be obtained for patients with undiagnosed bony pain.

Patients with persistent pain and an equivocal bone scan should either be followed closely (every 2–3 weeks) or evaluated further with an MRI. While MRI is not the best initial screening test, it is a good study for all osteosarcomas in determining the exact extent of bony and soft tissue involvement. As a general rule, a CT scan is the preferred imaging technique for bony abnormalities, and MRI is clearly the best imaging study for soft tissue tumors.

5. How do you distinguish a simple bone cyst from a malignant bone tumor on plain x-rays?

I evaluate three x-ray characteristics: location, margin, and density of the lesion. The location of the lesion refers to its bony location (metaphyseal, epiphyseal, or diaphyseal) and whether the abnormality is centrally located or eccentric. The margin or bony interface refers to whether or not the tumor is surrounded by reactive bone. The density of the center of the abnormality refers to the radiographic appearance of the content of the lesion (lucent, empty, calcified, or osteoblastic). The anatomic location of the tumor will give some indication of which diagnosis is most likely (e.g., an eccentric cortical-metaphyseal lesion with a sclerotic margin is suggestive of nonossifying fibroma).

The bony margin reflects the interaction of the tumor with adjacent host bone. Slow-growing or inactive tumors will be surrounded by a sclerotic margin. Fast-growing tumors will have little to no surrounding bony margin or reaction because the tumor's growth rate is faster than the bony reaction. The density of the abnormality will give some indication of the contents of the tumor. Osseous tumors (osteoblastic), cartilage (calcified) lesions, and empty or cystic lesions (ABC, cystic) can be identified.

6. What is "staging" of musculoskeletal tumors?
The assessment of the extent of disease. For benign tumors, that refers to the local anatomic containment of a benign aggressive tumor or its degree of cellular activity. For malignant tumors, staging refers to the tumor's "containment via adjacent tissues," its degree of histologic activity (histologic "grade"), and whether or not there is metastatic disease.

7. What laboratory tests are useful for making the diagnosis of osteosarcoma?
Blood studies are an essential part of the work-up of bony pediatric abnormalities. This is particularly true for children younger than the age or 10 years with bony abnormalities that include osteomyelitis in the differential diagnosis. Studies such as complete blood count, erythrocyte sedimentation rate, and C-reactive protein are important in the assessment of possible osteomyelitis.

The only blood test helpful at this point in time is alkaline phosphatase level, which is elevated in more than half of all patients with osteosarcoma. New molecular studies are receiving attention as diagnostic studies for some sarcomas.

8. How should I evaluate a child with a soft tissue "mass"?
Most soft-tissue masses in children are benign. Benign soft tissue masses are usually small, soft, and superficial. Soft tissue masses that are larger than 5 cm (in diameter), firmer than muscle, and deep are more likely to represent a sarcoma and should be evaluated with an MRI and biopsy. Small (smaller than 5 cm), soft, superficial soft tissue tumors are usually benign and may be excised with or without preoperative imaging. Masses that are 5 cm in diameter or larger should be evaluated with an MRI *prior* to biopsy or resection. Incisional or needle biopsy by a surgeon with experience in tumors is recommended *prior* to excision of these larger masses.

Soft tissue cysts are one of the more common soft tissue tumors in children younger than the age of 10 years. These cysts typically occur behind the knee or in the calf. They should be transilluminated to confirm that they are fluid filled. Masses that truly contain clear fluid are rarely malignant. The excision of these cysts is elective and not always indicated.

9. A patient has an MRI demonstrating a large (10-cm) soft tissue tumor. How should the patient be managed?
The patient should be managed with an open or needle biopsy done in the operating room by a surgeon with experience with soft tissue tumors. If that biopsy is diagnostic for a high-grade soft tissue sarcoma, careful consideration should be given to the delivery of preoperative chemotherapy prior to resection of the mass. The most common location for soft tissue sarcomas is the thigh, and teenagers are also at greater risk for developing soft tissue sarcomas than younger children. Benign or low-grade soft tissue tumors are appropriately managed with resection after frozen-section biopsy. Careful resection of benign soft tissue masses is important, since the risk of local recurrence is high.

10. What are the most common errors in diagnosing osteosarcoma?
(1) Failure to recognize the nature or anatomic location of persistent bony pain in an adolescent. (2) Failure to get good radiographs that are interpreted properly. (3) Failure to carry out an appropriate biopsy prior to resection.

Be aware of the risk of malignancies in all children with undiagnosed bony pain. Be careful with regard to the initial history and exam. These are probably the most important first steps leading to an accurate and early diagnosis.

BIBLIOGRAPHY

1. Downing JR, Khandekar A, Shurtleff SA, et al.: Multiplex RT-PCR assay for the differential diagnosis
   of alveolar rhabdomyosarcoma and Ewing's sarcoma. Am J Pathol 146(3):626–634, 1995.
2. Mankin HJ, Lange TA, Spanier SS: The hazards of biopsy in patients with malignant primary bone and
   soft-tissue tumors. J Bone Joint Surg 64A:1121–1127, 1982.
3. Schmale GA, Conrad EU, Raskind WH: The natural history of hereditary multiple exostoses. J Bone Joint
   Surg 76A(7):986–992, 1994.
4. Simon MA: Current concepts review. Causes of increased survival of patients with osteosarcoma: current controversies. J Bone Joint Surg 66A:306–310, 1984.

80. BONE TUMORS

James D. Bruckner, M.D.

1. What are the most common bone tumors in children younger than age 5?

Primary bone tumors are uncommon in children younger than the age of 5. The differential diagnosis of a destructive lesion of bone in this age group includes osteomyelitis, leukemia, Langerhans' cell hystiocytosis (eosinophilic granuloma), and metastatic neuroblastoma.

2. What are the most common bone tumors in children between the ages of 5 and 10?

The most common benign tumors are simple bone cyst, Langerhans' cell histiocytosis, and fibrous
dysplasia. The most common malignant bone tumors are Ewing's sarcoma and osteogenic sarcoma. Leukemia presenting as a metaphyseal destructive process and osteomyelitis must also be
kept in mind.

3. What are the most common bone tumors in children between the ages of 10 and 20?

The most common benign tumors are osteoid osteoma and osteoblastoma, aneurysmal bone cyst,
nonossifying fibroma, enchondroma, osteochondroma, and chondroblastoma. The most common
malignant bone tumors are osteosarcoma and Ewing's sarcoma.

4. What primary benign bone tumor occurs in the epiphysis or apophysis of the growing child?

Chondroblastoma.

5. Which bone tumors in children occur in the metaphysis of long bones?

Any of the benign and malignant bone tumors that occur in children can occur in the metaphysis
with the exception of chondroblastoma, although this tumor can cross the epiphyseal growth plate
into the metaphysis. Ewing's sarcoma occurs in the metaphysis in 10% of cases, presenting atyp-
ically as a geographic lytic process without a significant soft tissue mass.

6. Which bone tumors in children occur in the diaphysis?

Ossifying fibroma of Campanacci, Langerhans' cell histiocytosis, osteoid osteoma or osteoblastoma, and Ewing's sarcoma.

7. What are the four "classic questions" of Enneking with regard to the radiologic evalu-ation of any bone tumor?

Where is the lesion? What is it doing to the bone? What is the bone doing to it? Are there any intrinsic clues to the histologic diagnosis?

8. What are the common benign bone-forming lesions in children?
Osteoid osteoma and osteoblastoma.

9. What are the common malignant bone-forming tumors in children?
Osteosarcoma.

10. What are the benign cartilage-forming tumors in children?
Enchondroma, periosteal or juxtacortical chondroma, osteochondroma, chondromyxoid fibroma, and chondroblastoma.

11. What are the common malignant cartilage-forming tumors in children?
Malignant cartilage-forming tumors in children are extraordinarily rare.

12. What are the common fibrous and fibrohistiocytic tumors in children?
Nonossifying fibroma, fibrous cortical defect (metaphyseal fibrous defect), fibrous dysplasia, and osteofibrous dysplasia.

13. What are the common tumors of vascular tissue in children?
Benign lesions include hemangioma and lymphangioma. Malignant lesions include hemangioendothelioma, angiosarcoma, and hemangiopericytoma.

14. What are the common hematopoietic tumors in children?
Benign lesions include the entire spectrum of Langerhans' cell histiocytosis. Malignant lesions include Hodgkin's disease and leukemia.

15. What are the common tumors of neural origin in children?
Benign lesions include neurofibroma, neurilemoma, and neurofibromatosis. Malignant lesions include malignant schwannoma, Ewing's sarcoma, and primitive neuroectodermal tumor (PNET).

16. What are the common malignant tumors of muscle in children?
Rhabdomyosarcoma.

17. What are the common tumors of adipose tissue of children?
Lipoma and angiolipoma.

18. What are the bone tumors of unknown origin that occur in children?
Simple bone cyst and aneurysmal bone cyst.

19. How does one establish a differential diagnosis for any lesion of bone in a child?
Based on the age of the child, the bone involved, the geographic location of the lesion within the bone, and the radiographic characteristics of the lesion as determined by Enneking's four "classic questions."

20. What is the typical clinical presentation of a unicameral (simple) bone cyst?
A well-marginated lucent lesion of bone occurring most commonly in the metaphysis of the proximal humerus or femur in children between the ages of 5 and 20. The lesions are painless unless a pathologic fracture has occurred or weightbearing bone is involved.

21. What is the typical diagnostic radiographic feature of a unicameral bone cyst?
The fallen fragment sign. If a pathologic fracture has occurred, a small piece of cortex may break loose and fall to the dependent portion of the lesion, confirming its fluid-filled nature.

22. What is the differential diagnosis of a unicameral bone cyst?
Aneurysmal bone cyst is typically a more aggressive benign lesion that is refractory to the conservative treatment methods usually employed in the management of simple bone cysts.

23. What is the treatment of a unicameral bone cyst?
If a pathologic fracture has occurred, the cyst should be allowed first to heal. Then treatment is begun. A large number of surgical and nonsurgical treatments have been employed for this lesion in the past. Regardless of treatment selected, local recurrence rates are high. The most popular nonsurgical treatment is dual-needle cyst aspiration and steroid injection. Surgical treatment of a simple bone cyst refractory to nonsurgical management is curettage, cryosurgery, and grafting with autologous or allogeneic cancellous bone.

24. What other important clinical ramifications do these lesions have in growing children?
Simple bone cysts have been associated with limb undergrowth when they abut the epiphyseal plate, regardless of treatment or presence of pathologic fracture.

25. What is the typical clinical presentation of a nonossifying fibroma?
A male or female between the ages of 10 and 20 with an asymptomatic, often incidentally found metaphyseal eccentric lucent lesion, most likely in the distal femur, distal tibia, or proximal tibia. Multiple lesions may be present. There is almost universally a sclerotic rim with a periosteal shell. Lesions may present in various stages of healing. Pathologic fractures can occur if lesions are large enough.

26. What is the treatment of nonossifying fibroma?
Most nonossifying fibromas can be observed if they are asymptomatic. Large lesions occupying more than 30% of the diameter of the bone involved, particularly if they are elongated and show no evidence of healing, should be considered at risk for pathologic fracture and treated. Symptomatic lesions of any size should be treated. Treatment consists of curettage and grafting with autologous or allogeneic cancellous bone. Adjuvant cyrosurgery or phenolization is not necessary.

27. What are the three diseases that compose the clinical spectrum of Langerhans' cell histiocytosis?
Eosinophilic granuloma, Hand-Schüller-Christian disease, and Letterer-Siwe disease.

28. What is a typical clinical presentation of eosinophilic granuloma?
Painful permeative lytic lesion of bone involving any bone of the body in any location in the bone, often associated with "onionskin" periosteal reaction. The skull is commonly affected. Lesions are polyostotic in 15–20% of cases. Most common in the first and second decades, they can be seen up to age 60.

29. What is the approiate initial evaluation of a patient presenting with an apparent eosinophilic granuloma?
Technetium bone scan, skull x-ray, and careful physical examination for evidence of organomegaly or diabetes insipidus.

30. What is the typical clinical presentation of eosinophilic granuloma in the spine?
Vertebra plana.

31. What is the differential diagnosis of vertebra plana in a child?
Eosinophilic granuloma and Ewing's sarcoma.

32. What are the distinguishing characteristics of eosinophilic granuloma and Ewing's sarcoma when they present as vertebra plana?

Eosinophilic granuloma presenting as vertebral plana typically does not have an associated soft tissue mass. Ewing's sarcoma rarely presents as vertebra plana. When it does, it typically has an associated soft tissue mass. Vertebra plana consistent with eosinophilic granuloma does not routinely require biopsy, while vertebra plana associated with a soft tissue mass does.

33. What is the treatment of eosinophilic granuloma in the extremities?

Local curettage is usually curative. Recurrence rates are less than 10%.

34. What is the treatment of eosinophilic granuloma presenting as vertebra plana?

In the thoracolumbar spine, if symptoms are minimal, observation is indicated and spontaneous resolution is the rule. In the cervical spine, low-dose radiation therapy is usually recommended.

35. What is the typical clinical presentation of Hand-Schüller-Christian disease?

A child age 3–10 presenting with a single lesion or multiple osseous lesions, hepatosplenomegaly, anemia, exophthalmos, and possibly diabetes insipidus.

36. What is the typical clinical presentation of a child with Letterer-Siwe disease?

A child younger than the age of 3 with progressive multisystem involvement including hepatosplenomegaly, pulmonary disease, and anemia, usually leading to death.

37. What is the treatment of a patient with Hand-Schüller-Christian or Letterer-Siwe disease?

Chemotherapy and corticosteroids.

38. What are the classic histologic features seen in eosinophilic granuloma?

Langerhans' cell histiocytes are large cells with an indented or folded nucleus and abundant pale eosinophilic cytoplasm. Eosinophils are also seen.

39. Describe the typical clinical presentation of osteoid osteoma or osteoblastoma.

Most commonly, a male presenting with a characteristic history of osseous pain, typically pain at rest and at night, that is relieved by aspirin or nonsteroidal anti-inflammatory medication.

40. What are the typical radiographic findings in osteoid osteoma?

Fusiform cortical thickening and sclerosis with a tiny central lucency (the nidus).

41. What other diagnostic modalities are useful in the evaluation of this osseous lesion?

Technetium bone scan and high-resolution CT will often reveal the nidus if it is not visible on plain x-ray. Radionuclide uptake in the technetium bone scan is usually intense.

42. What is the treatment of osteoid osteoma?

En bloc excision of the radiolucent nidus with bone grafting when indicated.

43. How does the clinical presentation of osteoblastoma differ from osteoid osteoma?

The central lucent nidus is larger, usually greater than 1 cm, and may contain a central density. This lesion is common in the spine, usually the posterior vertebral elements. It usually occurs in older teenagers or young adults.

44. What is the treatment of osteoblastoma?

Ideally, en bloc resection when possible. If this would lead to excessive morbidity, curettage and adjuvant local treatment with cryosurgery or phenolization followed by cancellous bone grafting are acceptable.

45. What is the typical clinical presentation and radiographic appearance of enchondroma?

Older teenager or young adult presenting with an asymptomatic lesion brought to attention by x-ray of a nearby symptomatic joint. The small bones of the hands, distal femur, and proximal humerus are the most common sites.

The typical radiographic appearance is a central geographic intramedullary lesion with occasional endosteal scalloping and intralesional calcifications. The lesion calcification pattern has been described as punctate, popcorn-like, and rings and arcs.

46. What is the treatment of enchondroma?

Observation. In the adult, these lesions must be distinguished from low-grade chondrosarcoma. This distinction is made based on evidence of lesional growth (which should not occur in adulthood) that is marked by increasing lucency in a previously mineralized tumor, cortical erosion, soft tissue mass, and pain. Biopsy is generally not helpful in distinguishing low-grade chondrosarcoma from enchondroma.

47. What is Ollier's disease?

Multiple enchondromatosis typically occurring in a unilateral distribution.

48. What is Maffucci's syndrome?

Multiple enchondromatosis associated with multiple soft tissue hemangiomas. Malignant degeneration of enchondromas into chondrosarcomas in adulthood is much more common in Ollier's disease and Maffucci's syndrome than in solitary enchondromas.

49. What is a typical clinical presentation of an aneurysmal bone cyst?

Painful lytic lesion occurring in almost any bone in the body, usually associated with swelling.

50. What are the distinctive radiographic features of an aneurysmal bone cyst?

A radiolucent lesion with ballooning or aneurysmal expansion of the affected bone. A thin rim of reactive bone is often seen. An aggressive destructive appearance is common in young children.

51. What pathologic features distinguish an aneurysmal bone cyst from a simple bone cyst?

Aneurysmal bone cysts contain hemorrhagic, fleshy, solid aggregates of tissue interspersed with cystic spaces containing blood. Simple bone cysts contain very little, if any, tissue about their reactive shell and are often filled with clear yellow fluid.

52. What highly malignant bone tumor in children can mimic the radiographic appearance of an aneurysmal bone cyst?

Telangiectatic osteogenic sarcoma.

53. What is the treatment of an aneurysmal bone cyst?

Curettage with local adjuvant therapy such as cryosurgery or phenol, and autograft or allograft reconstruction.

54. What is the typical clinical presentation of an osteochondroma?

A child, usually older than age 10 with a juxta-articular osseous mass. The most common locations are distal femur, proximal humerus, and proximal tibia. Pain may be present as a result of irritation of overlying tendons or muscles.

55. What are the diagnostic radiographic features of osteochondroma?

A pedunculated or sessile projection of bone from the metaphysis of a long bone. Continuity of cortical and cancellous bone of the lesion with that of the underlying metaphysis. This radiographic feature will distinguish exostosis from myositis ossificans and parosteal osteosarcoma.

56. What are the principal pathologic features of osteochondroma?
Normal cortical and cancellous bone structure with a thin cartilaginous cap.

57. What is the treatment of osteochondroma?
Observation unless the lesion is symptomatic. Lesions that are irritating overlying muscles or tendons may be treated by simple excision. Local recurrence will occur if the cartilage cap is incompletely excised. In the very young child, lesions occur very near the growth plate from which they arise. The cartilage cap may be in continuity with the growth plate. Injury to the growth plate must be avoided, and local recurrence rates are higher.

58. What is the typical clinical presentation of chondroblastoma?
A child older than the age of 10, and occasionally young adults, presenting with a painful lesion located in the epiphysis or apophysis of a long bone, most commonly the proximal humerus (Codman's tumor), distal femur, proximal tibia, or proximal femur. Trochanteric apophysis and triradiate cartilage occasionally give rise to these lesions.

59. What are the typical radiographic features of chondroblastoma?
Well-marginated geographic lytic lesion with a sclerotic rim, occasional expansion of the epiphysis or apophysis, and matrix calcification in 25% of cases.

60. What are the characteristic histologic features of this lesion?
Numerous ovoid polyhedral chondroblasts with multinucleated giant cells, islands of chondroid, and a characteristic pattern of matrix production by the chondroblasts, which gives rise to the so-called "cobblestone appearance." Mineralization of this matrix will lead to the observation of "chicken wire calcification."

61. What is the treatment of chondroblastoma?
Curettage with local adjuvant therapy such as cryosurgery or phenolization followed by bone grafting. Local recurrence rate is 10–20%.

62. What is the typical clinical presentation of fibrous dysplasia in the child?
A child older than the age of 10 presenting with a metaphyseal or diaphyseal lytic bone lesion characterized by cortical expansion, sharp margination, and occasionally deformity or pathologic fracture. Metaphyseal and diaphyseal long bones are commonly involved. Rib lesions are common. Polyostotic disease is common.

63. What is Albright's syndrome?
Polyostotic fibrous dysplasia associated with cutaneous pigmentation and precocious puberty in girls.

64. What is the treatment of fibrous dysplasia?
Observation for asymptomatic lesions. Symptomatic lesions or those associated with deformity may be treated by curettage and grafting, usually with a cortical allograft. Extensive involvement of long bones may be successfully treated with long-term intramedullary stabilization and osteotomy to correct deformity.

65. What is the typical clinical presentation of osteofibrous dysplasia in the child?
Pain and swelling in the leg in a child younger than age 10, occasionally associated with anterior bowing of the tibia. Occasionally associated with a soft tissue mass.

66. What are the classic radiographic features of osteofibrous dysplasia?
An intracortical diaphyseal tibial or, less commonly, femoral lesion associated with expansion and thinning of the cortex and multiple radiolucencies with intervening regions of sclerosis.

67. What are the classic histologic findings in osteofibrous dysplasia, and how do they differ from fibrous dysplasia?

Osteofibrous dysplasia is a hypocellular tumor with a storiform pattern of spindle cells and scattered bony trabeculae. There is prominent osteoblastic rimming about the bony trabeculae. This contrasts with fibrous dysplasia, in which the moderately cellular spindle-cell background is associated with a dense collagenous matrix and metaplastic bone formation in a pattern characteristically termed "alphabet soup" or "Chinese letters," seen under low-power magnification.

68. What is the treatment of osteofibrous dysplasia?

Observation for asymptomatic lesions. En bloc excision if feasible for large symptomatic lesions in children older than the age of 10. Curettage, cryosurgery, and grafting with autologous or allogeneic cancellous bone is an alternative approach. Local recurrence rates are 20–30% with intralesional resection compared with 5–10% with marginal resection.

69. What is the typical clinical presentation of classic high-grade osteogenic sarcoma?

Pain, often associated with a soft tissue mass, most commonly about the knee, in a teenage male slightly more frequently than in a teenage female. Radiographs reveal a destructive lesion with a variable amount of bone formation and a soft tissue mass, also with bone formation.

70. What is the treatment of classic high-grade osteosarcoma?

Neoadjuvant chemotherapy followed by wide surgical resection and limb salvage reconstruction, followed by adjuvant chemotherapy.

71. What is the expected survivorship of nonmetastatic classic high-grade osteosarcoma at presentation?

Five-year survival of 60–80%, depending on response to chemotherapy. The more rare variants of osteosarcoma, including pagetoid, postradiation, and telangiectatic osteosarcoma, have worse survival rates, approximately 30–50% at five years.

72. What are the common variants of osteogenic sarcoma?

Parosteal osteosarcoma, periosteal osteosarcoma, well-differentiated fibroblastic osteosarcoma, telangiectatic osteosarcoma, pagetoid osteosarcoma, and postradiation osteosarcoma.

73. Describe the classic features of periosteal osteosarcoma.

Typically, a juxacortical lesion with a large soft tissue mass occurring in the diaphyseal region of a long bone, as opposed to classic osteosarcoma, which occurs in metaphyseal long bones.

Histologically, these lesions demonstrate chondroblastic features. They may be difficult to distinguish from chondrosarcoma.

74. What is the treatment of periosteal osteosarcoma?

Low-grade chondroblastic histologic subtypes should be treated with wide surgical resection and limb salvage reconstruction. The chondroblastic component of these tumors fails to respond to neoadjuvant or adjuvant chemotherapy.

75. What are the local recurrence rate and overall prognosis in periosteal osteosarcoma?

Local recurrence rate is 5–10%, and overall prognosis is 75–80% 5-year survival.

76. Describe the classic clinical presentation of parosteal osteosarcoma.

A painful posterior distal femoral osteoblastic lesion in a teenager or young adult. Occasionally discovered incidentally, as an asymptomatic lesion. Radiographically, a juxtacortical dense osseous lesion. Histologically low grade.

77. What are the treatment, local recurrence rate, and overall prognosis of a parosteal osteosarcoma?
Treatment is wide resection and limb salvage reconstruction. Local recurrence rate is 5%. Overall prognosis is 80–90% survival at 5 years.

78. What is the differential diagnosis of parosteal osteosarcoma?
Atypical exostosis and myositis ossificans.

79. How is myositis ossificans differentiated from parosteal osteosarcoma?
The mineralization of myositis ossificans is more dense peripherally than centrally, whereas the mineralization of parosteal osteosarcoma is more dense centrally than peripherally. Additionally, myositis ossificans is usually characterized by a thin line of soft tissue separating the lesion from nearby cortex that may only be appreciated on CT scanning.

80. Describe the typical clinical presentation of Ewing's sarcoma.
A painful extremity typically associated with night pain or rest pain in a child between the ages of 5 and 20. There may be associated fever or an elevated erythrocyte sedimentation rate. An associated soft tissue mass is common. Diaphyseal long bones are typically affected. Involvement of the pelvis is common. Radiographically, a permeated poorly defined diaphyseal lesion associated with periosteal reaction and a soft tissue mass is seen.

81. What is the treatment of Ewing's sarcoma?
Neoadjuvant chemotherapy followed by limb salvage resection of the tumor followed by adjuvant chemotherapy and radiation therapy.
Alternatively, chemotherapy and radiation therapy may be employed for unresectable lesions, such as extensive lesions of the spine.

82. What is the 5-year survivorship of Ewing's sarcoma.
Survival rates are 50–60%. Late osseous and pulmonary metastases are not uncommon.

BIBLIOGRAPHY

1. Antman KH, Eilber FR, Shiu MH: Soft tissue sarcomas: current trends in diagnosis and management [review]. Current Probl Cancer 13:337–367, 1989.
2. Campanacci M, Ruggieri P: Osteosarcoma [review]. Bull Hosp J Dis Orthop Inst 51:11–11, 1991.
3. Marks KE, Bauer TW: Fibrous tumors of bone [review]. Orthop Clin North Am 20:377–393, 1989.
4. Jaffe N: Osteosarcoma [review]. Ped Rev 12:333–343, 1991.
5. Rosenthal HG, Terek RM, Lane JM: Management of extremity soft-tissue sarcomas [review]. Clin Ortho 289:66–72, 1993.
6. Mirra JM: Bone Tumors. Philadelphia, Lea & Febiger, 1989.

81. SOFT TISSUE TUMORS

Mark C. Gebhardt, M.D.

1. What are the most common causes of death in childhood?
Trauma is the most common cause, and cancer is the second most common cause of death in children up to the age of 15 years.

2. How common are soft tissue sarcomas in children?

Soft tissue sarcomas are an important, but not a common, cause of cancer in children. Surveillance, Epidemiology, and End Result (SEER) data indicate that soft tissue sarcomas occur in 8 in 100,000 children, which represents about 6% of childhood cancer.

3. Which are more common: benign or malignant lesions?

Benign lesions are much more common than malignant ones, but it may be difficult to distinguish between the two.

4. How frequent are pediatric soft tissue sarcomas in the United States?

There are about 420 new soft tissue sarcomas reported each year in the United States in children younger than the age of 15 years. In contrast, about 320 cases of bone sarcomas are reported per year.

5. How many deaths per year are due to soft tissue sarcomas?

Soft tissue sarcomas account for 110 deaths per year; bone sarcomas account for 85 deaths per year.

6. What is the cause of soft tissue sarcomas?

We do not know. Genetic alterations have been found in many, but not all, soft tissue sarcomas. They include clonal karyotype abnormalities such as translocations of parts of one chromosome to another, which in some instances are specific for a given histologic subtype. Recently, the fusion products of many of these newly formed genes have been sequenced and are believed to be related to the pathogenesis of the lesions. Genetic alterations in specific tumor suppressor genes (*p53*, *RB*) have been identified in soft tissue sarcomas and may be correlated with outcome. Chemical carcinogens and trauma have also been implicated in the development of sarcomas, but the exact mechanism is unknown.

7. Which are the different types of benign lesions of soft tissue in children?

The most common lesions are ganglions (including popliteal cysts), lipomas, and vascular malformations. Perhaps the most difficult to manage is the desmoid tumor or aggressive fibromatosis. In addition to presenting in teenagers as large masses that may mimic a soft tissue sarcoma, they may present in an infantile form or as plantar fibromatosis. Synovial chondromatosis, pigmented villonodular synovitis, and nerve sheath tumors are also seen. In addition, it is important to recognize that nonmalignant soft tissue lesions, such as myositis ossificans, can mimic soft tissue tumors.

8. Which are the different types of malignant tumors?

Rhabdomyosarcoma is the most common malignant soft tissue sarcoma in children, accounting for more than half of all soft tissue sarcomas. Nonrhabdomyosarcoma soft tissue sarcomas also occur, most commonly synovial sarcomas, malignant peripheral nerve sheath tumors, fibrosarcoma, and malignant fibrous histiocytoma. Finally, Ewing's sarcoma and peripheral primitive neuroectodermal tumors (PNETs) may present as soft tissue sarcomas.

9. What are the pathologic features of these lesions?

Rhabdomyosarcomas are "round cell tumors," meaning that under the microscope, they appear as sheets of homogeneous cells with large hematoxylin-staining nuclei and varying amounts of eosinophilic cytoplasm. Two subtypes occur in the extremity and trunk: embryonal (more common in young children) and alveolar (usually in the adolescent age group). Differentiation usually requires special studies such as immunohistochemistry, electron microscopy, and, at times, karyotype analysis. The t(2;13) translocation is specific for alveolar rhabdomyosarcoma. Other round cell sarcomas (Ewing's sarcoma and PNET) are part of the differential diagnosis and are distinguished from rhabdomyosarcoma by the findings on immunohistochemistry and electron microscopy. Ewing's sarcoma and PNET share a clonal t(11;22) translocation and are positive for the MIC2 antibody. The nonrhabdomyosarcomas are spindle cell neoplasms of either low or high grade. Again, immunohistochemistry is helpful in the differential diagnosis. It is essential that the pathologist be familiar with the clinical and radiographic presentation of all these lesions so that biopsy tissue can be properly processed.

10. What happens if these lesions are not treated?

Certain benign lesions such as a popliteal cyst may regress spontaneously. Others such as lipomas and vascular malformations remain relatively constant in size and are usually asymptomatic. Lesions such as pigmented villonodular synovitis and synovial chondromatosis continue to enlarge and become painful if not treated. Malignant lesions are to be taken much more seriously. Most sarcomas grow progressively and ultimately metastasize. The lung is the most frequent site of metastasis, but certain lesions such as rhabdomyosarcoma and synovial sarcoma may also spread to lymph nodes in about 15% of cases. Less commonly, they may spread to bone or bone marrow and rarely to other organs as well. Without treatment, they are invariably fatal. For reasons that are not well understood, synovial sarcoma may be present as an asymptomatic mass for a year or more before enlarging and becoming painful.

11. What are the clinical features of soft tissue lesions?

The sign that alerts the patient or parent to the problem is usually a mass of the involved extremity. In benign and some malignant lesions, the mass may be asymptomatic. Often, the recognition of the mass is preceded by an injury that may call attention to the lesion. Benign lesions are usually asymptomatic, but they may also be painful, especially if bumped or touched. Vascular malformations are painful, presumably because of venous stasis and thrombophlebitis within the vascular channels of the lesion. Popliteal cysts have smooth borders and are located most frequently near the medial gastrocnemius origin. Diagnosis can be confirmed by transillumination or ultrasonography. Lipomas have a characteristic doughy feel on palpation and have smooth lobular borders. Pigmented villonodular synovitis and synovial chondromatosis usually present with pain, limitation of motion, and swelling or effusion of a joint. It may be extremely difficult to distinguish a benign from a malignant mass. In general, benign lesions are small and superficial and malignant ones are large and deep, but malignant ones may also be tiny and located in the subcutaneous tissue. A mass larger than 5 cm that is deep to the fascia should be presumed to be malignant until proven otherwise!

12. What should be asked in the history?

The patient's age and the location of the mass are important. Embryonal rhabdomyosarcomas usually present in young patients (< 5 years of age), and alveolar rhabdomyosarcoma presents in older children. Infantile fibromatoses and fibrosarcomas present in the first year of life. The extremity and pelvis are common sites for soft tissue sarcomas. One should ascertain the nature of the pain and the length of time that symptoms have been present. Find out if symptoms began following an injury. Most benign lesions do not cause pain at rest or at night but hurt mainly following aggravation or with activity. The pain of a malignant lesion is usually constant, steadily worsens, and may cause symptoms at rest or at night. It is important to learn whether the lesion is enlarging. Are there predisposing conditions such as neurofibromatosis or familial cancer syndromes (Li-Fraumeni) that may alert the physician to the possibility of malignancy?

13. What are the physical findings with an extremity soft tissue lesion?

It is difficult to distinguish benign from malignant lesions with history and physical examination alone. A small smooth-bordered lesion on the wrist or in the popliteal fossa that transilluminates is almost certainly a ganglion or popliteal cyst. A smooth-bordered doughy subcutaneous mass is most likely a lipoma. Vascular malformations of the extremity often present as an ill-defined fullness that increases in size in the dependent position. At times, skin discoloration may be present. Bruits are seldom noted, since the majority of these are low-flow venous lesions. Schwannomas and neurofibromas present as smooth mobile masses aligned along nerves; these lesions are more likely in patients with café au lait markings and other findings of neurofibromatosis. There are no pathognomonic findings of an extremity or pelvic soft tissue sarcoma. At times, they may present as an asymptomatic superficial mass. Lesions that are painful to palpation, large (> 5 cm), and deep to the deep fascia should be presumed to be malignant, however (see Figure). Enlarging, painful "neurofibromas" in patients with neurofibromatosis should also be viewed with suspicion.

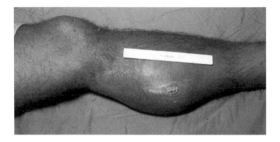

This 15-year-old boy had a mass on his thigh that was initially thought to be due to an athletic injury. Myositis ossificans was the provisional diagnosis because a radiograph showed calcifications of the posterior calf. He presented 6 months later with this large posterior compartment mass, which was firm and tender.

14. Which type of imaging is useful?

The most useful test for evaluating a questionable soft tissue lesion in an extremity or in the pelvis is magnetic resonance imaging (MRI). Although it will not give a definitive diagnosis, it does provide important clues such as the size, the depth, and the relationship of the mass to surrounding muscle and neurovascular structures. Certain lesions can be diagnosed with a degree of certainty. Lipomas can be distinguished by their signal characteristics, which are identical to those of fat. Vascular malformations can be distinguished from solid lesions and may demonstrate slow (venous) or fast (arterial) flow. Malignant lesions are characterized by a location deep to the fascia and usually well-defined borders with respect to the surrounding muscle (see Figure). It is not usually possible to distinguish one tumor type from another or benign or malignant status with assurance, but in combination with other historical and physical findings, the physician can usually identify worrisome lesions. Ultrasound is excellent for defining cystic and vascular lesions but in the author's experience is of little other value. Computed tomography (CT) scans provide information similar to that seen on MRI but with less distinction from normal tissues. It is essential to obtain CT scans of the chest for lesions suspected to be malignant. Plain films are of value in distinguishing lesions with mineralization (myositis ossificans, synovial sarcoma). Bone scans are obtained in children with soft tissue sarcomas to look for bony metastases.

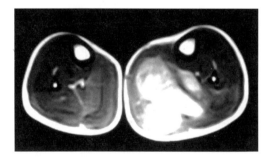

An axial T1-weighted MRI shows the extent of this mass in the musculature of the posterior calf. A biopsy showed synovial sarcoma, and chest CT showed multiple pulmonary metastases. Wide excision and radiotherapy achieved local control, but despite initial response with chemotherapy, he died 3 years later.

15. What type of laboratory studies are useful?

Other than excluding infection or hematopoietic malignancy (which rarely presents as a soft tissue mass) by means of a complete blood count and erythrocyte sedimentation rate, laboratory studies are not of diagnostic importance in the work-up of patients with a soft tissue mass.

16. Which lesions require treatment?

Lipomas, popliteal cysts, ganglions, and vascular malformations can be observed unless symptomatic. Pigmented villonodular synovitis and synovial chondromatosis require synovectomy and are associated with a relatively high local recurrence rate. Malignant lesions require biopsy to establish the diagnosis and appropriate local and systemic treatment.

17. Who should manage the malignant lesions?

These highly lethal tumors should be treated by a multidisciplinary team consisting of pediatric surgeons, orthopaedic surgeons, pediatric oncologists and radiotherapists, and pathologists and radiologists with expertise in this area. The biopsy should be performed by the surgeon who is capable of carrying out the definitive local treatment. The pathologist must be knowledgeable in handling the specimen for appropriate histology, immunohistochemistry, electron microscopy, and molecular studies. The multidisciplinary team makes the treatment decision relative to the combination of surgical resection, radiotherapy, and chemotherapy depending on the diagnosis and stage. Since these are rare lesions, they should be treated in clinical protocols so that advances in our ability to treat these patients can continue.

18. What is the prognosis?

The prognosis will vary with the grade, size, and clinical stage of the lesion, but tremendous advances have been made in our ability to achieve long-term survival in childhood soft tissue sarcomas. The third Intergroup Rhabdomyosarcoma Study demonstrated a 76% overall progression-free survival. Nonrhabdomyosarcomas that can be completely resected have an even better prognosis. It is important to note, however, that improper biopsy technique and delay in the diagnosis of these lesions can have a detrimental effect on eventual outcome.

19. What should I tell the family?

It is important not to frighten the patient and parents unnecessarily. It is best to tell them that you are concerned about this mass and would like to seek the opinion of an expert to decide whether a biopsy is indicated. You can point out that the likelihood of a benign mass is much greater than that of a malignant one, but that it is best to check it out. Most major medical centers have expertise in evaluating these lesions, so it is generally possible to schedule a referral to an orthopaedic or pediatric surgeon with expertise in oncology quickly.

20. What are the complications?

The complications of the untreated malignancy have already been discussed. The complications of surgical resection and chemotherapy are complex and are related to the location of the primary tumor and the specific treatment regimen. An unplanned excision ("shell out") or improperly done biopsy can be devastating and in many cases can lead to unnecessary amputation or poor disease outcome.

BIBLIOGRAPHY

1. Christ WM, Kun LE: Common solid tumors of childhood. New Engl J Med 324:461–471, 1991.
2. Conrad EU III, Bradford L, Chansky HA: Pediatric soft tissue sarcomas. Orthop Clinics North Am 27:655–664, 1996.
3. Letson GD, Greenfield CB, Heinrich SD: Evaluation of the child with a bone or soft tissue neoplasm. Orthop Clin North Am 27:431–452, 1996.
4. Miller RW, Young JL, Novakovic B: Childhood cancer. Cancer 75:395–405, 1995.
5. Parker SL, Tong T, Bolden S, Wingo PA: Cancer statistics, 1997. CA Cancer J Clin 47:5–27, 1997.
6. Pizzo PA, Poplack DG: Principles and Practice of Pediatric Oncology. Philadelphia, J.B. Lippincott Co., 1993.
7. Rao BN, Santana VM, Parham D, Pratt CB, Fleming ID, Hudson M, Fontanesi J, Philippe P, Schnell MJ: Pediatric nonrhabdomyosarcomas of the extremities: influence of size, invasiveness and grade on outcome. Arch Surg 126:1490–1495, 1991.
8. Smith JT, Yandow SM: Benign soft tissue lesions in children. Orthop Clinics North Am 27:645–654, 1996.
9. Young JL Jr, Gloeckler R, Silverberg BS, Horm JW, Miller RW: Cancer incidence, survival, and mortality for children younger than age 15 years. Cancer 58:598–602, 1996.

82. OSTEOMYELITIS

Walter B. Greene, M.D.

1. Can I skip this chapter?

Absolutely not. Although a missed diagnosis does no harm in most pediatric orthopaedic conditions, that is **not** the case in osteomyelitis. Indeed, even a 24- to 48-hour delay in diagnosis and proper treatment will significantly increase the risk of complications such as pathologic fracture, distant seeding of the infection, or the dreaded chronic osteomyelitis. Furthermore, it is important that **from the beginning**, primary care physicians and orthopaedic surgeons work together in the evaluation and management of osteomyelitis.

2. What is osteomyelitis?

Inflammation in the bone and medullary canal. The term is generally restricted to an infectious process and, unless specified, refers to a bacterial infection.

3. How common is osteomyelitis in children?

The problem is common, but the incidence has decreased over the past 20–30 years. In a study from Glasgow, Scotland, the incidence was 87 of 10,000 children in 1970 but had decreased to 42 of 10,000 in 1990. The reason for the decrease is uncertain but probably includes a combination of increased access to medical care, increased use of antibiotics at an early stage of other childhood illnesses, and further development of vaccinations (*Haemophilus influenzae*).

4. How does osteomyelitis in children differ from that observed in adults?

Acute osteomyelitis is significantly more common in children and in the pediatric age group is most secondary to a hematogenous cause. By contrast, adult osteomyelitis most often develops following direct penetration (open fractures).

5. What is the pathophysiology of hematogenous osteomyelitis in children?

The growth plate or physis is an avascular barrier to the terminal branches of the metaphyseal arteries. Therefore, these vessels must make a "U turn" at the physis. The resultant sluggish circulation in combination with transient bacteremia creates a set-up for bacteria to gain a "foothold." The columns of primary and secondary spongiosa also limit access of reticuloendothelial cells from the adjacent medullary canal.

The resultant infection spreads from its metaphyseal crypt (see Figure). Because pus under pressure takes the path of least resistance, the infection travels in two directions: down the medullary canal and through the relatively thin metaphyseal bone. The cartilaginous growth plate, however, is a barrier. Therefore, the physis and adjacent epiphysis are typically spared.

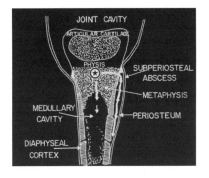

Spread of osteomyelitis in typical metaphysis.

In certain locations, the insertion of the joint capsule is below (distal to) the physis. At these sites, osteomyelitis perforating the metaphyseal cortex will cause concomitant **septic arthritis** (see Figure). This most commonly occurs with spread of osteomyelitis from the proximal femur to the hip joint.

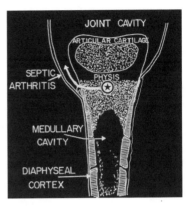

Spread of osteomyelitis when joint capsule inserts distal to metaphysis.

6. What determines the extent and nature of the disease?

The extent and type of osteomyelitis depend on the duration of the infection and the virulence of the infecting organism. Even with aggressive bacteria, however, if the infection is only of 24 to 48 hours' duration, the osteomyelitis is most likely confined to the medullary canal of the metaphysis. In the initial stage of the infection, recruitment of polymorphonuclear leukocytes is observed, but thrombosis of terminal vessels and necrosis of bone are limited. In essence, the early acute stage can be likened to a **cellulitis of bone**.

Left untreated, osteomyelitis progresses, with spread of the infection down the medullary canal and through the thin cortex of the metaphysis. Histologically, necrosis of bone and hordes of acute inflammatory cells are observed. Bone resorption is dramatic in acute osteomyelitis, progressing at a rate far surpassing the most aggressive malignancy. Radiographic evidence of bone resorption is demonstrated 8–12 days after onset of symptoms by irregular patches of radiolucency in the metaphysis.

When pus perforates cortical bone, the periosteum is elevated, and a **subperiosteal abscess** may subsequently develop. Periosteal elevation is radiographically demonstrated 10–14 days after onset of symptoms by an outside rim of reactive new bone formation.

Similar to other conditions, bone formation follows osteonecrosis and bone resorption. The initial bone formed is woven or immature bone, which is not as dense as lamellar bone. Therefore, new bone formation also contributes to radiolucent changes observed in the healing phase of osteomyelitis.

Chronic osteomyelitis represents a failure of therapy. As a result, a **sequestrum** forms (osteonecrotic bone surrounded by fibrous tissue). To decompress continued purulent drainage from the infected bone, a *sinus tract* often develops. These pathologic changes limit spread of the osteomyelitis, but the fibrous tissue is also a barrier to antibiotics and inflammatory cells. Therefore, eradicating chronic osteomyelitis requires surgical resection of the necrotic bone.

Subacute osteomyelitis is secondary to infection by a less virulent bacterium and a more effective response of the immune system. Histologically, subacute osteomyelitis is characterized by a greater proportion of granulation tissue, chronic inflammatory cells, and new bone formation. Two types of subacute osteomyelitis occur. **Cavitary** or cystic lesions are observed in the metaphysis or epiphysis. Subacute osteomyelitis can also simulate an **aggressive, neoplastic-like** lesion with periosteal elevation and new bone formation. This pattern is most often observed in the diaphysis.

7. What are the different types of osteomyelitis?

Acute osteomyelitis is generally defined as infection diagnosed within 2 weeks of the onset of symptoms. The boundary between early acute and **late acute** forms is less precise, but most agree that disease in patients presenting 4–5 days after onset of symptoms should be placed in the late acute category. A typical patient with early acute osteomyelitis presents within 24–48 hours of symptom development. Osteomyelitis in this situation responds readily to antibiotic therapy. On the other hand, children who present 4–5 days after onset of symptoms are more likely to have a subperiosteal collection of pus and to require surgical drainage. Because the history is not always reliable and because bacterial strains are different, it is not possible to determine optimal treatment solely from the duration of symptoms.

Subacute osteomyelitis presents after 2 weeks of symptoms, but generally the duration of symptoms is one to several months. Subacute osteomyelitis is categorized as either a *cavitary* or an *aggressive* lesion.

Chronic osteomyelitis represents a delay in diagnosis or a failure of treatment. In third world countries, chronic osteomyelitis in children is relatively common and typically follows inadequate treatment of hematogenous osteomyelitis. In industrialized countries, chronic osteomyelitis is uncommon in children and most often is a sequela of an open fracture.

8. What happens if the condition is not treated?

The infectious process spreads, causing more destruction. The risk of complications is significantly increased. Even a few hours' delay may be detrimental. Laboratory studies, radiographs, and cultures should be obtained expeditiously and intravenous antibiotics started promptly, using a maximum or near-maximum dosage.

9. What are the clinical features of the different categories of disease?

Acute osteomyelitis is more common in males (2:1 ratio), is most often monostotic (94%), and most often involves the lower extremity (90%). A limp or refusal to walk is a common complaint voiced by the parents.

Early acute osteomyelitis is characterized by a febrile illness of 24–48 hours' duration, generalized signs of acute infection, an avoidance of using the extremity, and localized tenderness and swelling.

Late acute osteomyelitis is more likely to occur in three groups of children: neonates, older children, and premature infants. Well neonates and older infants do not stress the limb with walking activities. Therefore, the diagnosis is more often delayed in this age group. At presentation, these children are more likely to have obvious swelling and painful movement of the involved extremity. In older children (> 9 years of age), the diagnosis may be delayed because this age group has better coordination and therefore limps less during the early stages of the infectious process. In premature infants who are relatively immobile and who have been in the neonatal unit for several weeks, the appearance of a mass may be the initial clue. Multifocal osteomyelitis is more common in premature infants.

Children who develop **subacute** osteomyelitis are typically older, ranging in age from 2–16 years of age. In addition, the sex ratio in this category is equivalent. The history is often vague with neither the parents nor the child being able to pinpoint onset of symptoms. Systemic signs such as fever are either mild or absent, and the physical exam either is within normal limits or demonstrates mild localized tenderness and swelling.

Likewise, children with **chronic** osteomyelitis may present with ill-defined symptoms or may only seek medical attention after spontaneous purulent drainage occurs.

10. What questions should be asked in the history?

Inquire about recent illnesses such as otitis media, pharyngitis, and impetigo. The vaccination status as well as recent temperature elevation should be noted. The onset of symptoms and the duration of limping should be recorded.

11. What are the physical findings?

These depend on the location, duration, and severity of the infection. Osteomyelitis in locations that are relatively superficial, e.g., the distal femur and proximal tibia, causes obvious swelling and localized tenderness. In deeper locations such as the proximal femur and proximal humerus, physical findings are limited to restriction of hip or shoulder motion, but this is not as severe as that observed in septic arthritis. A fever of 38°–39°C is typical in late acute osteomyelitis, but the temperature may be normal or elevated in the other categories of disease.

12. What laboratory studies should be obtained?

Routine studies include a complete blood count, erythrocyte sedimentation rate, AP and lateral radiographs of the affected area, blood culture, and aspiration of the affected area. The **white blood cell count** is most often elevated in late acute osteomyelitis but may be within normal limits in all groups. The **sedimentation rate**, a sensitive but nonspecific parameter of an inflammatory process, is usually elevated but may be within normal limits in early acute and subacute osteomyelitis. Initial **radiographs** in acute osteomyelitis are usually normal but may demonstrate contiguous soft tissue swelling.

Blood cultures identify the offending organism 50% of the time in acute osteomyelitis. Obtaining a positive blood culture is less likely in subacute and chronic osteomyelitis; in this situation, blood cultures are only requested when there is evidence of systemic toxicity (i.e., fever). **Aspiration of the bone** should be attempted. In patients with late acute osteomyelitis who have developed a subperiosteal abscess, the yield from aspiration will obviously be greater. After sterile preparation of the skin, a spinal needle is inserted into bone at the suspected area of infection. If aspiration does not yield diagnostic material (pus) in the subperiosteal space, the needle is inserted, if possible, into the metaphysis, and aspiration is repeated. With **blood culture plus aspiration**, the offending organism can be identified 70% of the time in acute osteomyelitis. In subacute osteomyelitis, cultures are less likely to grow or identify the infecting organism. In chronic osteomyelitis, surface swabs of sinus tract drainage are often contaminated by skin-surface contaminants. Therefore, obtaining a specimen of bone is often indicated to identify the bacteria responsible for the osteomyelitis.

13. What special imaging studies are useful?

A **technetium-99m bone scan** is a very sensitive and specific test for acute osteomyelitis; however, the test is not infallible (overall accuracy of approximately 90%). Furthermore, in most cases, a bone scan is not needed because results of this study would not alter treatment. A bone scan is useful when the diagnosis is unclear, however, as frequently occurs with an infection in atypical locations such as the clavicle, pelvis, or fibula. **Indium and gallium scans** are more sensitive but have the disadvantage of causing higher radiation exposure and requiring 24–48 hours for completion. **Magnetic resonance imaging** is the best special study, but owing to its cost and the frequent need for general anesthesia in children, it should be reserved for diagnostic purposes in unusual cases and to identify sequestrum and "map out" chronic osteomyelitis. Recent reports indicate that **ultrasound** is a good method of defining a subperiosteal abscess, but its best use is presently unclear. One study advocated immediate surgical drainage if the ultrasound study showed periosteal elevation of ≥ 2 mm; however, a subsequent report noted good results following a trial of antibiotic therapy even when the periosteum was elevated 3–4 mm.

14. What other conditions may be confused with osteomyelitis?

Cellulitis may restrict movement and cause the child to limp, but in most cases, swelling and erythema of the skin are obvious. If the infected bone is close to the skin (i.e., proximal tibia or first metatarsal) osteomyelitis may cause erythema of the adjacent skin; however, the changes in the skin are considerably less than those observed in cellulitis.

Septic arthritis is a consideration in locations such as the hip. In this situation, aspiration of the joint may be required to define the site(s) of infection.

Fractures also cause swelling and increased warmth of the extremity. The history and radiographs usually differentiate these two conditions; however, in occult fractures or in children with insensate lower extremities due to myelomeningocele or other paralytic conditions, fractures may create a clinical picture similar to osteomyelitis.

Neoplasms, especially leukemia and Ewing's sarcoma, may be confused with osteomyelitis. Children with leukemia have neoplastic infiltrates of the hematopoietic marrow and may present with pain in the extremity accompanied by a limp, lethargy, and even a fever. Radiographs in acute leukemia may also demonstrate osteopenia and lucent lesions. The diagnosis is made by the more gradual onset of symptoms in leukemia and other signs such as easy bruisability, night pain, pain at multiple sites, and a low leukocyte count. Subacute osteomyelitis in the diaphysis causing periosteal elevation may simulate Ewing's sarcoma. A biopsy will provide the correct diagnosis.

Bone infarction in conditions such as sickle cell anemia and Gaucher's disease causes pain in the extremity, fever, and an elevated white blood cell count and sedimentation rate. Frequently, there is enough difference in these signs and symptoms to differentiate osteomyelitis from a sickle cell or Gaucher's crisis, but sometimes a biopsy is required.

15. Does the condition require treatment?

Yes! Furthermore, if acute osteomyelitis is suspected, treatment with intravenous antibiotics should start immediately. To do otherwise permits spread of the infection and increases complications. Aspiration of the bone does not affect the bone scan, at least for 24–72 hours. Therefore, if osteomyelitis is suspected, do not delay therapy to obtain special imaging studies.

16. Pending a positive culture, what organisms should be covered by the antibiotic therapy?

Initial selection of antibiotic(s) is empiric. The choice depends on the age of the child and the type of osteomyelitis. For **acute osteomyelitis** in a child younger than 1 year of age, *Staphylococcus aureus* is the most common infecting agent, but group B *Streptococcus* and enteric organisms such as *Escherichia coli* are common enough that coverage of these organisms should be included pending a positive culture. Between the ages of 1 and 4 years, coverage of *S. aureus* and *Haemophilus influenzae* is presently recommended. With greater utilization of the H. **influenzae** immunization, that guideline may be amended. For children 4 years of age or older, initial antibiotic coverage is restricted to *S. aureus*, since that organism accounts for more than 90% of cases of acute hematogenous osteomyelitis in that age group.

For **subacute cavitary osteomyelitis**, a 6-week trial of oral antibiotic therapy effective against *S. aureus* should be initiated. Pending culture and biopsy results of an **aggressive-appearing** lesion, antibiotic therapy should be a drug effective against *S. aureus*. If cultures show no growth, then oral antibiotics should be continued 6 weeks.

A bone biopsy for culture should be obtained in children with **chronic osteomyelitis**. Because gram-negative bacteria are more common in chronic osteomyelitis, these organisms as well as *S. aureus* should be covered pending culture results.

17. What are the indications for surgical treatment?

Surgical intervention is rarely, if ever, needed for early acute osteomyelitis. In late acute osteomyelitis, most children can be treated with intravenous antibiotics for 24–48 hours before determining whether surgical drainage is indicated. If the child has persistent fever and swelling, the bone should be explored and the subperiosteal abscess decompressed. Some children with late acute osteomyelitis, particularly those diagnosed more than 1 week after onset of symptoms, present with an obvious subperiosteal abscess. These patients should be treated with immediate surgical decompression. To minimize the risk of avascular necrosis, septic arthritis of the hip secondary to osteomyelitis of the proximal femur should be treated with immediate surgical drainage.

Cavitary subacute osteomyelitis used to be treated with surgical exploration. It is now recognized that most of these children can be treated with a trial of antibiotics. If the cavitary lesion does not respond, operative débridement and curettage should be done.

Chronic osteomyelitis requires biopsy for culturing and removal of all necrotic bone and surrounding fibrous tissue.

18. How long should antibiotics be continued?

Generally, antibiotics are continued 6 weeks. A longer course of therapy may be needed if the infection has not completely resolved. In acute osteomyelitis, antibiotics are discontinued when there is no tenderness and when radiographs demonstrate an appropriate healing response. Lucent areas due to new bone formation and bone remodeling may still be present at 6 weeks; however, if the radiographic changes are consistent with a healing response and if the child is asymptomatic, the antibiotics may be discontinued. Likewise, in subacute and chronic osteomyelitis, the radiographs may not be normal after 6 weeks of therapy, but if the picture is consistent with a resolving process, therapy can be discontinued.

C-reactive protein levels and erythrocyte sedimentation rates may also be used to monitor response to therapy. C-reactive protein levels decline more rapidly than erythrocyte sedimentation rates, and therefore this test is a better marker of therapeutic response in the first week of therapy.

19. What are the complications?

Distant seeding is hematogenous spread of infection to another location. This complication is more likely in late acute osteomyelitis. Pneumonia and septic pericarditis are the most likely consequences of distant seeding, but any location is vulnerable, and the physician should continue to examine the child for a possible secondary infection.

Septic arthritis occurs in locations where the joint capsule inserts "below" the metaphysis, and therefore direct perforation of the metaphysis seeds the joint. This is most likely in the proximal femur but may also occur in the proximal humerus, proximal radius, and distal lateral tibia. If this occurs, the child typically presents with symptoms and signs more consistent with septic arthritis. The diagnosis of concomitant osteomyelitis is often made when lytic areas are observed on follow-up radiographs.

Pathologic fractures occur because the bone is weakened by osteonecrosis, bone resorption, and subsequent bone formation and remodeling. During the latter process, the infection with its associated local and systemic symptoms largely resolves. As a result, the child feels good and resumes normal activity. Unless the affected bone is protected, a fracture may occur through the site of osteomyelitis. This is most problematic with osteomyelitis involving the proximal femur. If the infection was diagnosed expeditiously, I have the child carried or placed in a wheelchair. A spica cast is often necessary to protect the proximal femur if the osteomyelitis is late acute type with extensive osteonecrosis.

Physeal bars are more common with severe late acute osteomyelitis. Damage to the growth plate with subsequent partial closure may not be apparent for several months. Therefore, I recommend follow-up exams for 2 years after onset of osteomyelitis. If the bar is central, growth is symmetrically tethered, and a leg-length discrepancy develops. If the bar has a peripheral location, asymmetric growth and an angular deformity develop.

Recurrent infection with resultant chronic osteomyelitis may not be apparent for several months. This problem most often results from a sequestrum or from foci of necrotic bone.

20. Who should manage the problem?

A primary care physician should initiate the diagnostic evaluation, select the appropriate method of antibiotic administration, monitor the child for distant seeding and work with the orthopaedic surgeon to determine whether surgical drainage is indicated. The orthopaedic surgeon should assist in the diagnostic evaluation and should aspirate the bone for culturing. The orthopaedic surgeon should apply appropriate forms of immobilization to minimize the risk of pathologic fracture and should determine when satisfactory resolution of infection and bone remodeling have occurred. The orthopaedic surgeon, in consultation with the primary care physician, should determine when and if surgical drainage should be done.

BIBLIOGRAPHY

1. Craigen MA, Watters J, Hackett JS: The changing epidemiology of osteomyelitis in children. J Bone Joint Surg [Br] 74:541, 1992.
2. Dagan R: Management of acute hematogenous osteomyelitis and septic arthritis in the pediatric patient. Pediatr Infect Dis J 12:88, 1993.

3. Hamdy RC, Lawton L, Carey T, Wiley J, Marton D: Subacute hematogenous osteomyelitis: are biopsy and surgery always indicated? J Pediatr Orthop 16:220, 1996.

4. Jaramillo D, Treves ST, Kasser JR, Harper M, Sundel R, Laor T: Osteomyelitis and septic arthritis in children; appropriate use of imaging to guide treatment. AJR 165:399, 1995.

5. Juhn A, Healey JH, Ghelman B, Lane JM: Subacute osteomyelitis presenting as bone tumors. Orthopaedics 12:245, 1989.

6. Mah ET, LeQuesne GW, Gent RJ, Paterson DC: Ultrasonic features of acute osteomyelitis in children. J Bone Joint Surg [Br] 76:969, 1994.

7. Ross ERS, Cole WG: Treatment of subacute osteomyelitis in childhood. J Bone Joint Surg [Br] 67:443, 1985.

8. Sonnen GM, Henry NK: Pediatric bone and joint infections. Diagnosis and antimicrobial management. Pediatr Clin North Am 43:933, 1996.

9. Unkila-Kallio L, Kallio MJ, Eskola J, Peltola H: Serum C-reactive protein, erythrocyte sedimentation rate, and white blood cell count in acute hematogenous osteomyelitis of children. Pediatrics 93:59, 1994.

10. Wong M, Isaacs D, Howman-Giles R, Uren R: Clinical and diagnostic features of osteomyelitis occurring in the first three months of life. Pediatr Infect Dis J 14:1047, 1995.

83. SEPTIC ARTHRITIS

Perry L. Schoenecker, M.D., and Scott J. Luhmann, M.D.

1. What are the joints most commonly affected by septic arthritis?

The most common site is the knee (41%), followed by the hip (23%), ankle (14%), elbow (12%), wrist (4%), and shoulder (4%). The remaining joints (of the hands and feet as well as the sacroiliac and acromioclavicular joints) comprise the remaining 2%. Classic suppurative septic arthritis involves a single joint in 94% of the cases.

2. What is the basic pathophysiology of septic arthritis?

Bacteria can be introduced into the joint through transient bacteremia, direct inoculation (i.e., puncture wound), or local extension (of osteomyelitis). Once a sufficient inoculum has been introduced into the joint, the bacteria colonize the vascular synovium and "culture tube-like" environment of the joint. Some bacteria (e.g., *Staphylococcus* and *Pseudomonas*) have an affinity for cartilage and directly attach to the chondral surface. Bacterial proliferation is possible owing to the relatively nonimmunogenic environment of the normal joint.

3. What is the causal relationship between osteomyelitis and septic arthritis?

The most common site of osteomyelitis in the skeletally immature patient is the metaphyses of long bones. Advanced metaphyseal osteomyelitis can directly decompress into (1) the hip joint from metaphyseal involvement of the proximal femur, (2) the shoulder from the proximal humeral metaphysis, (3) the elbow from the proximal radius, and (4) the ankle joint from the distal lateral tibia.

4. What is the most common age group to be affected by septic arthritis?

The peak age for presentation is younger than 3 years, but it can present in patients of any age.

5. What are the clinical hallmarks in a 15-month-old with septic arthritis?

Typically, the 15-month-old will be irritable and may limp with weightbearing or refuse to use the involved extremity. Fever is an inconsistent finding. In subcutaneous joints, one should be able to detect an effusion, increased warmth, soft tissue swelling, and possibly erythema. To a variable degree, all septic joints will have a painful, limited range of motion and will be tender to palpation. The joints will be held in position of maximal comfort (e.g., hip will be in flexion, abduction and external rotation; knee will be in slight flexion).

6. What might be the clinical findings in septic arthritis in a 6-day-old child in the neonatal unit?

The 6-day-old will exhibit irritability, lethargy, difficulty in feeding, and limb disuse or pseudoparalysis. Fever is an inconsistent finding in this age group. The inability to communicate makes rapid diagnosis difficult, often resulting in a delay in diagnosis.

7. How do you make a definitive diagnosis of septic arthritis?

The diagnosis is made by joint aspiration or identification of purulent effusion with or without identifiable pathologic comparison.

8. Does the history of trauma to the extremity rule out septic arthritis?

No, it is not infrequent for the caregivers to relate the child's complaints to a traumatic event. Minor trauma and falls are common in the peak age for septic arthritis and are frequently reported by parents. Nonpenetrating trauma is thought to play a potential role as well.

9. Are there any systemic conditions that are important to consider in the work-up and treatment of septic arthritis?

One must consider any factors that may make the child more susceptible to development of bacteremia. Recent systemic illness (i.e., chickenpox), infections (i.e., upper respiratory, urinary tract, or otitis media), indwelling intravenous catheters, and a positive exposure history have all been implicated in septic arthritis. In addition, suppression of the child's immune system, such as with steroid use or chemotherapy, must be noted, since this will have an impact on the choice of antibiotic therapy.

10. Why is the identification of a septic joint important?

The presence of bacteria and inflammatory mediators in the joint space elicits a proliferative response by the host immune system. Cartilage damage occurs secondary to the enzymes (proteases, peptidases, collagenases, elastases) released from both the endogenous cells (leukocytes and synovial cells) and the infecting organism. The initial damage is leaching of glycosaminoglycans (within 8 hours) from the cartilage with eventual degradation of collagen in advanced cases. The cartilaginous destruction that occurs even after destruction of live organisms not only is due to the release of enzymes but also is secondary to the immune response via an Arthus-type reaction.

11. What are the studies one should obtain in the work-up of septic arthritis?

Hematologic studies, plain radiographs, and joint aspiration are all mandatory for a complete work-up. The peripheral white blood cell (WBC) count with differential is not a reliable index in an early infection but usually will be elevated ($> 50,000/mm^3$) with a left shift after 24 hours. Erythrocyte sedimentation rate (ESR) is elevated only after 48–72 hours of symptoms, with 90% of those tested showing an ESR between 50 and 90 mm/hr. ESR will typically peak at 3–5 days. Be careful, since ESR is unreliable in the neonate, patients with hematologic disorders (sickle cell anemia), and patients on steroids. C-reactive protein (CRP) is used by some in the detection of early septic arthritis. It will be elevated 6 hours after onset (mean 90 mg/dl) and peaks on day two. Blood cultures are essential and will be positive in 30–50% of cases. Plain radiographs may show (especially in the hip) joint space widening, effusion, soft tissue swelling, or subluxation or dislocation of the joint. Comparison views of the contralateral joint may be useful. Normal hematologic and radiologic studies do not rule out septic arthritis.

12. Are MRI or bone scans useful?

Neither MRI nor bone scans are useful initially in the diagnosis of acute septic arthritis. If the patient's temperature remains elevated after irrigation and débridement, a bone scan can be helpful to evaluate possible involvement of the bone.

13. Is ultrasonography helpful?

Ultrasonography is an effective, safe, noninvasive imaging modality for the evaluation of the painful hip joint. It is the study of choice for assessing an effusion and can be used to compare the affected joint to the unaffected contralateral hip joint. In the work-up of septic arthritis, the presence of an effusion warrants hip arthrocentesis.

14. Should aspiration of a suspicious joint ever be delayed?

No, one should not delay arthrocentesis of suspected septic arthritis. It will not affect the results of further imaging studies (e.g., bone scan) if the arthrocentesis is "dry."

15. Can the joint aspiration be done at the bedside?

Joint aspiration is a meticulous procedure that must be performed in a controlled environment with adequate sedation. Use of a sufficient needle caliber (i.e., 18 gauge) will optimize the possibility of a successful aspiration. Aspiration of a knee, an ankle, or an elbow would be predictably done at bedside. On the other hand, aspiration of the hip joint must be done in a radiology suite under fluoroscopic guidance with needle position confirmed by arthrography.

16. What studies of the joint aspirate should be performed?

One should order a Gram's stain, aerobic and anaerobic cultures, and WBC count with differential for all joint fluid aspirates. Visually, the fluid is opaque, varying from a cloudy yellow to creamy white in color. Gram's stain will have positive findings in 30–40% of aspirates and can be helpful in diagnosing the gram-negative intracellular diplococci in gonorrheal septic arthritis. WBC count will be elevated within 24 hours of the onset of symptoms and will usually be greater than 50,000/mm^2. It is often greater than 100,000/mm^2 with a differential of more than 90% polymorphonuclear leukocytes.

Evaluation of Joint Fluid

	APPEARANCE	WBC COUNT	POLYMOR-PHONUCLEAR LEUKOCYTES (%)	GRAM'S STAIN	CULTURE
Normal	Clear/straw-colored	< 200	< 25%	Negative	Negative
Traumatic arthritis	Bloody	< 5000, many red blood cells	< 25%	Negative	Negative
Septic arthritis	Turbid/yellow-white	> 50,000	> 90%	Positive in 30–40% of cases	Positive in 50–70% of cases
Juvenile rheumatoid arthritis	Slightly cloudy/straw-colored	15,000–80,000	> 60%	Negative	Negative

17. Are there any special technical considerations in the handling of fluid from a suspected septic joint?

Fluid should be immediately transported to the laboratory and plated on the appropriate medium (agar). Several milliliters should also be injected into blood culture bottles, which may increase the possibility of positive identification of the pathogen. Joint aspirates of suspected cases of gonococcus need to be plated on chocolate agar to optimize yield. *Haemophilus influenzae* type B and gonococcus need to incubated in a CO_2 environment.

18. What is the likelihood of a positive culture of the joint aspirate?

Typically in the 60–80% range. For *Neisseria gonorrhoeae*, it is around 50%.

19. What are the most likely organisms causing septic arthritis?

Neonate: *Staphylococcus aureus*, enteric gram-negative organisms, group B *Streptococcus*

Child < 5 years old: *S. aureus, H. influenzae* type B, group A *Streptococcus, Streptococcus pneumoniae*

Child > 5 years old: *S. aureus*, group A *Streptococcus*

Adolescent: *S. aureus, N. gonorrhoeae*

Other less common organisms include *Kingella kingae, Salmonella* spp., *N. meningitidis,* and anaerobic bacteria.

20. What are the clinical and laboratory guidelines for differentiating toxic synovitis from acute septic arthritis?

Toxic synovitis is an acute inflammatory process typically seen in the 2 to 10-year-old patient. Findings on physical exam can include painful and limited hip range of motion, muscle spasm, refusal to bear weight on the limb, and low-grade fever. Overall, the physical signs are not as dramatic in toxic synovitis. Typically, the ESR is greater than 30 mm/hr in only 14% of patients with toxic synovitis (compared with 71% in septic arthritis). WBC count and differentials are not usually elevated. Ultrasonography of the affected hip will show no effusion in most patients and a slight increase in the minority of patients.

21. What are the three main therapeutic interventions?

Joint decompression and débridement, antibiotics, and initial joint immobilization (to decrease local irritation) followed by mobilization to decrease the development of fibrous adhesions and improve cartilage nutrition.

22. When should antibiotics be initiated?

Intravenous antibiotics should be started after the arthrocentesis. If started prior to joint aspiration, the chance of obtaining a positive culture is lessened. Recent antibiotic use for otitis media or upper respiratory infection should not dissuade one from performing an arthrocentesis, however.

23. What should the initial antibiotic regimen be?

Neonate: oxacillin plus cefotaxime or gentamicin

Child < 5 years old: oxacillin and cefotaxime; or cefuroxime

Child > 5 years old: oxacillin

Adolescent: ceftriaxone plus oxacillin or first-generation cephalosporin

24. What should the route of delivery of antibiotics be? How long should they be continued?

Initial delivery should be intravenous for a minimum of 1 week with conversion to oral antibiotics, if possible, for another 2–5 weeks. Oral antibiotics can be used if there is positive clinical improvement, the organism has been identified and is sensitive, the serum antibiotic level is adequate, the parents are reliable, there is no vomiting or diarrhea, and there is adequate surgical débridement. ESR or CRP levels can be used to monitor therapy. Antibiotics should be continued until ESR CRP values normalize.

25. What is the surest method of decompressing and débriding a septic joint?

Open arthrotomy with débridement is the surest way to irrigate and débride the joint. Arthroscopy and arthrocentesis have their supporters but tend to be associated with higher recurrence rates, do not allow vigorous débridement of potential loculi and thick fibrinous exudates, and have been shown to predispose to more long-term joint space narrowing.

26. How quickly does treatment need to be done?

In general, treatment of most joints should proceed as soon as it is safe for general anesthesia, which may take 6 hours if the child has recently eaten. Infection of the hip joint is a surgical emergency, however. Prolonged elevated intracapsular pressure in the hip can tamponade blood flow to the femoral head and increase the possibility of developing avascular necrosis.

27. Is there a role for intra-articular antibiotic infusion as definitive management?
No, this has not been found to alter the course of septic arthritis. It has been implicated as being irritating to synovium and could exacerbate the inflammatory process. Antibiotics are delivered into the joint in sufficiently high bacteriocidal concentrations intravenously via the joint synovium.

28. What are the complications of missed septic arthritis?
Aggressive surgical treatment of suspected septic arthritis might result in the occasional unnecessary arthrotomy of joints suspected of being infected. The potentially disastrous results of improperly diagnosed or inadequately treated septic arthritis, however, make occasional overtreatment acceptable and an overall low risk for the child. Occurrence of avascular necrosis of the femoral head with secondary limb-length discrepancy (due to proximal femoral physeal closure), coxa magna, pathologic dislocation, and osteomyelitis can be minimized with appropriate surgical intervention.

29. What are the most important factors in determining long-term prognosis?
There are four main factors: time from onset to irrigation and débridement, the joint involved, the presence of associated osteomyelitis, and the age of the patient. The goal of diagnosis and treatment is rapid clearance of the intra-articular chondrolytic process; delays of more than 5 days lead to uniformly poor long-term results. Involvement of the hip can lead to avascular necrosis because the main blood supply to the femoral head is intra-articular. Effusions of the hip can impair blood flow to the femoral head, leading to total head necrosis. Associated osteomyelitis (in 10–16% of children with pyogenic arthritis) that has decompressed into the hip implies extensive involvement of the proximal femur with sequestrum. This can lead to significant pain and functional problems for the patient. Neonates often have a worse prognosis due to a delay in diagnosis. The morbid sequelae of septic arthritis may not be obvious until years after the occurrence of the acute infection. Therefore, long-term follow-up (> 10 years) is necessary to assess the effect of other surgical or medical treatment.

30. What are the characteristic findings in gonococcal septic arthritis?
This typically afflicts the teenager or preteenager who is sexually active. Gonococcal (GC) arthritis involves multiple joints (average is 2.6 joints) in 60% of cases and is the most common cause of polyarthritis in this age group. In 80%, there will be a history of migratory polyarthralgias. Fever is present 60% of the time and skin lesions 45% of the time. Genitourinary symptoms are present in 80% of males and 50% of females. GC arthritis occurs in 5% of patients with gonorrhea. This is most commonly seen in the hands (especially the dorsum), wrists, ankles, and feet. Joint aspirates usually average 48,000/mm^2. One needs to culture all orifices if GC arthritis is suspected owing to the growth of gonococcus in culture in only 50% of cases. If one is suspicious of GC arthritis, the pharynx, anorectal areas, blood and skin lesions need to be cultured.

31. What is definitive treatment for gonococcal septic arthritis?
Antibiotics. Specific antibiotic treatment depends on patient age and chronicity of symptoms. Joint irrigation and débridement are not necessary owing to the rapid response of the infection to antibiotics. In addition, the gonococcus has less damaging effect on the joint; long-term cartilage damage is not seen until late in the process.

BIBLIOGRAPHY

1. Chung WK, Slater GL, Bates EH: Treatment of septic arthritis of the hip by arthroscopic lavage. J Pediatr Orthop 13:444–446, 1993.
2. Goldstein WM, Gleason TF, Barmada R: A comparison between arthrotomy and irrigation and multiple aspirations in the treatment of pyogenic arthritis. Orthopedics 6:1309–1314, 1983.

3. Green NE: Disseminated gonococcal infections and gonococcal arthritis. Instr Course Lect 32:40–43, 1983.
4. Green NE, Edwards K: Bone and joint infections in children. Orthop Clin North Am 18(4):555–576, 1987.
5. Gutierrez KM: Infectious and inflammatory arthritis. In Long SS, Pickering LK, Prober CG (eds): Principle and Practice of Pediatric Infectious Diseases. New York, Churchill Livingstone, 1997, pp 537–580.
6. Jackson MA, Nelson JD: Etiology and management of acute suppurative bone and joint infections in pediatric patients. J Pediatr Orthop 2:314, 1983.
7. Morrissy RT: Bone and joint sepsis. In Morrissy RT, Weinstein SL (eds): Lovell and Winter's Pediatric Orthopaedics, 4th ed. Philadelphia, J.B. Lippincott Co., 1996, p 579.
8. Nelson JD: Antibiotic concentrations in septic joint effusions. N Engl J Med 284:349–353, 1971.
9. Skyhar MJ, Mubarak SJ: Arthroscopic treatment of septic knees in children. J Pediatr Orthop 7:647–651, 1987.

84. ATYPICAL INFECTIONS

Jack C.Y. Cheng, M.D.

1. What is the pathology of tuberculous infection?

Tuberculous infection typically appears histologically as tuberculous follicles with a mixture of endothelial cells, lymphocytes, and giant cells. With the enlargement of the follicle, central caseation may occur together with various degrees of destruction of the surrounding parent tissues. Acid-fast bacilli can be detected by the Ziehl-Neelsen stain and are usually found in large amount in the pulmonary TB tubercle follicles and in much smaller amount in the bone and joint aspirates or excised tissues. Culture using Lowenstein-Jensen medium gives the most definitive bacteriologic diagnosis. Culturing usually takes at least 4–6 weeks, however, and will not be positive when the number of bacteria is low, such as in the case of spinal TB.

2. How serious is the problem of TB?

The incidence is rising, not only in endemic areas like Asia and Africa but also in more developed countries in Europe and North America. It is estimated that every year about 20 million individuals will develop overt TB infections.

3. What are the types and common clinical presentations of TB?

The types are pulmonary and extrapulmonary TB. The relative frequency ratio varies from place to place. In endemic areas, the ratio can be 1:1. The extrapulmonary lesions include TB meningitis, TB lymphadenitis, and infections of the gastrointestinal, genitourinary, and musculoskeletal systems. The most severe form of infection is miliary TB, which can affect all tissues and organ systems of the body. Multifocal infections are being increasingly reported in patients with human immunodeficiency virus infection and other immunodeficiency diseases.

4. How can the diagnosis be made?

It can be a problem in nonendemic areas because the presentation is usually nonspecific and the disease is often missed. The diagnosis depends on a high level of suspicion in the higher risk groups of patients. Histologic and bacteriologic diagnosis can be made from tissues or fluids obtained by aspiration, needle biopsy, or open biopsy. TB has a typical appearance on radiologic and other imaging techniques such as ultrasonography, bone scan, CT scan, and MRI. Immunologic diagnosis and DNA probe study done on joint fluid aspirates and cerebrospinal fluid have also been used by some centers as adjunctive diagnostic techniques.

5. What is the role of skin testing in diagnosis?

The tuberculin skin test has been used to demonstrate a nonspecific type of delayed hypersensitivity to mycobacteria. It is not very useful, since positive test results are present in at least 40–50% of the population after the first 3–4 years of life. A negative test result also does not preclude active bone or joint infections.

6. What is the role of bacillus Calmette-Guérin vaccination?

Bacillus Calmette-Guérin (BCG) has been given in endemic areas to newborns, and revaccination is given again at early school age. The vaccine has been recognized for its protective effect, in particular against the disseminated forms of TB in children, including TB meningitis and miliary TB. There is no conclusive evidence that BCG revaccination confers additional protection against TB or that it prevents other milder forms of TB infections, however.

7. Are drugs effective in treating TB infections?

The penetration of antituberculous drugs into the tubercles and abscesses has been proven to be adequate in many pharmacokinetics studies. The bacilli are usually smaller in number and slower growing when compared with other typical bacterial infections. The drug therapy program would have to be given for much longer periods of time to "sterilize" the lesions. Classically, triple therapy including streptomycin, isoniazid, and para-aminosalicyclate (PAS) was given for a period of 18 months. The more recently developed short course of therapy utilized four bactericidal drugs, including isoniazid, rifampin, pyrazinamide, and ethambutol for 4 months and then 2 months of isoniazid and rifampin, and was shown to be highly efficacious for treating pulmonary TB. For bone and joint infections, the recommended period of treatment is a minimum of 9 months using a similar regimen.

8. What is it so difficult to eradicate TB?

Apart from a small number of drug-resistant cases, the most difficult problem is the default treatment rate. Owing to the long period required for multiple drug therapy, many patients would fail to comply with the follow-up or the drug intake. It was found that well-organized supervised treatment was necessary to insure that every dose of the correct medication was taken by the patient under direct supervision of the health care workers.

9. What are the common orthopaedic manifestations of TB infection?

Of all the extrapulmonary TB infections, about 20–25% will involve the musculoskeletal system. TB can affect virtually every part of the skeleton, but the most common site is the spine, followed by the major limb bones and joints. Among the joints infected, the hip and the knee joints are most commonly affected. The infection can present as chronic osteomyelitis and arthritis or as a silent "cold abscess" that may be drained spontaneously through the overlying skin, forming chronic sinuses. Pure tenosynovitis can also occur along tendon sheaths; in the hand and wrist, this can present as a compound ganglion.

10. How does TB arthritis present clinically?

TB infections of the joint typically present as nonspecific monoarticular chronic synovitis. They are characterized by the presence of a significant amount of hypertrophic synovial proliferation and progressive destruction of the articular surfaces and the underlying bone. The blood chemistry results are nonspecific. The definitive diagnosis relies on tissue examination with either needle or, more often, open biopsy.

11. How does spinal involvement present clinically?

The spine can be infected in all age groups. The thoracic and upper lumbar spine is more commonly affected. Early presentations are localized pain with or without systemic symptoms of malaise, low-grade fever, and weight loss. Later, kyphus deformities may be detected, and in adults, a large "cold abscess" may be found. The cold abscess can appear in the loin region just below the spinal involvement or may track down along the psoas muscle sheath and appear as a mass in the groin region. Some cases can present as Pott's disease with paraparesis or paraplegia as a result of significant destruction of the vertebra, leading to compression of the spinal cord or direct involvement of the dural sheath.

12. What are the radiologic features of spinal involvement?

The lateral plain radiograph of the thoracolumbar spine shows the characteristic appearance of destruction of two or more adjacent vertebral bodies and the intervertebral disks (see Figure). Additional imaging techniques such as CT scanning allow better visualization of the degree of destruction of the vertebral body, the extradural extension, the extent of adjacent soft tissue involvement, and the large and multiloculated psoas abscess formation.

13. What causes atypical mycobacterial infection?

More than 40 mycobacterium species have been described. The more common species causing atypical infections in humans are *Mycobacterium marianum, M. ulcerans, M. chelonei, M. xenopi,* and *M. fortuitum.*

14. How do atypical mycobacterial infections present clinically?

This heterogeneous group of opportunist mycobacteria can cause infection and ulceration of the skin, the hand, and the fingers as well as cervical lymphadenitis. Deep bone and joint infections can also develop in immunologically compromised individuals, although infection of the spine is very rare. High-risk patients are those with HIV infection, those receiving oral steroids for a long period, renal dialysis patients, and patients undergoing intra-articular steroid injections.

15. How does one treat atypical mycobacterial infections?

In general, they do not respond to the conventional antituberculous drugs. Their heterogeneous nature makes the selection of drugs difficult. The site of infection, the sensitivity of the cultured bacilli, and the immunologic status of the affected patient must be considered. Some may response

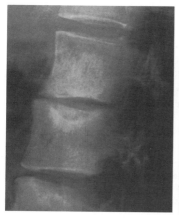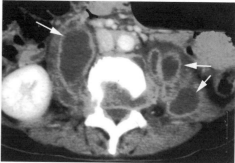

Left, Lateral plain radiograph of the thoracolumbar spine shows the characteristic appearance of destruction of two or more adjacent vertebral bodies and the intervertebral disc. *Right,* Additional imaging techniques such as CT scanning allow better visualization of the degree of destruction of the vertebral body, the extradural extension, and the extent of adjacent soft tissue involvement as well as the large and multiloculated TB psoas abscess formation *arrows.*

to conventional antibiotics (e.g., *M. fortuitum* is sensitive to aminoglycosides). In other instances, deep infections of bone and joint can be resistant to multiple chemotherapeutic agents. For those who respond to the antibacterial agents, long-term treatment is often not necessary. Surgical treatment may be necessary as well.

16. What is chronic multifocal osteomyelitis?

This is a poorly understood rare condition thought to be due to an infectious agent. In 25% of cases, an association with group A α-hemolytic stretococcal sore throat and elevated antistreptolysin O titer was found. Biopsy findings show nonspecific subacute and chronic osteomyelitis.

17. How does chronic multifocal osteomyelitis present clinically?

The condition affects mainly young children and young adults and affects the tibia, clavicle, femur, fibula, hand, and foot. The clinical course is often characterized by bouts of exacerbation and remission. Diagnosis is made by means of bone scan, MRI, and direct bone biopsies.

18. How is it treated, and what is the expected outcome?

Culture of the biopsy material and blood culture are nearly always negative in this condition. In the acute phase, response to conventional antibiotics is often good. After a variable period from one year to many years, complete resolution usually results.

19. Who is most likely to get fungal infections?

Most fungal infections are opportunistic infections in patients with immunodeficiency or in those receiving immunosuppression, prolonged potent broad-spectrum antibiotics, or long-term steroid therapy.

20. Which types of fungi cause bone and joint infections and how do they present clinically?

The most commonly reported fungal infections are candidiasis, cryptococcosis, aspergillosis, coccidioidomycosis, sporotrichosis, and blastomycosis. In recent years, however, an increasing number of very rare saprophytic opportunist fungal infections such as phaeohyphomycosis, trichosporosis, and Fusarium and Pseudallescheria infections have been reported. Many of the infections present as nonspecific osteomyelitis or arthritis. The spine and the knee joint are most frequently affected. Certain fungal infections are endemic in certain areas, for example, coccidioidomycosis is virtually limited to the southwestern United States and northern Mexico. Knowledge of the specific epidemiology would be of considerable importance to the attending clinician.

21. How does one diagnose fungal infection of the bone and joints?

A high index of suspicion should always exist for high-risk patients. An unusual bone or joint infection should be thoroughly investigated, including biopsy. Immunodiagnostic techniques are now available for a limited number of fungal infections, such as *Candida albicans*, but for most infections, they are still not specific and sensitive enough.

22. How should one treat a fungal infection of bone and joints?

The lesion should be covered aggressively with antifungal agents before the final histologic or microbiologic proof is available, since testing may take a few weeks. The mortality and morbidity in immunocompromised patients are very high, in some reports up to 50%. The most commonly used antifungal agents are amphotericin B alone or in combination with the newer drugs like flucytosine, ketoconazole, and itraconazole. Aggressive surgical treatment may be necessary if the response to drug treatment is not satisfactory.

23. What causes brucellosis?

Brucellosis in humans is most commonly caused by the gram-negative intracellular coccobacillus *Brucella melitensis*. Other species such as *B. suis*, *B. canis*, and *B. abortus* have also been reported in human infections. The disease is a worldwide public health problem and a significant cause of loss of domestic livestock. In one series, 92% gave a history of animal contact, usually with sheep or goats, or of ingesting raw milk, milk products, or raw liver. A brucellar cause should be considered in any child from an endemic area who has osteoarticular manifestations.

24. What is the clinical presentation, and how is it diagnosed?

Brucellosis can be either insidious or abrupt in onset and can affect virtually every organ system; skeletal involvement (spondylitis, arthritis) is the most frequent metastatic complication. In the acute phase, clinical features include pyrexia, arthralgia, hepatosplenomegaly, and lymphadenopathy. A subacute presentation with peripheral monoarthritis predominantly affecting hips or knees is common. Involvement of the spine is either focal or diffuse, with a predilection for the lumbar region. Erosions and sclerosis of vertebral end plates with intact disks are typical with the focal form. In diffuse brucellar spondylitis, osteomyelitis of neighboring vertebrae, involvement of the intervening disk, and moderate epidural extension may be found. Children with osteoarticular brucellosis have a higher relapse rate and a longer hospital stay.

For diagnosis, a high index of suspicion is important. The agglutination titers are usually elevated, with positive blood culture results in less than 50% of patients. Histologic diagnosis and culture of infected tissues are necessary in chronic cases.

25. What is the preferred drug for treatment of brucellosis?

Single-drug therapy with ciprofloxacin, tetracycline, or co-trimoxazole, although effective for the acute symptoms, is associated with an appreciable rate of relapse. A combination of two or more drugs (rifampicin, co-trimoxazole, tetracycline, and streptomycin) for 4–6 weeks is associated with a much lower recurrence rate.

26. How does Lyme disease appear clinically? How does one confirm the diagnosis?

Three stages of Lyme disease have been described: stage I, characterized by erythema chronicum migrans and flulike symptoms; stage II, characterized by dermatologic, ophthalmologic, neurologic, and cardiac disorders; and stage III, characterized by arthritis, a multiple sclerosis-like syndrome, psychiatric disorders, and a chronic fatigue syndrome. The clinical presentation of Lyme arthritis in children is different from that in adults (e.g., a preceding erythema migrans is very rare). The diagnosis of Lyme arthritis requires the exclusion of other diseases and positive findings on serologic testing for IgG antibodies to *Borrelia burgdorferi*. Enzyme-linked immunosorbent assay, immunoblotting, and polymerase chain reaction techniques to identify infection by *B. burgdorferi* are also used.

27. What is the preferred treatment for Lyme disease?

Therapy with penicillin or tetracycline for a period of 10 days to 3 weeks is usually effective in the treatment of stage 1 symptoms. Later stages of Lyme arthritis can be treated with 1-month courses of oral doxycycline or amoxicillin or with 2- to 4-weeks courses of intravenous ceftriaxone. A safe vaccine for the prevention of Lyme disease in humans has been developed, and clinical vaccine efficacy trials are currently underway.

BIBLIOGRAPHY

1. Benjamin B, Annobil SH, Khan MR: Osteoarticular complications of childhood brucellosis: a study of 57 cases in Saudi Arabia. J Pediatr Orthop 12(6):801–805, 1992.
2. Broner FA, Garland DE, Zigler JE: Spinal infections in the immunocompromised host. Orthop Clin North Am 27(1):37–46, 1996.
3. Mousa AR, Muhtaseb SA, Almudallal DS, Khodeir SM, Marafie AA: Osteoarticular complications of brucellosis: a study of 169 cases. Rev Infect Dis 9(3):531–543, 1987.
4. Nemir RL, O'Hare D: Tuberculosis in children 10 years of age and younger: three decades of experience during the chemotherapeutic era. Pediatrics 88(2):236–241, 1988.
5. Rose CD, Fawcett PT, Eppes SC, Klein JD, Gibney K, Doughty RA: Pediatric Lyme arthritis: clinical spectrum and outcome. J Pediatr Orthop 14(2):238–241, 1994.

6. Rowe JG, Amadio PC, Edson RS: Sporotrichosis. Orthopedics 12(7):981–985, 1989.
7. Steere AC: Musculoskeletal manifestations of Lyme disease. Am J Med 2498(4A):44S–48S, 1995.
8. Upaahyay SS, Seji MJ, Sell B, Hsu LC: Controlled trial of short-course regimens of chemotherapy in the ambulatory treatment of spinal tuberculosis. Results at three years of a study in Korea. Twelfth report of the Medical Research Council Working Party on Tuberculosis of the Spine. J Bone Joint Surg [Br] 75(2):24–28, 1993.
9. Upaahyay SS, Sell P, Saji MJ, Hsu LC: Surgical management of spinal tuberculosis in adults. Hong Kong operation compared with debridement surgery for short and long term outcome of deformity. Clin Orthop 302:173–182, 1994.
10. Yao DC, Sartoris DJ: Musculoskeletal tuberculosis. Radiol Clin North Am 33(4):679–689, 1995.

85. CEREBRAL PALSY

Eugene E. Bleck, M.D.

1. What is cerebral palsy?
A group of nonprogressive disorders in young children in which disease of the brain causes impairment of motor function. Motor disorders that are transient or the result of progressive brain disease or spinal cord impairment are excluded. Some neurologists prefer the term "static encephalopathy."

2. What are the motor manifestations of cerebral palsy?
- **Spastic:** increased stretch reflexes in the muscles.
- **Athetoid:** takes various forms. *Ballismus*—uncontrolled involuntary motion of the proximal joint; *chorea*—involuntary jerking of the distal joints (e.g., the fingers); *rigidity*—leadpipe type, characterized by continuous resistance to passive motion, and cogwheel type, which has discontinuous resistance to passive motion; *dystonia*—intermittent distorted posturing of the limb, neck, and trunk; and *tension athetosis*—usually extension patterns that can be broken by repetitive motion of the involved joint.
- **Ataxic:** lack of balance and uncoordinated movement.
- **Tremor:** intentional or nonintentional, rhythmic or nonrhythmic
- **Atonia:** rarely persists beyond infancy. Hypotonic infants usually evolve to having athetosis.
- **Mixed types:** we try to avoid this classification. Most often disequilibrium (i.e. lack of balance reactions) is found in children with the spastic type and athetosis.

3. How is the geographic involvement of the paresis classified?
- **Hemiplegia:** arm and lower limb affected only on involved side.
- **Diplegia:** major spasticity in the lower limbs and minor (usually lack of fine motor coordination) in the upper limbs.
- **Paraplegia:** involvement only in the lower limbs is probably not cerebral palsy but is rather a hereditary spastic paraplegia or is due to spinal cord disease or spinal abnormalities.
- **Triplegia:** three-limb involvement.
- **Quadriplegia:** four limbs. Quadriplegia is no longer used to describe the usual child who has this much involvement. The head, neck, and trunk are generally always affected. We prefer "total body involved."

4. Are there associated defects due to brain dysfunction in cerebral palsy?
Yes, we see *visual disturbances* such as esotropia in spastic diplegia associated with prematurity; blindness is now rare since high concentrations of oxygen are no longer given to newborns presumed to be at risk. Perceptual problems are common in many children. Paralysis of the upward gaze is common in athetosis due to kernicterus (hemolytic anemia of the newborn, erythroblastosis fetalis).

Loss of hearing was characteristic of the rubella syndrome but is rarely encountered today owing to rubella immunization.

Speech delay and difficulties in articulation are found in many children who have cerebral palsy. Those whose total body is involved are often nonverbal but may have inner language.

Convulsive disorders occur mainly in spastic hemiplegia and are usually late in onset.

Sensory loss of shape and recognition (astereognosis) is common in the hands in spastic hemiplegia and may be seen in diplegia and in those with the total body involved. The sensory loss will also be found in two-point discrimination. Thus, the hand function particularly in spastic hemiplegia will depend on visual feedback.

Mental retardation occurs frequently in the patient with the total body involved with spasticity. Children who have athetosis, even though nonverbal, can have normal intelligence. In general, children with spastic diplegia and hemiplegia have normal intelligence, but some may lack the ability of abstract reasoning, and others may have dyslexia.

5. What are the major causes of cerebral palsy at or around the time of birth?

The leading cause in the Western world is *premature birth* and a birth weight of less than 2500 grams, the progressively higher prevalence in decreasing birth weights. The disease of the brain in premature birth has been defined as periventricular atrophy suggestive of leukomalacia due to ischemic damage and intraventricular hemorrhage. Recent MRI studies suggest that prenatal factors are probably responsible for cerebral palsy rather than perinatal complications.

Birth trauma and asphyxia were formerly blamed for cerebral palsy, but such causation is rare today.

Erythroblastosis fetalis and kernicterus as a cause of cerebral palsy with chorea-athetosis have fallen dramatically owing to the widely used prophylaxis with anti-D immune globulin G in the Rh-negative mother, intrauterine intravascular transfusion of the fetus, and phototherapy.

Other etiologic risk factors are familial inheritance, teratogenic factors, congenital infections, rubella, cytomegalic inclusion disease, and genetic glucose-6-phosphate dehydrogenase (G6PD) deficiency.

6. What is the prognosis for walking in the child who has cerebral palsy?

After the age of 12 months, the persistence of infantile reflexes and automatisms and the failure to develop can determine walking prognosis in 95%. There are five major tests.

1. Persistence of the neck righting reflex. With passive head turning, the infant can be rolled over and over, as rolling a log.

2. Persistence of the fully developed, imposable, and obligate tonic neck reflex. When the infant's head is turned to one side, the upper and lower limbs flex on the occiput side and extend on the face side (fencing position).

3. Moro's reflex. A sudden loud noise or jarring of the table causes the full-blown response of abduction of the arms followed by the embrace. A startled reaction is not a Moro's reflex.

4. Extensor thrust. The baby is held erect by the trunk, and the feet are lowered to the tabletop. progressive extension of the lower limbs is abnormal at any age.

5. Absent parachute reaction. When the baby is held prone and suddenly lowered to the table, the normal response is automatic hand placement, a protective reflex we keep for life when we fall (see Figure).

If two of these are present or if the parachute reaction is absent, the prognosis for walking is poor. Most of these infants will have cerebral palsy with total body involvement of either the athetoid or the spastic type. Those who have hemiplegia generally all walk by the age of 18 months; most who have diplegia will walk at the mean age of 36 months; with pure ataxia, walking will be delayed usually to age 4–5 years.

Inability to sit unsupported after the age of 4 years predicts the inability to walk. Another predictor is head balance. Those who develop head balance by 9 months are able to walk either independently or with external support. Those who have no head balance at 20 months are unable to walk. Sitting by 24 months is a good prognostic sign. Mental retardation alone or with a motor disability does not affect the ability to walk.

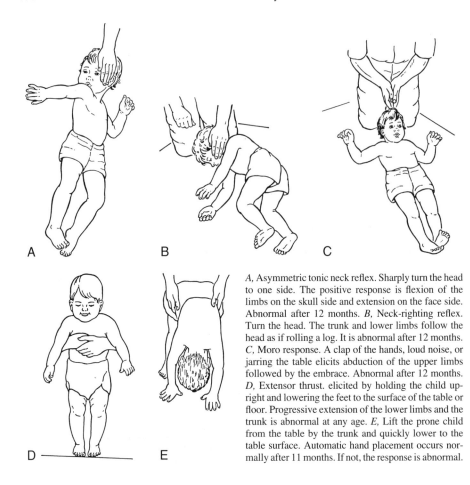

A, Asymmetric tonic neck reflex. Sharply turn the head to one side. The positive response is flexion of the limbs on the skull side and extension on the face side. Abnormal after 12 months. B, Neck-righting reflex. Turn the head. The trunk and lower limbs follow the head as if rolling a log. It is abnormal after 12 months. C, Moro response. A clap of the hands, loud noise, or jarring the table elicits abduction of the upper limbs followed by the embrace. Abnormal after 12 months. D, Extensor thrust. elicited by holding the child upright and lowering the feet to the surface of the table or floor. Progressive extension of the lower limbs and the trunk is abnormal at any age. E, Lift the prone child from the table by the trunk and quickly lower to the table surface. Automatic hand placement occurs normally after 11 months. If not, the response is abnormal.

7. Which children need crutches or walkers?

External supports are needed not to compensate for muscle weakness but because of lack of balance reactions (disequilibrium). When able to stand alone, the child can be tested by gently pushing him or her side-to-side and then anteriorly and posteriorly. These children lack a stepping response and fall over like a felled tree. If the balance is poor side-to-side but good anteriorly, crutches will be needed. If poor side-to-side, anteriorly, and posteriorly, a walker is necessary. If the reactions are good side-to-side and anteriorly but absent posteriorly, they can walk independently but will fall backwards easily and often in a crowd (characteristic of spastic diplegia) with slight perturbation of their balance.

8. When should a wheelchair be prescribed?

When the prognosis for walking is poor and the child is at the developmental age when mobility for exploring is paramount (18 months or older), a wheelchair should be considered. Because most of those with a poor walking prognosis are the total body involved and have limited upper limb use, we prescribe a motorized wheelchair. Even children who are struggling to walk with walkers or crutches will find a motorized wheelchair a boom to their development and mobility. Trying to walk against the spasticity or athetosis is so energy consuming that they cannot cope with or progress in education and social development.

9. Is there a treatment for cerebral palsy?

There is no specific treatment for the loss of neurons in the central nervous system. Various therapy methods claim great success if begun in an "infant-at-risk" at a very early age, e.g., 6–8 months. It is well established that you cannot even diagnose cerebral palsy before the age of 12 months in most cases, however. In addition, even infants-at-risk can "outgrow" neurologic signs of cerebral palsy.

"Systems of therapy" such as Bobath neurodevelopment, Votja, sensory integration, patterning, Rolfing, and neuromuscular facilitation as well as physical therapy have had claims of success. "Conductive education" and the Portage Project have been popular, but these are not treatment methods. Rather they are systems of education and child development. Brain surgery and cerebrellar stimulation have been found ineffective.

10. What about drug therapy?

None of the oral "muscle relaxants" has been efficacious in alleviating the spasticity of the muscles, and there are no drugs that have helped athetosis or ataxia. This class of drugs acts on the brain to depress its function. Most patients do not like the effects of central nervous system depression, and long-term use is generally abandoned. Diazepam (Valium) seems to help severe athetosis by relieving anxiety and tension in some patients. It has been useful postoperatively for a few days after orthopaedic surgery.

Intrathecal baclofen (Lioresal), originally used for spasticity of the lower limbs in multiple sclerosis, has been used in the past few years with some success in those with total-body-involved cerebral palsy.

Botulinum toxin, type A (Botox) injected into the muscles to block neuomuscular transmission was originally used for strabismus. In the past few years, it has been tried in cerebral palsy to reduce spasticity in the limb muscles selectively. Its effect is not permanent, but the duration of action is much longer than with 45% alcohol injections. Currently, its major use has been to block spasticity in the calf muscles to overcome dynamic equinus of the ankle in children with spastic diplegia and hemiplegia. As with alcohol, it might help decide the effects of proposed surgery of the adductor muscles, calf muscle, and hamstrings. The advantage of botulinum toxin is that there is little or no postinjection pain in the muscle. It is hoped that recurrent blocking of the spastic muscle will allow its antagonist to grow stronger and thus overcome the bad effects of the stronger agonist, but this has yet to be demonstrated.

11. Are orthotics useful?

There have been no studies that show long-term reduction in contractures of joints in the lower limb with the use of orthotics (such as the plastic ankle-foot orthosis) to correct, control, and prevent spastic equinus, pes varus, or pes valgus). The ankle-foot orthosis is most often used in the young child who has spastic equinus as a temporizing method in the hope that with the establishment of better balance reactions, the equinus will be minimized. Orthotics do not correct actual contractures. The problem with orthotics for the hands and wrist in cerebral palsy is that they barricade sensory input and are usually used only when the child is at school or in a therapy unit.

12. What about rhizotomy?

The basis for cutting 30–40% of the lumbar posterior rootlets (rhizotomy) is reduced inhibition of muscle contraction via descending tracts from the brain when the neurons are damaged. This damage causes excessive spinal anterior horn cell activity with resultant spasticity. Cutting the posterior root afferents to the spinal cord reduces the facilitatory influences on the anterior horn cell motor neuron. From its original implementation in 1982, the indications for this procedure have been refined. The best candidates seem to be children with spastic diplegia, good balance reactions, no major or severe muscle contractures, and voluntary control of muscle function. Hemiplegics are excluded as well as those who have athetosis. The lower limbs are flail after the procedure and then gradually recover. Several months of physical therapy consisting of active and resistive exercises and muscle rehabilitative measures are necessary postoperatively.

13. Does rhizotomy eliminate the need for orthopaedic surgery?
No. Rhizotomy will not correct contractures of the muscles or joints or structural joint changes. It cannot correct progressive subluxation of the hip, pes valgus, or femoral antetorsion or prevent scoliosis. We have seen reports that subluxation of the hip and severe lumbar lordosis have been seen postoperatively. Some believe both rhizotomy and orthopaedic surgery are indicated and are not mutually exclusive.

14. What should the physician prescribe?
Manual stretching and night splints or braces have had no effect in stemming the development of contractures and secondary skeletal changes.

Therapeutic exercise (active and resistive) does have some rationale, since the muscles are both spastic and weak. Designing and implementing sports for the disabled have been extremely valuable. For those who are confined to wheelchairs, getting out of the sitting position regularly and doing floor and mat activities seem to alleviate stiffness and postural contractures. Swimming and exercise in a heated pool with supervision have been a boon and are enjoyable to most.

15. What are the most important functions for the child who will become an adult?
(1) Communication (which also implies education), (2) activities of daily living (eating, dressing, personal hygiene, and grooming), (3) mobility (getting from here to there), and (4) walking.

16. How are functional goals implemented?
Assistive technology has been accepted as a way to compensate for lost or deficient functions (e.g., communication devices for the nonverbal child, motorized chairs with electronic interfaces and controls for mobility, adaptive toilet equipment, wheelchair inserts to compensate for loss of sitting balance, and adaptive clothing and shoes). Incidentally, feeding devices have not been very successful. For the person who is severely disabled, precluding effective hand use, the only times of the day when he or she has human contact are at meals. Thus, mechanical feeding devices and robots are received unenthusiastically.

17. What is the prognosis for hand function?
Obviously the ability to pinch, grasp, and release is essential in at least one hand for most tasks of daily living. If there is no early lateralization (dominance) of hand use and if the hands do not cross the midline, the prognosis for hand function is poor.

18. What is the prognosis for communication?
Good if the child makes recognizable sounds before the age of 2 years. Speech pathologists and engineers can assess the potential for nonverbal communication methods and devices.

19. What can we tell parents about their child's future?
Our experience is that goals can be set as early as the age of 4 years if we have reasonably good predictions of eventual function. In setting advanced goals for optimum independent living, we need to emphasize that the child with cerebral palsy becomes the adult with cerebral palsy. In spastic hemiplegia and diplegia, we can be optimistic that the child will be able to blend in with the community as a productive person, barring severe mental retardation. Today, this group of children is integrated into the regular school, and quite a few attend college. Most whose total body is involved can achieve to the limits of their intellectual ability and have a life of friendship and achievement. They will need adaptive equipment, sometimes special housing arrangements, and sometimes attendant care.

We can also emphasize that on long-term follow-up, children with cerebral palsy who have been manipulated into doing unproven therapies often face a crisis of a lost childhood in later adolescence and early adult life. Nervous breakdown and psychiatric care may ensue.

20. Are there structural skeletal changes?

In the spastic type, the muscles will contract and produce joint deformities. The most devastating one is dislocation of the hip, which can lead to eventual painful degenerative joint disease. Knee flexion contractures will compromise efficient walking and over a period of years will cause knee pain due to osteoarthritis. Retropatellar pain is usually the first symptom of cartilage degeneration. Contracture of the calf muscles causes fixed equinus with resultant excessive toe pressure and pain. Foot deformities, varus (inversion deformity) in hemiplegia and valgus (eversion deformity) in diplegia, will cause unequal weight bearing and painful calluses and will affect shoe wear and fitting. Scoliosis is common in the total body involved and compromises sitting.

21. Can orthopaedic surgery prevent hip subluxation and eventual dislocation?

Hip subluxation and dislocation are seen almost exclusively in the nonwalking child, in those whose total body is involved, or in those who walk with crutches or walkers. It is rare in hemiplegia and in those who have diplegia and walk independently. Orthopaedic surgery (iliopsoas tenotomy and adductor myotomy) can prevent dislocation of the hip if done early, certainly before the age of 5 years and preferably earlier. In older children, femoral (mainly subtrochanteric derotation) and pelvic osteotomy (Dega in the growing child or Chiari in the skeletally mature) are also necessary.

PERCENT OF SUBLUXATION

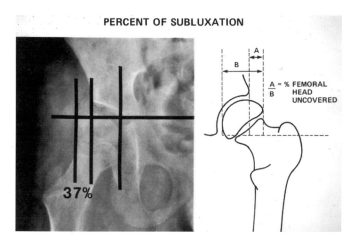

$\dfrac{A}{B}$ = % FEMORAL HEAD UNCOVERED

37%

Measurement of the migration percentage of the femoral head on the AP x-ray. Normal up to 15%. **Note:** In paralytic subluxation of the hip, in contrast to congenital dislocation, there is no acetabular dysplasia. In acquired subluxation, acetabular dysplasia develops later in childhood.

22. Why is the Salter innominate osteotomy or its variations not indicated for acetabular dysplasia in spastic paralytic subluxation or dislocation?

In most cases of spastic paralytic subluxation and dislocation of the hip, the acetabulum is more deficient posteriorly than anteriorly. The Salter and similar pelvic osteotomies uncover the hip posteriorly. Therefore, other acetabular reconstructive procedures should be considered.

23. What surgery is indicated for scissoring during gait?

Scissoring during gait due to adductor spasticity can be relieved by adductor longus and gracilis tenotomy. Anterior-branch obturator neurectomy in the ambulatory child is now avoided because this nerve also innervates the adductor brevis, a major hip stabilizer during the stance phase of gait. Transfer of the origins of the adductor muscles seems to offer no advantage over simple myotenotomy.

24. What is the rationale for surgical correction of a hip flexion deformity in the child who walks?
Since 60% of the gait cycle is stance, limited hip extension greatly affects the efficiency of walking. Hip flexion contractures are compensated for by anterior inclination of the pelvis and lumbar lordosis. Generally, hip flexion contractures of more than 15° need surgical correction by iliopsoas tenotomy at the pelvic brim, Z-lengthening, or recession. Currently, tenotomy at the pelvic brim seems to be favored.

25. What is the best way to measure the degree of hip flexion contracture?
In cerebral palsy, the traditional Thomas test is inaccurate owing to the usual concomitant spastic contracture of the hamstrings. The best measurement method is Staheli's, in which the patient is placed prone with the limbs hanging over the edge of the table. With the examiner's fingers on the posterior superior iliac spines, one limb is gently and slowly brought into extension. The point at which the pelvis rotates anteriorly is the degree of contracture measured against the horizontal plane.

26. What surgery can correct the hip internal rotation during gait?
The best method to correct the gait pattern is subtrochanteric femoral derotation osteotomy using internal fixation with a compression nailplate. Other surgeons use crossed Steinmann's pins to hold the osteotomy secure, but this demands spica plaster immobilization. Still others like a supracondylar femoral derotation osteotomy, but I find that immobilizing the knee in plaster postoperatively risks knee stiffness and prolongs the time to restoration of knee function.

27. Can the patient's gait be made worse with derotation osteotomy?
If a femoral derotation osteotomy is done when there is compensatory external tibial-fibular torsion, the result will be functionally and subjectively worse, and the child will walk like a duck. Then only additional internal rotation osteotomies of the tibia and fibula can be offered.

28. Can you overcorrect femoral torsion?
If all hip internal rotation is eliminated, then the femur cannot externally rotate as it should at midstance of the gait cycle. With no internal rotation, pelvic rotation substitutes. Save 20°–30° of passive internal rotation at the time of osteotomy.

29. Should additional hip surgery be done at the time of femoral derotation osteotomy?
If the iliopsoas has not been previously lengthened (tenotomy at the pelvic brim or Z-lengthened or recessed) and if there is a hip flexion contracture, iliopsoas lengthening should be done at the time of the osteotomy. Not to do it invites an increased hip flexion contracture.

30. What is normal torsion?
Two standard deviations above or below the norm for the anterior twist of the proximal end of the femur. In the child who has a spastic flexion contracture of the hip from birth, femoral anteversion exceeds the normal range (mean at birth is 31°; declines to a mean of 15° at maturity).

31. Are imaging studies essential to measure anteversion of the femur in cerebral palsy?
Probably not. Numerous published studies show that excessive femoral anteversion persists in the majority of children who have spastic hip muscles.

32. In the examination of the ambulatory patient, how do you diagnose femoral antetorsion (excessive femoral anteversion)?
Measure the passive range of femoral rotation with the patient prone and the knees flexed 90°. If the range of internal rotation is greater than 60° and the external rotation is less than 30°, femoral torsion is the explanation for the internally rotated hip gait pattern. Most patients with cerebral palsy will have passive internal rotation greater than 75° and less than 20°.

33. What surgery is done for the flexed-knee gait?

Fractional semimembranosus aponeurosis and biceps aponeurosis fractional lengthening and semitendinosus tenotomy. A long-standing knee flexion posture leads to contracture of the posterior knee joint capsule. Fifteen degrees of knee flexion contracture is within the physiologic range for function. If a knee flexion contracture is present, posterior capsulotomy of the knee is necessary followed by a slow correction in wedging casts.

34. Is there an indication for additional surgery for the flexed-knee gait pattern?

Cospasticity of the quadriceps is present in most children who have flexed-knee gait patterns and limits knee flexion on the swing phase of gait. For cospasticity of the quadriceps, rectus femoris distal tendon transfer to the sartorius or stump of the semitendinosus can be done at the same time or deferred until later to overcome lack of sufficient knee flexion in the swing phase of gait (normal initial swing = 35°; complete swing = 70°).

35. What is the most common foot deformity in spastic hemiplegia?

Pes varus is due to major spasticity of the posterior tibial muscle.

36. What is the most common foot deformity in spastic diplegia?

Pes valgus is seen mainly in spastic diplegia.

37. What are the current popular operations for pes valgus in the skeletally immature child?

The open-wedge interfacet calcaneal osteotomy (Mosca) and the subtalar extra-articular arthrodesis. In the latter, I prefer the method of screw fixation of the talus to the calcaneus with a bone graft in the sinus tarsi. Crawford has had success using staples to fix the subtalar joint with the foot in the corrected position.

38. What are the indications for triple arthrodesis?

Fixed varus or valgus in the skeletally mature child.

39. Is there a problem with triple arthrodesis for pes valgus?

It often fails to correct the deformity. To correct it, you have to bring the talus out of its plantar flexed position and in alignment with the navicular. To do this, a screw from the talar neck to the calcaneous is needed to keep the corrected position while the denuded joints are fusing. Equinus of the calcaneus is impossible to correct in mature feet. Posterior capsulotomy and Achilles lengthening do not help. When the talus is in the long-standing equinus position, limited anterior articular surface develops, which blocks sufficient dorsiflexion.

40. What is the most effective and simple operation for the tiptoeing child who has the spastic type of cerebral palsy?

Equinus of the ankle due to a contracture of the calf muscles best responds to a sliding Achilles tendon lengthening. Many experienced orthopaedic surgeons favor the percutaneous method of lengthening the tendon with two cuts halfway through medially, one proximal and one distal in the tendon, separated by a cut halfway through laterally between the two medial ones.

41. What is a major pitfall in Achilles tendon lengthening, and how can it be avoided?

A calcaneus postoperatively is an undesirable result. It is due to over lengthening of the Achilles tendon. Care should be taken not to push the foot into dorsiflexion beyond neutral position after the incision in the tendon is completed. The tendon will be overlengthened with resultant irretrievable calcaneus deformity and a much less functional gait.

42. What is the function of the gastrocnemius?

The gastrocnemius prevents forward progression of the tibia in stance phase. If it is overly weakened by Achilles tendon lengthening, a knee-flexed gait posture will result.

43. When is cast immobilization indicated after surgery?

After iliopsoas and adductor tenotomy for early subluxation of the hip, a spica cast with the hips in a comfortable 45°–60° of abduction for 6 weeks should be sufficient. Abduction splinting for several months postoperatively is recommended by many surgeons worried about recurrence. After femoral and pelvic osteotomies, spica cast immobilization for 6 weeks followed by mobilization exercises is usual.

After iliopsoas pelvic brim lengthening or recession, no spica cast is necessary if this is the only procedure. Bed rest and hip abduction and extension isometric exercises done in bed for 3 weeks appear satisfactory. Sitting should be avoided to prevent recontracture.

After a subtrochanteric femoral osteotomy with internal fixation for intoed gait, no cast immobilization should be necessary. If bilateral, the child can use the wheelchair and bed regimen until healing occurs, usually for 8 weeks.

After hamstring lengthening with a cylinder cast, standing and walking within a day or two and continuing for 3 weeks are sufficient. If a rectus femoris transfer has been done, a reinforced fabric knee immobilizer that can be removed for daily intermittent exercise is used.

After foot tendon surgery, 6 weeks of short-leg cast immobilization and weight-bearing to tolerance seem to offer an uncomplicated postoperative course in most children. No special orthoses or shoes should be required.

After Achilles tendon lengthening, a long-leg walking cast allowing weight-bearing has not compromised the final result. After 3 weeks, the cast can be cut down to below the knee and walking continued for an additional 3 weeks before removal. No postoperative orthoses or special therapy has been required. The children can wear ordinary sports or tennis shoes.

44. When should surgery of the lower limbs be done?

Generally, surgery is done in spastic diplegia and hemiplegia once the gait pattern is established and the child is walking. This is usually between the ages of 5 and 7 years. Femoral osteotomies for internal rotation gait can be deferred until age 10 or older.

45. Is instrumented gait analysis essential in selecting the surgical procedure in cerebral palsy?

Without a doubt, the science of gait analysis has deepened our understanding of the gait cycle. Whether it is essential depends on the surgeon's experience in observational gait analysis. At the minimum, the observer should describe the gait of the patient in terms of stance and swing phases in the sagittal plane and rotation in the frontal plane. Electromyogaphy is not quantitative, but it does tell what muscles are firing out of phase or are prolonged in phase.

Kinematics will measure stride length and ranges of joint motion during the cycle and can help one decide what value is out of the functional range. It is an important assessment tool but cannot be the whole story of how that patient functions in daily life.

Gait analysis does not measure the influence of disequilibrium or demonstrate specific structural deformities in the foot or their potential for passive correction.

46. How and when should scoliosis be treated?

Scoliosis is common in the nonwalking patient. Often, pelvic obliquity is evident, since the pelvis really is part of the curve. Orthoses or special seating pads and adjustments are useless to prevent progression or hold the curve. Correction should be in early adolescence when there is not much potential for additional major growth of the spine. Once the curves are at 40° or more and are approximately 50% passively correctable, fusion with instrumentation using a form of the Luque unit rod, the Galveston pelvic fixation method, and interlaminar wiring is the best method. The idiopathic type of curve will occasionally be seen in the ambulatory patient and should be treated the same as in the child with no paralysis.

If the curve resists passive pre-operative correction, anterior disk excision and fusion without interval fixation are required. A week to 10 days separating the anterior from the posterior procedure is safe and entails no special holding orthodics or casts. A postoperative removable shell thoracolumbar spinal orthosis can be used while fusion is occurring for the ensuing 6–8 months. Some surgeons do both anterior and posterior surgery at the same stage.

47. Can scoliosis be prevented by correcting the adduction contracture of the hip or the subluxation and dislocation that also result in a pelvic obliquity?

No. Scoliosis has no relationship to these disorders.

48. Is there a place for hand surgery in cerebral palsy?

Only in spastic paralysis. While the results can look good, function is compromised by the common lack of stereognosis in the child with hemiplegia. Improved appearance of the involved hand in hemiplegia is much valued by the patient, however.

49. What is the most common upper limb deformity in the spastic type, and what methods can be used to correct it?

The thumb-in-palm deformity can be disabling. Correction entails release of the adductor pollicis at its insertion, release of the first dorsal interosseous muscle, fixation or fusion of the hypermobile metacarpal phalangeal joint, and rerouting of the extensor pollicis longus tendon.

50. What can be done for the fisted hand and wrist in spastic hemiplegia.

Finger flexion contractures can be relieved by selective myotendinous lengthening in the forearm. Finger and wrist extension can be improved by transfer of the flexor carpi ulnaris to either the extensor carpi radialis brevis or the common finger extensors. Sectioning of the profundi above the wrist and suturing to the distal cut ends of the superficialis tendons can result in too much weakness of finger flexion and the subsequent development of an intrinsic-plus deformity. Similarly, lengthening of the profundi risks the same undesirable result.

51. How do you decide which surgery to do on the upper limb?

All contemplated upper limb surgery in cerebral palsy demands detailed and frequent preoperative analysis. At times, infiltration of a local anesthetic or botulinum A toxin into the offending flexor muscle belly and observation of the potential for active voluntary finger extension are a help in deciding the appropriate procedure.

52. Is there a trap in assessing a spastic-appearing hand for surgery?

The trap is failing to distinguish dystonic posturing from spastic paralysis. Dystonic posturing will be revealed when you get the patient to relax. Then there are no contractures. The minute they attempt to move the hand, however, the posture returns. Tendon transfer or lengthening in dystonia will result in a reverse posture, from flexion to extension posturing.

53. What can be done for the pronated forearm in spastic hemiplegia?

For the pronation contracture of the forearm, if passively correctable and if there is some active voluntary supination, simple excision of the pronator teres tendon at its insertion on the radius can be successful. Voluntary supination is needed for a good result. Transfer of the flexor carpi ulnaris to the extensor carpi radialis brevis to correct the wrist flexion posture and restore active supination by itself has not been that successful. In most cases, release of the pronator teres has also been done. Transfer of the flexor carpi ulnaris demands considerable dissection of the muscle from the ulna in order to gain length. If there is no wrist flexion posture, this is more surgery than needed to restore only supination. Fixed pronation of the forearm is not so bad and is functional, while fixed supination is dysfunctional.

54. Should wrist arthrodesis be considered for the flexed wrist?
Wrist arthrodesis is avoided unless the patient is skeletally mature and wants the fixed wrist flexion corrected for a better appearance and to overcome a barrier to employment.

55. Should surgery, particularly of the lower limbs, be "staged"?
If you have examined and reexamined the patient in detail, doing all the surgery at one time has been found to be feasible and effective in the usual patient with spastic diplegia. Bony surgery of the foot might be deferred until the indications for it become more certain.

BIBLIOGRAPHY

1. Campos da Paz A Jr, Miranda Burnett S, Willandiono Braga L: Walking prognosis in cerebral palsy: a 22 year retrospective analysis. Dev Med Child Neurol 36:130, 1994.
2. Hagberg B, Hagberg G: Prenatal and perinatal risk factors in a survey of 681 Swedish cases. In Stanley F, Alberman E (eds): The Epidemiology of the Cerebral Palsies. Clinics in Developmental Medicine No. 87. New York, Cambridge University Press, 1984.
3. Milani-Comparetti A: Priorities in rehabilitation: a progress report on a community program. Omaha, NE, Mary Elaine Meyer O'Neal Award Lectureship in Developmental Pediatrics, 1979.
4. Nelson KB, Ellenberg JH: Apgar scores as predictors of chronic neurologic disability. Pediatrics 68:36, 1981.
5. Nelson KB, Ellenberg JH: Children who "outgrew" cerebral palsy. Pediatrics 69:529, 1982.
6. Nelson KB, Ellenberg JH: Antecedents of cerebral palsy. N Engl J Med 315:81, 1986.

86. SPINA BIFIDA

Richard E. Lindseth, M.D.

1. What is myelomeningocele?
A malformation at the base of the spine consisting of a cyst of the meninges and of the spinal cord. The cyst is often open to the outside of the body and leaks cerebrospinal fluid. It is the most common of the neural tube defects.

2. Is the neurologic abnormality limited to the end of the spinal cord?
No. Malformations occur throughout the central nervous system. This disorder is usually associated with hydrocephalus and other malformations of the brain and brain stem. There is herniation of the brain stem into the cervical spine, which is called an Arnold-Chiari II malformation. The central canal of the cord remains open and communicates with the fourth ventricle, which can lead to hydrosyringomyelia. The base of the spinal cord is attached to the sacrum, preventing the cord from migrating upward and leading to a tethered cord syndrome. There also is an abnormality of pituitary function; most of these children have growth hormone deficiency.

3. What causes it?
The cause of myelomeningocele is probably multifactorial. There is a definite inheritance pattern. If a first-degree relative has a neural tube defect, the incidence of myelomeningocele increases from 1:2000 live births to 1:50 live births. The inherited abnormality appears to be a decreased ability to metabolize folic acid.

The environmental cause appears to be an insufficient amount of folic acid within the fertilized egg at the time of the development of the spinal cord. The spinal cord develops between days 21 and 26; therefore, if folic acid supplementation is to be used to prevent myelomeningocele, it should be given preconception. Once the pregnancy test has been obtained and is positive, the

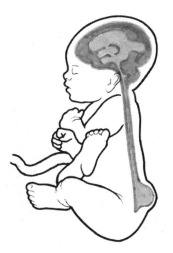

The relationship between hydrocephalus, hydromyelia, and myelomeningocele.

neural tube has already formed, and supplementation at that time is too late. The amount of folic acid necessary for prevention is controversial. For women whose babies who have a high risk of developing myelomeningocele, 0.4 mg, the amount contained in the usual vitamin pill, is probably insufficient unless there is a considerable normal intake of folic acid in the diet. It appears that at least 0.8 mg is needed to overcome the genetic abnormality in these children. It should be noted that valproic acid, an antiseizure medication, interferes with folic acid metabolism and has been found to cause myelomeningocele.

Maternal diabetes is another cause, although it usually forms a different type of abnormality, sacral agenesis.

4. Can myelomeningocele be diagnosed prenatally?
Myelomeningocele can be diagnosed with ultrasound examination at about 12 weeks' gestation. Amniocentesis evaluation will show serum α-feto protein at 21 weeks' gestation to be elevated and will indicate the likelihood of a neural tube defect.

5. What is the benefit of prenatal diagnosis?
If prenatal diagnosis is made during the second trimester, several options are available. The first is to abort the child and try to conceive again, this time with prenatal vitamin supplementation. If this is unacceptable, there is a second option for an improved outcome. Studies have shown that the parents can be prepared for the child. As soon as the child has developed sufficiently that fetal lung disease will not develop, delivery by cesarean section will decrease the neurologic injury to the open neural tube and will decrease the amount of paralysis. If delivery by cesarean section is not performed, the family must plan for this child and seek out expert care for the child prior to delivery.

6. What are the neurologic abnormalities?
Neurologic abnormalities involve the entire central nervous system. Owing to the hydrocephalus and Arnold-Chiari malformation, there are perceptual motor abnormalities and attention deficit disorder. There are abnormalities of the cervical, thoracic, and lumbar cord due to the hydrosyringomyelia. There is injury to the end of the spinal cord caused by the myelomeningocele itself. The neurologic abnormality at the meningocele is primarily sensory in nature. The anterior horn cell and motor pathways are usually intact. This means that reflex activity and uncontrolled and nonpurposeful movements may occur. The posterior columns, which involve sensation and proprioception, are most likely to be injured. A classification of paralysis should be done on the intact neural arc. Spontaneous purposeful movements will

demonstrate the level of paralysis as the child develops. A simple examination can give a good estimate of the level of paralysis.

Vertebrae involved	Corresponding movement
T12–L1	Flex the hips.
L2	Adduct the hips.
L3	Extend the knee.
L4	Flex the knee through the medial hamstrings.
L5	Dorsiflex the foot and dorsiflex the toes.
S1	Plantar flex the toes. There will be marked weakness in the gluteus maximus and gastrocnemius. These children usually have claw toe and cavus deformity.

In most cases, the sacral roots are absent, which means that there is a lack of bladder and bowel control.

7. What is the treatment for hydrocephalus?

Most of these children require a shunt extending from the ventricles to the peritoneal cavity.

8. What are the symptoms of shunt malfunction?

There is an increase in occipital-frontal circumference (OFC), bulging fontanelle, and irritability. There may be papilledema. Arnold-Chiari symptoms may become worse, which would cause sleep apnea, difficulty in swallowing, and other cranial nerve symptoms.

When the child is older and is in the upright position (either sitting or standing), the symptoms become less acute. The cerebrospinal fluid in the brain is decompressed by the connection of the fourth ventricle to the central canal of the cord. Therefore, in older children, the symptoms are often of spinal cord dysfunction rather than of brain dysfunction. The spinal cord symptoms include increasing paralysis, change in bowel and bladder function, and scoliosis. All these abnormalities can be reversed by the prompt reinsertion of the shunt.

9. What are the symptoms of Arnold-Chiari malformation?

The symptoms of an Arnold-Chiari malformation are primarily related to brain stem function. They involve breathing and swallowing disturbances, hyperactive protective sensation of the mouth, and upper extremity weakness.

10. What are the signs and symptoms of hydrosyringomyelia?

These depend to a large extent on which area of the spinal cord has developed the syrinx. In most cases, the worst symptoms are at the base of the spinal cord and would involve bowel and bladder function and an increasing level of paralysis. Very often, the first symptom to appear is scoliosis. The scoliosis is usually in the area of the thoracolumbar spine above the level of paralysis. It is often uncompensated. In some individuals, the syrinx may form in the cervical spine, producing upper extremity weakness and pain.

11. What are the causes and symptoms of a tethered cord?

The cause of the tethered spinal cord syndrome is undetermined. At the time of the initial closure, the cord is released and may migrate proximally; however, it usually becomes reattached. Most affected children do not develop symptoms from the tethered cord. The symptoms may vary somewhat based on the cause of the syndrome, which is thought to be due to stretching of the filum terminale, decreased circulation to the cord, and perhaps pressure on the spinal cord caused by the last intact arch. Most children have a change in bowel and bladder function. Many will have a change in their level of paralysis, very often associated with increasing spasticity and decreased voluntary function. Many, if not all, of the children will have pain in the back or in the legs, often in an area where they do not normally have sensation. There usually is an increasing lumbar lordosis and lumbar scoliosis.

12. What should be evaluated at each office visit?
There is a tendency for worsening of neurologic functioning throughout the patient's lifetime. Therefore, these changes should be looked for at each office visit, even though the patient is also being seen by a neurosurgeon and an orthopaedist. Their visits are often few and far between, and significant changes can appear in the nervous system before the child is reevaluated. During each visit, there should be a brief neurologic evaluation of the lower extremities to see if there is a change in muscle function, strength, or sensation. Often, observation of walking ability is sufficient to determine whether there has been a change. The parents or the patient can often relate whether there has been a change in ability to function. Symptoms of hydrocephalus should be evaluated by examining for changes in mental function, presence of a headache, or changes in upper extremity function. The spine should also be examined for scoliosis.

13. What are the metabolic abnormalities?
All the metabolic abnormalities have not been determined. Almost all these children have growth hormone deficiency and are short in stature. Most of the children are obese. Attempts to limit caloric intake to decrease the amount of obesity have resulted in decrease in growth. The obesity is not necessarily related to decreased activity or excessive caloric intake.

14. What are the spine deformities?
At least 86% of children with spina bifida will have a spine abnormality. Usually, this is scoliosis. Ten percent will have severe kyphosis, particularly in the lumbar spine. Severe lordosis with associated scoliosis of the lumbar spine is also very common.

15. Why are spine deformities important?
The scoliosis is usually uncompensated and progressive. Although idiopathic scoliosis may stop progressing when the child becomes mature, in myelomeningocele, scoliosis progression may continue throughout life and may lead to difficulties with sitting balance and to pressure sores under the prominent ischium. In the adult, pressure sores are one of the more common causes for hospitalization.

Kyphosis in the lumbar spine is almost always progressive and may develop into extreme deformity equaling 140°–150° of curvature. Kyphosis decreases the ability to eat and survive. It decreases the ability to breathe and may require the child to be on a respirator. It also can make it difficult for the child to lie down because of pressure on the back, causing pressure sores over the gibbus.

16. What should I look for?
From the side, there should be a normal S-shaped contour of mild kyphosis in the dorsal spine and lumbar lordosis. From the back, the head should be centered over the pelvis. There should be equal weight on both ischia. This is observed while the child is sitting. If there is any question about scoliosis or kyphosis, a sitting AP and lateral spine x-rays should be obtained. Because of paralysis, standing x-rays are usually not possible.

17. What causes hip deformity?
Hip deformity is very common. Most of the deformities are related to muscle imbalance. In almost all children, the sacral nerve roots are absent, which means that there is no muscle power in the gluteus maximus and weak or absent muscle power in the hip abductors. The hip flexors and adductors are innervated, which causes a flexion/adduction contracture of the hips. Typically, this leads to dislocation of the hip.

18. Are the hip deformities important?
The flexion contractures interfere with the ability to lie down and stand. The hip dislocation per se does not cause difficulties.

19. Can a child go to school and participate in therapy with a dislocated hip?

Yes. The dislocated hip is not painful and does not interfere with activities. There have been studies that have shown that a child walks with or without a dislocated hip.

20. Should a hip dislocation be treated?

The treatment of hip dislocation is controversial. Historically, treatment of hip dislocation has often resulted in a stiff hip, which was more disabling that a mobile dislocated hip. Reduction of the hip is important if there is sufficient muscle activity around the hip to benefit from having the hip located. Unless muscles can be transferred to the hip or there are already sufficient muscles around the hip to make it functional during walking, attempts to reduce the hip are probably not warranted. Children who have good knee control because of function of the quadriceps and hamstrings are candidates to have the hip reduced with muscle transfers to help control the dislocation. In children who are paralyzed at a higher level and who do not have knee control, reduction of the hip is probably ill advised.

21. When should foot deformities be treated?

Almost all children with myelomeningocele have foot deformities. These rarely respond to cast treatment in the newborn period. Anesthesia of the skin around the foot increases the possibility of pressure sores. Most fixed deformities of the feet will require surgical correction. This should be performed when the child has progressed sufficiently in developmental skills to be ready to stand and make use of the feet. Otherwise, there is a tendency for the deformity to recur. In most circumstances, the surgery is performed somewhere between 15 and 24 months of age.

22. What do braces do?

Braces substitute for the absent muscles and sensation by stabilizing joints that the child cannot control. They do not prevent or correct deformity, but are used to maintain function after surgical correction of the deformity. For example, most affected children have paralysis of their foot and ankle muscles. An ankle/foot orthosis is used to give stability to the ankle because of lack of muscle power and sensation in that area. If the knee does not have quadriceps and hamstring control, the brace must be extended above the knee. If there is lack of hip control, the brace must be extended above the hip.

23. What determines whether a child will walk or will use a wheelchair?

The biggest determination is the level of muscle paralysis. If the child has the ability to flex and extend the knee, there is a good chance that he or she will be a walker in the community as a young adult. If they do not have knee control, they will probably be in a wheelchair. During the school-aged years, most children can be made to walk in braces and crutches or a walker. For thoracic and upper lumbar levels of paraplegia, however, the usual age which the child quits walking is around 8 or 9 years. Many adults will quit walking because the energy required to walk is much greater than that used to manipulate a wheelchair. We are also beginning to find an increasing frequency of degenerative joint disease, particularly of the knees, in midlumbar-level paraplegics who are still walking in their twenties.

Whether children who do not have knee control should be put into braces and urged to walk during childhood is controversial. Some treatment centers state that it is a waste of time and money to get the children into a situation in which they are destined to fail. These centers will place them into a wheelchair right away. Other centers feel that it is beneficial psychologically to get the children upright, even though later on, they may elect to use the wheelchair. There are no good studies to justify favoring one approach over the other.

24. Why do these children fracture their legs so frequently?

Between the ages of 2 and 12 years, these children are very prone to fracture of their legs. This is especially true after postsurgical immobilization. Many studies have been performed, but no metabolic abnormalities have been identified. There is no question that this is associated with decreased muscle tone and stress on the bones to maintain mineralization. These fractures can often appear with minimal stress, such as turning over in bed or a sibling falling on the patient's leg when playing games.

25. How do the signs and symptoms of fracture in myelomeningocele differ from the signs in normal children?

Because of the lack of sensation, these children usually do not complain of pain. They may or may not have instability of the fracture. There usually is severe swelling of the leg along with increased temperature and redness in the area. The disorder resembles cellulitis and not a fracture. The child may run a temperature of 39°C. Because of the appearance of infection, antibiotics may mistakenly be prescribed.

A fracture should be suspected whenever a red, warm, swollen leg is encountered. X-rays will usually identify the fracture. If the fracture has existed for a week or two, there will be excessive callus formation, which may resemble an infection. A diagnostic difference is that the bone changes will be too far advanced to be caused by osteomyelitis. The fever does not respond to antibiotics and usually promptly drops to normal as soon as the leg is immobilized.

26. What is the treatment of fracture?

These fractures cannot be treated the same as fractures in a normally innervated child. If the leg is placed in a cast, further osteoporosis will develop. As soon as the cast is removed, usually another fracture will promptly develop. There has been instances in which a child has experienced multiple fractures, in one case as many as 22, before it was decided that another method of treatment was indicated.

If the fracture is in the tibia, all that is required in most instances is to wrap the extremity in a bulky soft dressing, such as multiple layers of cast padding, until the padding is an inch thick, followed by application of a nonlatex elastic bandage for compression. If the fracture is in the femur, I prefer to place additional padding (such as a blanket) between the legs, wrap the legs in a nonlatex elastic bandage, and use the well leg as a splint. This splinting can be removed for catheterization and hygiene. The leg is then rewrapped to provide splinting of the fracture. Fractures usually heal in approximately 3–4 weeks, after which further immobilization is not indicated.

In some parts of the world, different types of soft splinting have been used, including a sheepskin wrap. The important thing to remember is that a rigid dressing, such as a plaster or fiberglass cast, is probably contraindicated. Internal fixation, as one would use in osteogenesis imperfecta, is very rarely indicated.

27. What is the problem with latex hypersensitivity?

A high percentage of these children have hypersensitivity to latex. Typically, these are children who have undergone multiple surgical procedures during infancy, but it can occur in the older child as well. In some areas, the incidence is greater than 30%. A latex-free environment is advisable for all children who have myelomeningocele. If there is a history of allergic reaction, a latex-free environment becomes essential.

BIBLIOGRAPHY

1. American Academy of Allergy and Immunology: Task force report on allergic reactions to latex. J Allergy Clin Immunol 92:16, 1993.
2. Carter CO: Spina bifida and anencephaly—a problem in genetic-environmental interaction. J Biosoc Sci 1:71, 1969.
3. Centers for Disease Control and Prevention: Recommendations for the use of folic acid to reduce the number of cases of spina bifida and other neutral tube defects. MMWR 41(RR-14):1–7, 1992.
4. Kumar SJ, Cowell HR, Townsend P: Physeal, metaphyseal, and diaphyseal injuries of the lower extremities in children with myelomeningocele. J Pediatr Orthop 4(1):25, 1984.

5. Lawrence KM: Clinical and ethical considerations on alphafetoprotein estimated for early prenatal diagnosis of neural tube malformations. Dev Med Child Neurol 16(suppl 32):117, 1974.
6. Lindseth RE: Myelomeningocele. In Morrissy RT, Weinstein SL (eds): Pediatric Orthopaedics. Lippincott-Raven, 1996, pp 503–536.
7. McLone DG, Herman JM, Gabrieli AP, Dias L: Tethered cord as a cause of scoliosis in children with a myelomeningocele. Pediatr Neurosurg 16(1):8, 1990.
8. Seller MJ, Nevin NC: Periconceptional vitamin supplementation and the prevention of neural tube defects in southeast England and north Ireland. J Med Genet 21:325, 1984.
9. Toriello HV, Higgins JV: Occurrence of neural tube defects among first, second, and third degree relatives of proband—results of a USA study. Am J Med Genet 15:601, 1987.
10. Tosi LL, Slater JE, Shaer C, Mostello LA: Latex allergy in spina bifida patients—prevalence and surgical implications. J Pediatr Orthop 13:709, 1993.

87. MUSCULAR DYSTROPHY

Michael D. Sussmann, M.D.

1. What is Duchenne's muscular dystrophy?

Duchenne's muscular dystrophy is the most common heritable disease of muscle. In this condition, the muscle shows progressive characteristic deterioration histologically as well as functionally with the passage of time.

2. What is the difference between muscular dystrophy and myopathy?

In dystrophies, there is a progressive deterioration of muscle function, whereas in a myopathy, the muscle has both histologic and functional abnormalities that are nonprogressive.

3. What is Becker's muscular dystrophy?

Becker's muscular dystrophy is also a heritable dystrophic disease of muscle in which the histologic changes are identical to those seen in Duchenne's muscular dystrophy but affected patients run a much milder clinical course. In Duchenne's muscular dystrophy, patients lose the ability to walk at about age 10, whereas in Becker's muscular dystrophy, patients may walk well into their third decade.

4. What is the inheritance pattern of Duchenne's muscular dystrophy?

Duchenne's muscular dystrophy is an X-linked condition with a 15% spontaneous mutation rate. A female carrier will pass the disease to half her male children and the carrier state to half her female children. Many of the spontaneous mutations have been found to occur originally in the gonadal cells of the maternal grandfather.

5. What is the pathophysiology of Duchenne's muscular dystrophy?

Both Duchenne's and Becker's muscular dystrophy are due to abnormalities in the protein *dystrophin.* Dystrophin is one of a family of proteins that stabilize the cell membrane. This is a very large protein with a molecular weight of 427 kD, and its gene constitutes a full 1% of the X chromosome. The dystrophin protein constitutes only 0.001–0.01% of total muscle protein, however. In Duchenne's muscular dystrophy, there are a variety of different deletions, many of which are quite large, in the dystrophin gene. These deletions cause a break in the normal reading frame of the triplet coding sequence. Therefore, when the gene is respliced after a deletion has occurred, the triplet sequence will have shifted so that all the downstream nucleotides are no longer in normal sequence and nonsense protein is produced that is either not completely synthesized or rapidly degraded. Therefore, in Duchenne's muscular dystrophy, no dystrophin seen in either immunohistochemical sections or Western blot analysis. On the other hand, in Becker's dystrophy, although there are also significant deletions, they do not disrupt the normal reading frame. A dystrophin protein is synthesized that is smaller than the normal dystrophin, is produced in much lesser quantity, and clearly does not provide the same stability as normal dystrophin. This leads to a less severe disease than when dystrophin is completely absent.

6. How does the knowledge of the dystrophin abnormality affect the clinical management of these patients?

The major impact at this time is in the realm of diagnosis. DNA from any source will reflect the deletion in the dystrophin gene on the X chromosome. Therefore, blood cells from patients can be used to show these deletions, the patterns of which correlate with the Duchenne's or Becker's type of involvement. In about one third of patients, however, the genetic abnormality is a very small deletion or point mutation, so that the DNA screening test is not informative. Therefore, in the two thirds of patients who have a large deletion, one can make an *absolute* diagnosis of Duchenne's or Becker's muscular dystrophy on the basis of DNA analysis of blood. If the test is negative, however, this does not rule out Duchenne's or Becker's muscular dystrophy.

In those patients in whom test results are positive, genetic counseling of family members (such as sisters of the mother of the patient) is facilitated, since definite identification of carriers can be ascertained.

7. What is the incidence of Duchenne's muscular dystrophy?

One in 3500 male children.

8. Does dystrophin affect other organ systems in addition to skeletal muscle?

Yes. Dystrophin is also found in smooth muscle, cardiac muscle, and neural tissue and in small amounts in other tissues. This explains the abnormalities found in some of these other organ systems, such as cardiomyopathy, delayed gastric emptying, and chronic constipation (seen in older patients).

9. What are the clinical signs of Duchenne's muscular dystrophy?

Because of the relative rarity of this condition, the clinician must have a high index of suspicion to make the diagnosis. In those families with a positive family history, the index of suspicion will be relatively high and the diagnosis will be made early in life. In those patients without a family history, however, diagnosis may be significantly delayed. It has been shown by Galasko that the mean delay between the time that patients present to the orthopaedic surgeon and the time when the diagnosis is made averages 2 years.

The disease should be suspected in any male child who does not walk by the age of 18 months and in whom there is no other obvious reason, such as cerebral palsy, to explain delay in developmental milestones. One also sees enlargement of the calves, known as pseudohypertrophy. Patients will show not only delayed walking but also delayed acquisition of other motor skills such as ascending and descending steps, and they will walk with a wide-based gait. They will use the Gowers' maneuver in rising from the floor. Unlike in diseases that involve neuronal or neural tissues, deep tendon reflexes will be present and will continue to be present until the muscle becomes too weak to respond.

10. What is the Gowers' maneuver, and what does it indicate?

The Gowers' maneuver is the motor process used by a child with weak musculature to arise from a sitting position on the floor. This involves several components.

1. The sitting child will assume the prone position on hands and knees.

2. The child will then extend the knees and, with the hands still on the floor, will assume a quadriped type of position.

3. Following this, to bring the trunk into the upright position as well as to help maintain knee extension, the child will use the hands to "walk up" the leg until the upright position is finally achieved.

It may be very difficult to do manual muscle testing on young children, and the Gowers' maneuver is an excellent screening test for significant muscle weakness. It is found universally in boys with Duchenne's muscular dystrophy; however, it is not specific for muscular dystrophy and may be seen in other conditions causing weakness of the proximal muscles. "Wheelbarrow" walking provides similar information about the upper extremities.

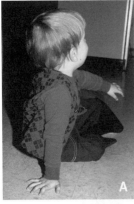
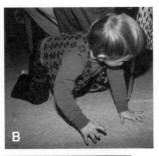
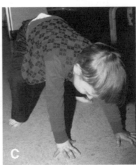
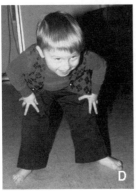
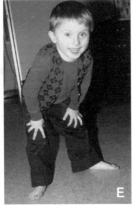

The Gowers' maneuver. *A*, Patient sitting on floor. *B*, Patient rolls over into the prone position on hands and knees. *C*, Patient up in the "bear" position. *D*, Patient uses upper extremities to keep the knees extended and move the trunk upright on the lower body. *E*, Patient finally achieves the upright position.

11. What laboratory studies are required for diagnosis?

- *Creatine kinase (CK)*. If muscular dystrophy is suspected, blood should be drawn and levels of creatine kinase should be measured. In most laboratories, the normal CK range is 0–250. In affected patients, levels will be 5000 or greater. Equivocal elevations of CK are not significant. The CK test is not absolutely diagnostic, but these tremendously elevated levels are found essentially only in inflammatory muscle disease and Duchenne's and Becker's muscular dystrophy.

- *DNA studies*. As mentioned previously, DNA studies using peripheral blood will identify two thirds of patients and allow one to make a definitive diagnosis. Therefore, if these studies are positive, no further diagnostic studies will be necessary.

- *Electromyography (EMG)*. EMG studies may provide significant diagnostic information. They may be quite uncomfortable, however, because the test does involve needle placement. Therefore, these studies should be done only by electromyographers skilled in dealing with children.

- *Muscle biopsy*. In those cases in which the DNA studies are not informative, in order to make an absolute diagnosis, muscle biopsy will need to be done (see Fig. on next page). Needle biopsy may be used by those skilled in the technique, including both the physician taking the biopsy and the pathologist reading it. If these skills are not available, an open biopsy of the rectus femoris should be done. This is most efficaciously done under general anesthesia, avoiding agents that incite malignant hyperthermia such as succinylcholine and halothane. Conscious sedation of these patients may be difficult to obtain and is actually quite risky. Muscle must be processed immediately by a lab experienced in analysis of muscle disorders. The specimen must not be placed in formalin, since histochemical stains such as adenosine-triphosphatase are most informative. Absolute diagnosis may be made in all cases of

Duchenne's and Becker's dystrophy by immunohistochemical staining for dystrophin as well as biochemical assay of dystrophin by Western blot testing of the muscle tissue.

12. What is the differential diagnosis for a 3- to 5-year-old boy with significant muscle weakness?

- *Duchenne's muscular dystrophy*
- *Spinal muscular atrophy.* This is an autosomal recessive condition due to an abnormality of the survival motor neuron gene and related genes, all located together on chromosome 5. In this condition, anterior horn cells are progressively lost, resulting in progressive flaccid muscle weakness. Involvement may vary from very severe, with death in the first year or two of life, to relatively mild, compatible with normal survival. Diagnosis may be made by DNA testing, which is 80–95% accurate. Patients will show atrophy rather than pseudohypertrophy and will also have loss of reflexes early. In addition, because of muscle irritability, spontaneous contractions occur. These can be most readily seen in the tongue as constant fasciculations (and are seen on EMG as fibrillations).
- *Dermatomyositis.* Dermatomyositis is an inflammatory disease of muscle of unknown cause. Unlike the insidious onset of Duchenne's dystrophy, it tends to have a relatively acute onset of muscle weakness. It is associated with a malar rash, and these patients frequently have an elevated erythrocyte sedimentation rate. Specific abnormalities will be seen on EMG. Absolute diagnosis may be made by skin and muscle biopsy, which will show the characteristic changes of perivascular inflammation and muscle necrosis. Patients may have a markedly elevated CK level. Many of these patients have spontaneous remission or respond to corticosteroid treatment. This disease does not have any genetic implications.
- *Emery Dreifuss dystrophy.* These patients may appear very similar to those with Duchenne's dystrophy but will have normal dystrophin and will not show the characteristic muscle changes of patients with Duchenne's dystrophy. They do tend to run a more benign course but will present within the first decade of life with progressive weakness. They will develop plantar flexion contractures at the ankles, flexion contractures at the elbows, and extension contractures in the posterior cervical area, causing progressive neck extension with loss of neck flexion. This is also an X-linked condition, and it has been shown to result from abnormalities in the muscle cell nuclear membrane associated protein emerin.
- *Limb-girdle muscular dystrophy.* These patients tend to present in the second decade of life with progressive muscle weakness. They will have a mildly elevated CK level but will not show histologic changes characteristic of Duchenne's dystrophy. These patients also have normal dystrophin levels, but many show abnormalities in other muscle cell membrane associated proteins, such as adhalin and the sarcoglycans, which can be of diagnostic significance. This is an autosomal recessive condition.
- *Other myopathies.* There are a variety of myopathies that have characteristic changes on either standard histologic or ultrastructural studies and that demonstrate weakness, but they are generally nonprogressive.

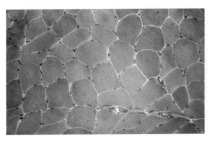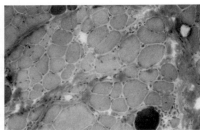

A, Section of normal muscle. *B*, Section of muscle from patient with relatively advanced Duchenne's muscular dystrophy showing irregularity in diameter of muscle fibers, central nuclei, evidence of necrosis, and intramuscular fibrosis.

13. Is there any medical treatment for Duchenne's muscular dystrophy?

- *Corticosteroids.* There are several studies demonstrating that corticosteroid administration may statistically delay the loss of muscle strength in patients with Duchenne's muscular dystrophy. These drugs, however, do not completely eliminate the deterioration but only slow it a relatively modest amount. It must be remembered that these medications have significant side effects, which include weight gain, mood changes, and osteoporosis. Therefore, the relatively modest benefits must be weighed against the significant side effects. I personally counsel patients not to use these medications because of these potentially significant side effects. A corticosteroid known as Deflazacort, which is not available in the United States, has been particularly advocated as having the most beneficial effects with the fewest side effects. This has not been verified in clinical trials, however.
- *Gene replacement therapy.* There is a tremendous amount of work in progress to develop techniques to try to correct the dystrophinopathy by introduction of the dystrophin gene into the muscle of affected patients. This has been successfully done in zygotes of affected mice, but effective gene replacement therapies have not yet been developed for humans.
- *Other.* In addition to efforts to replace dystrophin genetically, efforts are being made to determine if the introduction of other dystrophin-associated proteins may adequately stabilize the cell membrane. There are also a variety of other approaches being considered that use pharmacologic strategies to stabilize the cell membrane in the absence of dystrophin.

14. What is the initial role of the physician once the diagnosis has been made?

Boys who are 4–8 years old should be given stretching exercises for the heelcords and hamstrings to help prevent contractures and should use a nighttime ankle-foot orthosis (AFO) to help prevent heelcord contracture. Ambulatory AFOs should be avoided, since they interfere with balance and will make walking difficult. In addition, families should be counseled regarding appropriate recreational outlets, keeping in mind that in addition to demonstrating muscle weakness, these patients also have a much higher incidence of long bone fracture than their able-bodied peers.

15. What is the cognitive level of boys with Duchenne's muscular dystrophy?

The mean IQ of these patients is the low 80s. There is still a bell-shaped distribution, however, and some patients on the high end of the curve may be quite bright, although severe mental retardation is infrequent. Low IQ levels may represent learning disabilities, particularly in the area of communication skills, rather than true retardation.

16. When and why do patients lose the ability to walk?

Between the ages of 8 and 12, patients will develop progressive weakness of their hip and thigh musculature, particularly the hip extensors and the quadriceps, and will also begin to develop flexion contractures of the knees and hips as well as plantar flexion contractures at the ankles. Some develop weakness without the superimposition of these contractures; these patients tend to be able to stand and walk for a longer period of time. Once the quadriceps develop significant weakness and knee flexion contracture develops, patients are no longer able to support themselves unless a knee-ankle-foot orthosis (KAFO) is used. The loss of walking ability can be predicted within 6 months to 1 year of losing the ability to walk up and down steps and rise from a chair. This will correlate with the development of an extensor lag at the knee. Once this extensor lag approaches 30°–45°, quadriceps weakness is usually such that frequent falling will progress to total inability to stand.

17. How can walking be prolonged in patients with Duchenne's muscular dystrophy?

- When patients develop significant quadriceps weakness and are falling frequently, application of lightweight KAFOs may allow household ambulation and standing to be prolonged several years.

- If contractures develop along with the muscle weakness, release of contractures by tenotomy of the iliotibial band, hamstrings, and Achillis tendons may allow patients to have their legs braced in full extension in order to maintain their standing ability.
- Progressive equinovarus deformities occur even after tendo Achillis tenotomy and create problems for the sitting patient because of abnormal pressure on the feet and inability to get the feet into adequate shoes. This may be prevented by tibialis posterior transfer to the middorsum of the foot through the interosseous membrane at the time of Achilles tendon lengthening. I am also assessing the role of tibialis posterior tenotomy along with tenotomy of the flexor hallucis longus and flexor digitorum longus at the time of tendo Achillis lengthening as a simpler alternative. Long-term follow-up is not yet available for this approach, however.

18. When should a wheelchair be ordered for these patients?

When patients begin to experience significant fatigue with walking, a manual wheelchair should be acquired. This may only need to be used for longer trips but allows the patient to participate in activities that they would be excluded from otherwise. When the patient begins to experience more significant difficulty in walking, a power chair will be the only effective means of ambulation, since the upper extremities will not be powerful enough to propel a manual chair.

19. What happens to pulmonary function in patients with Duchenne's muscular dystrophy?

Patients begin to experience significant decline in pulmonary function at the beginning of the second decade. This is due to weakness and contracture of respiratory muscles and is aggravated by spinal deformity. This may lead to problems with clearing secretions; thus, pulmonary or upper respiratory infections in these patients may lead to severe clinical problems. Without ventilatory support, respiratory failure will occur at the end of the second decade. Death may occur owing to progressive pulmonary failure, or more frequently, owing to the acquisition of an upper respiratory infection that the patient is unable to clear and that leads to rapid respiratory failure.

20. What is the incidence of spinal deformity in these patients?

Most (90–95%) patients will develop progressive scoliosis early in the second decade. This will aggravate pulmonary dysfunction as well as lead to inability to sit unsupported and results in severe functional problems.

21. What is the role of spinal bracing in the treatment of scoliosis in these patients?

Spinal bracing will only delay curve progression in a patient who is simultaneously experiencing progressive pulmonary and metabolic deterioration. Since the natural history of these curves is inexorable progression, the earlier these patients receive definitive treatment for their spine, the better. The optimal treatment is spinal fusion and segmental instrumentation from the upper thoracic area to L5 prior to the development of severe pulmonary insufficiency or severe curvature.

22. Should this spinal fusion extend to the pelvis?

It is my feeling (which is substantiated by clinical follow-up) that when patients are operated on before deformities become severe (less than 30°) and before the onset of significant pelvic obliquity, then fusion to the pelvis can be avoided and fusion to L5 is sufficient. Fusion should extend completely to L5, however, or late pelvic obliquity may occur.

23. Are there any patients who will maintain straight spines?

Yes. The 5–10% of patients who do not develop spinal curvatures tend to develop a total thoracolumbar lordotic pattern. This pattern seems to lock the spine and prevent the development of scoliosis. A variety of techniques have been tried to induce the development of this pattern but have been unsuccessful.

24. What are the surgical risks for these patients, and how can these be minimized?

- *Malignant hyperthermia*. Patients with muscular dystrophy have an increased incidence of malignant hyperthermia. Therefore, inciting agents, particularly succinylcholine, need to be avoided. Patients should be continually monitored for evidence of early malignant hyperthermia, such as ventricular arrhythmia.
- *Cardiac dysfunction*. Patients with Duchenne's muscular dystrophy may have cardiomyopathy and therefore should have a complete cardiac evaluation preoperatively. This should include not only electrocardiography but also echocardiography to assess the thickness of the left ventricular wall and the ventricular ejection fraction.
- *Pulmonary dysfunction*. Because of their muscle disease, patients will have pulmonary dysfunction, and the greatest postoperative risk is that of pulmonary problems. These patients experience prolongation of the effects of muscle relaxants and should be assessed carefully prior to extubation. Patients whose functional vital capacity is greater than 50% have a relatively small risk of postoperative pulmonary problems, whereas those with vital capacities of less than 35% are at significant risk.
- *Excessive blood loss*. Owing to the intramuscular fibrosis, tissues can be rather difficult to dissect and quite rigid. In addition, these tissues seen to bleed excessively, perhaps owing to inability of small vessels to constrict appropriately. This can be avoided by careful dissection and adequate blood and volume replacement.
- *Postoperative gastrointestinal problems*. Owing to the lack of dystrophin, gastric emptying may be delayed, and generalized ileus may be prolonged. Therefore, nasogastric suction should be used in the initial postoperative period, and oral feeding should be delayed until active bowel function has returned.

Many of these complications may be avoided by performing the spinal surgery early, at around age 12, at the first evidence of a curvature. Since the natural history is quite clear, there is no advantage to waiting, because once a curve appears it will not stabilize but will continue to progress. The longer one waits, the more metabolically fragile the patient will be.

25. Are there any disadvantages to spinal fusion in the patient with Duchenne's muscular dystrophy?

Although patients will achieve better sitting balance and will be able to sit for longer periods of time comfortably, because of the loss of trunk mobility they may actually lose some ability to provide a few self-care skills, such as self-feeding. An elevated tray that allows them to slide the arm easily horizontally or a ball-bearing type of feeding assistive device may be beneficial.

26. How long must patients be hospitalized following spinal fusion, and when can they return to school?

When patients with Duchenne's dystrophy undergo spinal fusion at approximately age 12, the mean length of hospital stay is in the range of 7–10 days. Patients can usually return to school and resume normal activities within 1–2 weeks of returning home.

27. What are the other problems of the teenager following successful spinal fusion?

Following spinal fusion, patients will be able to maintain their sitting balance for a long period of time. Because of the inability to shift their weight, however, they should have a well-made seat cushion, such as a "Jay" cushion, which distributes pressure throughout the buttock area. A chair that tilts back electrically is also of some benefit. Patients will continue to lose skills that provide them independence in daily life and will become totally dependent on others. Some of these skills may be provided by adaptive equipment; however, these patients will progress to the need for totally assisted transfers. Transfer to the toilet or into the bathtub is particularly difficult, in part owing to the small size of most bathrooms. Patients also have difficulty moving at night and may have to be shifted 5–10 times a night in bed to maintain their comfort.

28. What is the expected life span of patients with Duchenne's muscular dystrophy?

Most patients succumb to pulmonary problems by the time they reach 20 years of age.

29. Is there any means of prolonging the life span of these patients?

Yes. If ventilatory support is provided, patients may live into the third or fourth decade. Initially, this may consist of only nighttime ventilatory support with use of a nasal mask, but ultimately it will progress to full-time ventilatory support by means of tracheostomy. These patients, however, are very fragile and require a full-time aide. They will remain mentally alert and in the proper setting can lead a productive life. Although a small percentage of patients will have severe cardiomyopathy, in most patients cardiac function is sufficient.

30. Do the female carriers of the dystrophin gene show any signs or symptoms?

Occasionally, a female carrier may show mild weakness (manifesting heterozygote), although many will show histologic changes on muscle biopsy. A very recent report has shown clinically significant cardiomyopathy in a large percentage of adult female carriers.

BIBLIOGRAPHY

1. Dubowitz V: Muscle Disorders in Children. London, Wolfe Medical Publishers Ltd., 1989.
2. McKusick, VA (ed), Online Mendelian Inheritance in Man (OMIM), http://www3.ncbi.nlm.nih.gov/omim/searchomim.html.

88. ARTHROGRYPOSIS MULTIPLEX CONGENITA

George H. Thompson, M.D.

1. What is arthrogryposis multiplex congenita?

A congenital nonprogressive disorder in which there are multiple joint contractures. It is a diagnosis of exclusion, since there are 150 different disorders or syndromes that have joint contractures as part of their manifestations. The term "amyoplasia" is frequently used to refer to the disease in those children with no abnormalities other than joint contractures.

2. Describe the typical features of the arthrogrypotic limb.

The extremities are described as featureless with a tubular shape and absent skin creases. There can be either flexion or extension contractures.

3. Describe the topographic classification of arthrogryposis multiplex congenita.

The topography of involvement is classified as quadrimelic (all four extremities), bimelic (upper or lower extremities only), or monomelic (one extremity). Approximately two thirds of involved children have quadrimelic involvement (see Figure on following page). The majority of the others have bimelic lower extremity involvement. Bimelic upper extremity and monomelic involvement are rare.

4. What is the characteristic posture of the shoulders?

The shoulders are adducted and internally rotated. There is typically weakness of the deltoid muscles.

5. Which is more common in the elbow, extension or flexion contracture?

Extension contracture. This is due to weakness of the biceps and brachialis muscles and to a secondary posterior elbow capsule and triceps contracture. Flexion contractures occur much less frequently.

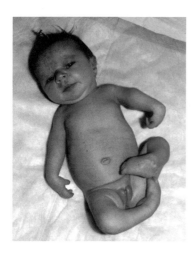

A 1-month-old female with the quadrimelic form of arthrogryposis multiplex congenita. Note the flame nevus of the forehead.

6. Describe the typical position of the wrist, fingers, and thumb.
The wrist is typically flexed and in ulnar deviation due to contracture of the flexor carpi ulnaris. The thumb is adducted, assuming a thumb-in-palm position. There is a contracture of the adductor pollicis muscle and the first web space. The fingers are typically flexed at the metacarpophalangeal, proximal interphalangeal, and distal interphalangeal joints. Active and passive motion is limited.

7. What is the incidence of teratologic hip dislocation in arthrogryposis multiplex congenita?
Approximately two thirds of involved infants will have either hip dysplasia or dislocation. This is a teratologic disorder, since the dislocation occurs prior to birth. The hip examination of an involved newborn will typically demonstrate flexion, abduction, and external rotation contractures.

8. Which is the most common knee deformity, flexion or extension contracture?
A flexion contracture is most common and occasionally is associated with a pterygium. This contracture is due to quadriceps weakness. Occasionally, the knees will be contracted in extension. This produces much less functional impairment, especially if the child is a walker. In nonwalkers the extension contracture can be problematic and can interfere with sitting. This may require treatment.

9. What is the most common foot deformity?
Congenital talipes equinovarus (clubfoot) is the most common foot deformity. Other less common deformities include congenital vertical talus and calcaneovalgus foot.

10. Describe the typical facial appearance in these infants and children.
The head and face are usually not dysmorphic, but there may be micrognathia and microstomia due to lack of mandibular motion. The latter can result in difficulty in feeding, respiratory infections, and a failure to thrive. There is frequently a midline facial hemangioma, termed a flame nevus (see above figure).

11. What viscera are involved?
There are no visceral abnormalities. There may be labial hypoplasia in females and an increased incidence of inguinal hernias in males.

12. Describe the clinical criteria for diagnosis.
The characteristic limb appearance and position, lack of visceral involvement, lack of significant dysmorphic facial features, and a negative family history.

13. What form of arthrogryposis multiplex congenita has a genetic basis?

Distal arthrogryposis, which includes involvement of the face, hands, and feet, is inherited as an autosomal dominant trait. All other forms of arthrogryposis are sporadic.

14. What are the two neuromuscular forms of arthrogryposis multiplex congenita?

This disorder may be divided into neuropathic and myopathic forms. The neuropathic form, which involves dysgenesis of the anterior horn cells, is the most common, accounting for 95% of cases. The myopathic form occurs in approximately 5% of cases.

15. Describe the typical muscle histopathologic findings in the neuropathic form.

The muscles are denervated and partially replaced by fat and fibrous tissue. The remaining muscle tissues will show fiber type disproportion and increase in the number of neuromuscular junctions. There will also be electron microscopic abnormalities. There is periarticular fibrosis due to an increase in collagen formation. This leads to joint contractures.

16. List the treatment goals for upper extremity deformities.

Self-care and mobility skills. Selfcare typically involves feeding and toileting. It is usually best to have one extremity in flexion for feeding and the other in extension for toileting. The extremities should be able to meet in the midline for coordinated functions. Mobility skills include the use of crutches and wheelchairs and assistance in arising from a chair.

17. What are the treatment goals for lower extremity deformities?

Alignment and stability to achieve maximum ambulatory potential. Treatment is directed at joint stability and alignment in the upright or standing position.

18. What are the general concepts in the management of arthrogryposis?

(1) Physical and occupational therapy, (2) orthotics, and (3) surgery. The latter includes both soft tissue releases and osteotomies. Usually, soft tissue releases are performed early, while osteotomies are performed in later childhood and adolescence.

19. What procedures are beneficial in the correction of shoulder adduction and internal rotation?

Usually, treatment of this deformity is not necessary, since it produces minimal functional impairment. Occasionally, a derotation proximal humeral osteotomy can be performed to place the extremity in a more functional position.

20. What procedures are beneficial in the correction of an elbow extension contracture?

A transfer of the pectoralis major muscle to the biceps tendon tends to produce the best functional results. It allows an acceptable range of elbow flexion with fair strength. This procedure is frequently performed in conjunction with triceps lengthening and posterior elbow capsulotomy. Triceps transfer or a Steindler flexorplasty can be considered but are usually not as strong. Occasionally, a distal humeral flexion and derotation osteotomy may be performed to salvage a very contracted elbow deformity.

21. What procedures are beneficial in the correction of wrist flexion and ulnar deviation deformities?

Flexor carpi ulnaris to extensor carpi radialis brevis transfer and a volar capsulotomy can be beneficial in improving the position of the wrist. Occasionally, in very stiff deformity, a proximal row carpectomy can be performed. Wrist fusion can be considered in an adult.

22. What procedures are beneficial in the correction of thumb-in-palm and finger flexion deformities?

Adductor pollicis lengthening and deepening of the first web space can be useful for the thumb-in-palm deformity. A volar release and skin grafts are occasionally necessary for proximal interphalangeal joint contractures. This will not improve motion. Arthrodeses can also be considered.

23. What treatment may be best for moderately flexible bilateral teratologic hip dislocations?
In this situation, leaving the hips dislocated may be preferred. Reduction of the hips may result in stiffness and subsequent difficulties in standing or sitting. Hip mobility is of major importance.

24. Describe the management of unilateral teratologic hip dislocation.
Closed reduction is usually unsatisfactory. Open reduction through a medial or an anterior approach is effective. The anterior approach also allows an acetabuloplasty to be performed to correct coexistent acetabular dysplasia. In the older child, a pelvic osteotomy and a proximal femoral varus osteotomy with shortening and derotation may be beneficial in achieving a stable hip.

25. What procedures are beneficial in the treatment of knee flexion contractures?
Initially, passive range-of-motion therapy and nighttime splinting may be attempted. If this is unsatisfactory, hamstring release and posterior knee capsulotomy are commonly performed. Extension supracondylar osteotomy of the distal femur can be considered. The deformity tends to recur with growth, however. In the older child or adolescent, anterior distal femoral hemiepiphysiodesis may be beneficial in achieving correction with growth.

26. What procedures are beneficial in the correction of knee extension deformity?
This deformity does not require treatment. Physical therapy will usually allow a satisfactory range of motion for comfortable sitting in nonwalkers. Occasionally, quadriceps lengthening in nonwalkers may be beneficial in achieving 90° of knee flexion.

27. At what age is talipes equinovarus best treated with a complete soft-tissue release?
Clubfeet are usually treated surgically at 12–18 months of age. It is important that the child be ready to assume an upright posture with or without orthoses shortly after the feet have been corrected. Early operative intervention predisposes to recurrent deformities.

28. List three procedures for treatment of recurrent clubfeet in young children.
Repeat complete soft-tissue release, talectomy, and Verbelyi-Ogston procedure (decancellation of the talus and cuboid).

29. What is the incidence of scoliosis in arthrogryposis multiplex congenita?
Approximately one third of involved children will develop a progressive spinal deformity.

30. Describe the management of progressive arthrogrypotic scoliosis.
Scoliosis in arthrogryposis multiplex congenita has the same general characteristics as other neuromuscular spinal deformities. The curves tend to progress steadily throughout growth and development. They respond poorly to orthotics. Early surgical intervention is the best method of management. This may consist of a posterior spinal fusion with segmental spinal instrumentation or occasionally a combined anterior and posterior spinal fusion with segmental spinal instrumentation.

BIBLIOGRAPHY

1. Atkins RM, Bell MJ, Sharrard WJW: Pectoralis major transfer for paralysis of elbow flexion in children. J Bone Joint Surg 67B:640–644, 1985.
2. Banker BQ: Neuropathologic aspects of arthrogryposis multiplex congenita. Clin Orthop 194:30–43, 1985.
3. Bennett JB, Hansen PE, Granberry WM, Cain TE: Surgical management of arthrogryposis in the upper extremity. J Pediatr Orthop 5:281–286, 1985.

4. Carlson WO, Speck GJ, Vicari V, Wenger DR: Arthrogryposis multiplex congenita. A long-term follow-up study. Clin Orthop 194:115–123, 1985.
5. Daher YH, Lonstein JE, Winter RB, Moe JH: Spinal deformities in patients with arthrogryposis. A review of 16 patients. Spine 10:609–613, 1985.
6. Dias LS, Stern LS: Talectomy in the treatment of resistant talipes equinovarus deformity in myelomeningocele and arthrogryposis. J Pediatr Orthop 7:39–41, 1987.
7. Goldberg MJ: Syndromes of orthopaedic importance. In Morrissey RT, Weinstein SL: Lovell and Winter's Pediatric Orthopaedics, 4th ed. Philadelphia, Lippincott-Raven, 1996, pp 255–360.
8. Gross RH: The role of Verebelyi-Ogston procedure in management of the anthrogrypotic foot. Clin Orthop 194:99–103, 1985.
9. Guidera KJ, Drennan JC: Foot and ankle deformities in arthrogryposis multiplex congenita. Clin Orthop 194:93–98, 1985.
10. Hall JG: Genetic aspects of arthrogryposis. Clin Orthop 194:44–53, 1985.
11. Heydarian K, Akbarnia BA, Jabalameli M, Tabador K: Posterior capsulotomy for the treatment of severe flexion contractures of the knee. J Pediatr Orthop 4:700–704, 1984.
12. Hoffer MM, Swank S, Eastman F, Clark D, Teitge R: Ambulation in severe arthrogryposis. J Pediatr Orthop 3:293–296, 1983.
13. Palmer PM, MacEwen GD, Bowen JR, Mathews PA: Passive motion therapy for infants with arthrogryposis. Clin Orthop 195:54–59, 1985.
14. St. Clair HS, Zimbler S: A plan of management and treatment results in the arthrogrypotic hip. Clin Orthop 194:74–80, 1985.
15. Sarwark JF, MacEwen GD, Scott CL Jr: Current concepts review. Amyoplasia (a common form of arthrogryposis). J Bone Joint Surg 72A:465–469, 1990.
16. Shapiro F, Specht L: Current concepts review. The diagnosis and orthopaedic treatment of childhood spinal muscular atrophy, peripheral neuropathy, Friedreich ataxia, and arthrogryposis. J Bone Joint Surg 75A:1699–1714, 1993.
17. Sodergard J, Ryoppy S: Foot deformities in arthrogryposis multiplex congenita. J Pediatr Orthop 14:768–772, 1994.
18. Sodergard J, Ryoppy S: The knee in arthrogryposis multiplex congenita. J Pediatr Orthop 10:177–182, 1990.
19. Solund K, Sonne-Holm S, Kjolbye JE: Talectomy for equinovarus deformity in arthrogryposis. A 13 (2–20) year review of 17 feet. Acta Orthop Scand 62:372–374, 1991.
20. Staheli LT, Chew DE, Elliott JS, Mosca VS: Management of hip dislocations in children with arthrogryposis. J Pediatr Orthop 7:681–685, 1987.
21. Swinyard CA, Bleck EE: The etiology of arthrogryposis (multiplex congenita contracture). Clin Orthop 194:15–29, 1985.
22. Thomas B, Schopler S, Wood W, Oppenheim WL: The knee in arthrogryposis. Clin Orthop 194:87–92, 1985.
23. Thompson GH, Bilenker RM: Comprehensive management of arthrogryposis multiplex congenita. Clin Orthop 194:6–14, 1985.
24. Williams P. The management of arthrogryposis. Orthop Clin North Am 9:67–88, 1978.
25. Yonenobu K, Tada K, Swanson B: Arthrogryposis of the hand. J Pediatr Orthop 4:599–603, 1984.

89. POLIOMYELITIS

Hugh G. Watts, M.D.

1. Since the vaccine was developed 40 years ago, poliomyelitis has disappeared. Why do I need to read about it now?

Poliomyelitis has *not* disappeared. In the Western hemisphere, the World Health Organization claims that there have been no new wild cases since the early 1990s, but in the rest of the world, particularly in Africa, poliomyelitis is widespread. The most recent reports show about 100 new paralytic cases a day worldwide, and there is an estimate that only one in 10 cases is reported.

2. But I live in the United States and don't plan to practice elsewhere, so why should I read this?

The world is a small place, made smaller by rapid airplane travel and immigration. This brings children who have had the disease to the United States. Furthermore, the vaccine occasionally causes a clinical episode of poliomyelitis either in the vaccinated child or in the vaccinated child's parents.

3. What is poliomyelitis?

The poliomyelitis virus is an enterovirus. When poliomyelitis is contracted, the anterior horn cells of the spinal cord may be destroyed with permanent loss of muscle activity.

4. What kinds of clinical poliomyelitis are there?

Abortive poliomyelitis: a brief febrile illness with anorexia, nausea, vomiting, headache, and sore throat as well as coryza, cough, pharyngeal exudate, and diarrhea.

Nonparalytic poliomyelitis: These children have the same symptoms but they also will have headache, nausea, and vomiting, which are more intense. There will be soreness and stiffness of the muscles, particularly in the back of the neck, as well as in the trunk and limbs.

Paralytic poliomyelitis: These children will have all the symptoms just described as well as weakness or paralysis of the trunk and extremities. The spinal form is the most common and involves the neck, trunk, and extremities. The bulbar form can involve one or more of the cranial nerves. There may be a combination of bulbar and spinal forms.

5. Why don't we see more children with the bulbar form of the disease?

These patients frequently die of respiratory failure.

6. How is the poliomyelitis virus spread?

Man is the only natural host of the poliomyelitis virus, and it is spread from person to person by fecal and oral routes.

7. What is the pathophysiology of poliomyelitis?

The poliomyelitis virus multiplies and kills the anterior horn cells. Some of the injury to the nerve cells may be reversible.

The neural lesions occur chiefly in the anterior horn cells of the spinal cord but to a lesser extent in the intermediate and dorsal horn cells, and the dorsal root ganglia as well. The cerebral cortex (but not the motor areas of the cerebral cortex) is spared, as is the cerebellum (except the vermis and deep midline nuclei).

8. What other diseases might be confused with an acute poliomyelitis infection?

The most common by far would be postinfectious polyneuropathy, better known as the Guillain-Barré syndrome. Generally, the headache and meningeal signs are less striking. The paralysis tends to be symmetric, and sensory changes and pyramidal tract signs are common (but absent in poliomyelitis).

Guillain-Barré usually becomes apparent about 10 days following a nonspecific viral infection. Spontaneous recovery begins usually at 2–3 weeks and in most situations is complete. There is a chronic or intermittent recurrent form affecting about 7% of children, however. Children with this may be hard to distinguish from those with the chronic residua of poliomyelitis.

9. What kind of vaccines are available to prevent poliomyelitis?

The oral, living attenuated virus (Sabin) and the injectable, killed virus (Salk).

10. Which poliomyelitis vaccine is best?

The living attenuated vaccine is cheap, is easy to administer, and has the added advantage of secondarily spreading the vaccine through fecal contamination from actively vaccinated children.

This makes it especially useful for gaining herd immunity in the event of an epidemic. This vaccine is readily inactivated by heat, however, which makes its care more precarious.

The oral vaccine, in addition, may cause a clinical case of paralytic poliomyelitis in about one in five million children who are vaccinated (or in the child's parents).

This is why the injectable vaccine is important. It is particularly indicated for pregnant women or children who are compromised in their immune status owing to chronic illness.

11. What are the chronic residua of poliomyelitis?
Muscle weakness, growth disturbance, and deformity.

12. What sort of problems would you expect a child to have as a result of muscle weakness?
Obviously, this is going to depend on how severe the muscle weakness is and which muscles are involved as well as what the balance is between opposing muscles.

13. How weak is "weak"? How do you test muscle strength?
Manual muscle testing was developed for the management of poliomyelitis. The possible strength of a muscle is divided into six grades.
Zero: there is no muscle twitch at all.
Grade 1: the muscle twitches and can be felt by your palpating hand, but no useful motion is generated.
Grade 2: the muscle is able to power the joint through a *full range of motion with gravity eliminated*.
Grade 3: the ability of the muscle to carry the joint through a *full range of motion against gravity*.
Grade 4: is a muscle that is able to go through a full range of motion not only against gravity but also against added resistance.
Grade 5: normal.

14. How reproducible is this grading system?
It depends on the part of the scale that we are discussing. There is clearly an age-related factor in determining what normal muscle strength is.

Below grade 4, the muscle testing is remarkably reproducible. One has to take care that the muscle assigned a grade of 2 or 3 is able to carry the limb through the *full* range of motion. If there are contractures that limit the range, then the strength is determined by the muscle's ability to carry the limb through the *possible* range.

15. Does a grade of 3 (out of 5) mean that the muscle has 50% of the strength of normal?
Definitely not! It depends, in part, on which muscle is in question. For example, for the quadriceps, it takes about 10% of normal muscle strength to be able to extend the knee a full range of motion against gravity (i.e., grade 3). It takes about 5% of muscle strength to extend the knee its full range of motion with gravity eliminated (i.e., grade 2). This means that it only takes a small percentage loss of muscle strength to go from a situation where you can walk (because your quadriceps can hold your knee straight) to the point where you can't walk without a brace.

16. What does this tell you about the so-called "post-poliomyelitis syndrome"?
If you had poliomyelitis and had a grade 3 quadriceps as a teenager, you would be able to walk around without a brace. As you got a bit older, however, and lost an additional 5% of normal muscle strength, you would have to wear a brace to be able to walk. This has nothing to do with recrudescence of the virus but is an effect of getting older.

17. What muscles are needed to support the knee when walking?
The quadriceps is needed, but if the quadriceps is absent, the gluteus maximus or soleus muscle can take its place.

18. How can another muscle take the place of the quadriceps?

To explain this, stand up. Now lean forward a bit at your waist and reach down and grasp your patella between your thumb and your index finger. As you lean forward, you can wobble your patella from side to side. This tells you that your quadriceps isn't doing any work. You are actually standing up without using your quadriceps.

19. How does that work?

Because your center of gravity falls in front of your knee joint, gravity is working to extend your knee. The ligaments at the back of the knee are preventing the knee from hyperextending, thereby supporting your weight. Now with your thumb and index finger wobbling your patella, gradually flex your knees. You will see that you come to a point, when your knee is flexed about 10°–15°, where you can't move your patella. That's the point where the quadriceps start doing their work.

You can see that anything that brings your center of gravity in front of your knees will allow you to stand on your leg without using your quadriceps. Now you can see that the gluteus maximus, by pulling the femur posteriorly, brings the knee behind your center of gravity. The soleus does the same thing.

20. What happens if I have a weak gluteus maximus? How can I stand up?

When you lean backward and get your center of gravity behind the axis of the hip joint, the trunk wants to fall backward but can't because of the tight ligaments in front of the hip joint. The Y ligament of Bigelow prevents your hip from hyperextending and allows you to stand up.

21. What happens if both my gluteus maximus and my quadriceps are weak?

You need to lean forward to get your weight anterior to your knee and you need to lean backward to get your weight posterior to your hip. With a little cleverness and a certain amount of breath holding you *can* precariously balance that way. The smarter thing to do is to use a brace that prevents the knee from flexing and then stand by leaning backward at the hip. This kind of a brace we would call a KAFO (knee-ankle-foot orthosis).

22. How does poliomyelitis affect the growth of a limb?

When there is no normal muscle activity across a joint, the cartilage cells of the physis are not stimulated to grow normally, and a short leg is a common result.

23. What happens if one leg is too short?

Keep in mind that if the child has poliomyelitis, you don't necessarily want the legs to end up being of equal length. The weight of the brace, the thickness of the brace on the sole of the foot, and the muscle weakness may make it hard to swing the leg forward when walking if the legs are exactly equal. This is particularly true if the child is wearing a long-leg brace (KAFO) with the knee locked and fully extended.

24. How does the muscle weakness of poliomyelitis result in deformity?

Deformities due to muscle weakness can be a result of the imbalance of muscles or fibrosis of the dead muscle.

For example, if the posterior tibialis muscle of the leg were absent and the peroneal muscles were normal, the heel of the foot would be pulled into eversion. If the foot is allowed to grow with this imbalance, the bones will gradually become misshapen.

Lack of muscle pull can also alter the shape of a bone. For example, a weak gluteus medius will give less pull on the apophysis of the greater trochanter, leading to a valgus shape of the upper end of the femur as growth progresses.

25. How did the muscle become fibrotic?

When the nerve to a muscle dies, the muscle gradually becomes atrophic and is replaced by fibrous tissue. This fibrous tissue can work as a very tough band preventing a joint from going through its full range of motion. The most common example of this is the tensor fasciae latae muscle and its extension down the leg. The fibrosis of the tensor fasciae latae can cause an abduction contracture of the hip. Since the muscle is anterior to the axis of the hip joint, it can cause a hip flexion contracture as well. The continuation of the fasciae latae to the tibia is posterior to the knee joint, so fibrosis can lead to a flexion deformity in the knee. Furthermore, the fasciae latae across the knee joint is inserted laterally on the proximal tibia, which can lead to a rotational deformity as the tibia grows.

26. Is there anything special about the physical examination of a child with poliomyelitis?

Yes. The mechanics of walking requires a subtle alignment of the center of gravity in relation to the joints. What is happening in one part of the body, such as the ankle, can make a big difference in what happens in another part, such as the knee. A classic example is the effect of an equinus deformity (i.e., a plantar flexion contracture at the ankle) on support of the knee. Remember we talked about keeping the axis of the knee joint posterior to the center of weightbearing. The soleus muscle can do that, but so can an equinus contracture.

27. How does that happen?

If the ankle is in equinus when the foot comes forward and touches the ground, the weight of the body pushes the foot flat onto the ground. The tibia cannot move forward (because the ankle is fixed in equinus from the contracture), and as the inertia carries the body forward, the knee stays posterior. That may be obvious to you now, but is not always obvious to the surgeon, who may decide to lengthen a tight heelcord and find to his dismay that the child is now unable to stand and walk without using a long-leg brace. This means that a physical examination of *all* parts of the body, including manual muscle testing is a necessary minimum for evaluating a child with poliomyelitis.

28. Who should treat a child with the residua of poliomyelitis?

Most characteristically, the treatment falls to the orthopaedic surgeon. This is because management often involves both bracing and surgery. The physical therapist is usually an important member of the treating team. The orthotist (i.e., the brace maker) will usually be involved as well.

29. With so many different areas of weakness, where do I begin?

The problem is best managed by setting priorities. Initially, the priority should be to get the child walking. This can be done with fairly simple bracing. Getting the child to fit into a brace may require some simple surgical releases at the hips, knees, or ankles.

The second priority is to correct the factors that are liable to create deformities with further growth. Later, one can focus on surgical treatments to reduce the extent of bracing or the necessity for crutches. This is followed by attention to the loss of function in the upper extremities and correcting problems in the spine (i.e., scoliosis).

30. What can be done to correct contractures?

If a child is very young (< 3 years), exercises may be enough to stretch out contractures. As the child gets older and the joint contractures become stiffer, the contractures may be amenable to serial casting, in which a cast is put on with the limb as straight as possible. Usually over the next week or two, the contracture will relax a little bit while inside the cast, allowing a new cast to be applied with the joint about 10° straighter than it was. While this has the advantage of not requiring surgery, it can be a considerable hassle for the child and the child's family. It may be simpler to do soft tissue releases surgically. In later years, during adolescence and young adulthood, it may be simpler just to correct the deformity by cutting the bone (an osteotomy) and straightening the limb.

31. What can be done to correct an imbalance of muscle pull across a joint?

Sometimes, this can be managed by providing a brace to replace the missing muscle strength. The simplest example of this would be in a child who has plantar flexors of the ankle but no dorsal flexors. This could be managed with a simple brace to hold the foot from going into equinus.

At other times, it may be possible to transfer a muscle so that its tendon insertion is put in a more advantageous location. For example, if a child has a weak gastrocsoleus muscle but has intact peroneus muscles, it is possible to move the direction of the peroneal tendons back to the heel to give sufficient strength (if not good push-off) to prevent deformity in the shape of the os calcis.

32. Is there any penalty to transferring a muscle?
When a muscle is transferred, it characteristically loses one grade of strength. In addition, moving a muscle may make the joint that it originally controlled unstable. When the peroneal muscle is moved back to the os calcis, this may make the subtalar joint unstable. In that case, the problem might be managed by fusing the subtalar joint to take away the need for the peroneal muscles.

33. Do you find that parental and social attitudes toward children with poliomyelitis are different from attitudes toward those with other chronic diseases of childhood?
Yes. Because poliomyelitis does not affect mental status or the cerebellum, these children function remarkably well. Furthermore, because the disease is acquired, parents seem to feel that there is less reflection on the family genes. In addition, there have been prominent people who have had the disease, the most well-known being Franklin D. Roosevelt.

BIBLIOGRAPHY

1. Beaty JH: Poliomyelitis. In Crenshaw AH (ed): Campbell's Operative Orthopedics, 8th ed. St. Louis, C.V. Mosby Co., 1992, pp 2383–2431.
2. Cherry JD: Enteroviruses. In Berhman RE (ed): Nelson Textbook of Pediatrics, 14th ed. Philadelphia, W.B. Saunders Co., 1992, pp 823–831.
3. Drennan JC: Poliomyelitis. In: Morrissy R. (ed): Lovell and Winter's Pediatric Orthopaedics, 3rd ed. Philadelphia, J.B. Lippincott Co., 1990, pp 406–436.
4. Watts HG, Gillies H: A Practical Guide To The Orthopedic Management of Children With The Residua Of Paralytic Poliomyelitis. Orthopedics Overseas Publication. New York, Bobit Publishing, 1992.

90. LIMB DEFICIENCY

Robert Gillespie, M.D., Ch.B., FRCS(C), FRCS (Ed)

1. What is limb deficiency?
Part of a limb or limbs is missing. The missing part may be at the end of the limb (e.g., congenital amputation), leaving a simple "stump." The proximal bones may be absent with foreshortening of the limb, as in phocomelia. A distal bone may be absent in the radius or fibula with shortening and deformity of the hand or foot.

2. What causes it?
The cause is usually unknown, especially in isolated single-limb anomalies in an otherwise normal child. The classic exception was multilimb deficiency caused by the drug thalidomide. There are other exceptions, particularly tibial defects, which are known to be heritable. Same rare syndromes involving limb deficiency and facial abnormality have been reported as being genetic, in some cases inherited from diabetic mothers.

3. How is it classified?

Classification of congenital limb deficiency is a serious problem because of variable international nomenclature and because specific terms for the more common anomalies have been established in the literature (see figure).

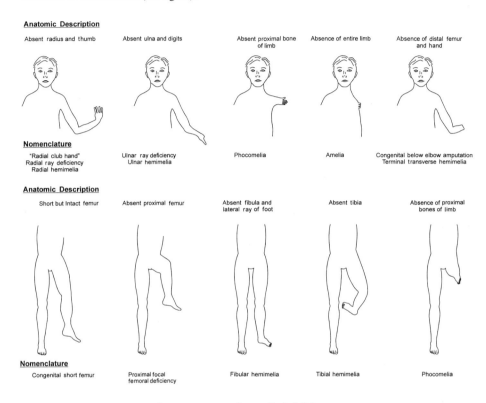

Anatomic Description

| Absent radius and thumb | Absent ulna and digits | Absent proximal bone of limb | Absence of entire limb | Absence of distal femur and hand |

Nomenclature

| "Radial club hand" Radial ray deficiency Radial hemimelia | Ulnar ray deficiency Ulnar hemimelia | Phocomelia | Amelia | Congenital below elbow amputation Terminal transverse hemimelia |

Anatomic Description

| Short but intact femur | Absent proximal femur | Absent fibula and lateral ray of foot | Absent tibia | Absence of proximal bones of limb |

Nomenclature

| Congenital short femur | Proximal focal femoral deficiency | Fibular hemimelia | Tibial hemimelia | Phocomelia |

Common patterns of upper limb deficiency.

4. How likely is it to happen again in the same family?

Very unlikely. An increasing number of reports of genetic transmission, however, make genetic counseling a wise step.

5. What is the most common type?

A left below-elbow transverse hemimelia (i.e., a congenital below-elbow amputation).

6. Is it associated with other syndromes or congenital defects?

Radial deficiencies in particular are associated with a number of syndromes.
- Blood dyscrasia
    Fanconi's anemia
    Thrombocytopenic purpura (TAR syndrome)
- Congenital heart defect
- Holt Oram syndrome (anterior septal defect and radial clubhand, less commonly with tetralogy of Fallot).
- Vertebral and other defects, as in the VATER syndrome (vertebral anomaly, tracheoesophageal fistula, anal atresia, renal anomalies, and radial clubhand).

These associations rarely occur in other multilimb deficiencies.

7. Who should be referred to a geneticist?
All affected children.

8. Who is the ideal person to look after these patients.
A pediatric orthopaedist who works in a special children's amputee clinic with a dedicated prosthetist and therapist.

9. How early should these children be seen by a pediatric orthopaedist?
As soon after birth as possible to allow the parents to have accurate information and reasonable expectations right from the beginning.

10. Is there an indication for surgery for these cases?
With the exception of simple transverse congenital amputations, which can be fitted with a prosthesis easily, most cases need some surgical modification to maximize function.

11. In general, what is the role of amputation and prosthetic fitting?
In the more severe lower limb deficiencies, the limb is unreconstructable, and the best functional result is obtained by amputation of the foot, which is often deformed, and prosthetic fitting. This is particularly true in fibular and tibial hemimelia. An excellent functional and cosmetic result can be achieved by this technique. The surgery is best done at age 9 months.

12. What are the surgical principles of reconstructive amputation for limb deficiency?
Reconstructive amputation provides an ideal end-bearing stump to facilitate prosthetic replacement in an otherwise unreconstructable limb. Invariably, this applies only to the lower limb, usually for fibular hemimelia, tibial hemimelia, and some cases of proximal focal femoral deficiency.

The overriding principle is *never* to amputate through the shaft (diaphysis) of a bone but to disarticulate at the joint level (usually the ankle) to retain the distal epiphysis for growth and the ability to bear weight on the end of the stump, which greatly simplifies the prosthetic fitting. Another enormous advantage is the avoidance of terminal spiking (see question 32).

13. What are the principles of management of upper limb versus lower limb deficiencies?
Prosthetic replacement of the upper limb is infinitely less satisfactory than the lower. Almost any hand remaining is more functional than a prosthesis. Amputation in upper limb deficiencies is never indicated, whereas surgery to improve function often is.

14. Can these limbs be lengthened?
In carefully selected cases. Limb lengthening is difficult and trying for both patient and surgeon and very complication prone. New technology has improved the situation, however. In some cases, particularly with congenital short femurs and some lesser degrees of fibular deficiency, lengthening can be very successful.

15. When is amputation preferred to limb lengthening?
In most cases of deficiency below the knee (fibular or tibial), the foot is ill formed and the ankle is unstable. In these situations, a lengthened and reconstructed limb is much less functional than an end-bearing below-knee prosthesis.

16. What are the complications of amputation and prosthetic fitting?
Very few. The cost of the prosthesis and the need for regular replacement in the growing child can be a financial problem in some situations.

17. What are the complications of limb lengthening?
Unfortunately, there are many. Subluxation of joints, especially the knee, and deformity and fracture of the lengthened bone are common. Six to 12 months of careful management are often necessary, and the patient and family can face a great deal of stress.

18. What are the most common indications for reconstructive surgery in limb deficiency?

Congenital short femur   Radial clubhand (radial hemimelia)
Proximal focal femoral deficiency   Tibial deficiency (tibial hemimelia)

19. What can be done for proximal focal femoral deficiency?
In this condition, the femur is extremely short and its substance is defective, usually at the proximal end. There are varying degrees of formation of the hip joint. It is sometimes possible to reconstruct the proximal femur and provide much better hip stability, improving gait.

The knee in these cases is usually dysplastic and flexed. The limb is so short that the foot lies at the level of the normal knee.

Prosthetic fitting and function can be improved by fusing the knee to produce a straighter and stronger lever arm for the prosthesis. Occasionally, there is an indication to rotate the limb 180° to allow the ankle to function as a knee in the prosthesis (the van Ness rotationplasty). Otherwise, amputation of the foot provides a functional stump that can be fitted like a knee disarticulation.

20. What can be done for congenital short femur?
If the lower limb is normal and the femur is 60% or more of the length of the normal femur, femoral lengthening can be considered.

21. What can be done for radial clubhand?
In ideal circumstances, the hand can be stabilized on the end of the ulna (ulnar centralization). Because these children always have a missing thumb, the index finger can be moved to function as a thumb by pollicization.

22. What can be done for tibial hemimelia?
Often, there is a proximal tibia present, and the fibula can be fused to it to provide a long functional below-knee stump. If not, rarely the fibula can be transferred to form a knee under the femoral condyles (the Brown procedure). Otherwise, a knee disarticulation is necessary.

23. What functional result can be expected in a child with unilateral ankle disarticulation?
Excellent. These kids have function close to normal and are capable of competing equally with their peers in most sports.

24. What functional result can be expected in a child with a unilateral through-knee or above-knee amputation?
Loss of the knee joint greatly diminishes function, but modern prosthetics allow a good gait with only a slight limp. Complete independence in school and job can be expected, but the higher energy costs of walking and running greatly limit sports participation.

25. What about functional expectations in a multilimb deficiency?
Infinitely variable. A bilateral below-knee amputee can achieve independence. A bilateral through-knee amputee with normal upper limbs will usually have limited outside independence and will use a wheelchair for speed and distance. If all four limbs are seriously deficient, independence is lost and a great deal of help is needed. Toileting can be a special problem.

26. How good are prosthetic lower limbs?

Generally excellent at through-knee and below-knee levels. Better suspension and socket-lining technology as well as better prosthetic feet (Seattle, energy-storing) have improved function in recent years. Replacing the limb after a high-thigh or hip disarticulation remains less satisfactory.

27. How good are prosthetic upper limbs?

Always disappointing. The fine manipulative, proprioceptive, and sensory functions of the hand are irreplaceable. Children with a unilateral upper limb prosthesis will often reject it. Purely cosmetic hands are often well accepted in later adolescence. Bilateral below-elbow amputees will often prefer a standard split-hook device for function and biofeedback.

28. What are the advantages and disadvantages of myoelectric prostheses?

The advantages are fairly good cosmesis and excellent grip strength. The disadvantages are weight, cost, breakdown, and the difficulty in cleaning and maintaining the glove. They are very useful in older unilateral below-elbow amputees in aiding bimanual work.

29. What are the psychologic effects of limb deficiency, amputation, and prosthetic reconstruction?

The birth of a baby with a significant limb deficiency is devastating to the parents. Very early consultation with an expert will help promote understanding and acceptance. In some cases, amputation as a therapeutic step will be rejected, and well-chosen second opinions are necessary. Once surgery is over and function has been established, parents become very positive and proud of their child's achievements. For the most part, the children themselves are very accepting and untroubled by the limb defect, unlike children suffering amputation due to trauma or malignancy.

30. Is a child with a traumatic amputation different?

Absolutely. The psychologic injury to both the child and the parents is severe and permanent. In North America, these injuries are often associated with a component of parental or guardian guilt as in lawn mower, snowblower, and agricultural equipment accidents.

31. What are the surgical issues in traumatic amputation in childhood?

Preservation of length and growth. Children heal so well that length can often be maintained by patience, secondary wound closure, and skin grafting. Great efforts to preserve distal epiphyses are worth it to provide growth and end bearing.

"Terminal spiking" is a process by which a transected bone end in young children elongates and becomes pointed, often protruding through the skin of the stump. Sometimes called "terminal overgrowth," this unhappy state of affairs can lead to multiple stump revision procedures.

32. Can anything be done to prevent terminal spiking?

In some cases, yes. The most common incidence is in below-knee amputations because the fibula is particularly prone to overgrow and protrude through the skin. Fusion of the end of the fibula to the tibia with free transfer of the proximal fibular epiphysis to the end of the tibia often is successful in prevention of further spiking.

BIBLIOGRAPHY

1. Aitkin GT. Amputation as a treatment for certain lower extremity congenital abnormalities. J Bone Joint Surg 41A:1267–1285, 1959.
2. Frantz CH, O'Rahilly R: Congenital skeletal limb deficiencies. J Bone Joint Surg 43A:1202, 1961.
3. Gillespie R, Torode IP: Classification and management of congenital abnormalities of the femur. J Bone Joint Surg 65B:557, 1983.
4. McBride WG: Thalidomide and congenital abnormalities. Lancet 2:1358, 1961.

91. SYNDROME EVALUATION

Jon M. Aase, M.D.

1. What is a "dysmorphic child"?
Any child born with structural abnormalities (birth defects) or with a disease that alters body structure after birth (such as the osteochondrodystrophies). Roughly 3 in every 100 babies will be found to have a *major* congenital anomaly.

2. What is a major congenital abnormality?
In general terms, a major birth defect is one that if uncorrected or uncorrectable will significantly impair normal function or reduce normal life expectancy. There are dozens of such anomalies, including cleft palate, ventricular septal defect, imperforate anus, and phocomelia. Surgical procedures can correct or alleviate some of these abnormalities and may be required soon after birth to permit survival.

3. Do minor abnormalities mean anything?
Sometimes. Isolated minor abnormalities such as birthmarks, preauricular pits, and clinodactyly of the fifth fingers usually are of only cosmetic importance. The presence of *three or more* such minor defects is rare in normal children, however, and may be an indication of a dysmorphic *syndrome*.

4. What is a dysmorphic syndrome?
Syndromes are simply recognizable patterns of abnormality. In dysmorphology, a syndrome usually denotes a distinctive, rare combination of major and minor physical anomalies. Some syndromes can be linked to a specific causative agent, such as a gene mutation, a chromosomal aberration, or an environmental teratogen. Others are purely descriptive, serving as handy "bookmarks," a convenient way to refer to a complex clinical disorder. There are thousands of dysmorphic syndromes, with more being added continually.

5. Does every child with multiple birth defects have a dysmorphic syndrome?
No. Sometimes congenital anomalies occur together by chance alone, or one underlying anomaly may cause a "sequence" of abnormalities in other structures (e.g., lung hypoplasia in a fetus with renal agenesis). To add to the confusion, some congenital abnormalities seem to occur together more often than would be expected by chance but not in the consistent pattern of a syndrome. For now, these nonrandom clusters of anomalies are called "associations."

6. What causes birth defects?
The majority of structural abnormalities we see at birth result from *intrinsic* developmental aberrations, in which cell functions and interactions are thrown off track by erroneous genetic instructions. When this involves tissues in a localized region of the body, a true *malformation* occurs. *Dysplasias* are caused by genetic errors that affect one specific type of tissue everywhere it occurs in the body.

Birth defects also can result from *extrinsic* influences on normal tissues. *Deformations* are caused by abnormal mechanical stress, usually as the result of intrauterine constraint. *Disruptions* involve localized tissue destruction, either by mechanical forces, as in the case of amniotic bands, or by insults resulting from vascular compromise or infection.

7. Which major birth defects are most common?
Localized abnormalities that affect just one body structure ("single-system anomalies") occur most frequently. This category makes up more than 60% of all birth defects and includes club-foot, cleft palate, congenital heart disease, cleft lip, neural tube defects, pyloric stenosis, and con-

genital hip dislocation. Congenital heart malformations affect about 8 of every 1000 babies, while each of the other anomalies occurs individually about once in every 1000–2000 births. Happily, almost all are correctable, with an excellent outlook for survival and function. The major exception is open neural tube defects, which usually produce some residual disability even with the very best treatment.

8. What is the difference between a malformation and a deformation?

Deformations are simply distortions of the shape of otherwise normal structures. They usually involve bending or compression of bone or cartilage and stretching of connective tissue. Once the deforming force has been removed, continuing growth will tend to restore the structure to a more normal form.

In contrast, true malformations come in a number of different flavors. Using the development of the fingers as an example, malformations can be manifested in the following ways.

Total failure of development—absence of the central ray (ectrodactyly)
Partial failure of development—short distal phalanx (acrobrachyphalangy)
Diminished relative size—short fingers (brachydactyly)
Excessive relative size—localized gigantism (macrodactyly)
Partial or total duplication—supernumerary finger (polydactyly)
Failure of normal developmental cell death—webbed fingers (syndactyly)
Aberrant tissue location—digital nevus (capillary angioma)

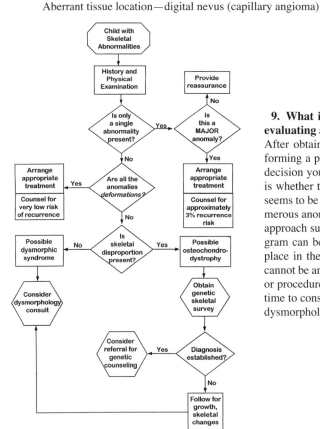

9. What is a good starting place for evaluating a dysmorphic child?

After obtaining a good history and performing a physical examination, the first decision you will probably need to make is whether the abnormality is isolated or seems to be part of a larger pattern. If numerous anomalies are present, a stepwise approach such as that outlined in the diagram can be of help. When you reach a place in the algorithm where a question cannot be answered or special counseling or procedures are required, it is probably time to consider referring the patient to a dysmorphologist or clinical geneticist.

10. What laboratory tests should I order?

There is no universal "screening" test for children with dysmorphologic disorders, and only a small minority of birth defect syndromes can be confirmed with laboratory studies. As a rule, lab testing is reserved for confirmation of a diagnosis once the possibilities have been narrowed down to two or three overlapping conditions. Since many of these specialized tests can be quite expensive, it is important to have a clear idea of which study to order and of what difference the results will make in the care, treatment, or counseling of the patient.

Metabolic tests may be indicated in some forms of bone dysplasia (such as the mucopolysaccharidoses), in the different forms of hypophosphatasia, and in children with short stature.

Chromosome studies usually are appropriate only in situations where the patient has multiple unrelated abnormalities together with mental deficit or growth retardation.

Specific gene testing has become available for several genetic diseases in the past few years, but most dysmorphic syndromes still cannot be confirmed by DNA analysis. Things are moving very rapidly in this field, however, and newly recognized gene mutations are announced almost weekly. The best source of information about possible testing for specific genetic disorders would be the nearest genetic clinic or counseling center.

11. Are there any strictly orthopaedic clues that suggest the diagnosis of dysmorphism?
Each of the skeletal abnormalities listed in the Table raises suspicion of an underlying dysmorphic abnormality. Further investigation of any of these might include a genetic skeletal survey or consultation with a dysmorphologist or clinical geneticist.

Orthopaedic Abnormalities Found as Components of Dysmorphic Syndromes

ABNORMALITY	EXAMPLES OF DYSMORPHIC DIAGNOSES
Short limb segments	
Short proximal segment (rhizomelia)	Achondroplasia, chondrodysplasia punctata, femoral hypoplasia, unusual facies syndrome
Short middle segment (mesomelia)	Leri-Weill, Robinow, Schinzel-Gideon syndromes
Short distal segment (acromelia)	Achondroplasia, Down syndrome, fetal warfarin syndrome
Disproportion between trunk and limb length	
Short trunk, relatively normal limbs	Jarcho-Levin syndrome, Kniest dysplasia, Morquio syndrome
Short limbs, relatively normal trunk	Achondroplasia, spondyloepiphyseal dysplasia
Asymmetric limb size	Klippel-Trenaunay-Weber syndrome, Russell-Silver syndrome
Absence of one or more skeletal elements	Amniotic band sequence, ectrodactyly, VATER association
Duplication of one or more skeletal elements	Trisomy 13, Bardet-Biedl, Meckle-Gruber syndromes
Bone fragility, repeated fractures	Osteogenesis imperfecta (types I & II), hypophosphatasia, osteopetrosis
Multiple enlarged joints	Kniest syndrome, Stickler syndrome
Joint contractures	Arthrogryposis (several types), Hurler syndrome, oligohydramnios sequence, fetal alcohol syndrome
Joint hypermobility/laxity	Down syndrome, Marfan syndrome, Ehlers-Danlos syndrome, Metatropic dysplasia

12. What is a genetic skeletal survey?
Many skeletal dysplasias can best be diagnosed by x-ray evaluation, but one does not have to see every bone in the body to accomplish this. The characteristic radiographic changes usually will be evident in several different skeletal elements. In the interest of minimizing costs and radiation exposure, the following limited set of films should be sufficient for diagnosis in almost every case:

AP view of one arm from midhumerus to wrist   AP and lateral views of pelvis
AP view of one leg from midfemur to ankle   AP and lateral views of thoracolumbar
PA view of one hand   spine

In smaller children, some of these views can be combined on a single film.

13. What do I tell the parents?

When a baby is born with congenital anomalies, the parents can be expected to experience the classic sequence of emotions in response to loss: fear, anger, guilt, and sadness. Each of these phases may last days, months, or even years. I feel that the best way to help the parents through each stage is to tell them everything I know abut their child and not to hesitate in telling them when I *don't* know. Keeping them informed about what's *right* with the child and updating them on the results of any tests (as well as what's to be expected next) help to demystify the diagnostic process. The goal is to allow them to focus on their child, not his or her abnormalities.

14. If there is no way to "cure" a child's birth defects, why bother trying to make a diagnosis?

Probably the greatest value of an accurate diagnosis is to provide answers to important questions for the parents, such as:

> What will my child's life be like? Will he need surgery? Is something else wrong that we haven't found out about? Will she grow up to have children of her own? Will they have the same problems? What caused this in the first place? Was it something I did wrong during the pregnancy? Can my wife and I have normal children in the future? How about our other children's children?

Once a definitive diagnosis has been established, these and many other concerns can be addressed in a meaningful and supportive way. It is at this point that a genetic counselor can provide a great deal of help for the family.

BIBLIOGRAPHY

1. Aase JM: Diagnostic Dysmorphology. New York, Plenum Medical Book Company, 1990.
2. Aase JM: Dysmorphologic diagnosis for the pediatric practitioner. Pediatr Clin North Am 39:135, 1992.
3. Graham JM: Smith's Recognizable Patterns of Human Deformation, 2nd ed. Philadelphia, W.B. Saunders Co., 1988.
4. Jones KL: Smith's Recognizable Patterns of Human Malformation, 5th ed. Philadelphia, W.B. Saunders Co., 1997.

---

92. SHORT STATURE EVALUATION

Michael J. Goldberg, M.D.

---

1. What are the causes of short stature?

Causes include *endocrine* disorders such as growth hormone deficiency or hypothyroidism, *metabolic bone diseases* such as rickets, and *chronic diseases* such as renal failure or congenital heart disease. Some children are small and *fail to thrive* because of feeding disorders or as a result of psychologic deprivation. Short stature is a feature of a number of well-recognized *syndromes*. These can be *chromosomal disorders* (such as Turner syndrome or Down syndrome), a *single gene disorder* (such as familial dysautonomia or the mucopolysaccharidoses), disorders caused by an *intrauterine teratogen* (such as fetal alcohol syndrome), or a *dysmorphic syndrome* of yet-to-be determined cause (such as de Lange or Rett syndrome). Short stature may also be the result of a primary disorder of bone and cartilage growth. These are called *skeletal dysplasias*. Some children are short because they come from short families. Stature has a strong genetic influence. This is known as *constitutional* short stature, or normal-variant short stature. Indeed, from a practice point of view, more than 80% of short people fall into this category, where work-ups yield no specific cause of the short stature.

2. How are children with short stature evaluated?

History-taking is particularly important and must include a prenatal history to see if growth retardation began prior to birth. Intrauterine growth retardation is a feature of many genetic syndromes. Some children are small right from the start and stay small. Children with skeletal dysplasias are an example. Other children grow normally for a while and then fall below the growth curve and continue to drop further below the normal percentile. This occurs in those who develop endocrine disorders such as growth hormone deficiency. It is important to know the heights of the parents and of other family members. Standardized growth tables are available in every pediatric textbook. Remember that most of these growth charts were derived from a caucasian United States population and are less accurate for certain ethnic and racial groups.

In addition to a general physical examination, look specifically for congenital anomalies that may suggest a syndrome (unusual facial features, mental retardation, or subtle deformities of the hands or feet).

Assess the signs and stages of puberty (Tanner stages). It is somewhat easier to do this in girls.

3. How are children measured?

Standard growth charts for boys and girls with percentile markings spanning either birth to 36 months or 2–18 years are available in every pediatric text.

In infants, measure recumbent height and weight, and also measure head circumference. In children, measure standing height and weight. Sitting height may also be important. Sitting height establishes the ratio between the trunk and the limbs and helps determine if stature is in proportion or not. The ratio or percentage of sitting height relative to total height changes with age. At birth, trunk length is about 70% of total height; by age 3 it is about 60%; and at adolescence it is very close to 50%.

4. Why is the ratio between trunk length and limbs length important?

In general, children with short stature fall into two groups: proportionate and disproportionate. In children with proportionate short stature, the relationship between their trunk length and their limbs is identical to that of a child of normal stature, except that these children are small. Proportionate short stature is typical of endocrine disorders such as absent growth hormone, metabolic disorders such as rickets, and failure to thrive due to chronic disease. Disproportionate short stature is characteristic of skeletal dysplasias (dwarfism). Disproportionate short stature may consist of either short limbs in relation to the trunk (such as achondroplasia) or a short trunk in relation to limbs (such as spondyloepiphyseal dysplasia).

Technical tip: The fingertips of children with proportionate stature fall midway between the anterior superior iliac spine and the patella. In children who have disproportionate short stature, the fingertips are at hip level. In those with disproportionate short trunk, the fingertips are low, close to the patella.

5. What is skeletal dysplasia?

Skeletal dysplasia is a generalized developmental disorder that affects both bone and cartilage.

6. How common are skeletal dysplasias?

Individually, each diagnosis is rare. The most common skeletal dysplasias are multiple hereditary exostosis (1:18,000 live births) and achondroplasia (1:26,000 live births). When both lethal and nonlethal forms of skeletal dysplasia are included, the incidence is about 5 affected fetuses in 10,000 pregnancies.

7. What are the clinical findings in skeletal dysplasia?

The child is abnormally short, below the third percentile. The child has disproportionate short stature and dysmorphic facial features. Since skeletal dysplasias affect both bone and cartilage, there are often abnormalities in the facial structures.

8. What imaging is needed to determine if skeletal dysplasia is present?

Most skeletal dysplasias can be diagnosed from a limited skeletal survey that includes a lateral x-ray of the skull, an AP x-ray of the pelvis, an AP x-ray of the knee, a lateral x-ray of the spine, and an AP x-ray of the hand and wrist.

9. Why x-rays of the hand and wrist?

First, this gives some idea of the morphology of the bones and their growth centers. The configuration may be suggestive of skeletal dysplasia. Second, the child's skeletal age can be read from the hand x-ray, thus providing a clue to an endocrine basis for short stature.

10. What is skeletal age?

The degree of bone maturation is due to factors other than just the age of the child. Hormones (thyroid, growth, and sex) have a significant effect on the maturation of bone. Thus, children with the same chronologic age may have a different skeletal age.

Greulich and Pyle serially x-rayed the hands of children at various ages and established the most common x-ray appearance for each age. This is known as the bone age. By comparing the patient's hand x-ray to the x-ray in the Greulich and Pyle atlas, one can determine the patient's bone age. Thus, a child may have a chronologic age of 8 but a skeletal age of only 5. Delayed bone age is typical of short stature due to endocrinopathies. Bone age corresponds well with the development of secondary sexual characteristics. There is considerable interobserver variability, however. There are wide standard deviations (variations) among normal children, and different genetic populations have different rates of maturation.

11. How are children with short stature treated?

Treatment depends on the cause of the short stature. For children with an endocrinopathy such as growth hormone deficiency, replacement therapy with genetically engineered recombinant human growth hormone is very effective. Similarly, recombinant human growth hormone is effective for certain chromosomal disorders such as Turner syndrome. Girls with Turner syndrome have short stature and delayed secondary sexual characteristics. A combination of sex hormone replacement and recombinant human growth hormone accelerates the rate of growth and also results in an increased ultimate height. The use of growth hormone for children of short stature who are not growth hormone deficient is controversial, with conflicting data reported on growth velocity and effect on ultimate height. Growth hormone is not effective for children with skeletal dysplasias.

12. How can the stature of children with skeletal dysplasias be increased?

There is no evidence that children with skeletal dysplasias are deficient in growth hormone or have other endocrine or metabolic abnormalities. Thus, the use of human growth hormone in disorders such as achondroplasia has no scientific basis, although it continues to undergo clinical trials.

Children with short stature can be made taller by elongation of the long bones in the leg (femur and tibia) and elongation of the humerus so that the children look in proportion. Gradual distraction of the bone using special fixators, either circular ring frames (Ilizarov) or unilateral frames, has resulted in substantial elongation of up to 30 cm in overall height between femur and tibia. The technique involves performing an osteotomy through the bone and then distracting the bone slowly as the new bone (callus) is formed. Distraction is 1 mm a day, so the procedure takes considerable time.

13. Why is skeletal elongation controversial?

The proponents of skeletal elongation argue that disproportionate short stature poses both physical and emotional handicaps for the child. The person is stigmatized and impaired in activities of daily living because of the standard height of countertops and workbenches. Elongation offers psychologic benefits and a more normal appearance. In addition, angular malalignments of the legs are present in many skeletal dysplasias; during elongation, these deformities can be straightened. This realignment of the joints may prevent precocious arthritis. In certain dysplasias such as achondroplasia, skeletal elongation of the femur appears to improve the swayback (lumbar lordosis) characteristic of this disorder.

Those opposed to skeletal elongation argue that average adult height is rarely achieved and that a normal proportional ratio of limbs to trunk is very difficult to accomplish. In addition, they argue that from the child's perspective, undergoing the prolonged surgical procedures results in the child feeling psychologically rejected by the parents. The procedure takes substantial time and is carried out in a child who usually has no symptoms. Often, there is a significant loss of school time and socialization. In addition, experimental lengthening in immature dogs has demonstrated damage to the growth plate from compressive forces as well as compression across the articular cartilage, predisposing to arthritis. The procedure is extraordinarily expensive and fraught with complications (although complications of lengthening skeletal dysplasias seem to be fewer than those of lengthening congenitally short limbs). There are no long-term outcome studies that establish the benefits of lengthening dwarfs.

14. What is achondroplasia?
Achondroplasia is the most common form of short-limb dwarfism. Affected individuals have the characteristic appearance of a large head with frontal bossing, a depressed nasal bridge, and short limbs that are even shorter in their proximal segments (rhizomelia). Trunk length is nearly normal.

15. What medical problems are faced by people with achondroplasia?
In the child, the most significant problem is narrowing of the foramen magnum, leading to respiratory distress, apnea, hypotonia, and delayed achievement of developmental milestones. In the adult, there is narrowing and stenosis of the lumbar spine leading to back pain, claudication, weakness, and paralysis in the legs. Other associated abnormalities include internal hydrocephalus, dislocated radial heads at the elbow, and bowed legs.

16. What is the cause of achondroplasia?
Achondroplasia is an autosomal dominant disorder. There is a mutation in the fibroblast growth factor receptor 3 gene located on the tip of the short arm of chromosome 4. It is a remarkably constant mutation, the same nucleotides being affected in all patients. Thus, all patients with achondroplasia look nearly identical.

BIBLIOGRAPHY

1. Bassett GS: The osteochondrodysplasias. In Morrissy RJ, Weinstein SL (eds): Lovell & Winter's Pediatric Orthopaedics, 4th ed. Philadelphia, Lippincott-Raven, 1996, pp 203–254.
2. Bell DF, Boyer MI, Armstrong PF: The use of the Ilizarov technique in the correction of limb deformities associated with skeletal dysplasia. J Pediatr Orthop 12:283–290, 1992.
3. Chipman JJ: Study design for final height determination in Turner syndrome: pros and cons. Horm Res 39 (suppl 2):18–22, 1993.
4. Cuttler L, Silvers JB, Singh J, Marrero V, Finkelstein B, Tanin G, Neuhauer D: Short stature and growth hormone therapy. A national study of physician recommendation patterns. JAMA 276:531–537, 1996.
5. Francomano CA: The genetic basis of dwarfism. N Engl J Med 332:58–59, 1995.
6. Furlanetto RW and the The Drug and Therapeutics Committee of the Lawson Wilkins Pediatric Endocrine Society: Guidelines for the use of growth hormone in children with short stature. J Pediatr 127:857–867, 1995.
7. Greulich WW, Pyle SI: Radiographic atlas of skeletal development of the hand and wrist. Stanford, CA, Stanford University Press, 1959.
8. Lavini F, Renzi-Brivio L, DeBastiani G: Psychological, vascular, and physiologic aspects of lower limb lengthening in achondroplastics. Clin Orthop 250:138–142, 1990.
9. Tanner JM, Davies PSW: Clinical longitudinal standards for height and weight velocity for North American children. J Pediatr 107:317–329, 1985.

93. OSTEOCHONDRODYSPLASIA

Mohammad Diab, M.D.

1. Distinguish dwarf from midget, dysplasia from dysostosis, deformity from malformation.

1. A midget demonstrates proportionate short stature, whereas in dwarfism the parts of the body are disproportionate.

2. Dysplasia represents systemic disease, whereas dysostosis indicates involvement of a single bone or a group of physically or functionally related bones.

3. Malformation describes primary disease, whereas deformity occurs as a secondary phenomenon.

2. How are the osteochondrodysplasias classified anthropometrically and radiographically?

Disproportionate involvement of the trunk is known as microcormia. Disproportionate involvement of the limbs is known as micromelia. Micromelia may be subdivided into rhizomelia, indicating that the humerus or os femoris is affected; mesomelia, indicating that the radius and ulna or the tibia and fibula are affected; and acromelia, indicating that the hands or feet are affected.

The radiographic classification is based on the region of bone principally affected, such as epiphysis, metaphysis, or diaphysis. The convenience of this system has led to its wide adoption by clinicians. However, it is simplistic, bears no relationship to morbidity, and frequently suggests a connection between entities where there is none.

3. Define collagen.

Collagen is the name given to a family of proteins that comprise the principal constituents of the extracellular matrix of tissues of the musculoskeletal system. The collagen molecule is composed of three polypeptide chains, each assigned the Greek letter α, and is therefore a trimer. Although the primary structure of each polypeptide chain differs among collagen types, a repeating three-amino-acid motif is strictly preserved.

At least 15 genetically distinct types of collagen have been identified. Each is given a Roman numeral indicative of the order of discovery.

4. Define proteoglycan.

Proteoglycan (PG), formerly known as protein polysaccharide or mucoprotein, refers to a molecule of "protein and sugar." It has three components.

1. Glycosaminoglycan (GAG), formerly known as mucopolysaccharide. This represents an unbranched chain of repeating disaccharide units, of which one is an amino sugar. With the exception of hyaluronic acid, the GAGs carry a high negative charge due to the sulfate and carboxyl groups added to their sugar residues.

2. Link protein. This interacts noncovalently to stabilize the bond formed between each GAG and protein core.

3. Protein core.

The major proteoglycan of cartilage is aggrecan. Cartilage also contains small nonaggregating proteoglycans, including decorin and biglycan. The molecular structure and negative charge of PGs enable them to occupy a large volume for mass and to attract water according to the Gibbs-Donnan equilibrium. They form a porous hydrated gel that resists compression and regulates the passage of molecules and cells through the extracellular matrix.

5. What is the clinical ramification of epiphyseal diseases compared with those that affect the metaphyses and diaphyses of long bones?

The former results in osteoarthritis.

6. **Describe the type II collagenopathies.**

- **Achondrogenesis.** Perinatal lethal, hydrops fetalis, and retarded ossification (in particular of sacrum and spine), with unossified bodies and ossified pedicles of vertebræ.
- **Spondyloepiphyseal dysplasia.** Associated with skeletal disease, including of the spine, with scoliosis, kyphosis, and lordosis; hypo- or aplasia of the dens axis with atlantoaxial instability and ovoid vertebræ; and epiphyseal degeneration, in particular of the proximal os femoris, resulting in coxa vara. Ocular disease, including myopia and retinal detachment, is also present.
- **Kniest dysplasia.** Associated with skeletal disease, including joint contractures, clubfoot, cuneiform vertebræ, and "Swiss cheese" or cystic degeneration of epiphyseal cartilage with metaphyseal widening to produce osteoarthritis, coxa vara, and "dumbbell" long bones. Cleft palate, sensorineural and conductive hearing loss, and inguinal hernia are also seen.
- **Stickler disease (arthro-ophthalmopathy).** Associated with skeletal disease, including osteoarthritis, vertebral end plate irregularity, and articular hypermobility. Ocular disease, including myopia, retinal detachment, and vitreous degeneration; cleft palate; and sensorineural hearing loss are seen.
- **Autosomal dominant spondyloarthropathy.** Associated with mild short stature, premature osteoarthritis, and limited range of motion of the joints.

7. **Give characteristic features of diastrophic dysplasia. What mutation has been identified in this disorder?**

Characteristic features include kyphosis, scoliosis, clubfoot resistant to nonoperative treatment and demonstrating a high recurrence rate following operation ("twisted" spine and feet), calcification of the auricular cartilage (producing "cauliflower ears") and of costal cartilage, shortening and abduction of the first metacarpal (producing "hitchhiker thumb"), and periarthric contractures associated with osteoarthritis.

Positional cloning by fine-structure linkage disequilibrium mapping has located the diastrophic dysplasia gene to human chromosome 5q approximately 70kb proximal to the *CSF1R* locus. The gene encodes a novel sulfate transporter, and fibroblasts from a diastrophic individual demonstrate significantly diminished sulfate uptake. While the disease affects principally cartilage and bone, the sulfate transporter is ubiquitously expressed. This may reflect the high sulfate requirement of chondrocytes when compared with other cell types for the synthesis of proteoglycans. The sulfate groups confer a negative charge essential to their function in the extracellular matrix. Abnormality of type IX collagen has been observed in hyaline cartilage from a diastrophic individual. Several forms of type IX collagen have been identified. One bears a chondroitin sulfate glycosaminoglycan on the $\alpha 2$ chain and is therefore a proteoglycan.

Mutations in the diastrophic dysplasia sulfate transporter gene have been identified in atelosteogenesis type II and achondrogenesis type IB. In both, abnormal sulfation of proteoglycans has been demonstrated.

8. **Define fibroblast growth factor receptor (FGFR).**

Nine genetically distinct fibroblast growth factors (FGFs) have been identified in mammals. Their pleiotropic effects, which include mitogenesis, differentiation, and chemotaxis, are mediated by fibroblast growth factor receptors (FGFRs). Four FGFRs have been identified in mammals. They belong to the tyrosine kinase family of receptors. Their common structural features include a split intracellular tyrosine kinase domain, a transmembrane domain, and two or three extracellular immunoglobulin-like domains. FGFRs are expressed at different stages of development and are located on the surface of several cell types, including chondrocytes during endochondral ossification and cells of the embryonic central nervous system.

9. **Name three osteochondrodysplasias caused by FGFR mutations.**

1. Achondroplasia. This is the most common osteochondrodysplasia, occurring once in every 15,000 live births. Features include relative macrocephaly with narrow foramen magnum, micromelia, spina gibba, lumbar spinal stenosis secondary to hypoplasia of vertebral pedicles and reduced interpedicular distance, periarthric contracture, prolonged fibulæ, retarded growth of the triradiate cartilage producing a "champagne pelvis," and "trident hand" anomaly.

2. **Thanatophoric dysplasia.** So named because it is "death-bearing" in the perinatal period. Features include kleeblattschädel, or cloverleaf skull, as a result of hydrocephalus and sutural synostosis; narrow thorax with short horizontal ribs and hypoplastic scapulæ; "telephone-receiver" ossa femorum; and platyspondylia.

3. **Hypochondroplasia.** This presents a spectrum ranging from severe disease, which is indistinguishable from achondroplasia, to mild, which approaches the normal.

10. With what sclerosing bone dysplasia was the French impressionist painter H. M. R. de Toulouse-Lautrec-Monfa said to have been affected?

Pyknodysostosis, which is characterized by micromelia, craniofacial dysmorphia, acroosteolysis, and spinal anomalies such as morbid curvature, olisthy, and atlantoaxial failure of segmentation. It shares several features with osteopetrosis, including generalized sclerosis, which leads to cortical thickening and increased osseous density on radiography, and a propensity to fracture.

In pyknodysostosis, there is normal demineralization but abnormal degradation of the organic component of bone by osteoclasts.

11. For which osteochondroplasia is mutation of type IX collagen responsible?
Mutation within the gene that encodes the α2 chain of type IX collagen, *COL9A2,* has been identified in multiple epiphyseal dysplasia (MED). MED is characterized by a normal facies, micromelia, precocious osteoarthritis, joint contractures, brachydactyly, "slanting" of the proximal articular surface of the tibia, and osteochondritis dissecans of the knee. Symmetric involvement of femoral capital epiphyses and a stable clinical presentation in the setting of other epiphyseal irregularities distinguishes MED from Legg-Calvé-Perthes disease. Relative sparing of the spine contrasts with spondyloepiphyseal dysplasia, while relative sparing of the pelvis contrasts with pseudoachondroplasia.

12. For which osteochondrodysplasia is mutation of type X collagen responsible?
Mutation within the gene encoding type X collagen, *COL10A1,* causes metaphyseal chondrodysplasia, type Schmid (MCDS). Features of this disorder include micromelia, distal greater than proximal metaphyseal irregularity of the os femoris and tibia, coxa vara, and anterior cupping, splaying, and sclerosis of the ribs. The hands, spine, and pelvis are spared. Several mutations in *COL10A1* that result in a reduction of type X collagen synthesis do not cause MCDS, which argues against haploinsufficiency as the underlying mechanism.

13. For which osteochondrodysplasia is mutation of cartilage oligomeric matrix protein responsible?
Mutations in the cartilage oligomeric matrix protein (COMP) gene cause pseudoachondroplasia (PSACH) and some types of multiple epiphyseal dysplasia (MED). The underlying mechanism appears to be deposition of abnormal, or reduction of, COMP in the extracellular matrix, resulting in impairment of calcium binding. PSACH is characterized by micromelia with epiphyseal as well as metaphyseal malformation, in particular in the hands and feet; articular laxity; precocious osteoarthritis; retarded and irregular pelvic maturation; and mild vertebral malformation with abnormal spinal curvature and atlantoaxial instability. The craniofacial skeleton is unaffected.

14. For which osteochondrodysplasia is mutation of cartilage-derived morphogenetic protein responsible?
Mutation in this protein causes acromesomelic chondrodysplasia. This resembles murine brachypodism, which is produced by a null mutation in growth differentiation factor 5. It is characterized by micromelia, in particular brachydactyly; articular dislocations; lumbar kyphosis with dis-

tal reduction in interpedicular distance; and acetabular dysplasia. There is relative sparing of the craniofacial and axial skeletons.

15. Parathyroid hormone-related protein, parathyroid hormone–parathyroid hormone-related protein receptor, and Indian hedgehog are responsible for which disease?

Because of homology between amino-terminal domains, parathyroid hormone (PTH) and parathyroid hormone-related protein (PTHrP) bind the same receptor (PTH-PTHrP receptor), through which they exert similar effects on calcium and phosphate homeostasis and skeletal development and turnover. Indian hedgehog (Ihh) belongs to a family of conserved molecules that serve as signals during organogenesis in the embryo. Ihh and PTHrP participate in a negative feedback loop that controls the temporal and spatial sequence of differentiation of chondrocytes from proliferative to hypertrophic state during endochondral ossification.

Mutation in the gene encoding parathyroid hormone–parathyroid hormone-related protein (PTH-PTHrP) receptor has been identified in metaphyseal chondrodysplasia, type Jansen (MCDJ). This is characterized by micromelia; joint contractures, especially of the hips and knees; waddling gait; brachydactyly; and osteopenia. There is hypercalcemia and hypophosphatemia in the setting of normal parathyroid glands and normal levels of PTH and PTHrP. The skeletal manifestations resemble those of hyperparathyroidism. The underlying mechanism in MCDJ involves ligand-independent activation PTH-PTHrP receptor, leading to abnormal endochondral ossification.

16. Name three characteristic spinal deformities in achondroplasia.

1. A reduction in interpedicular distance in the lumbar spine. This may lead to clinically significant spinal stenosis. Affected children assume positions in which the lumbar spine is flexed to obliterate lordosis and expand the capacity of the spinal canal. Neurologic embarrassment necessitates operative intervention. This consists of decompression with arthrodesis in the setting of associated thoracic kyphosis.

2. Thoracic kyphosis. This is evident in the sitting child. With ambulation, the majority of such deformities resolve spontaneously. Those that persist (beyond age 5 years) and are significant ($> 40°$) require anterior and posterior arthrodesis with instrumentation that does not occupy the spinal canal.

3. Narrowing of the foramen magnum occipitale. This produces compression of the upper part of the cervical division of the spinal cord. Manifestations include respiratory compromise and motor retardation. Decompression is an accepted though risky surgical treatment.

17. What are the characteristic spinal deformities in diastrophic dysplasia?

Spina bifida occulta.

Cervical kyphosis. Typically, there is spontaneous resolution. Progressive deformity produces anterior spinal cord compression. Treatment consists of posterior decompression and arthrodesis with or without anterior arthrodesis.

Thoracic kyphoscoliosis.

Lumbosacral lordosis.

18. What spinal anomaly has the greatest potential for morbidity in spondyloepiphyseal dysplasia?

In spondyloepiphyseal dysplasia, hypoplasia of the dens axis leads to atlantoaxial instability. This may necessitate posterior arthrodesis. Atlantoaxial or occipitoaxial arthrodesis may be required in the event that the posterior arch of the atlas has not ossified.

BIBLIOGRAPHY

1. Beighton P: McKusick's Heritable Disorders of Connective Tissue. St. Louis, Mosby-Year Book, 1992.
2. Bellus GA, McIntosh I, Smith EA, et al.: A recurrent mutation in the tyrosine kinase domain of fibroblast growth factor receptor 3 causes hypochondroplasia. Nat Genet 10:357, 1995.

3. Briggs MD, Hoffman SMG, King LM, et al.: Pseudoachondroplasia and multiple epiphyseal dysplasia due to mutations in the cartilage oligomeric matrix protein gene. Nat Genet 10:330, 1995.
4. Diab M, Wu J-J, Eyre DR: Collagen type IX from human articular cartilage: a structural profile of inter-molecular cross-linking sites. Biochem J 314:327–332, 1996.
5. Gelb BD, Shi G-P, Chapman HA, et al.: Pycnodysostosis, a lysosomal disease caused by cathepsin K deficiency. Science 273:1236, 1996.
6. Hästbacka J, de la Chapelle A, Mahtani MM, et al.: The diastrophic gene encodes a novel sulfate transporter: positional cloning by fine-structure linkage disequilibrium mapping. Cell 78:1073, 1994.
7. Hästbacka J, Superti-Furga A, Wilcox WR, et al.: Atelosteogenesis type II is caused by mutations in the diastrophic dysplasia sulfate transporter gene (DTDST): evidence for a phenotypic series involving three chondrodysplasias. Am J Hum Genet 58:225, 1996.
8. Muragaki Y, Mariman ECM, van Beersum SEC, et al.: A mutation in the gene encoding the $\alpha2$ chain of the fibril-associated collagen IX, COL9A2, causes multiple epiphyseal dysplasia. Nat Genet 12:103, 1996.
9. Rousseau F, Saugier P, Le Merrer M, et al.: Stop codon FGFR3 mutations in thanatophoric dwarfism type 1. Nat Genet 10:11, 1995.
10. Schipani E, Kruse K, Jüppner H: A constitutively active mutant PTH-PTHrP receptor in Jansen-type metaphyseal chondrodysplasia. Science 268:98, 1995.
11. Shiang R, Thompson LM, Zhu Y-Z, et al.: Mutations in the transmembrane domain of FGFR3 cause the most common genetic form of dwarfism, achondroplasia. Cell 78:335, 1994.
12. Spranger J, Winterpacht A, Zabel B: The type II collagenopathies: a spectrum of chondrodysplasias. Eur J Pediatr 153:56, 1994.
13. Supert-Furga A, Hästbacka J, Wilcox WR, et al.: Achondrogenesis type IB is caused by mutations in the diastrophic dysplasia sulphate transporter gene. Nat Genet 12:100, 1996.
14. Thomas JT, Lin K, Nandedkar M, et al.: A human chondrodysplasia due to a mutation in a TGF-β superfamily member. Nat Genet 12:315, 1996.
15. Vortkamp A, Lee K, Lanske B, et al.: Regulation of rate of cartilage differentiation by Indian hedgehog and PTH-related protein. Science 273:613, 1996.
16. Wallis GA, Rash B, Sykes B, et al.: Mutations within the gene encoding the $\alpha1$ (X) chain of type X collagen (COL10A1) cause metaphyseal chondrodysplasia type Schmid but not several other forms of metaphyseal chondrodysplasia. J Med Genet 33:450, 1996.

94. NEUROFIBROMATOSIS

Alvin H. Crawford, M.D., F.A.C.S.

1. What is neurofibromatosis?

Peripheral neurofibromatosis, von Recklinghausen's disease (NF-1), is a multisystemic disease that primarily affects cellular growth of neural tissue. It is an autosomal dominant disorder.

2. How common is neurofibromatosis?

NF-1 has been found to affect one in 4000 individuals. It is one of the most common dominantly inherited gene disorders in humans. The gene locus of NF-1 in humans has been identified (characteristically localized to chromosome 17) and cloned.

3. What are the causes?

Approximately 50% of all cases are new mutations, which is one hundredfold higher than the usual mutation rate for a single locus and may reflect the huge size of the NF-1 locus (estimated at 350,000 base pairs). Prenatal testing is now possible in some families but is not very useful, because in most patients mutations have not been easy to identify. The manifestations of NF-1 vary from one person to another, but each individual who carries the gene will eventually show some clinical features of the disease, the penetrance of NF-1 being close to 100%.

4. What is the pathophysiology?

Patients with NF-1 may develop Schwann's cell tumors called neurofibromas and pigmentation abnormalities. The orthopaedic manifestations and especially the complications after treatment are frequent.

5. What are the criteria for diagnosis?

The consensus development conference on NF-1 held at the National Institutes of Health in 1987 concluded that the diagnosis of NF-1 could be assigned to a person with two or more of the following criteria: (1) More than 6 café au lait spots, at least 15 mm in their greatest diameter in adults and 5 mm in children. (2) Two or more neurofibromas of any type or one plexiform neurofibroma. (3) Freckling in the axillary or inguinal regions. (4) Optic glioma. (5) Two or more Lisch nodules (iris hamartomas). (6) A distinctive bony lesion, such as sphenoid wing dysplasia or thinning of the cortex of a long bone with or without pseudarthrosis. (7) A first-degree relative with NF-1.

These criteria have been shown to be very useful even in young children. Since the consensus panel meeting, specific kinds of learning disabilities and MRI abnormalities (especially in children) have also been specifically associated with NF-1.

6. What are the different types?

Neurofibromatosis can be divided into several categories; however, most common is NF-1, which can be clearly distinguished from central neurofibromatosis (NF-2). The latter is also an autosomal dominant disorder but occurs less frequently (estimated to affect 1 in 100,000 individuals). Characteristically, in NF-2, there are bilateral schwannomas of the vestibular portion of the eighth cranial nerve, but schwannomas of other peripheral nerves, meningiomas, and ependymomas are also common. Eighth cranial nerve tumors are not found in NF-1. The gene for NF-2 has been localized on the long arm of chromosome 22, and the gene has recently been cloned.

7. What happens if the condition is not treated?

Once the clinical manifestations of NF-1 have been noted, it appears as though a progressive deterioration of the area occurs over time. If treatment is not effective, significant disability occurs.

8. What are the clinical features?

The dermatologic features include **café au lait spots,** which are present in more than 90% of patients with NF-1. The pigmentation is melanotic in origin and is located both in the basal layers of the epidermis and in melanocytes of upper layers. The lesions are usually found in the skin areas not exposed to the sun, such as the groin or inguinal and axillary regions. **Fibroma molluscum** are small neurofibromas in the subcutis. Neurofibromas are mixed-cell tumors rich in Schwann's cells but also including fiberglass, endothethial cells, and glandular elements. The primary cell responsible for tumor formation is unknown.

Plexiform neurofibroma is a subcutaneous neurofibroma that has a "bag of worms" feeling and is very sensitive. It is often found underlying an area of cutaneous hyperpigmentation. When the pigmentation approaches or crosses the posterior midline of the body, it appears that the tumor may be aggressive and may originate from the spinal canal. It is known that a plexiform neurofibroma has the potential to become malignant. **Elephantiasis** is another dermatologic manifestation of the disease, which is characterized by large soft tissue masses with a rough raised villous type of skin. Attempts to resect sizable portions of the soft tissue have met with limited success. There is dysplasia of the underlying bone when the lesions occur in an extremity. **Verrucous hyperplasia** is an infrequent and unsightly cutaneous lesion of NF-1. There is tremendous overgrowth of the skin with thickening, but also with a velvety soft papillary quality. The lesion is geographic, develops most often in a unilateral fashion, and is considered to be one of the most grotesque cutaneous lesions found in humans. **Axillary and inguinal freckles** are diffuse small hyperpigmented spots of 2–3 mm in diameter. They are found in the armpits and inguinal region and, if present, are helpful diagnostic criteria. About 40% of patients with NF-1 have axillary freckling.

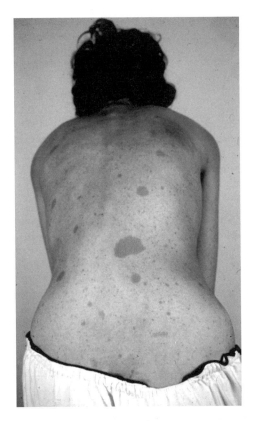

Multiple café au lait spots in a young patient with spinal deformity. Note the variation in size and shape of the lesions. These lesions tend to increase in size and number as the child matures. Reprinted with permission from Crawford AH: Neurofibromatosis in the pediatric patient. Othop Clin North Am 9(2):11, 1978.

Ophthalmologic **Lisch nodules** are slightly raised, well-circumscribed hamartomas in the iris and are present in more than 90% of patients with NF-1 who are 6 years of age or older. Other centers report more than 50% involvement by 5 years old, 90% at adulthood. The lesions are thought to be specific for NF-1. Although **optic gliomas** account for only 2–5% of all brain tumors in childhood, as many as 70% of these are found in persons with NF-1. In some patients, these tumors change little in size over many years.

9. What should be asked in the history?
The primary questions are whether there is a family history of the clinical manifestations of NF-1 and whether there are relatives with significant birthmarks similar to the dermatologic examples just listed. The mother or father may only have dermatologic lesions and none of the orthopaedic or neurologic manifestations, whereas the child and siblings may show all the manifestations of NF-1.

10. What spinal deformities are associated with neurofibromatosis?
The primary spinal deformity is scoliosis and appears to be the most common osseous defect associated with NF-1. It may vary in severity from mild nonprogressive forms to severe curvatures. The cause of dystrophic NF-1 spinal deformity is unknown, but it has been suggested to be secondary to osteomalacia, a localized neurofibromatous tumor eroding and infiltrating bone, endocrine disturbances, or mesodermal dysplasia.

In a general orthopaedic clinic, 2% of the population with scoliosis will have NF-1, whereas in a population with NF-1, perhaps 10–20% of patients will have some disorder of the spine. The majority of patients will have nondystrophic spinal deformities. The dystrophic or classic spinal deformities include short, segmented, sharply angulated curvatures in which there appear to be scalloping of the posterior vertebral margins, severe rotation of the apical vertebrae, widening of the spinal canal, enlargement of the neural foramina, defective pedicles, the presence of a paraspinal mass, spindling of the transverse process, and rotation of the ribs, resembling a twisted ribbon. There is invariably thoracic lordosis associated with this deformity.

There may also be nondystrophic spinal deformities, not unlike idiopathic scoliosis. These nondystrophic idiopathic-appearing deformities have the tendency to become dystrophic with time or following spinal fusion. Pseudarthrosis following spinal surgery is common in NF-1, and as a result, there is a growing trend toward performing anterior and posterior fusion in these patients to prevent pseudarthrosis.

Cervical spine deformities as well as kyphotic deformities and spondylolisthesis secondary to pathologic involvement of the pedicles and pars interarticularis are seen somewhat uncommonly in NF-1. Most often, the deformity or appearance of dysplasia has to do with bone erosion from adjacent neurofibromas.

All patients with NF-1 who undergo surgery require endotracheal anesthesia and halo traction or, if they present with neck tumors, should undergo a cervical spine x-ray series. Widening of the neural foramina on oblique views may represent "dumbbell lesions" characteristic of neurofibromas as they extrude from the spinal canal. If there is any suspicion of subluxation, then tomography, CT, and MRI are appropriate studies. Other reasons for obtaining cervical spine x-rays include torticollis and dysphagia.

Dural ectasia, meningocele, pseudomeningoceles, and dumbbell lesions are all related to the presence of neurofibromas or abnormal pressure phenomena in and about the spinal canal neuraxis. High-volume myelography or MRI should be used in the investigation of all dystrophic curves prior to initiating treatment.

11. What tibial disorders are seen?

Congenital bowing and pseudarthrosis of the tibia are rare problems that occur in 1:140,000 liveborn children but 1–2% of the time in NF-1. The bowing associated with NF-1 is always anterolateral. The deformity may present before other manifestations such as café au lait spots. It is usually evident within the first year of life, with a fracture not uncommonly occurring before 1–3 years of age.

There are two types of bowing: nondysplastic and dysplastic. In **nondysplastic** (type I) bowing, there is anterolateral bowing with increased bony density and sclerosis of the medullary canal. This type may convert to dysplastic bowing following osteotomy to correct the angulation. In **dysplastic** (type II) anterolateral bowing, there is a failure of medullary canal tubulation, anterolateral bowing with cystic prefracture or canal enlargement due to previous fracture, and frank pseudarthrosis and atrophy with "sucked candy" narrowing of the ends of the two fragments.

The most effective treatment to date has been chronic bracing initiated at the time of diagnosis. Other forms of treatment include **pulsating electromagnetic fields, surgical bone grafting, vascularized autogenous graft, Ilizarov callotasis** (compression, transplantation, and distraction histogenesis), and **amputation.**

The quality of life associated with numerous unsuccessful operative procedures makes chronic bracing the reasonable alternative. The high incidence (25%) of subsequent central nervous system neoplasms should cause one to consider whether attempts at bony synostosis should be continued after three or four procedures. By the age of 7 years, the benefit to the child of further procedures as opposed to amputation should be very strongly scrutinized.

Posterior medial congenital bowing (kyphoscoliosis tibia) is a benign condition associated only with occasional limb-length inequality. Tibial bowing associated with skin dimples, bilateral presentation, ring constrictions, and foot deformities is rarely associated with NF-1.

12. What are the disorders of bone growth?

Segmental hypertrophy and subperiosteal bone growth and proliferation.

Overgrowth of an extremity is not a rare complication of NF-1 and may be related to changes in the soft tissues, i.e., hemangiomatosis, lymphangiomatosis, elephantiasis, or beaded plexiform neuromas. The zones of overgrowth in bone and soft tissue are usually unilateral, involving the upper or lower extremities or the head and neck. These osseous changes characteristically cause the bone to elongate with a wavy irregularity or thickening of the cortex. There is a higher incidence of neoplasia associated with this segmental hypertrophy than with other lesions.

Subperiosteal bone proliferation is another of the manifestations of multiple NF-1. Most cases are initiated by minor fractures with subperiosteal bleeding followed by osseous dysplasia of the subperiosteal hematoma. The early onset of subperiosteal hematoma may be identified on technetium bone scanning by the presence of a "doughnut sign," a peripheral realm of increased activity surrounding a relatively photopenic center appearing in the blood pool and in delayed imaging. Aggressive aspiration of the lesion may prevent the development of the dysplasia.

13. What type of imaging is useful?

For scoliotic lesions, the primary imaging modality is PA and lateral thoracolumbar spine films. If there is evidence of significant dysplasia or neurologic clinical involvement, then an MRI is recommended. As previously stated, soft tissue neurofibromas and spinal cord dural ectasia or hydrostatic expansion of the dural sac may be responsible for some of the bony deformities. These could be identified more readily with MRI.

Plain x-rays are usually utilized to determine the characteristics of the anterolateral bowing associated with congenital pseudarthrosis tibia. MRI has recently been used to determine whether healing is occurring in the area of pseudarthrosis.

For disorders of bone growth, plain x-rays and radioisotope scintigraphy (bone scan) are usually adequate to identify the lesions and their level of activity.

14. Are laboratory studies useful?

Serologic laboratory studies are rarely useful. Prior to the identification of the gene for NF-1, genetic and karyotypic analyses were carried out on all patients in an effort to identify the gene. To date, amniocentesis and prenatal screening for NF-1 have not been carried out.

15. With what other conditions may neurofibromatosis be confused?

McCune-Albright syndrome, Watson syndrome, and Proteus syndrome. The contour of café au lait spots associated with Albright's fibrous dysplasia has historically been identified as irregular, as opposed to the smooth edges in NF-1. This finding does not always bear out clinically.

16. Does the condition require treatment?

All the conditions associated with NF-1 require monitoring for evidence of progression. If there is progression, active treatment is recommended.

17. Who should manage the problem?

Since NF-1 is a multisystemic multidimensional problem, it is most important that the patient be managed by a team. We propose that the team consist of a primary care physician, a geneticist, an orthopaedist, a neurologist, and a social worker. Consultation should be readily available with ophthalmology, general surgery, and neurosurgery. The condition can best be managed by recognition of the manifestations of the disease and a complete evaluation of the patient and family, with involvement of a multidisciplinary team according to the nature of lesions present. Most important is specific treatment of individual lesions based on careful judgment, especially concerning radical operative procedures. Thereafter, continuing observation of the patient for the remainder of life is required.

18. What is the prognosis?

In a 250-patient series of individuals with disseminated NF-1, 41% were asymptomatic, 35.2% had neurologic problems, and 13.2% had disfigurement. Orthopaedic manifestations were found in 6.8% and sarcomatous changes in 3.6%. There is little doubt that NF-1 predisposes one to an increased risk of certain malignancies. Underrecognition of this relationship may occur when the cutaneous signs of NF-1 are overlooked or are not yet apparent in young children. Neurofibrosarcoma, childhood leukemia, rhabdomyosarcoma of the urogenital tract, and Wilms' tumor have all been reported.

19. What should I tell the family?

The family should be informed of the multifaceted nature of NF-1 when the child is first diagnosed. A good basic physical examination as well as indicated x-rays, auditory brain evoked potentials, and a CT or MRI scan of the skull should be obtained as a part of the initial work-up. The family should be informed of the possibility of progression of all the lesions noted in NF-1 and emphatically encouraged to maintain continuous follow-up.

20. What are the complications?

Although there are significant osseous as well as neurologic complications associated with NF-1, the majority of patients do not have them. Our NF-1 multidisciplinary center started off attracting mostly the worse cases of musculoskeletal problems because of our interest in complex cases.

It is important that the reader be aware that 25% of all affected patients with NF-1 have café au lait spots as the only manifestation of the disease, and less than 10% of patients will ever require orthopaedic treatment.

BIBLIOGRAPHY

1. Cohen MM Jr: Further diagnostic thoughts about the elephant man. Am J Med Genet 29:777–782, 1988.
2. Crawford AH: Neurofibromatosis. In Weinstein SL (ed): Pediatric Spine; Principles and Practice. New York, Raven Press, 1994.
3. Crawford AH: Neurofibromatosis in children. Acta Orthop Scand 57(suppl):218, 1986.
4. Crawford AH: Orthopaedic complications of von Recklinghausen's disease in children. Current Orthop 10:49–55, 1996.
5. Goldberg NS, Collins FS: The hunt for the neurofibromatosis gene. Arch Dermatol 127:1705–1707, 1991.
6. Mandell GA, Harcke HT: Subperiosteal hematoma another scintigraphic "doughnut." Clin Nucl Med 11:35–37, 1986.
7. National Institute of Health Consensus Development Conference Statement: Neurofibromatosis. Neurofibromatosis 1:172, 1988.
8. Riccardi VM: Type I neurofibromatosis and the pediatric patient. Curr Probl Pediatr 66:106, 1992.
9. Sirois JL, Drennan JC: Dystrophic spinal deformity in neurofibromatosis. J Pediatr 10:522–526, 1990

95. OSTEOGENESIS IMPERFECTA

Paul D. Sponseller, M.D.

1. What is osteogenesis imperfecta?

Osteogenesis imperfecta (OI) is a genetically transmitted disease resulting in fragility of the entire skeleton. It is seen with varying degrees of severity, from an infant with multiple fractures to a child who has only a few fractures before maturity. The clinical variation is due to differences in the mutation. The incidence of OI is about 1:20,000 in the population. Intelligence is not affected.

2. How is the diagnosis made?

By a combination of clinical and radiographic findings. In most cases, OI is not readily confused with other entities. Clinically, the patients usually have short stature. The sclerae may be blue in many but not all cases. The dentin of the teeth may be abnormally thin in some cases. Deformities of the long bones on both sides of the body usually develop. The ligaments are usually slightly lax. Hearing may be impaired owing to defects in the bones of the middle ear. In some patients, there may be a positive family history.

Radiographically, the bones usually demonstrate osteopenia. In most patients this is evident from visual inspection, but in even the mildest cases of OI, densitometry studies show at least a 25% decrease in mineralization. The bone cortices are usually thin, and trabecular patterns are not well developed. The long bones may be thin and bowed. The pelvis may show acetabular protrusion. The vertebrae may be biconcave.

3. What is the cause of osteogenesis imperfecta?

OI has been identified as a defect in type I collagen. Type I is the collagen that makes up most of the organic scaffolding for bone. It is a triple helix, composed of two alpha-I chains and one alpha-II chain. Glycine, the smallest amino acid, composes every third amino acid and is critical to the coiling of the collagen chains. Mutations of various amino acids result in OI of varying degrees of severity, depending on how much collagen exists and how functional it is. Since glycine is so crucial to the structure of collagen, mutations involving glycine substitution often produce severe forms of osteogenesis imperfecta. Other mutations have been found, however. Since type I collagen also plays a role in other components of connective tissue, such as ligament and tendon, it is not surprising that patients with OI have ligamentous laxity as well. Type I collagen is also a constituent of dentin and sclerae, thus explaining involvement of these tissues in some patients with OI.

4. Is there a test for osteogenesis imperfecta?

Genetic analysis of collagen from dermal fibroblasts will many times identify an abnormality in type I collagen. There are many false negatives with this test, however. It is not routinely recommended, especially since clinical exam is diagnostic in many cases.

5. How are the various forms classified?

There are many different classification systems. The most commonly used is that of Sillence, which includes four types.

Type I: mild OI, blue sclerae, normal teeth, autosomal dominant
Type II: perinatal lethal OI; rarely survive infancy
Type III: severe, progressively deforming OI; dentinogenesis imperfecta; neonatal fractures
Type IV: moderately severe OI; sclerae fade from blue to white

6. What is the differential diagnosis?

Nonaccidental injury, or child abuse, is the most important thing to rule out. Also note that juvenile osteoporosis may present with spontaneous or pathologic fractures but is usually a transient, self-limited disorder. Fibrous dysplasia may exhibit bone deformities and fractures, but the bones are not as tapered and thin as in OI, and many of the bones in an affected patient are totally free of the disease. Metabolic disorders may occasionally present with pathologic fractures. On in utero ultrasonography, the reduced size and limb flexion of camptomelic dysplasia may resemble OI.

7. How is child abuse distinguished from OI?

Usually on clinical grounds; rarely by skin biopsy. Clinically, a witnessed injury caused by low force and the presence of abnormalities of the teeth, sclera, or hearing may suggest OI. A skeletal survey should be done, looking for thin gracile diaphyses, "wormian" (inclusion) bones in the cranial sutures, acetabular protrusion, or multiple vertebral compressions (codfish vertebrae). The pattern of fracture is not diagnostic, unfortunately. In some cases, a fibroblast biopsy may be helpful if positive. A negative test, however, does not rule out OI.

8. What are the gross and histologic characteristics of bone in OI?

In general, the bone in OI is coarse in external texture. It is not cylindrical in shape like normal bone but is flattened or irregular in cross section. It often has a crumbling, pumice-like texture. The cortices are thin. The medullary cavity may be flattened or obliterated, which explains the difficulty with rod stabilization. Histologically, the trabecular network is often random and poorly developed.

The bone is highly cellular. The trabeculae have been compared to Chinese letters. The bone is mostly woven in nature with little lamellar bone, especially in the more severe varieties of OI.

9. What is the natural history?

In type II of Sillence, most die in early infancy. Most patients with other types live indefinitely. Intelligence is not affected, and most patients are quite resourceful. The use of powered personal transportation has greatly increased mobility. Most patients are employed and independent. Medical problems that may cut short the life span of a person with OI include restrictive lung disease as well as brain stem compression or basilar invagination.

10. Is there a medical treatment for OI?

Many different agents have been attempted, but none is widely accepted. Calcium and phosphorus intake has no beneficial effect. Growth hormone and calcitonin have been shown to increase bone mineral density. Bisphosphonates have been suggested in clinical trials to have a protective effect, but research is still ongoing. Bone marrow transplant is being tried by a few early investigators for the most severe cases in young infants. In the long run, an effective medical treatment seems likely. In the short term, the best advice is to think preventively and eat a regular diet.

11. What are the main orthopaedic sequelae?

Bowing of the long bones due to fractures and microfractures, scoliosis, basilar invagination, spondylolisthesis, protrusion acetabula, and degenerative joint disease. Ligamentous laxity exists but rarely causes problems owing to the limited activity of the patients. Limb-length inequality may develop owing to symmetric fractures.

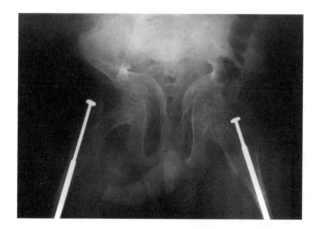

Severe protrusion acetabula in 10-year-old with type III OI. Limitation of motion and constipation were the results.

12. Does orthotic treatment play a role in the management of OI?

Braces for the lower extremities may help young patients to stand before they are able to do so on their own. Lightweight hip-knee-ankle-foot braces or pneumatic trousers may prevent fractures in patients who are at risk but who have not had rod stabilization. Ankle-foot orthoses may help those with unstable or valgus ankles. Bracing for scoliosis or basilar invagination has a small but definite role.

13. Is bone healing in OI delayed or normal?

Bone healing is usually biologically normal. It may be disturbed by mechanical factors, however, such as severe bowing at the site of fracture, which leads to tension in the callus. In one survey, more than 20% had at least one nonunion. Therefore, the fractures in these patients should be treated by immobilization, even though they are low-energy injuries.

14. What are the indications for straightening and rodding the long bones?

In the late 1950s, Sofield described his technique of correcting the bowing of OI with multiple osteotomies and intramedullary rod fixation. He divided the bowed segment of the bone into multiple straight smaller segments and realigned them over the rod. An improvement was introduced in 1963 when Bailey and Dubow developed a telescoping pair of rods that could be anchored in each epiphysis of a long bone and would then expand with growth.

This may be indicated in patients with severe diaphyseal bowing that prevents standing. Usually, this involves anterolateral bowing of the femur and anterior bowing of the tibia. Another indication is the occurrence of multiple fractures in a given region, which the rods can help markedly reduce. The technique may also be used effectively in the upper extremities, with rods inserted in the humerus or the ulna.

A prerequisite for this procedure is a reasonable size of the bones and the presence of at least a visible cortex, which some patients do not have. Care should be taken to use multiple hook-fixation points. The curve should not be corrected excessively, or else hooks will cut through bone and all will be lost. Special care should be taken not to correct much kyphosis if the patient has this. Some authors have recommended the use of methyl methacrylate to reinforce the hook purchase sites. The rods should be slightly flexible to allow assembly without undue stress on the hooks. The surgeon should prepare for more bleeding than is seen in idiopathic scoliosis. Mean long-term correction is only about 20%, but the important goal is to prevent or minimize progression.

15. What is basilar invagination?

Basilar invagination or impression is the settling of the cranium upon the cervical spine, producing an infolding of the base of the skull with pressure on the neurologic structures in this region. It occurs owing to mechanical forces, with the deformable bone of OI unable to withstand the increasing weight of the head. Compressive structures include the ring of the atlas, the clivus, and the odontoid process (see Figure). Basilar invagination is present if the tip of the odontoid extends more than 7 mm above MacGregor's line (drawn from the hard palate poste-

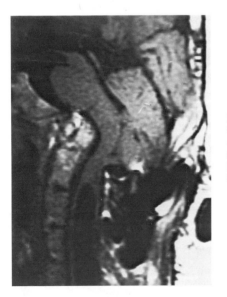

Basilar invagination in a 25-year-old male with type IV OI. Note compression from both anterior and posterior edges of the foramen magnum. Anteriorly, the compression is due to the clivus, atlas, and dens. Note also the hydrosyringomyelia of the cervical spinal cord. The patient had spasticity, weakness, and apneic spells.

riorly to the lowest point on the occiput). It is present radiographically in up to one quarter of patients with OI. Surprisingly, it is most common in the mild type IV B. Symptoms may include cranial nerve palsies, headaches, respiratory depression, spasticity, nystagmus, or weakness. It may be responsible for some of the early mortality seen in young adults with OI.

16. How is basilar invagination treated?
There is no completely satisfactory treatment for this condition. Conservative treatment has been reported, with full-time use of a brace (sterno-mandibular-occipital variety) followed by partial relief of symptoms. Surgical therapy is also an option. For very mild early cases of symptomatic basilar invagination, if the compression is not significant anteriorly, posterior decompression and fusion in situ with posterior instrumentation may possibly be effective in preventing future subsidence, if an abundant base of support is constructed posteriorly.

If significant bony compression anteriorly is seen, anterior transoral decompression must be considered. This is done as a combined effort by a neurosurgeon, an otolaryngologist, and an orthopaedic surgeon. The tongue, mandible, and maxilla may be divided for exposure, and resections performed of the clivus, anterior atlas, and odontoid. Then posterior fusion with plate fixation is performed from the occiput to the upper or middle cervical spine. Posterior decompression may be needed as a well.

17. Are other neurologic problems common in OI?
Hydrosyringomyelia and communicating hydrocephalus are seen in a significant minority of patients. Macrocephaly is common. Seizures are more common than in the general population.

18. Why is there increased incidence of constipation in OI?
In some patients with bilateral severe protrusion acetabula, the pelvic outlet may be critically narrowed such that mechanical difficulty with bowel movements occurs. Symptoms may include vague chronic abdominal pain. Use of a bowel program to soften the stools and promote regular elimination usually leads to relief of symptoms.

19. How does one handle chronic pain?
Chronic pain is seen with increasing frequency as age increases. The cause is multifactorial. Treatable orthopaedic causes should be ruled out, such as stress fractures and degenerative joint disease. If none can be found, safe physical modalities may be helpful. Antidepressants may be needed. Referral to a multidisciplinary pain clinic is justified, where a combination of behavioral therapy, counseling, and long-acting analgesics may be worked out.

BIBLIOGRAPHY

1. Cole WG: Etiology and pathogenesis of heritable connective tissue diseases. J Pediatr Orthop 13:392–403, 1993.
2. Gamble JG, Rinsky LA, Strudwick J, Bleck EE: Non-union of fractures in children who have osteogenesis imperfecta. J Bone Joint Surg 70A:439–443, 1988.
3. Harkey HL, Crockard HA, Stevens JM, Smith R, Ransford AO: The operative management of basilar impression in osteogenesis imperfecta. Neurosurgery 27(5):782–786, 1990.
4. Lee JH, Gamble JG, Moore RE, Rinsky LA: Gastrointestinal problems in patients who have type III osteogenesis imperfecta. J Bone Joint Surg 77A:1352–1356, 1995.
5. Elongating intramedullary rods in the treatment of osteogenesis imperfecta. J Bone Joint Surg 59A:467–472, 1977.
6. Moorefield WG, Miller GR: Aftermath of osteogenesis imperfecta: the disease in adulthood. J Bone Joint Surg 62A:113–119, 1980.
7. Ring D, Jupiter JB, Labropoulos PK, Guggenheim, JJ, Stanitsky DF, Spencer DM: The treatment of deformity of the lower limb in adults who have osteogenesis imperfecta. J Bone Joint Surg 78A, 220–225, 1996.
8. Stott NS, Zionts LE: Displaced fractures of the apophysis of the olecranon in children who have osteogenesis imperfecta. J Bone Joint Surg 75A:1026–1103, 1993.

96. RICKETS AND METABOLIC DISORDERS

James Aronson, M.D., and Elizabeth A. Tursky, R.N.P., B.S.N.

1. What is metabolic bone disease?

Impairment in the shape, strength, and composition of bone due to altered bone mineral homeostasis. The major factors affecting this homeostasis can be thought of as the **"three 3s"**: intra- and extracellular levels of **three ions** (calcium, phosphorus, and magnesium), which are regulated by **three hormones** (parathyroid hormone, calcitonin, and 1,25-dihydroxyvitamin D) and act upon **three tissues** (bone, intestine, and kidney). Of course, other minerals, hormones, and target tissues are involved as well, making this disease category a complex interaction of many exogenous and endogenous factors, calling for a team approach in coordinating care. Frequent clinical features include electrolyte disturbances, fractures, bone deformity, abnormal gait, and short stature.

2. What are common forms of metabolic bone disease in children?

The most commonly encountered forms of metabolic bone disease in children are the various types of rickets and renal osteodystrophy. Nutritional rickets, the historical counterpart, is much less commonly seen today owing to improved diets and supplementation of foods with calcium and vitamin D, but it can occur in socially depressed areas such as inner cities. Other less common but important pediatric metabolic conditions include osteoporosis and hypophosphatasia.

3. What is the pathophysiology of the bone disease in these metabolic disorders?

Although there are multiple types of **rickets,** the basic pathogenesis is a relative decrease in calcium, phosphorus, or both, of large enough magnitude that it interferes with physeal growth and normal mineralization of the skeleton of the growing child. This decrease in calcium or phosphorus may be due to inadequate intake or impaired absorption of phosphorus or vitamin D, decreased conversion of vitamin D to its active form, end-organ insensitivity, impaired release of calcium from bone, or phosphate wasting. In addition, there is evidence that insufficient vitamin D may interfere with mineralization independent of calcium and phosphate levels.

In **renal osteodystrophy,** glomerular damage leads to phosphate retention, and tubular injury causes decreased production of the active form of vitamin D (1,25-dihydroxyvitamin D). These two factors severely inhibit the gut's ability to absorb calcium. The resultant hypocalcemia triggers secondary hyperparathyroidism, which remains ineffective in increasing intestinal absorption of calcium. Therefore, the body's only means of increasing serum calcium levels is by bone resorption.

In patients with **osteoporosis,** the bone is made normally but reduced in overall amount. In children, osteoporosis may be idiopathic, as in juvenile osteoporosis, or due to disuse or chronic corticosteroid administration. The pathophysiology of idiopathic juvenile osteoporosis is unclear, but various theories include increased bone resorption versus decreased bone formation (possibly due to deficient 1,25-dihydroxyvitamin D or calcitonin or due to a fundamental disturbance in the transduction of mechanical forces that stimulate new bone formation). In disuse osteoporosis, the lack of stress across bone results in a net decrease in bone mass. The precise link between mechanical force and cell physiology is not clear, however, Glucocorticoids decrease bone mass through suppression of osteoblast function as well as decreased intestinal absorption of calcium, resulting in increased PTH secretion and enhanced osteoclast activity.

Hypophosphatasia results from a genetic error in the synthesis of alkaline phosphatase, an enzyme necessary for the maturation of the primary spongiosa in the physes. This results in normal production of bone (osteoid) but inadequate mineralization, with resultant skeletal deformities that mimic rickets.

4. How much do I have to know about calcium, vitamin D, and phosphorus metabolism to be able to manage effectively the orthopaedic needs of these patients?

Just the basics. Healthy bone requires constant calcium and phosphorus concentrations within the serum. These concentrations are normally maintained in a steady state through an elaborate system involving the kidney, gut, and skeleton. Low levels of calcium stimulate the release of parathyroid hormone (PTH), which stimulates the synthesis of the active form of vitamin D. Together, these two hormones act to increase intestinal absorption, renal tubule reabsorption, and bone resorption of calcium with a resultant increase in serum levels. Activated vitamin D is a necessity in facilitating calcium transportation across the gut. PTH also works independently to stimulate osteoclasts to resorb bone. The net effects on the skeleton are decreased mineralization, decreased amount of bone, and altered structure and integrity of bone. Calcitonin works in the opposite way to decrease serum calcium concentrations.

Normal serum calcium and phosphorus levels are required to maintain bone homeostasis. Hypocalcemia will result (and potentially cause metabolic bone disease) if there are abnormalities in any of the following.

Calcium: Inadequate dietary intake, insufficient intestinal absorption (due to either deficient activated vitamin D or PTH or, in cases of steatorrhea where calcium binds with free fatty acids, formation of an insoluble compound that cannot be absorbed), or reduced renal reabsorption.

Vitamin D: Lack of sufficient amounts of the activated form. This deficiency can occur owing to insufficient dietary intake (nutritional rickets), decreased intestinal absorption (as with steatorrhea, since vitamin D is fat soluble, or in certain genetic forms of rickets where the end-organ gut cell is insensitive to vitamin D) or insufficient conversion of vitamin D to its active form owing to lack of ultraviolet light exposure, hepatic disease, or especially renal tubule dysfunction, since the sequential and essential sites of conversion are the skin, the liver, and the kidney. The ingested provitamin ergosterols are stored in the skin and, in the presence of ultraviolet light, are converted to ergocalciferol (vitamin D_2) and cholecalciferol (vitamin D_3). After transportation to the liver, they are converted to 25-hydroxyvitamin D. The final and most critical conversion occurs in the kidney, where 25-hydroxyvitamin D is converted to either the less active 24,25-hydroxyvitamin D or the highly active 1,25 hydroxy form.

Phosphorus: Hyperphosphatemia, which occurs in renal osteodystrophy due to glomerular damage, "turns off" the system that actively transports calcium out of the gut into the extracellular space, resulting in inability to absorb calcium from the intestinal tract. It also shunts renal conversion of 25-hydroxyvitamin D into the less active 24,25-hydroxy form. Conversely, hypophosphatemia, which occurs in several forms of rickets, also causes skeletal abnormalities, since adequate phosphorus is required for normal mineralization.

5. What is the difference between rickets, osteomalacia, and renal osteodystrophy?

Anatomically, **rickets** and **osteomalacia** are both characterized by the presence of excessive amounts of unmineralized osteoid, resulting in skeletal deformity. **Rickets** occurs only in the growing skeleton, however, and is further characterized by deficient mineralization and excess cartilage accumulation in the growth plates at the site of enchondral bone formation. **Osteomalacia** is the adult counterpart of rickets, occurring only after the physes have closed. It lacks the growth abnormalities.

Osteodystrophy is a syndrome of four pathologic entities that occur in response to the profound hypocalcemia of renal disease: (1) rickets or osteomalacia, with deficient mineralization of osteoid; (2) osteitis fibrosa cystica, a condition associated with severe lytic changes in the skeleton due to overproduction of PTH; (3) osteosclerosis, which occurs in about 20% of patients with osteodystrophy (especially in the spine and occasionally the long bones), owing to increased numbers of bony trabeculae rather than increased mineralization; and (4) ectopic calcification or mineralization, which occurs owing to precipitation of calcium salts (in the corneas, conjunctivae, skin, arteriolar walls, and periarticular soft tissues) if calcium levels increase to normal with dietary indiscretion, spontaneous improvement, or dialysis.

6. Are X-linked (hypophosphatemic) and vitamin D-resistant rickets the same thing?

This is a trick question. First, hypophosphatemia is a common denominator in many forms of rickets. Second, although "X-linked" and "vitamin D-resistant" are terms often used interchangeably to describe a relatively common inherited form of rickets, there are multiple other types of vitamin D-resistant rickets. This common form of vitamin D-resistant rickets has also been called refractory rickets, familial hypophosphatemia, familial vitamin D-resistant rickets, and phosphate diabetes. It is caused by a genetic (X-linked dominant) error in phosphate transport, probably located in the proximal nephron, although there is increasingly strong evidence that the defective tubular reabsorption of phosphate in this disease is not intrinsic to the kidney but is instead due to an unidentified circulating humoral agent. It is fully expressed in hemizygous male patients. Isolated hypophosphatemia may signify the presence of the trait in heterozygous females. With full expression, the condition consists of hypophosphatemia, lower limb deformities, and stunted growth. Although the hypophosphatemia is present shortly after birth, the skeletal deformities and short stature really do not become evident until the child begins walking and the deformities progress beyond the physiologic range.

7. How does the nonorthopaedic management vary among the different types of rickets?
The mainstay of medical management is replacement of phosphate, although some forms respond to administration of vitamin D, most commonly in the form of calcitriol (1,25-dihydroxyvitamin D_3).

8. What are the clinical features of rickets?
>   **General:** Irritability or apathy; short stature, often under the third percentile; muscle weakness.
>   **Skull:** Frontal bossing and enlargement of the suture lines.
>   **Dental anomalies:** Delayed dentition, enamel defects, and extensive caries.
>   **Trunk:** Enlargement of the costal cartilages ("rachitic rosary"), long thoracic kyphosis (rachitic "catback" deformity), protuberant abdomen.
>   **Extremities:** Ligamentous laxity; long-bone deformities, including bowing and shortening; apparent enlargement of the elbows, wrists, knees, and ankles. A general guideline is that if the disease manifests during the stage of physiologic bowing (ages 1–2), the result will be varus, while active disease during the stage of physiologic genu valgus (ages 2–4) produces valgus.

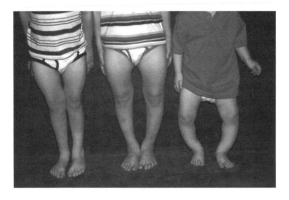

Three brothers with vitamin D-resistant hypophosphatemic rickets demonstrating typical skeletal deformities. Note the valgus deformity in the oldest child and varus in the youngest boy. The two older children have previously undergone osteotomy for severe deformity.

9. What other conditions should be considered in the differential diagnosis of rickets?
Physiologic genu varus or valgus; Blount disease; metaphyseal, epiphyseal, or other skeletal dysplasias; achondroplasia or hypochondroplasia; fibrous dysplasia; enchondromatosis.

10. What should be asked in the history?
>   **Past medical:** Renal or hepatic abnormalities, use of anticonvulsants, growth and development, previous fractures, reduced sunlight exposure.
>   **Dietary:** Malabsorption syndromes, milk allergy, or other reason for reduced dietary intake of calcium.

Family: Short stature, lower limb deformities, frequent fractures, or bone dysplasias.
Dental: Delayed eruption or excessive caries.

11. What imaging studies are useful?

Plain radiographs are the most useful, with classic findings seen in florid rickets. In milder forms of rickets, x-ray findings may be subtle. A bone scan may be useful in these cases to delineate increased activity over the shafts of long bones, ribs, and skull, and especially at the sites of fracture.

12. What findings can be seen on the plain radiographs?

General findings include osteopenia, thin cortices, and small trabeculae with overall decreased bone mass. The osteopenia is more marked in the metaphyses, contributing to a "washed-out" appearance. The cortices, vertebral end plates, and trabeculae often appear fuzzy and indistinct. Classic findings, most often seen with florid rickets, include irregular widening or cupping of the physes (see Figure). Looser's lines (also known as Milkman's pseudofractures) are ribbonlike radiolucencies extending transversely from one cortex across the medullary canal. They represent areas of weakening or incomplete fracture and are pathognomonic for rickets and osteomalacia. The most common sites include the concave side of long bones, especially the femoral neck, ischial and pubic rami, ribs, clavicles, and axillary borders of the scapulae.

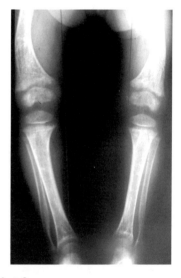

Classic radiographs appearance of the lower extremities in rickets. Note the widened physes, cupped metaphyses, and diaphyseal bowing.

13. What laboratory tests can be useful to screen for rickets?

The main tests are serum calcium, phosphate, and alkaline phosphatase levels. Other helpful laboratory tests include serum 25-hydroxyvitamin D (which is low in vitamin D-deficient rickets) and parathyroid hormone levels. In infancy, abnormal lab values may be the only findings in a child with rickets. In vitamin D-resistant (hypophosphatemic) rickets, abnormal laboratory findings include normal or slightly low serum calcium, low serum phosphate, low serum alkaline phosphatase, and elevated urine phosphate levels. Administration of vitamin D does not produce a response in these individuals.

14. When is orthopaedic treatment (bracing or surgery) indicated?

In the presence of fracture or when deformity exceeds the physiologic range and predisposes the individual to progressive deformity, altered mechanical alignment, or degenerative joint disease. With advances in medical management of this condition, orthopaedic intervention in the form of bracing or surgery is much less commonly needed.

15. If surgery is needed, what can I expect regarding bony healing in patients with rickets?
With adequate medical management, bony healing occurs, although some studies have found it to be delayed. After surgery, these patients should be watched carefully, since the prolonged immobilization due to hospitalization or casting may lead to hypercalcemia.

16. After orthopaedic treatment of rachitic deformities, what can I tell the parents about prognosis and risk of recurrence?
With all forms of rickets, the likelihood of recurrence is increased in cases of inadequate medical control. Compliance must be stressed, since lapses in the medication regimen will result in recurrent rickets and skeletal deformities. With X-linked hypophosphatemic rickets, recurrent deformity and short stature are more common despite adequate medical management and may necessitate reosteotomy or growth hormone therapy. Continued medical mangement (phosphate and vitamin D replacement) after physeal closure is controversial, since rachitic deformities of the skeleton do not tend to occur in adulthood and continued treatment carries a risk of nephrocalcinosis. Proponents of phosphate and vitamin D replacement in adult patients with rickets believe that it may reduce the risk of bone pain, stress fractures, osteoarthritis, and dental abscesses.

17. What are some radiographic findings in renal osteodystrophy that differentiate it from rickets and osteomalacia?
  • Changes due to osteitis fibrosa cystica are unique to renal osteodystrophy and include "salt-and-pepper" skull, absence of the cortical outline of the outer centimeter of the clavicles, and subperiosteal resorption of the ulnas, terminal tufts of the distal phalanges, and medial proximal tibias.
  • Brown tumors appear as expanded destructive lesions and are usually round or ovoid with indistinct margins. They are due to secondary hyperparathyroidism and are most common in cases of severe and long-standing renal osteodystrophy. Brown tumors may be present in the long bones or pelvis and, when associated with thinning or expansion of the cortex, may be the site of pathologic fractures. These lesions sometimes resemble primary or metastatic bone tumors.
  • Slipped epiphyses.

18. What are the most common sites of epiphyseal slipping in renal osteodystrophy?
The proximal femur is by far the most common site. Other reported sites include the proximal humerus, distal femur, and distal tibia. Slippage of the distal radial and ulnar epiphyses occurs almost exclusively in older (prepubertal and adolescent) children and may lead to ulnar deviation of the wrists.

19. What is the cause of the epiphyseal slipping in this disease?
It is due to profound hyperparathyroidism, which results in resorption of metaphyseal bone. This weakening of the metaphyseal area in combination with the chronic nature of the disease results in epiphyseolysis. Studies have shown that the risk of slippage is increased during periods of rapid growth or in cases of untreated renal disease and severe hyperparathyroidism. Treated renal disease with more normal parathyroid levels does not cause epiphyseal slippage.

20. What are the clinical features of idiopathic juvenile osteoporosis?
Bone and joint pain in previously healthy children, with onset usually between the ages of 8 and 14. Later symptoms include growth arrest, osteopenia of varying severity, collapse of the vertebral bodies, and metaphyseal fractures. The condition may be limited to the spine or may also involve the long bones, with bone loss more marked in the metaphyses than the diaphyses.

21. What differential diagnoses should be considered before making the diagnosis of idiopathic juvenile osteoporosis?
Because this is a rare disorder and a diagnosis of exclusion, other conditions resulting in osteopenia and bone fragility must be ruled out. These include osteogenesis imperfecta, hemato-

logic malignancies, thyroid disorders, Cushing's disease, steroid-induced osteopenia, and disuse osteopenia. Rapid progression after many years of normality differentiates idiopathic osteoporosis from osteogenesis imperfecta.

22. What studies are useful in evaluating idiopathic juvenile osteoporosis?
Laboratory and histomorphometric studies are difficult to interpret and not very helpful in evaluating this condition. Radiographs demonstrate decreased bone mass (osteopenia), especially in the metaphyseal regions; quantitative computed tomography and dual-photon densitometry can help measure decreases in bone density, but age-appropriate controls are limited.

23. What is the natural history of idiopathic juvenile osteoporosis?
This is a self-limited disorder that tends to resolve spontaneously within 2–4 years or after puberty. The completeness of the resolution depends on the age of onset and is related to the amount of growth potential remaining after the process stops. It has been difficult to demonstrate the efficacy of any treatment regimen in altering the natural history of this disease. Prolonged disuse or immobilization can worsen the osteoporosis and clinical symptoms, however.

24. Which anticonvulsants cause osteomalacia, rickets, and calcium metabolism disturbances?
Primarily phenytoin. Carbamazepine alone does not seem to cause significant osteomalacia or calcium metabolism disturbances, but when used in conjunction with valproate or phenytoin, it may enhance their adverse effects. Data are conflicting regarding valproate, with some studies showing no effect on the skeleton and others demonstrating clear decreases in bone density with valproate therapy. Phenobarbital does not affect hepatic metabolism of vitamin D but has been shown in some studies to reduce bone density; other studies have shown that overall plasma levels are not reduced and the skeleton is not affected. Clinically significant effects on bone due to anticonvulsants are very rare in noninstitutionalized, normally active patients.

25. How are the orthopaedic problems associated with anticonvulsants managed?
Although the exact pathogenesis of the osteomalacia or rickets varies with different drugs, most anticonvulsants appear to increase the daily vitamin D requirement. The orthopaedic manifestations of this increased requirement are more severe in patients with already reduced vitamin D levels (such as in institutionalized patients with reduced sunlight exposure or dietary supply) or in those with concomitant disuse osteopenia. Treatment is aimed at prevention of orthopaedic problems and includes ensuring adequate sunlight exposure and normal dietary intake of vitamin D, avoidance of disuse osteopenia through weightbearing activites, and, when possible, switching to an anticonvulsant with fewer skeletal manifestations. Administration of additional vitamin D may improve biochemical abnormalities in calcium metabolism but has not been shown to reverse cortical bone loss. The use of prophylactic vitamin D in patients receiving anticonvulsants remains controversial.

26. Which endocrine problems commonly cause orthopaedic manifestations in the pediatric population?

HORMONE	EXCESS OR DEFICIENCY	ORTHOPAEDIC MANIFESTATIONS IN CHILDHOOD
Parathyroid	Excess	Increased osteoclast activity with bone resorption and skeletal pain
	Deficiency	Increased bone density and soft tissue calcification; main clinical symptoms are systemic due to hypocalcemia
Thyroid	Deficiency	Delayed bone age and growth retardation, late appearance of the secondary ossification centers with occasional stippling, slipped capital femoral epiphyses
Androgens	Excess	Precocious puberty with initial accelerated growth but early growth plate closure and ultimate short stature
	Deficiency	Initial delayed bone age but late physeal closure and final height above average

(Continued on following page)

HORMONE	EXCESS OR DEFICIENCY	ORTHOPAEDIC MANIFESTATIONS IN CHILDHOOD
Estrogen	Excess	Enhanced epiphyseal maturation with reduced cell proliferation, resulting in short stature
	Deficiency	Increased bone resorption and osteoporosis
Glucocorticoids	Excess	Suppression of growth hormone synthesis with short stature, profound and irreversible osteopenia with possible vertebral and other compression fractures, osteonecrosis of the secondary ossification centers

ACKNOWLEDGMENT

The authors wish to thank A. Michael Parfitt, M.D., for his expert advice in the preparation of this chapter.

BIBLIOGRAPHY

1. Apel DM, Millar EA, Moel DI: Skeletal disorders in pediatric renal transplant population. J Pediatr Orthop 9:505, 1989.
2. Chung S, Ahn C: Effects of anti-epileptic drug therapy on bone mineral density in ambulatory epileptic children. Brain Dev 16(5):382, 1994.
3. Favus MJ (ed): Primer on the Metabolic Bone Diseases and Disorders of Mineral Metabolism, 2nd ed. New York, Raven Press, 1993.
4. Gough H, Goggin T, Bissessar M, Baker M, Crowley M, Callaghan N: A comparative study of the relative influence of different anticonvulsant drugs, UV exposure and diet on vitamin D and calcium metabolism in out-patients with epilepsy. Q J Med 59(230):569, 1986.
5. Latta K, Hisano S, Chan JCM: Therapeutics of X-linked hypophosphatemic rickets. Pediatr Nephrol 7:744, 1993.
6. Mankin HJ: Rickets, osteomalacia and renal osteodystrophy. An update. Orthop Clin North Am 21(1):81, 1990.
7. Sheth RD, Wesolowski CA, Jacob JC, Penney S, Hobbs GR, Riggs JE, Bodensteiner JB: Effect of carbamazepine and valproate on bone mineral density. Pediatrics 127(2):256, 1995.
8. Stanitski DF: Treatment of deformity secondary to metabolic bone disease with the Ilizarov technique. Clin Orthop 301:38, 1994.
9. Zaleske DJ, Doppelt SH, Mankin HJ: Metabolic and endocrine abnormalities of the immature skeleton. In Morrissey RT (ed): Lovell and Winter's Pediatric Orthopaedics, 3rd ed. Philadelphia, J.B. Lippincott Co., 1990, pp 203–261.

97. HEMATOLOGIC DISORDERS

David Keret, M.D., and Shlomo Wientroub, M.D.

HEMOPHILIA

1. What is the genetic picture of hemophilia and which musculoskeletal problems are associated with it?

A sex-linked (expressed mainly in males) recessive gene located on the X chromosome causes this disease. Hemophilia occurs in 1 in 10,000 of the population. The characteristic musculoskeletal manifestations in hemophilia are most common in patients with deficits of either factor VIII (classic hemophilia or hemophilia A) or factor IX (Christmas disease or hemophilia B). Partial thromboplastin time (PTT) and specific factor assays are the definitive diagnostic laboratory studies. The blood level of the factors VIII and IX (or their percent activity of the normal) is divided according to the severity of the clinical manifestations: 50–200% = within the normal limits, 25–50% =

essentially normal, 5–25% = mild form, 1–5% activity = moderate and <1% of normal factor level = severe hemophilia. In the severe deficits spontaneous bleeding into joints or tissues may occur; in the moderate form the bleeding usually follows minor trauma and patients with mild factor deficiency will rarely develop hemarthrosis after major trauma or surgical interventions.

2. What is the advantage of MRI in choosing treatment?
MRI presents details of soft tissue and articular cartilage better than plain radiographs. It is also helpful in decision-making regarding surgical synovectomy.

3. Which are the commonly affected skeletal sites in hemophiliacs and how is this related to the patient's age?
The knee, ankle, and elbow. In small children, the ankle is the most commonly affected because of the relatively greater amount of jumping. The knee is most commonly affected after the age of 5 years. Of great concern are the deep soft tissue hemorrhages occurring particularly in the calf, thigh, iliopsoas muscle, and upper extremities.

4. What are the physical findings of minor hemarthrosis?
Swollen and warm joints. In the older child, pain or discomfort can precede the swelling.

5. What are the modes of treatment in major hemarthrosis? Which is the most crucial one?
Major hemarthrosis is the result of major trauma or recurrent bleeding into a joint already affected with synovitis. The treatment of painful minor intra-articular hemorrhage begins with early aspiration at the same time as or shortly after factor transfusion. This is followed by short-term compression dressing and splinting in the most comfortable position, rehabilitation exercises (with splints in between), and continuous concentrate transfusions to reduce the risk of synovitis. The most crucial therapeutic measure is the evacuation of the intra-articular massive bleeding by aspiration. It usually prevents a possible synovitis and recurrent hemarthrosis. The decompressing aspiration of the joint leads to dramatic relief of pain. It also reduces the chances of infection by removing the clot or blood that may serve as a medium for bacterial growth. The treatment for hemarthrosis in advanced arthropathy is limited to concentrate transfusions in all painful episodes, splinting, and nonsteroid anti-inflammatory agents.

6. What about prophylactic transfusions for hemophiliacs?
Prophylactic transfusion is indicated during recovery from major hemarthrosis. The concentrates are transfused every 48 hours until the factor exceeds a level of more than 1%. This level is sufficient to prevent a possible hemorrhage from minor trauma. The prophylactic treatment is usually given 14 days following a major bleeding episode. This period of time enables absorption of the excessive intraarticular iron by the chondrocytes and synoviocytes, thereby preventing synovitis.

7. What are the clinical features and treatment choice in hemophilic synovitis?
In hemophilic synovitis, the joint is swollen and is usually *not* painful or restricted in its range of motion unless there had been a recent hemarthrosis. Prophylactic concentrate transfusions prevent a possible hemarthrosis and a consequent synovitis, and refrain from weight bearing and steroids for 1 week. The joint is protected in orthosis and muscle strengthening is advised.

8. Is synovectomy an option in hemophiliacs?
Synovectomy reduces the incidence of chronic or recurrent hemarthrosis. Its use is controversial in hemophiliacs because of an uncertain influence on the progression of the arthropathy and it is undecided whether to use arthroscopic synovectomy, an open synovectomy, or medical synovectomy. The use of continuous passive motion (CPM) post arthroscopic synovectomy has improved the results, but arthroscopy is demanding, it lacks hemostasis, and it is usually not possible to perform a total synovectomy. The open technique is less traumatic and more comprehensive. Medical synovectomy is less effective than surgical synovectomy.

9. How is elbow synovectomy performed in children and adolescents?

While elbow synovectomy usually includes radial head excision in older adolescents and adults, this is contraindicated in children for whom arthroscopic synovectomy is the treatment of choice.

10. What is the outcome following ankle synovectomy?

The rate of recurrent hemarthrosis is reduced from 3.4 per month to 0.1 per month. The range of motion is also improved by an average of more than 10°.

11. What are the advantages and disadvantages of radioactive synovectomy?

Radioactive synovectomy is the only option in patients with factor VIII inhibitors. Its advantages include low cost, the use of out-patient facilities, and only short-term transfusion of the expensive concentrates. The disadvantages include possible chromosomal changes, toxic effect on the articular surface, and a higher rate of recurrent hemarthrosis than that following surgical synovectomy.

12. What are the clinical features and sites of muscle hemorrhages in hemophiliacs?

Muscle hemorrhages are common in severely affected hemophiliacs and are usually the result of minor trauma or occur spontaneously. They occur mainly in the calf, forearm, iliopsoas, and quadriceps. Bleeding is characteristically deep and within the body of the muscle. Presenting symptoms can range from vague pain on motion to pain at rest. The significant hemorrhages into the compartments may result in fibrosis, contractures of muscles and stiffness of the joints across which the muscles act. To prevent compartment syndrome and contractures, treatment is primarily nonsurgical and includes ice packs, elevation, compression, dressings, and splints.

13. What are the treatment modalities for compartment syndrome post muscle bleedings in hemophiliacs with or without inhibitors?

General treatment includes appropriate replacement treatment and physical therapy to restore the normal range of motion and avoid fibrosis of the muscles. In patients with compartment syndrome and no inhibitors, the factor must be first raised to 100% and then an appropriate surgical procedure such as fasciotomy is carried out. (It is highly recommended that this be done within 24 hours). In patients with high titer inhibitors, treatment consisting of alternative transfusions must be initiated as early as possible.

14. What is the treatment for equinus contracture following hemorrhage into the gastrocnemius soleus muscle?

Hemorrhage into the calf muscles can result in an equinus deformity. Aggressive treatment with serial casting and splinting is recommended as soon as possible after a single factor replacement transfusion. The ankle joint is held in a cast in a maximum dorsiflexion position. Surgery may be indicated in resistant deformity.

15. How are iliopsoas hemorrhage and hemarthrosis of the hip joint differentiated?

A patient with an iliopsoas hemorrhage presents with vague symptoms of lower abdominal pains or upper thigh discomfort. The hip is flexed and externally rotated. The hip cannot be extended on examination because of pain, but internal and external rotation of the hip joint are normal. In hemarthrosis of the hip joint, the rotational movements are painful and limited.

16. What is a common complication of iliacus hemorrhage and how it is treated?

Distension of a hemorrhage of the iliacus muscle distally underneath the inguinal ligament may compress the femoral nerve. This can progress to complete femoral neuropathy in 60% of iliacus bleeding. The treatment of choice is bed rest and analgesics, physical therapy to avoid hip flexion contracture, and continuous factor replacement to the level of at least 50% for 7–14 days.

17. What is a significant complication of knee flexion contracture and what is the best way to treat it?

Severe and long-lasting knee contracture can result in posterior subluxation of the tibia. In such patients (mainly in those with inhibitors), traction and casting are aimed at reducing the knee flexion contracture to 5–10° at most. The correction is maintained with long-term bracing and physiotherapy.

18. What is the pathophysiology of hemophilic cyst (pseudotumor) and how is it recognized radiologically?

Hemophiliac cyst may arise from either intramuscular, intraperiosteal, or intraosseous bleeding. A pseudocapsule is formed around a blood clot and the blood is gradually catabolized and transformed into necrotic tissue. This clot gradually becomes enlarged secondary to bleeding or oozing from the small vessels lining the pseudocapsule. It can also be related to intracapsular hyperosmotic pressure, which results from blood catabolism. An expanding pseudotumor with periosteal attachment may cause erosion and cortical thinning of bone. The result may be a fracture of the involved bone or impingement on vital structures.

Findings of pseudo-tumor include soft tissue mass, calcifications, cortical thinning, bone destruction, and new bone formation. Differential diagnosis includes osteomyelitis, aneurysmal bone cyst, and bone sarcomas. Femur and pelvis are affected with the highest incidence in adults. Calcaneus and bones of the hand, foot, and leg were also reported to be affected.

Factor replacement with excision is carried out where possible. Delayed excision or no treatment of the pseudotumor will allow its further expansion and destruction of the surrounding structures.

19. What and where are typical fractures in hemophiliacs and how are they treated?

Fractures occur most frequently in the lower extremities, with femoral supracondylar and femoral neck fractures being the most common. Immediate adequate factor replacement, open reduction, and internal fixation may be used as for nonhemophilic patients. When a fracture can be treated noninvasively, transfusion protocol is individualized depending on the fracture location and the estimated amount of bleeding.

THROMBOCYTOPENIA WITH ABSENT RADIUS SYNDROME (TAR)

20. What are the characteristics of upper extremity deficiencies in TAR and its early treatment?

The pathognomonic upper extremity deficiencies are bilateral absence of radii with all five fingers present, although the thumbs are sometimes hypoplastic flexed and clasped. The rest of the upper extremity is frequently involved. The hands may also be shortened or there may be an absence of the middle phalanx of the fifth finger, clinodactyly, or partial syndactyly. In almost half of the patients, the forearm abnormalities may be manifested in an absent or shortening and/or bowing of the ulna and deficient extensor tendons. The humerus is affected in one-third of the patients, with short or absent humeri. The ulnar and humeral defects are bilateral in 90% of the patients.

Early prolonged splinting and daily careful stretching to avoid bleeding is mandatory to prevent soft tissue contractures. Centralization of the hand or wrist over the distal ulna is delayed until the thrombocytes return to normal or is prevented by the shortening of ulna and humerus. Tendon transfers are indicated in cases of recurrent deformity. Replacement of the radius with vascularized fibular graft is an optional treatment.

21. What are the typical lower extremity abnormalities in TAR?

Extensive lower limb abnormalities occur in 40% of the patients and are mainly at the knee joint. They include deformed, subluxed, or hypoplastic knees; dislocated hips and knees or patellae; varus or valgus rotation at the hips, knees, or feet; and short legs with absent tibiae and/or fibulae and absent or hypoplastic patellae and menisci. The most common skeletal defect in the lower limbs is genu varum with flexion contracture and internal tibial torsion. After skeletal maturity there is usually minimal progression of the surgically treated lower extremity.

22. When should these skeletal deformities be surgically corrected?
The timing is decided individually and is usually possible between 6 months and 6 years of age, or when the thrombocytes are elevated and bleeding tendencies are minor.

SICKLE CELL ANEMIA

23. What are the different sickle cell disorders (SC)?
Hemoglobin S differs from the normal adult hemoglobin (HgA) by the substitution of valine for glutamic acid in the sixth amino acid position in each of the two beta-polypeptide chains. HgS results from an abnormal β globulin gene on chromosome 11. Hemoglobin C occurs when lyssin is substituted for the same glutamic acid that is affected in HgS.
- A homozygous state for the abnormal hemoglobin S (HgS-S): this is the classic type, sickle cell anemia (sickle cell - hemoglobin's disease). It is a chronic hemolytic anemia.
- A heterozygous state for hemoglobin S (HgS-A): this is the disease trait and these patients have no clinical problem under physiologic conditions.
- A heterozygous state for one other variant: this type is also expressed as SC.

SC includes a group of other conditions: sickle cell HgC disease, sickle cell β-thalassemia disease, and sickle cell hemoglobin D or E diseases. Sickle cell *diseases* are also chronic hemolytic anemia with less or equal severity as sickle cell anemia.
- In sickle cell β-thalassemia, the β-thalassemia gene is responsible for the reduced synthesis of the β-globine polypeptide.
- Other conditions in which the abnormal hemoglobin S is combined with other types of abnormal hemoglobin, such as D and E

If no HgA (normal hemoglobin) is produced, the patients are $S\beta^0$ and have clinical problems similar to those in sickle cell anemia (SS). If there is some production of HgA, the patients are listed as $S\beta^+$ and have milder clinical manifestations such as those in SC. Patients heterozygous for HgS and β-thalassemia have different clinical manifestations, depending on the gene's output. In SC the patients are heterozygous for one HgS and one HgC gene. It is the second most common type of sickle cell disorder in the U.S. There are fewer complications associated with SC than with SS.

24. What is the ethnic distribution of the gene for hemoglobin S and what is the resultant incidence of sickle cell anemia?
The gene for hemoglobin S occurs in 8–10% of blacks in the U.S., in up to 40% in some ethnic groups in Central Africa, and in 0.8% in the non-black persons. A sickle cell *trait* appears in about 20% of the populations of Central Africa, and sickle cell *anemia* appears in approximately 1% to 2%. In the black population in the U.S., SS is less frequent and occurs in 14% per thousand of the population. The incidence of sickle cell *disease* and its variants is 7.7% in the African-American community.

25. What are the most common conditions in the triggering of HgS changes and what causes the hematologic manifestations?
Low oxygen tension or reduced blood flow are the most common conditions initiating the pathologic changes. The HgS polymerizes and the soluble HgS is changed into a gel. This results in distorted and fragile erythrocytes that are rapidly destroyed. The erythrocytes are more fragile and rigid and viscous. These changes will result in increased hemolysis and in small vessel occlusion and infarcts. Two separate pathologic abnormalities cause the clinical manifestations in sickle cell disorders: (1) sickling of the red cell, producing vaso-occlusion and thromboembolic bone infarcts, and (2) increased destruction of sickle cell red cells, producing hemolysis, an increased erythroblastic activity, and expansion of the bone marrow activity.

26. What are musculoskeletal problems which result from (1) vaso-occlusion in sickle cell disorders and (2) from hemolytic anemia?

1. Dactylitis, avascular necrosis (particularly in the femoral head), osteomyelitis, retardation of height and growth, septic arthritis, reactive arthritis, and leg ulcers.

2. Hyperplasia of the bone marrow will result in increased size of the medullar cavity, osteoporosis, thinning of the bone cortices, and biconcavity of the vertebrae. It accounts for the tendency to spontaneous fracture.

27. What are the causes and incidence of dactylitis (hand-foot syndrome) in sickle cell disorders and what is a characteristic expression?

Dactylitis is usually manifested between 6 and 12 months of age, when hemoglobulin F is replaced by hemoglobulin S. The syndrome affects the short tubular bones of the hands and feet. A representative case is a child below the age of 2 years with swollen, tender, and painful hand and/or foot. The symptoms are usually triggered by cold weather and last for 1–2 weeks. The incidence of dactylitis was reported to be 45% in patients with sickle cell disorders and 41% of the affected patients suffer from recurrent episodes. The hands and feet are spared after the age of 6 years due to the disappearance of the hematopoietic marrow activity in them.

28. What other conditions may be confused with dactylitis and how are they best recognized?

Osteomyelitis resembles dactylitis since both present clinically as localized soft tissue swelling and tenderness with systemic fever and leukocytosis. Radiographs yield similar findings in the two conditions, such as patchy areas of bone destruction, subperiosteal bone reaction and, finally, bone reformation. Aspiration of the affected bone is the best way to differentiate between the two, while bone scan is not adequately informative. The bony resolution after 4–8 week differs in the self-limiting nature of dactilities from osteomyelitis.

29. Describe the most common cause and site of extremity pain in SC.

Sickle cell crises, usually occurring between 3–4 years of age and lasting from 3–5 days, cause the accumulation of sequestrated sickle cells in the vascular canals leading to a localized area of bone marrow infarction or soft tissue crisis. The secondary inflammatory response will contribute to the process by causing a rise in the intramedullary pressure and its resulting severe pain. The most common sites are the long bones such as the humerus, tibia, and femur, whose growing ends are particularly involved. The physical findings are mild swelling, limitation of the range of motion, and low elevation of temperature.

30. What is the average rate of sickle cell crisis requiring I.V. steroid therapy?

The rates are: 0.8/year in sickle cell anemia (SS), 1.0/year in the $S\beta^\circ$ and 0.4/year in SC and $S\beta^+$. When the fetal hemoglobin (HgF) is elevated, the rate of crisis is low. Infarction occurs in 20–60% of patients with the hemoglobin C variant. High doses of intravenous corticoids will significantly reduce the severity of the pain and its duration.

31. What are the growth disturbances in SC children?

Retardation of growth is common. In SS children, weight and height are significantly low before 2 years of age. Skeletal maturity is also significantly retarded in SS children, and pubertal development is delayed. Chronic anemia, infections of the epiphysis or osteomyelitis can be the possible etiologic factors.

32. What are the common radiographic features in SC?

In the skull, the calvarium is thickened, the diploic space is widened and the bony texture has an agranular appearance. These changes occur in one-third to one half of the patients with sickle cell disease.

In the long bones, there is patchy osteosclerosis with focal radiolucency, cortical thinning, widening of the medullary canal, and mild periosteal elevation.

Cortical bone infarction with dense amorphous chalky zones and sclerosis are among the most common and typical radiological feature of sickle cell disorders.

The combination of new layers of repair bone with an infarcted cortex occasionally creates a "bone within a bone" pattern. Vertebral deformity occurs in as many as 70% of the patients.

Typically, the center of the subchondral bone plate is compressed and forms a sharp dip ("step deformity") while the periphery retains its normal contour. These changes usually occur in children older that 10 years of age and they differ from osseous disk herniation, osteoporotic fractures, or changes in multiple myeloma.

33. What are the possible reasons for elevated infection rate in sickle cell disorders?

Patients with sickle cell disorders are more susceptible to infection because of hyposplenism, reduced liver functions, interference with the reticuloendothelial system functions, suppressed clearing of the organisms from the blood, and abnormal opsonizing and complement functions. The infarcted bone marrow will add to the risk by serving as a preferred site for the organisms colonization.

34. What are the most common bacterial organisms which cause osteomyelitis in patients with sickle cell anemia?

Salmonella and its related species ($\geq 50\%$) have been considered the most common bacterial agents but there have been reports changing the infection profile to putatively implicate Klebsiella. Capillary occlusion secondary to intravascular sickling may infarct the bowel and permit the spread of the bacterial agent.

35. What is the rate of polyostotic involvement and why is this significant?

The rate of multifocal osteomyelitis, often symmetric, can range from 12 to 47%. It can be associated with some life-threatening disorders.

36. Why is it difficult to differentiate bone infarction from osteomyelitis?

- The clinical manifestations of fever, pain, and swelling can overlap
- The initial radiographs do not show abnormalities in either disorder
- The erythrocyte sedimentation rate is unreliable in sickle cell disorders because of the change in the shape or the erythrocytes
- Bone scan with Technetium-99m or Gallium-47 does not distinguish between them
- Both may involve multiple long bones, and boys are more susceptible in both
- Sickle cell crisis is 50 times more common than bacterial osteomyelitis

37. What are the modes of differentiating between these two pathologies and what are their limitations?

Combined technetium and gallium scintigraphy and technetium sulphur colloid bone marrow scan and gadolinium-data-enhanced MRI may help distinguish osteomyelitis from infarction in patients with SC. The relative limitation is the fact that the patterns of infarction may not differ from osteomyelitis after 7 days from the onset of symptoms. Recently, third generation cephalosporins have replaced chloramphenicol in the management protocol

38. What is the recommended antibiotic therapy if osteomyelitis is a possibility?

Osteomyelitis is best managed when chloramphenicol, ampicillin, and trimethoprim/sulfamethoxazole, which are used to cover the Salmonella. Oxacillin is provided to protect against *S. aureus,* and the new generation of cephalosporin is used for the resistant Salmonella species.

39. When and why is surgery the preferred treatment when the diagnosis of osteomyelitis has been delayed?

Surgical intervention is indicated when a delay in diagnosis of chronic infection with sequestrum-formation has led to the necessity for drainage of the resultant abscesses. The procedure is coupled with long-term parenteral antibiotic therapy. Some recommend that the wound should be left open when there is an extensive abscess, while others advise an immediate wound closure with closed suction perfusion irrigation.

40. What is the most common complication of long bone osteomyelitis is sickle cell patients?
Pathologic fractures are the most common complication of osteomyelitis in long bones. In patients with sickle cell disorders (in about 10% of the patients with osteomyelitis), these fractures are usually complicated by nonunion, delayed union, and malunion and joint stiffness.

41. Can septic arthritis be expected in sickle cell disorders?
Septic arthritis is uncommon is SC but the knee joint is most often involved when it is present. The causative organism is usually *not* Salmonella. Septic arthritis carries a poor prognosis and often requires aggressive surgical intervention. It can be complicated by avascular necrosis or dislocation in the hip joint.

42. What are the typical features of reactive arthritis in children with SC anemia and what is the treatment?
Reactive arthritis usually presents as an acute joint pain and moderate effusion in one or more joints (polyarthritis), and severe muscular spasm and tenderness may also accompany it. Analysis of the joint fluid reveals a low grade inflammation (less than 20,000 leukocytes in mm^3). The arthritis can last from a few days to 2 months. During the phase of acute arthralgia, the treatment is molded splints and analgesics.

43. What is the incidence and the prognosis of femoral head osteonecrosis in SC anemia and on what factors does it depend?
The prevalence and incidence of osteonecrosis in patients with sickle cell disorders older than 5 years of age was found to be 9.8% (in another smaller study the prevalence was significantly greater, 41%). Prevalence depends upon the age of onset and the different variants of the sickle cell disorders. For example, in the sickle cell disorder with the α-thalassemia gene, the risk for osteonecrosis and its extension is significantly higher due to vaso-occlusion. It is more common in children with hemoglobin C disease. It is rare in children with HgS disease because of their short life span.

Bilaterality occurred in 54% of the patients with osteonecrosis without relation to the type of sickle cell disorder. Patients with frequent painful crises are at highest risk for femoral head osteonecrosis. The prognosis is better in young children because of their superior potential for healing, but it is guarded in older children.

44. How useful is MRI in demonstrating avascular necrosis in SC?
It showed no advantage over radiography. It is helpful, however, in detecting the extent of the osteonecrosis and the developmental sequence of the different femoral head segmental infarctions.

45. What primary finding determines the management of avascular necrosis (AVN) and what are treatment options?
The identification of the lateral pillar is crucial for selecting treatment of femoral head osteonecrosis. If the lateral pillar is intact, conservative treatment is effective. In total head involvement and deficiency of the lateral pillar, surgical management is indicated, such as rotation upper femoral osteotomy, pelvic osteotomy, core decompression (in early AVN) or cement injection.

In children younger than 10 years, the use of crutch ambulation or abduction bracing is an optional treatment. Loss of motion and total head involvement will change the mode of treatment.

Total hip replacement yields poor results and prognosis because of the risks of infection, high blood loss, early aseptic loosening, and intra-operative femoral fracture and perforation.

Intraoperative consideration includes the use of tourniquets, oxygenation, maintenance of blood volume, and avoidance of hypothermia. Post-operative considerations are maintenance of intravascular volume and appropriate oxygenation.

46. Which is the second most common location of osteonecrosis in SC anemia?
Osteonecrosis of the humeral head. The incidence rate of radiographic evidence for the osteonecrosis is 5–6%. As for the femoral head, the prevalence rates are related to the child's age and the type of SC. Bilateral involvement was recorded in 67% of the patients with humeral osteonecrosis. Involvement of the non-weight bearing shoulder leads to less disability and pain, and 79% of the patients are asymptomatic at diagnosis. The typical radiographic appearance includes the crescent sign and collapse of the humeral head, which usually begin in the superior medial quadrant. Further fragmentation will lead to pain and stiffness. Good function can be often sustained in 12–24 months, and there is no need for joint replacement.

47. How common is cerebral infarction in SC anemia?
The incidence of cerebral infarction is about 8% of the patients with SC disorders. It may result in spastic hemiplegia in children.

48. What is current status of bone marrow transplantation (BMT) in patients with SC?
BMT in patients with SC is still in early stages. The complication rate is reduced in young patients free of major organ dysfunction and with healthy HLA-identical donors.

49. What are the differences between Perthes' disease and avascular necrosis in SC?
Perthes' disease occurs in young children between 3 and 10 years old, whereas avascular necrosis in sickle cell disorders usually occurs in the second decade of life or later. Perthes' disease is 10 times more common in white children and five times more common in boys. Hemoglobinopathic avascular necrosis has equal distribution between the sexes and is common among the black race. In Perthes' disease the methaphysis is involved, whereas in SC the metaphysis is almost never involved.

THALASSEMIA

50. What are the pathology and the clinical features in thalassemia major (Cooley's anemia or β-thalassemia, or Mediterranean anemia)?
The severe form of this disease is secondary to homozygous mutation of the β-globulin gene. The result is absent or severe deficiency of the β-polypeptide chain. The hemoglobin molecule is mainly composed of unpaired α-chains. This molecule is insoluble and causes intracellular precipitates. The hematologic findings include severe hypochromia, distorted erythrocytes, target cells, microcytosis and very low hemoglobin levels. There are large HgF (fetal) molecules in the red cells. The clinical manifestations are severe anemia (less than 5 gm/dL), growth and development retardation, hepatosplenomegaly and bone marrow expansion with related skeletal changes secondary to the intense hematopoietic activity. Infants with severe anemia who are not treated during their first months of life will die before 5 years of age from infections and cardiac failure.

51. What are the characteristic skeletal involvements and most common complications in thalassemia?
The main skeletal abnormalities are secondary to the hyperplasia and intramedullary excessive hematopoietic activity which cause expansion and widening of the marrow space, rarefaction of the bone trabeculae, and resorption of the central bone, thinning of cortical bone, perpendicular periosteal spicules, and severe osteoporosis. The earliest changes are in the hands and feet: the marrow cavities are widened in the metacarpals, metatarsals, and phalanges. There are several abnormalities in the skull, such as osteopenia overgrowth of facial bones, widening of the diploic space, and radial striations which give a "hair standing on end" appearance. The long

bones demonstrate cortical thinning with multiple circumscribed osteolytic areas that have a punched-out appearance.

Aseptic necrosis of the femoral head can complicate thalassemia.

Fractures are a frequent complications (one in three patients) and usually occur after minor trauma at an average age of 10 to 16 years. A hypertransfusion regimen with chelation therapy reduces osteoporosis, decreases the incidence of this complication and strengthen the bone. The treatment is also helpful in reducing the time needed for healing the fracture, a process which is improved with the supplement of vitamin C.

52. What is the rate of premature physeal closure in thalassemia patients?

Premature fusion of the epiphysis is seen in 15–20% of the patients and is responsible for the high incidence of deformities. It is very common in the proximal humeral physis. Its pathogenesis is obscure. It is more severe and frequent in patients older than 12 years in whom there had been a delay in initiating treatment with transfusions.

GAUCHER'S DISEASE

53. How common is Gaucher's disease?

Gaucher's disease, the most frequent lysosomal storage disorder, with an incidence of 1/40,000, is caused by a deficiency of the enzyme glucocerebroside β-glucosidase.

54. What are the pathology and the different types of Gaucher's disease?

The deficient enzyme results in reduced degradation and hydrolization of the glucocerebroside (an essential component of the cell wall), thus leading to its gradual accumulation in the macrophages of the reticuloendothelial system. These abnormal accumulations of Gaucher cells result in organ dysfunction.

There are three distinct clinical forms. In Type I, the chronic non-neuronopathic and most common type, the hematologic findings are mostly confined to viscera (spleen and liver), while bone involvement dominates the clinical picture. Most (60%) of the patients are Ashkenazi Jews. Type II, an acute neuropathic disease or infantile type, is rare. The severe involvement of the central nervous system leads to an early death (before 2 years of age). Type III, a subacute neuronopathic (juvenile) type, is a mixture of Types I and II.

55. How is the genetic pathology correlated with the clinical presentation?

The genotype causes a variable deficiency of the enzyme and it is best correlated with clinical severity and age at presentation. The most common symptom at presentation is a bleeding tendency (epistaxis, ease of bruising) from thrombocytopenia, which is the result of hypersplenism. The clinical signs include skin pigmentations, deposits in the scelera, hepatosplenomegaly, anemia, and bleeding disorders. Growth retardation is a prominent feature. Bone pain caused by small bone infarcts is usually reported in the femur or proximal tibia.

56. How common is skeletal involvement?

Bone complications are common, and 75%–90% of the patients have skeletal changes. The most frequent and characteristic one is the Erlenmeyer flask deformity of the distal femur. Its characteristic radiographic appearance is an abnormal expansion of the distal femoral metaphysis. The pathology is a result of fusiform widening of the relatively thin metaphysis cortices by the Gaucher cell infiltrate and the failure of trabeculation and modeling. The typical metaphyseal flaring can also occur in the proximal tibia and proximal humerus. In addition, there may be metaphyseal flaring, loss of bone density (osteopenia), thinning of the cortex, medullary expansion, loss of the normal trabeculations, patchy myelosclerosis, bone crisis (infarct), osteonecrosis, bone marrow hemorrhagic cysts mixed with sclerotic areas, and pathologic fractures. These skeletal involvements are secondary to the Gaucher cell's infiltration of the bone marrow in the medullary cavity.

The osteopenia is mainly located in the vertebrae and in the long bones of the proximal limbs (femora and humeri) where there is major hematopoietic activity. The infiltration of the marrow by Gaucher cells produces osteopenia, cortical thinning, and weakening of the bone, which can lead to the complication of pathologic features.

57. What is the pathophysiology of Gaucher crisis and what are the presenting signs and symptoms?

Gaucher crisis, or pseudomyelitis, is the product of an intramedullary hemorrhage of a large bone segment which can also affect the subperiosteal space. Accumulation of blood under the confinements of the bony, nonexpanding walls creates excessive pressure which can explain the intense pain of the crisis. The skeletal complaint of Gaucher crisis is usually acute onset of severe pain localized to the distal femur, proximal tibia, and proximal femur. Other localized signs are heat, redness, swelling, tenderness, and limited function and motion of the affected limb. The leukocyte count and the ESR are elevated. These signs and symptoms are very similar to those of osteomyelitis.

58. What are the typical radiographic and bone scan findings during the different stages of Gaucher crisis?

In the initial stage, the elevated intramedullary pressure creates ischemia of the bone. Radiographs are therefore normal while the bone scan demonstrates reduced uptake. A few weeks following the crisis, the remodeling and reconstitution of bone will be presented radiographically as periosteal elevation and lytic changes in the medullary canal. The radioisotope uptake of the lesion in the bone scan at this stage is increased and surrounds the photopenic sites. When the bone recovers several months later, the bone scan is normal again and radiographs show patchy myelosclerosis or osteonecrosis in the femoral head, tibial plateau, femoral condyles, or humeral head.

59. What characterizes osteomyelitis in Gaucher's disease?

Secondary infection of the bony infarct can lead to the rare complication of osteomyelitis in Gaucher's disease. The diagnosis is usually delayed and the causative bacteria is aerobic. Neither laboratory nor radiographic investigations can distinguish between the bone crisis and osteomyelitis. A biopsy or aspiration by strict aseptic technique can be helpful. Administration of antibiotics must be delayed until the bacteriologic diagnosis is made. A prolonged period of systemic antibiotics is required in Gaucher's infections because the infection is usually located in avascular bone.

60. Where do pathologic fractures usually occur in children with Gaucher's disease?

In the sites where the bone crisis altered the bony texture: the distal femur, proximal tibia, and femoral neck. Delayed union and non-union are frequent complications because of the change in the normal quality of bony repair. Treatment is usually conservative.

61. What are the causes for back pain in Gaucher's disease?

Severe back pain can result from bone crisis or pathologic fracture of the spinal vertebrae. Mild back pain can be secondary to osteopenia.

62. Where does osteonecrosis usually occur in Gaucher's disease and how is it treated?

The femoral head. Other sites are the femoral condyles, tibial plateau, and humeral head. In young patients, conservative treatment with bed rest and no weight bearing is recommended. Containment abduction bracing can be indicated when there is no collapse of the femoral head. If collapse had occurred in older adolescents or adults, partial or total hip replacement can be considered. Treatment of avascular necrosis in the shoulder is conservative unless the humeral head is destroyed.

63. What are the considerations before surgical intervention in Gaucher's disease?
Significant perioperative bleeding has to be considered. The thrombocytopenia secondary to hypersplenism and the clotting defects secondary to the liver involvement can be responsible for the bleeding.

64. What are the radiographic changes in Niemann-Pick?
Osteoporosis, widening of the metaphyseal-diaphyseal medullary canals, delayed bone age, and modeling defects. These changes are secondary to the accumulation of foam cells in the bone marrow. Findings also include delayed bone age, flaring of the distal metaphysis in the long bones, osteoporosis elongated vertebral pedicles (mainly in the lumbar region), widening of the metacarpal bones, kyphosis, and coxa valga.

LANGERHANS' CELL HISTIOCYTOSIS
(HISTIOCYTOSIS-X, EOSINOPHILIC GRANULOMA)

65. What is the unique structural aspect of Langerhans' cells?
The tubular or racket-shaped granules seen under electron-microscopy.

66. What is the histopathology of the classic bone lesion?
The classic bone lesion contains histocytes with acute and chronic inflammatory cells. The typical granules of Langerhans' cells are found in from 2% to 79% of the histocytes.

67. What are the ways to differentiate between the mature lesions of Langerhans' cell histiocytosis and subacute or chronic osteomyelitis?
The mature lesions of Langerhans' cells histiocytosis include foci of necrosis, granulomatous changes with fibrosis, and Langerhans' histiocytes. Differentiation is based on the use of electron-microscopy, which may demonstrate the typical granules.

68. What is the preferred classification of Langerhans' cell histiocytosis?
The classification is based on the presence of solitary or multiple bone involvement without soft tissue involvement, bone and soft tissue involvement, of soft tissue involvement alone. Organ dysfunctions (based on individual criteria) are determined and added to the classification.

69. What are the common sites of soft tissue involvement and what is the prognostic significance?
The skin, lungs, liver, spleen, pituitary gland, and bone marrow. Systemic skin involvement is a bad prognostic sign. The involvement of lungs, liver, spleen, and bone marrow can be the cause of death. Death can occur when the disease begins before two years of age but also may occur in late childhood, or even in adulthood.

70. How common are skeletal lesions and what are the common sites in Langerhans' cell histiocytosis?
80–97% of the patients have bony involvement while and 50–77% are free of visceral involvement. The typical skeletal sites are the skull, pelvis, spine, ribs, and femur.

71. What are the typical radiographic appearances of the different bony lesions?
In the skull the typical appearance is punched-out lesions. In the spine the vertebrae are collapsed (vertebra plana) with normal adjacent disc spaces. There is also metaphyseal or diaphyseal lytic with cortical thinning, widening of the medullary canal, endosteal scalloping, and occasional periosteal elevation.

72. How specific are bone scan, MRI, or CT in diagnosing bony lesion in Langerhans' cell histiocytosis?

Bone scan might detect early bony involvement not seen radiographically but it bears a high false negative rate. MRI bears the difficulties of differentiating eosinophilic granuloma from osteomyelitis and Ewing's sarcoma. MRI, CT, and bone scan can help in detecting the site of a lesion which may cause unexplained pain or spinal cord involvement.

73. What is the prognosis in the different types of patients with Langerhans' cell histiocytosis?

Patients with solitary bony lesions at presentation have the best prognosis with no fatal dissemination. Patients with organ dysfunction at disease onset have a 30% to 70% mortality rate. Multiple bone involvement without soft tissue involvement has a good prognosis. Evolution of soft tissue involvement, usually as diabetes insipidus, can occur in this group of patients. The mortality rate is low.

74. What are the presenting symptoms in patients with solitary bony lesions? What are the measures needed to rule out expanding involvement?

In solitary bone lesions the presenting complaints are swelling, pain, or limping. The possible expanding involvement can be detected by monitoring for the typical symptoms of the various organs' dysfunction, and physical examination with special assessment of the liver, spleen, spine, skull, and extremities. Lateral skull radiographs are a good screening test and there should be an additional survey of the chest skeleton. Laboratory tests are also useful for early detection of organ dysfunction.

75. What is the necessary measure to confirm the suspected diagnosis of Langerhans' cell histiocytosis?

Tissue biopsy is necessary to confirm the diagnosis. The skin lesions are the best sites for the biopsy. In bony lesions, Craig needle transcutaneous aspiration is optimal. Open biopsy is used when curettage of the lesion is indicated. Biopsy is not indicated in patients with well-defined multifocal radiographic involvement.

76. What is the treatment of bone lesions and what is its influence upon healing?

Methods of treatment for bony lesions without visceral involvement are observation, curettage, or steroid injection. The mode of treatment has no influence on the healing rate. In patients with painful lesions or with the imminent risk of fractures bone graft can be added to the protocol of curettage and open biopsy.

77. What are the clinical and radiographic features of spinal lesions? What is the treatment? What is the treatment of eosinophilic granuloma of the spine with neurologic deficit?

Spinal lesion is usually accompanied by pain and postural changes such as torticollis, kyphosis, or scoliosis. The typical radiographic changes are vertebra plana with intact posterior elements. In spinal involvement without neurologic deficit, conservative treatment with immobilization is sufficient. In the rare event of neurologic involvement, MRI and clinical examinations are needed for evaluation of nerve root or spinal cord compression. In nerve root involvement the treatment is usually rest, immobilization, and occasional steroid block. Surgical decompression is indicated in spinal cord compression. Radiotherapy may be the treatment of choice in disseminated spinal involvement.

78. What is the earliest radiographic finding seen in the healing of skeletal lesions?

The earliest sign is the return of the trabecular structure of the affected bone. This change can be detected 6 to 10 weeks after diagnosis, and complete healing is obvious after 36–40 weeks.

Radiography is recommended after 2 and 6 months from diagnosis. If no healing is evident after 4 months, additional therapy is indicated.

Additional radiologic surveys and physical examination are recommended every 6 months for 2 years or more.

LEUKEMIA

79. How common is leukemia among children?
Leukemia is the most common form of childhood cancer, accounting for 34% of the malignancies in white children and 24% in black children in the U.S. The most common type is acute lymphoblastic leukemia (ALL) which accounts for 70%–80% of the leukemias in children.

80. What are the musculoskeletal features of leukemia?
Bone and joint pain are the most common presenting complaint. Bone pain is diffuse, nonspecific and asymmetric, most frequently appearing in the metaphyseal region and may extend to the adjacent joints, hips, knees, ankles, and wrists. The incidence of these skeletal symptoms ranges from 10% to 32%. Back pain secondary to osteopenia, bone marrow infiltration, or fracture of the verebral body can be the initial complaint. Children presenting with bone and joint complaints can be misdiagnosed as having rheumatic fever, septic arthritis, osteomyelitis, juvenile rheumatoid arthritis, or polymyositis.

81. How common are radiographic changes and what are their characteristic findings? Which radiographic sign is most significant for the correct diagnosis of leukemia?
Children with leukemia may have significant symptoms and radiographic signs with a normal peripheral smear at the time of their presentation (10%).

The radiographic changes of all patients with ALL at the initial stage of the disease, with an incidence from 44% to 57%, are about twice as frequent as are the presenting musculoskeletal complaints. The percentage is higher in children below 1 year of age and is significantly lower after 10 years of age. The skeletal changes are most common in the long bones and skull. The characteristic findings are focal ("moth-eaten") or diffuse osteolytic lesions mainly in the form of bone resorption in the metaphysiodiaphyseal region, destruction and elevation of the periosteum with new bone formation, localized and generalized osteoporosis, radiolucent metaphyseal leukemic lines (bands), cortical defects, osteosclerosis, mixed osteolysis and sclerosis, permeated pattern of destruction, widening of the cranial sutures of the skull, and subcortical radiolucent zones in the vertebral body. Osteopenia is the most common radiographic findings in the spine and is the most significant sign for making the correct diagnosis. None of the radiographic findings is pathognomonic or typical to leukemia. Bone scan was not found to correlate with the clinical presentation and is unreliable in leukemia.

82. What is the debate about bone involvement at the onset of diagnosis being a prognostic factor?
Most authors report no prognostic significance for the presence of pathologic vertebral fracture or skeletal involvement at the onset of the disease. Other studies claimed that children without radiographic skeletal involvement and those with 5 or more skeletal lesions will have the same poor outcome as with an aggressive form of leukemia, while those with 1–4 lesions were considered to have an indolent form of short-duration leukemia. Another study found no significant correction between the survival time and the extent of skeletal involvement.

83. What are the possible musculoskeletal complications of chemotherapy?
- Steroid-induced osteopenia
- Steroid-induced osteonecrosis

- Pathologic fractures
- Bone and soft tissue infections
- Peripheral neuropathies

X-LINKED AGAMMAGLOBULINEMIA

84. What unique musculoskeletal problem is seen in hypogammaglobulinemia?

The unique and most common skeletal complication is aseptic arthritis, which is usually nonerosive, manifested as mono- or polyarticular, and affects mainly the knees, wrists, ankles and fingers. Treatment consists of gammaglobulin replacement. Some patients will develop chronic arthritis despite this treatment.

CHRONIC GRANULOMATOUS DISEASE

85. What is chronic granulomatous disease and what is the typical pathologic result?

A hereditary condition characterized by purulent granulomatous and eczematoid skin lesion, suppurative granulomatous lymphadenitis, pneumonia, and chronic osteomyelitis. Usually patients develop recurrent infections in very early childhood (with lymphadenopathy) from catalase-negative organisms (Staphylococcus), gram-negative bacteria, and fungi. The disease occurs in males who have a defective phagocytosis mechanism of polyphonuclear leukocytes. Osteomyelitis will result in 31–36% of the patients. The most common sites are the hands and feet.

86. What therapeutic measures are recommended for best results?

Preoperative bone scanning and imaging, avoidance of preoperative administration of antibiotics, intraoperative cultures, aggressive debridement of the infected bone and soft tissue, and leaving the wound open for secondary closure.

ACQUIRED IMMUNODEFICIENCY SYNDROME (AIDS)

87. What causes AIDS and what is the major source of AIDS in children today?

This is a retrovirus called the "human immunodeficiency virus" (HIV) of which there are at least two types, HIV-1 and HIV-2. Currently, most of the affected children are those born to HIV-infected mothers (in the U.S. this accounts for 80% of them). 25–30% of children born to HIV-infected mothers will become HIV seropositive children.

The main transmission routes of HIV to children are via transfusions of contaminated factor concentrates to hemophiliacs, through blood products of HIV-seropositive donors, and through intrauterine infection from HIV-infected mothers. Progress in the purification of the clotting concentrates and better screening of HIV carriers among blood donors have reduced the risk of such transmissions to a minimum.

88. What are the common musculoskeletal problems in HIV-infected children?

Musculoskeletal opportunistic infections are surprisingly uncommon. Septic arthritis can occur in joints which already suffer from arthropathy in children with hemophilia. Correct diagnosis might be delayed because of joint swelling, while pain might be suspected as being the result of the ubiquitous hemarthrosis. Since life expectancy is limited in HIV-infected children, treatment of the muscle and joint contractures following encephalopathy in mainly noninvasive and conservative.

89. How is recurrent hemarthrosis treated in hemophiliac children infected by HIV?

In HIV-infected hemophiliac children, for reasons yet to be discovered, the progress to AIDS is slower. Thus, synovectomy for recurrent hemarthrosis can be indicated.

BIBLIOGRAPHY

1. Anand AJ, Glatt AE: Salmonella osteomyelitis and arthritis in sickle cell disease. Semin Arthritis Rheum 24(3):211–21, 1994.
2. Benetrt OM, Namnyak SS: Bone and joint manifestations of sickle cell anemia. J Bone Joint Surg Br 72(3):494–9, 1990.
3. De Sanctis V, Pinamonti A, Di Palma A, et al: Growth and development in thalassemia major patients with severe bone lesions due to desferrioxamine. Eur J Pediatr 155(5):368–72, 1990.
4. Gallagher DJ, Phillips DJ, Heinrich SD: Orthopaedic manifestations of acute pediatric leukemia. Orthop Clin North Am 27(3):635–44, 1996.
5. Greene WF: Diseases related to the hematopoietic system. *In* Morissy R.T., Weinstein SL (eds.): Lovell and Winter's Pediatric Orthopaedics, 4th ed, Vol. 1. Philadelphia, Lippincott-Raven, pp 345–391, 1996.
6. Hernigou P, Bachir D, Galacteros F: Avascular necrosis of the femoral head in sickle-cell disease. J Bone Joint Surg Br 75(6):875–80, 1993.
7. Meehan PL, Viroslav S, Schmitt EW Jr.: Vertebral collapse in childhood leukemia. J Pediatr Orthop 15(5):592–5, 1995.
8. Moran MC: Osteonecrosis of the hip in sickle cell hemoglobinopathy. Am J Orthop 1995 24(1):18–24.
9. Nathan DG, Oski FA (eds.): Hematology of Infancy and Childhood, 4th Ed. Philadelphia W.B. Saunders, 1993.
10. Rivard GE, Girard M, Belanger R, et al: Synoviorthesis with colloidal 32P chromic phosphate for the treatment of hemophilic arthropathy. J Bone Joint Surg Am 76(4) 482–8, 1994. Comment in 77(5):807–8, 1995.
11. Tachdjian MO: Bone manifestations of hematologic disorders. In Tachdjian M.O. (ed.): Pediatric Orthopaedics, 2nd ed. Vol. 2. Philadelphia, W.B. Saunders, pp 1135–1150, 1990.
12. Timsit MA, Bardin T: Metabolic arthropaties. Curr Opin Rheumatol 6(4):448–53, 1994.
13. Zevin S, Abrahamov A, Hadas-Halpern I, et al: Adult-type Gaucher disease in children: genetics, clinical features and enzyme replacement therapy. Q J Med. 86(9):565–73, 1993.

INDEX

Page numbers in **boldface** type indicate complete chapters.